Cancer Treatment:
End-Point Evaluation

WILEY SERIES ON
NEW HORIZONS IN ONCOLOGY
Series Editor
Basil A. Stoll
(St Thomas' Hospital and Royal Free Hospital, London)

NEW HORIZONS IN ONCOLOGY

VOLUME 2

Cancer Treatment: End-Point Evaluation

Edited by

BASIL A. STOLL

Honorary Consulting Physician to Oncology Departments,
St. Thomas' Hospital and Royal Free Hospital, London

A Wiley Medical Publication

JOHN WILEY & SONS

Chichester · New York · Brisbane · Toronto · Singapore

Library of Congress Cataloging in Publication Data:
Main entry under title:

Cancer treatment: end-point evaluation

   (Wiley series on new horizons in oncology; v. 2) (A Wiley medical publication)
   Includes index.
   1. Cancer—Treatment.   I. Stoll, Basil Arnold.
II. Series.   III. Series: Wiley medical publication.
RC270.8.C384   1983   616.99′406   82–17492

ISBN 0 471 90080 X

British Library Cataloguing in Publication Data:

Cancer treatment:end-point evaluation—(Wiley series on new horizons in oncology)
   1. Cancer—Treatment
   I. Stoll, Basil A.
   616.99′406   RC270.8

ISBN 0 471 90080 X

Typeset by Photo-Graphics, Honiton, Devon.
Printed by Pitman Press Ltd., Bath, Avon.

Contributors

Malcolm Adams, MB, ChB, MRCOG, FRCR
Consultant in Radiotherapy and Oncology, Velindre Hospital, Whitchurch, Cardiff, UK

G. W. Barendsen, PhD
Professor of Radiobiology, University of Amsterdam, Radiobiological Institute, Rijswijk, The Netherlands

A. C. Begg, PhD
Research Scientist, Gray Laboratory, Mount Vernon Hospital, Northwood, Middlesex, UK

Bertil Björklund, MD
Chief, Cancer Immunology Section, National Bacteriology Laboratory, Stockholm, Sweden

C. M. L. Coppin, BM, FRCP(C), DPhil
Medical Oncologist, Cancer Control Agency of British Columbia, Vancouver, Canada

M. H. Cullen, BSc, MD, MRCP
Consultant Medical Oncologist, Queen Elizabeth Hospital, Birmingham, UK

J. E. Devitt, MD
Director, Continuing Medical Education, School of Medicine, Ottawa Civic Hospital, Ottawa, Ontario, Canada

D. R. Donaldson, BSc, FRCS, FRCS(E)
Department of Surgery, St James's University Hospital, Leeds, and Maelor General Hospital, Wrexham, UK

Edwin R. Fisher, MD
Director, Institute of Pathology, Shadyside Hospital, Pittsburgh, Pennsylvania, USA

G. R. Giles, MD, FRCS
Professor of Surgery, St James's University Hospital, Leeds, UK

J. L. Haybittle, MA, PhD
Lately Chief Physicist, Addenbrooke's Hospital, Cambridge, UK

Lucien Israël, MD
Professor, University of Paris, Chief of Medical Oncology, Hopital Avicenne, Bobigny, France

H. B. Kal, PhD
Research Scientist, Radiobiological Institute, Rijswijk, The Netherlands

Ian Kerby, MB, BS, FRCR
Consultant Radiotherapist, Velindre Hospital, Whitchurch, Cardiff, UK

Stephen Leveson, MD, FRCS
Senior Lecturer in Surgery, University of Leeds and Honorary Consultant Surgeon, St James's University Hospital, Leeds, UK

Santilal Parbhoo, PhD, FRCS
Senior Lecturer and Consultant Surgeon, Academic Department of Surgery, Royal Free Hospital and School of Medicine, London, UK

David F. Paulson, MD
Professor and Chief, Division of Urologic Surgery, Duke University Medical Center, Durham, North Carolina, USA

Alexander W. Pearlman, MD
Director, Radiation Therapy, Hospital for Joint Diseases and Associate Clinical Professor in Radiation Therapy, Mount Sinai Medical School, CUNY, New York, USA

Carol S. Portlock, MD
Associate Professor of Medicine, Section of Medical Oncology, Yale University School of Medicine, New Haven, Connecticut, USA

Oleg S. Selawry, MD
Medical Oncologist, Miami Cancer Institute, Florida, USA

Ian E. Smith, MD, MRCP
Consultant Medical Oncologist, Royal Marsden Hospital, London, UK

Basil A. Stoll, FRCR, FFR
Honorary Consulting Physician to Oncology Departments, St Thomas' Hospital and Royal Free Hospital, London, UK

K. D. Swenerton, MD, FRCP(C)
Medical Oncologist, Cancer Control Agency of British Columbia,Vancouver, Canada

Klaus-Rüdiger Trott, MD
Professor, University of Munich Medical Faculty, Radiobiological Institute, Munich, Germany

Ayad Wahba, MD FRCS
Associate Professor of Surgery, Faculty of Medicine, University of Suez Canal, Ismalia, Egypt

Harold J. Wanebo, MD
Professor of Surgery and Chief, Division of Surgical Oncology, University of Virginia Medical Center, Charlottesville, Virginia, USA

Contents

PART 2   PREDICTIVE VARIABLES AND MEASUREMENTS

PART 3   PREDICTIVE FACTORS AND SELECTIVE TREATMENT

Preface to Series

The series is intended to extend the horizons of the very large number of clinicians engaged in the management of the cancer patient. The books will provide a meeting ground between the scientist engaged in research and the practising clinician. The intention is to bridge their divergent philosophy and language so as to provide the clinician with an authoritative and balanced interpretation of new scientific findings and thinking, and to *orientate it specifically to its possible application to the clinical problem.*

Each volume will select a particular aspect of the cancer problem where recent research has suggested a pressing need for new perspectives in the clinical field. It is intended that each volume will be complete in itself.

Preface to Volume 2

It may be timely to examine our present methods of evaluating the results of cancer treatment. We now accept that even very prolonged recurrence-free survival after the primary treatment of cancer does not necessarily imply cure, and that decrease in size of a tumour after treatment does not necessarily imply that life will be prolonged as a result. It is recognized that the pattern of tumour behaviour is unique to each individual and largely reflects the biological characteristics of the tumour in relation to the host reaction.

Currently, there is an increasing trend to randomized trials of therapy which aim to define the method yielding the highest response rates in known subsets of cancer patients. Since our knowledge does not permit us to stratify the cases in the series according to *all* biologically important variables, the results do not identify those smaller subsets of patients in whom possible benefit is outweighed by damage to normal tissues and to the quality of life.

These reservations apply as much to trials of adjuvant systemic therapy in the high-risk patient as they do to comparisons of different forms of palliative treatment in advanced cancer. Overall advantage in a group in a randomized trial by no means implies that the treatment is the 'best buy' for an individual. Carefully planned prospective studies will no doubt throw light on presently unrecognized biological factors influencing prognosis, and randomized trials of therapy will elucidate further variables influencing response—but only if we record a more complete biological characterization of each patient's disease.

Individualization of treatment in the cancer patient will not be achieved until we can fully characterize each tumour biologically, and also quantitate the tumour load and its distribution in the body. Meanwhile, the natural history of each tumour and its tempo of growth need to be taken into account in selecting suitable treatment for each patient, and in not assuming that prolonged survival must necessarily result from a given treatment.

Treatment of the individual patient must continue to be based on an assessment of whether the risk/benefit ratio of a particular treatment justifies its use in the particular circumstances. Many clinical reports on trials in advanced cancer appear to be unclear as to the objectives of their treatment and of the end-points which measure these objectives. This book attempts to identify the problem areas so that we may find means of studying them scientifically.

We have a considerable accumulated knowledge of clinical and pathological prognostic variables for each type of cancer, and we have developed criteria which predict the likelihood of response to each type of treatment. The last section of the book illustrates the application of such factors to the selective treatment of the more common types of cancer.

I am indebted to the contributors for the enthusiasm with which they approached the challenge posed by the topic. Small points of overlap between chapters have been allowed, so that each is complete in itself.

London, 1983   BASIL A. STOLL

Part 1

End-points in treatment

Cancer Treatment: End Point Evaluation
Edited by B.A. Stoll
© 1983 John Wiley & Sons Ltd.

Chapter

1

J. L. HAYBITTLE

What is Cure in Cancer?

The question of whether cancer is curable has aroused considerable controversy. A number of authors in the 1950s (Park and Lees, 1951; McKinnon, 1954; Jones, 1956) took a very pessimistic view of the number of cancer patients that are cured, and even suggested that the effect of early diagnosis and treatment on survival time was negligible. The conclusions of these papers were criticized by other workers (Kraus, 1953; Angelm and Gray, 1961).

Jones (1956) and McKinnon (1954) did not deny that some treated series, when followed up for a long period, showed a residue of patients with death rates similar to the normal population. They maintained, however, that there was no accepted standard by which the malignancy of the original tumours in these 'cured' patients could be satisfactorily established. Their argument was almost a syllogism. Cancer is by definition incurable. Some patients appear to have been cured. Therefore they could not originally have had cancer! Such logic is difficult to counter.

In this chapter, end-points other than cure will first be discussed, followed by an analysis of the concept of cure according to three possible interpretations—statistical cure, clinical cure and personal cure. Each of these will then be dealt with separately in terms of its method of demonstration and the evidence for its achievement.

END-POINTS OTHER THAN CURE

The most commonly used end-point in the past has been the crude five-year survival rate, defined as the number of patients alive at least five years after treatment, expressed as a percentage of the total number of patients treated at least five years before the assessment date. Thus, a patient treated four years prior to the assessment date could not be included in the calculation even if his death had already been recorded.

The crude five-year survival rate has a number of limitations. No account is taken of causes of death: all deaths are included whether they are from cancer arising at the site in question or from intercurrent disease. The rate for an older age series will therefore tend to be lower because of an increased number of deaths from causes other than cancer. This defect can be remedied by calculating an age-corrected or relative survival rate, which is the crude rate divided by the expected fraction of survivors in a normal population of the same age and sex distribution as that of the treated series.

A second limitation of the five-year crude survival rate, which also applies to the corresponding age-corrected rate, is that only patients treated at least five years ago can be included, even though some information on deaths will be available on more recently treated patients. This can be overcome by using the life-table method (Stocks, 1950; Kaplan and Meier, 1958), which makes the maximum use of the available information and thus enables the five-year rate to be estimated with less uncertainty. It is inherent in the method that survival rates are calculated at intermediate times right up to the maximum follow-up time, and the resulting survival curve gives a fuller picture of the progress of the disease.

This also remedies the third limitation of the five-year rate, namely concentration on the result at a single point in time (five years) as a measure of treatment success. Figure 1 shows two survival curves for groups of patients followed up over 15 years. The one for patients with testicular tumours flattens out after an initial dip and in fact, from two years onwards, shows a death rate very similar to that of a normal population. Thus, a two – or three – year survival rate might well be a good indicator of treatment success

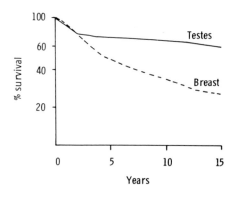

Figure 1. Survival curves for 124 cases of localized tumours of the testis and 1812 cases of cancer of the breast. (Reproduced from Easson and Russell, 1968, by permission of E.C. Easson and Pitman Medical Publishing Co. Ltd.)

in this group. By contrast, the curve for patients treated for cancer of the breast falls steadily throughout the 15-year period, and the five-year rate for these patients is an over-optimistic indicator of treatment success.

Instead of rates based on time from treatment to death, time to recurrence can be used as a measure of treatment success. Some difficulty arises in calculating a *crude* recurrence-free survival rate at say, five years because of patients who have died without recurrence but at a shorter time than five years. The concept of age correction is also inapplicable to recurrence-free survival rates. In general, recurrence-free (or relapse-free or disease-free) survival rates are best calculated by the life-table method in which a patient who dies from other causes without recurrence can be counted as a withdrawal (or as lost to follow-up) at the time of death.

Some assumption has to be made about patients who are reported to have died from their cancer, but with no earlier report of recurrence. Such patients are usually treated as recurrences at their time of death, but this will obviously give a favourable estimate of their recurrence-free times. Estimating time of recurrence in an individual patient (and hence allocating a recurrence-free survival time) is subject to much more uncertainty than estimating survival time to death. It can obviously be influenced by the sensitivity of the diagnostic techniques available and by the frequency of follow-up appointments; this added uncertainty should always be borne in mind when using recurrence-free survival rates for comparative purposes.

CONCEPTS OF CURE

The end-points discussed in the previous section do not answer the question: 'What proportion of patients with cancer at a particular site are cured by a particular treatment regime?' Before discussing methods that might answer such a question, it is necessary to clarify what is meant by the term 'cure' in cancer patients.

A layman's definition would probably be that cure means the complete elimination of disease, so that a patient 'cured' of cancer would be one whose subsequent medical history and length of life was completely unaffected by his having had cancer. In any single individual it would be impossible to assess a cure defined in such a way. Although the *average* life expectancy of a person of a given age is known, there is no means of telling how long a particular individual might have lived if he had not developed cancer. However, a person in whom the cancer had been completely eliminated would not be expected to have a higher risk of dying from that cancer than would persons of the same age and sex in the general population. Some evidence for this type of cure, which might be referred to as *clinical* cure, could be obtained from a study of causes of death in long-term survivors after treatment of cancer.

A patient would no doubt consider himself cured if he had no further symptoms from his cancer for the remainder of his life-time, however long or short he lived. This is obviously not the same as the complete elimination of disease or clinical cure, but, for the individual, would be a very satisfactory outcome and might be termed *personal* cure. Evidence for such cure can be provided not only by studying causes of death in treated series of patients, but also by national statistics of cancer incidence and mortality.

The more generally accepted concept of cure in cancer does not rely on such studies of causes of death with all their inherent uncertainty, and is applied to a group of patients rather than to an individual. It can be stated as follows: *if a group of patients subsequently show an annual death rate from all causes similar to that of a normal population of the same age and sex distribution, then this group can be said to be cured.*

This concept can be traced back to Berkson *et al.* (1952) who compared, on a semi-logarithmic plot, the survival curve of stomach cancer patients with that expected from a normal population of the same age and sex distribution. They showed that, after the seventh year, the annual death rate of cancer survivors became equal to the normal rate. In 1957 in a similar study on breast cancer (Berkson *et al.*, 1957) they commented on the parallelism of the survival curves and stated, 'These patients are "cured"—at least statistically speaking.'

Similar studies by Easson and Russell (1968) made this concept of cure more widely accepted. It is not the same as clinical or personal cure. The long-term survivors may well be subject to a higher risk of dying from cancer and may actually be doing so. It can perhaps be suitably referred to as *statistical* cure, in accordance with the quotation from Berkson *et al.* (1957) given above.

STATISTICAL CURE

Demonstration

The most common method of demonstrating statistical cure is illustrated in Figure 2. Curve A is the expected survival experience of a normal population of the same age and sex distribution as the treated cancer patients. If 30% of these patients are cured 'statistically', their survival experience will be represented by curve B which, since it is on a semi-logarithmic plot, will be parallel to curve A. (Curves which are parallel on a semi-logarithmic plot have the same death rate at any time, defined as $\Delta N/N\Delta t$ where N is the number alive at time t and ΔN is the number dying in the small interval t to $t+\Delta t$.) The remaining 70% who are uncured will have a much worse survival experience which is represented in Figure 2 by a decreasing exponential

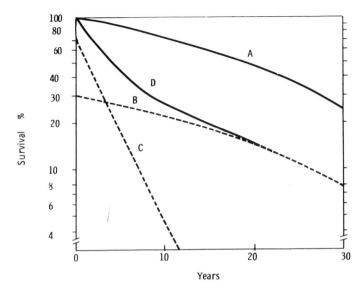

Figure 2 Demonstration of statistical cure. Curve A: expected survival cure of normal population of same age and sex distribution. Curve B: survival curve of 30% cured fraction. Curve C: survival curve of 70% uncured fraction. Curve D: observed survival curve of whole treated group. (Reproduced from Haybittle, 1983).

curve, C, but for the purpose of this illustration the actual form of the curve is unimportant. Curve D will be the survival which is actually observed in the whole group, and is the sum of B and C. In this particular case, the contribution of the uncured patients is insignificant after 20 years and curve D becomes parallel to A. If the uncured patients did much worse, i.e. curve C fell more rapidly, then the parallelism of curves A and D would be apparent earlier.

An alternative method of demonstrating the same point is to plot the age-corrected survival rates, in which case a cured group will be shown up by the curve becoming parallel to the time axis. A semi-logarithmic plot is not necessary for this demonstration.

The visual estimation of parallelism between curves (or between the curve and the time axis) is obviously rather subjective since the curve for the patient group will show irregular fluctuations due to the limited number of patients being observed at long follow-up. Cutler and Axtell (1963) suggested plotting interval survival ratios against time, where the interval survival ratio is defined as the observed conditional probability of surviving through the interval, divided by the conditional probability of surviving through the interval when subject only to normal mortality risks.

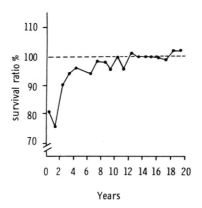

Figure 3 Plot of annual survival ratio for 198 cases of carcinoma of the cervix. After 12 years the ratio is about 100%, demonstrating that the death-rate in the survivors is similar to that in a normal population of the same age distribution. (Reproduced from Cutler and Axtell, 1963, by permission of the American Statistical Association.)

Figure 3 shows such a plot for a group of women treated for localized cancer of the cervix where the survival ratios are calculated in yearly intervals and expressed as percentages. As the mortality in the patient group approaches that of the normal population, the survival ratio approaches 100% and, if the graph then oscillates about this 100% level (as it does after 11 years in Figure 3), a statistically cured group is demonstrated.

A very similar procedure is to compare observed with expected deaths in time intervals, the expected deaths being calculated on the basis of the patient population being subject only to normal mortality risks. Figure 4 shows such ratios calculated in five-year time intervals for two breast cancer series (Langlands *et al.*, 1979; Brinkley and Haybittle, 1980). Statistical cure would be shown by the ratios falling to around unity, something which has not so far happened in either of the series in Figure 4.

Mathematical models have also been proposed for estimating statistical cure. In these models it is assumed that there is a fraction, c, of patients who are cured and only subject to normal mortality, and that the pattern of mortality in the uncured group is determined by a mathematical expression involving one or more parameters. The simplest model (Berkson and Gage, 1952) assumes an exponential mortality curve for the uncured group (as shown in Figure 2), the slope of the curve on a semi-logarithmic plot being determined by one parameter, β.

Boag (1948) showed that, in many series, the survival times of patients who died from cancer were distributed log-normally. His model therefore assumes

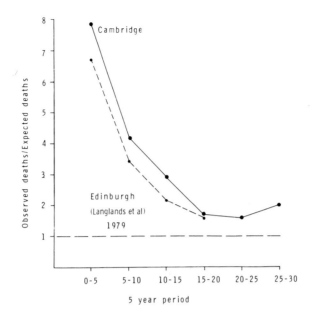

Figure 4 Ratio of observed to expected deaths in five-year periods for two series of cases of carcinoma of the female breast. Cambridge—704 cases reported by Brinkley and Haybittle (1980). Edinburgh—3878 cases reported by Langlands *et al.* (1979). (Reproduced from Haybittle, 1983).

a log-normal distribution of survival times in the uncured group, the mean and standard deviation of the distribution being μ and σ respectively. Haybittle (1959) proposed a model based on an exponential decrease with time of the mortality rate in the *whole* group. This also implies that there is a cured group, c, and only one other parameter, β, is required to determine the overall survival curve (Haybittle, 1965).

The method of maximum likelihood can be used to find the values of the parameters that give the best fit to the observed data and hence provides an estimate of c together with its standard error. If c is more than twice its standard error, then this will support the view that there is a cured fraction in the series.

Before leaving this section, one further comment should be made about the normal mortality rates with which the mortality in the treated series is compared. The normal survival curve is obtained by applying overall population mortality rates to a group of the same age and sex distribution as the initial treated series for the first five years, as the five-year survivors for the next five years, and so on (see Easson and Russell, 1968).

Population mortality rates vary not only from one country to another but also from one area to another within a country. For example, the rates tend to be higher in urban than in rural areas of the same country. It is important therefore to use mortality rates that are derived from the local area which has supplied the patient series, rather than those derived from the whole country. Even if this is done, the validity of the comparison still rests on the assumption that cancer patients differ from the normal population only in having cancer. This is obviously not always so, as instanced by lung cancer patients being more likely to be cigarette smokers and therefore to have a higher risk of death from other forms of disease.

Evidence for statistical cure

A comprehensive attempt to demonstrate cure over a wide range of sites was made by Easson and Russell (1968), who used data on patients treated at the Christie Hospital in Manchester from 1932 to 1949 inclusive, and followed up for a minimum of 15 years. They used the method of comparing curves on semi-logarithmic plots or of looking at age-corrected rates, and claimed to find evidence of curability in cancers of the tongue, mouth, antrum, cervix, testis and bladder, and in Hodgkin's disease and lymphoreticular sarcoma. Figure 5 shows their data for Hodgkin's disease where the age-corrected rates tend to flatten out after 12 years, with cure in about 40% of patients with localized disease.

A similar study of cancers at all sites has recently been published from Finland (Hakulinen *et al.*, 1981). The data are from the Finnish Cancer

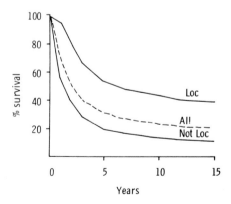

Figure 5 Plots of age-corrected survival rates for 103 localized and 216 non-localized cases of Hodgkin's disease. After 12 years the curves are parallel to the time axis, indicating statistically cured groups of about 40% of localized and about 10% of non-localized cases. (Reproduced from Easson and Russell, 1968, by permission of E.C. Easson and Pitman Medical Publishing Co. Ltd.)

Registry and are for patients registered in the period 1953–1974. Plots of interval survival ratios (Cutler and Axtell, 1963) are used to assess curability. The authors found evidence for cure at a large number of cancer sites, including corpus uteri and ovary, where Easson and Russell (1968) could not find convincing evidence, and also stomach and colon, which were not included in the Manchester survey. The actual proportion cured at these two latter sites was about 8% and 32% respectively, although if expressed as a percentage of patients presenting with localized disease, the figures were higher, about 22% and 57% respectively.

Berkson *et al.* (1952) also presented results from a large series of patients treated for cancer of the stomach and showed that, for those patients who had a total resection, the survival curve after the seventh or eighth year was parallel to that expected from a comparable normal population. About 35% of such patients were cured. Humphrey *et al.* (1979) obtained a similar result for men undergoing total resection, but with a cured group of 26%.

Statistically cured groups in patients treated for cancer of the cervix have been demonstrated by a number of authors, including Cutler and Axtell (1963), whose results were shown in Figure 3. Bush (1979) found that some 60% of a group of 688 patients treated at the Princess Margaret Hospital in Toronto had a normal survival experience up to 14 years. Parallelism of the survival curve of the whole patient series with that of the normal population was achieved from about eight years onwards. Cured groups were also demonstrated by Bush (1979) in patients with cancer of the ovary (31%) and with cancer of the endometrium (67%).

Survival of patients treated for cancers at other sites (lung, colon and rectum) were also studied by Humphrey *et al.* (1979), but in none of these groups were they able to observe a fraction subject only to normal mortality rates. They were however able to show that the survival curves could be represented by two exponential components, which they interpreted as partitioning the patient population into a high and low-risk group. Figure 6, from Humphrey *et al.* (1979), is for 1123 men who underwent resection for squamous carcinoma of the lung. The survival curve is split into two components, 56% dying with an annual mortality rate of 54.1%, and 44% with an annual mortality rate of 9.7%. The expected rate in a normal population would have been 4.2%.

This analysis of survival curves into two exponential components has also been made by other authors. Mueller and Jeffries (1975) and Fox (1979) have claimed that survival of patients treated for cancer of the breast can be represented by two exponential curves. As recognized by Humphrey *et al.* (1979), the finding that survival curves may be fitted by two exponential death rates does not prove that such a model is a correct one. It is unwise, therefore, to try to translate this mathematical finding into evidence for the existence of two biologically distinct populations.

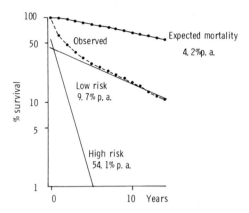

Figure 6 Survival curve for 1123 cases of cancer of the lung, together with that of a normal population of the same age distribution. The two straight lines show how the lung cancer curve may be split into two exponential components, one with a high rate of mortality and the other with a lower rate which is still more than twice that in the normal population. (Reproduced from Humphrey *et al.*, 1979, by permission of the Franklin H. Martin Memorial Foundation, publishers of *Surgery, Gynecology and Obstetrics.*)

Figure 7 illustrates the difficulty of distinguishing a two-exponential model from a more complicated one. The points on the curve would result from a five-component exponential model with the annual mortality rates of each component represented by the dashed lines in the diagram. Looking at the near-linearity of the curve between 15 and 20 years, one might well resolve the whole curve into two components, 55% dying with an annual mortality rate of 4.5%, (the low-risk group), and 45% dying with an annual mortality rate of 27% (the high-risk group). In fact, at no time up to 20 years does the surviving fraction calculated from this model differ from that calculated from the five-component model by more than 0.8%.

Biological data tend not to fit into well defined distinct compartments. A smooth spectrum of risk throughout a patient group seems more plausible, and this is not disproved by the two-component analysis presented in the literature.

The female breast is one of the sites which has received the most attention in the search for evidence of cancer cure. Most of the studies with follow-up of 20 years or less have not been able to demonstrate that the mortality rate for the treated patients became equal to that for a normal population (Jones, 1956; Myers *et al.*, 1966; Mueller and Jeffries, 1975; Langlands *et al.*, 1979; Fox, 1979; Hakulinen *et al.*, 1981).

Studies with longer follow-up have also been reported. Berkson *et al.* (1957) constructed a survival curve for 9477 patients with a maximum

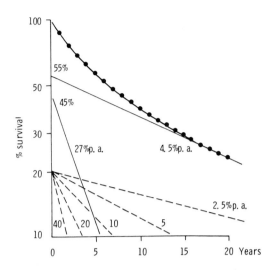

Figure 7 Hypothetical survival curve which can equally well be represented either by two exponential components (55% and 45% each) or by five exponential components each of 20%.

follow-up of 30 years. At about 20 years this curve was parallel with that of a normal population, but as the authors did not extend this latter curve beyond 20 years, it is difficult to judge whether this parallelism was maintained throughout the third decade.

Myers (1973) published a curve of relative survival rate against time up to 25 years for 4675 patients treated in 1940–1944. Between 20 and 25 years this curve was still falling, showing that the observed mortality was higher than that of a normal population. Adair *et al.* (1974) claimed that 21% of their patients in a series, all followed up for at least 28 years, 'must be considered to be practical cures' and no deaths from breast cancer were reported from year 29 to year 33. Unfortunately the authors did not give data from a normal population to demonstrate cure.

Brinkley and Haybittle (1975, 1977) followed up 704 cases from the Cambridge area for a minimum of 22 years and concluded that parallelism of the survival curve with that of the normal population was first evident between 21 and 25 years. A more recent follow-up of this series (Brinkley and Haybittle, 1980), which extends the curves to 30 years, shows that between 25 and 30 years the mortality rate in the breast cancer patients still exceeds that expected in a normal population (Figure 8).

The long-term follow-up studies do not therefore provide convincing evidence of statistical cure in cancer of the breast, although they show a substantial number of survivors free from disease at 20 years or longer after

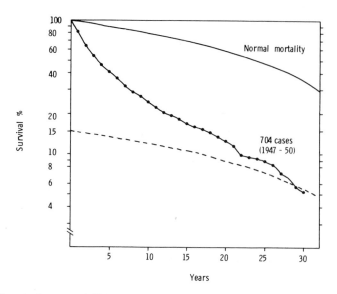

Figure 8 Survival curve of 704 cases of cancer of the breast. Even after 25 years the curve seems to be falling slightly more steeply than that of a normal population of the same age distribution. (Reproduced from Haybittle, 1983)

initial treatment. It has been pointed out elsewhere (Haybittle, 1983) that in cancer of the breast, if none of a series were cured but a fraction of the patients were subject to only a small excess mortality from their cancer, it might be impossible until well after 30 years follow-up to distinguish the survival curve for such a series from one for a series containing a cured fraction.

Use of mathematical models

The estimation of cure by the fitting of mathematical models to survival data has not been as popular as the methods referred to in the previous section.

If the cured fraction in Berkson and Gage's exponential model is zero, then the survival curve is a single exponential with normal mortality superimposed upon it. Jones (1956) and Metcalfe (1974) have claimed that a number of series can be fitted in this way, while Myers *et al.* (1966) and Byar *et al.* (1974), after dividing their series of breast cancers and prostatic cancers into subgroups according to prognostic information, were able to fit single-exponential curves to the survival data for each individual subgroup. In these cases, as demonstrated in Figure 7, the survival curve for the whole group would not be exponential.

Results of using the Berkson and Gage model with a finite value for the fraction cured are not common in the literature. They appear mostly in papers where the behaviour of the model is being compared with the log-normal and exponential model (Haybittle, 1959, 1963; Mould and Boag, 1975). It has been found that the single-exponential model does not always give as good a prediction of long-term survival, and does not represent the true state of affairs in the period immediately after treatment when the death rate is not necessarily a maximum as required by the model.

Boag (1948, 1949) initially demonstrated the use of his log-normal model on small series of cancer of the tonsil and cancer of the breast. Haybittle (1959) also used the log-normal model on three breast cancer series, but claimed some advantages for his own extrapolated actuarial model. A more recent example of the application of the log-normal model has been published by Maetani *et al.* (1980), who estimated that 31% of their series of 1026 patients with gastric cancer were cured.

The extrapolated actuarial model has also been applied to patients with cancer at a number of different sites (Haybittle, 1960) including cervix (Haybittle, 1964, 1965) and Hodgkin's disease (Haybittle, 1963). The most recent use of this model is by Gore *et al.* (1982) who estimated a cured group of 27% in the breast cancer series reported by Langlands *et al.* (1979). Like the Berkson and Gage model, the extrapolated actuarial model has the disadvantage of requiring the maximum death rate to occur in the period immediately after treatment. Gore *et al.* (1982) used it only for fitting the data from five years onwards.

All the papers referred to give results of mathematical model analyses in which a cured fraction is estimated which is greater than twice its standard error, and is therefore significantly different from zero. The validity of the estimates depends, however, on the length of follow-up and on how well the model is likely to fit the long-term survival. For a series of cervix cases (Sorensen, 1958) which were collected over eight years, analyses by all three models at three years after the end of the collection period gave estimates of the fraction cured which were not significantly different from the value of 18% obtained after 25 years follow-up (Haybittle, 1964).

On the other hand, the first analysis by the extrapolated actuarial model of the Cambridge breast cancer series (Figure 8), when all the patients had been followed up for at least seven years, gave an estimate of the fraction cured, c, as 0.242 ± 0.031 (Haybittle, 1959). When repeated after a minimum follow-up of 22 years (Brinkley and Haybittle, 1975), the analysis gave a value of $c = 0.176\pm 0.013$. The earlier analysis was almost certainly too optimistic and even the later result may turn out to be a little high in the light of the more recent follow-up shown in Figure 8.

In summary, although mathematical model analysis enables predictions of cure to be made after relatively short follow-up these predictions may not always be reliable and are unlikely to provide completely convincing evidence of statistical cure.

CLINICAL CURE

Demonstration

The concept of clinical cure introduced earlier requires that a group of long-term survivors shall have no higher risk of dying from cancer of the type for which they were originally treated than have persons of the same age and sex in the general population. Parallelism of survival curves will not show this as, although a group may be statistically cured, they may still be subject to a greater death rate from cancer.

Demonstration of clinical cure must therefore rely on information about individual causes of death, and this can often be obtained only from death certificates. The unreliability of information recorded on death certificates casts considerable doubt on their usefulness in long-term follow-up studies, and this may account for the limited amount of such evidence in the literature.

Evidence for clinical cure

In breast cancer it has been shown that although the survival curves approach parallelism after 20 years or so (Figure 8), the rate of dying from breast cancer in the long-term survivors was still much higher than would have been expected in a normal population. Brinkley and Haybittle (1977) found the mortality from breast cancer in their 20-year survivors to be at least 12 times as high as expected, and a more recent analysis of deaths between 20 and 30 years (Brinkley and Haybittle, 1980) found this ratio had increased to 16. They also found a significantly increased number of deaths from cancers at other sites.

Ederer *et al.* (1963) reported that, in treated breast cancer patients dying between 15 and 20 years after treatment, deaths from cancer of the breast were 16 times the expected number and deaths from cancer at other sites were 1.5 times the expected number. This latter ratio was not significantly different from unity, and two of the authors (Ederer and Goldenburg, 1961) noted in a subsample of the patients that death certificates of breast cancer patients, particularly long-term survivors, tended to underestimate breast cancer mortality and overstate mortality from other forms of cancer. Thus the finding of excess deaths from other cancers may be an artefact.

Humphrey *et al.* (1979) found that, for cancer of the lung and also for cancer of the colon and rectum, the death rate in long-term survivors was greatest for cancer of the original organ, being approximately 10 times the expected rate in a normal population. By contrast, in cancer of the stomach, where they were able to demonstrate a statistically cured group, there was no excess death rate from cancer of the stomach after eight years. Thus, in this one series, clinical cure does seem to have been achieved, but other evidence is scanty and must await further studies on causes of death together with more reliable death certification.

PERSONAL CURE

Demonstration

Any treated cancer patient who dies from other causes without any signs or symptoms of his original cancer is a demonstration of personal cure as defined earlier. More generally, such cure may be demonstrated by a study of nationally collected figures of cancer incidence and mortality. Such data have the advantage of being based on very large numbers, but are subject to inaccuracies due to misdiagnosis of cause of death, and possible underestimation of incidence due to inefficient coverage by cancer registries. Nevertheless, the figures can be used to shed some light on the proportion of patients with cancer at a given site who are registered as dying of some other cause. These will not *all* have achieved personal cure, as some may have had overt symptoms of their cancer present at death, even though it was not a contributory cause.

If a disease is treated successfully, then the annual number of deaths reported from that disease will be small compared with the annual number of patients presenting with the disease. On the other hand, if a disease is almost invariably followed by death from that disease, then the annual number of such deaths will approximate to the annual incidence. Since deaths will usually occur in years subsequent to the year of incidence, this equivalence will apply only if the annual incidence is constant and an equilibrium situation has been reached. For a slowly changing annual incidence, a comparison of incidence with deaths T years later (where T is the median survival time for patients with the disease in question) will give a good indication of the proportion achieving personal cure.

Evidence for personal cure

Figure 9 shows the data on annual registrations and deaths since 1962 for England and Wales for four cancer sites. Deaths and registrations are almost equal for cancer of the trachea, bronchus and lung throughout the period, and both have been increasing. This would be consistent with very few personal cures for patients with cancer at these sites, i.e. nearly all patients die with their cancer after a short survival time. By contrast, the data for cancer of the breast, although showing a slow increase in both deaths and registrations, consistently shows the curve for deaths well below that for registrations. The

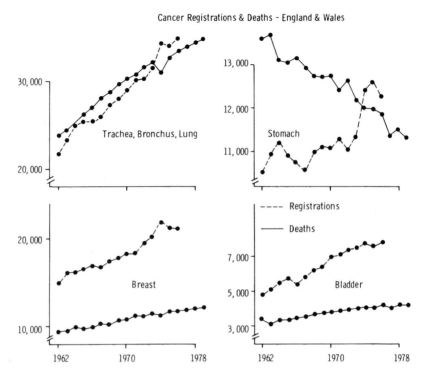

Figure 9 Comparison of cancer registrations and deaths in England and Wales for four cancer sites.

ratio of deaths to registrations four years earlier (the approximate median survival time for all breast cancer), is about 0.65 which could be interpreted as 35% of breast cancer patients achieving personal cure.

Similar data for cancer of the breast from Finland, Sweden and New York State suggest higher figures (from 45% to 60%) for the proportion achieving personal cure (Haybittle, 1983). The differences between the results in the different areas may largely be due to the wide geographical differences in stage distribution at presentation.

The results for England and Wales for cancer of the bladder (Figure 9) show a similar picture to that for cancer of the breast, with the implication that about 40% of such cases achieve personal cure.

The picture for cancer of the stomach is anomalous. Between 1962 and 1973, deaths from cancer of the stomach were well above registrations suggesting that quite large errors occurred either in initial diagnosis or in death certification, or in both. Throughout the period, deaths were falling while incidence was rising, suggesting that the liability to error was also changing. The figures are probably too unreliable to deduce anything about personal cure in cancer of the stomach. There are certainly no signs of a personally cured group corresponding to the statistically cured groups demonstrated by Berkson *et al.* (1952) and Humphrey *et al.* (1979).

CONCLUSION

Measures of treatment success, such as survival or relapse-free time, are obviously of value in comparing the results of different treatment modalities, but do not give information about cure. Of the three concepts of cure discussed in this chapter, clinical cure (i.e. the complete elimination of cancer from the patient) would be the most satisfying to the clinician but is in fact the most difficult to establish. The evidence for it is sparse and, relying as it does on accurate knowledge of causes of death, may not be forthcoming in practice.

Statistical cure can be demonstrated at a number of sites, and at many others the mortality rate in long-term survivors is not very much greater than the expected rate in a comparable normal population. Even if the percentage statistically cured is satisfying, it is still very disappointing to a clinician (and a reflection on the choice of treatment) if a long-term survivor suffers recurrence and death from his original cancer.

There is little doubt that a large number of treated cancer patients will experience personal cure in that they live symptom-free from their cancer until they die from some other cause. In the case of breast cancer, where evidence in favour of clinical and statistical cure is still very inconclusive, about 30% of all cases in England and Wales (and even higher percentages in Scandinavia) may be personally cured.

Perhaps too much emphasis in the past has been placed on clinical and statistical cure, the final proof of which could be very elusive at some sites. What matters to the patient is the length of recurrence-free survival without morbidity. New treatment methods that can increase this time will increase the number of patients experiencing personal cure, since they will on average be exposed for a longer period of time to the competing risks of death from other causes.

REFERENCES

Adair, F., Berg, J., Lourdes, J., and Robbins, G. F. (1974). Long-term follow-up of breast cancer patients: the 30–year report. *Cancer*, **33**, 1145–1150.

Angelm, T.J., and Gray, E.B. (1961). Cancer of the breast and biological predeterminism: a re-evaluation. *Cancer*, **14**, 1122–1126.

Berkson, J., and Gage, R.P. (1952). Survival curves for cancer patients following treatment. *J. Am. Stat. Assoc.*, **47**, 501–515.

Berkson, J., Harrington, S.W., Clagett, O.T., Kirklin, J.W., Dockerty, M.B., and McDonald, J.R. (1957). Mortality and survival in surgically treated cancer of the breast: a statistical summary of some experience of the Mayo Clinic. *Proc. Staff Meet Mayo Clinic*, **32**, 645–670.

Berkson, J., Walters, W., Gray, H.K., and Priestly, J.T. (1952). Mortality and survival in cancer of the stomach: a statistical summary of the experience of the Mayo Clinic. *Proc. Staff Meet. Mayo Clinic*, **27**, 137–51.

Boag, J.W. (1948). The presentation and analysis of the results of radiotherapy. *Br. J. Radiol.*, **21**, 128–138, 189–203.

Boag, J.W. (1949). Maximum likelihood estimates of the proportion of patients cured by cancer therapy. *J. R. Stat. Soc. B*, **11**, 15–44.

Brinkley, D., and Haybittle, J.L. (1975). The curability of breast cancer. *Lancet*, **ii**, 95–97.

Brinkley, D., and Haybittle, J.L. (1977). The curability of breast cancer. *World J. Surg.*, **1**, 287–289.

Brinkley, D., and Haybittle, J.L. (1980). The concept of cure in breast cancer. Paper read before a meeting of the Yorkshire Breast Cancer Group.

Bush, R.S. (1979). *Malignancies of the ovary, uterus and cervix*. London: Edward Arnold.

Byar, D.B., Huse, R., and Bailar III, J.C. (1974). An exponential model relating censored survival data and concomitant information for prostatic cancer patients. *J. Nat. Cancer Inst.*, **52**, 321–326.

Cutler, S.J., and Axtell, L.M. (1963). Partitioning of a patient population with respect to different mortality risks. *J. Am. Stat. Assoc.*, **58**, 701–712.

Easson, E.C., and Russell, M.H. (1968). *The curability of cancer in various sites*. London: Pitman Medical.

Ederer, F., Cutler, S.J., Goldenburg, I.S., and Eisenberg, H. (1963). Causes of death among long-term survivors from breast cancer in Connecticut. *J. Nat. Cancer Inst.*, **30**, 933–947.

Ederer, F. and Goldenburg, I.S. (1961). An inquiry into the accuracy of the statement of causes of death on the death certificates of breast cancer patients. *Methodological notes* no.16, End Results Evaluation Section, National Cancer Institute.

Fox, M.S. (1979). On the diagnosis and treatment of breast cancer. *J. Am. Med. Assoc.*, **241**, 489–494.

Gore, S., Langlands, A., Pocock, S., and Kerr, G. (1982). Natural history of breast cancer. Recent Results in Cancer Res., **80**, 134–141.

Hakulinen, T., Pukkala, E., Hakama, M., Lehtonen, M., Saxen, E., and Teppo, L. (1981). Survival of cancer patients in Finland in 1953–1974. *Ann. Clin. Res.*, 13, Suppl. 31.

Haybittle, J.L. (1959). The estimation of the proportion of patients cured after treatment for cancer of the breast. *Br. J. Radiol.*, **32**, 725–733.

Haybittle, J.L. (1960). The early estimation of the results of treatment for cancer. *Br. J. Radiol.*, **33**, 502–506.

Haybittle, J.L. (1963). Cure of Hodgkin's disease. *Br. Med. J.*, **2**, 933.

Haybittle, J.L. (1964). The cured group in series of patients treated for cancer. *Anglo-German Med. Rev.*, **2**, 422–436.

Haybittle, J.L. (1965). A two-parameter model for the survival curve of treated cancer patients. *J. Am. Stat. Assoc.*, **60**, 16–26.

Haybittle, J.L., (1983).The evidence for cure in female breast cancer. In *Commentaries on research in breast disease* (eds R.D. Bulbrook and D.J. Taylor). New York: Alan R. Liss.

Humphrey, E.W., Higgins, G.A., and Shields, T.W. (1979). The long term survival of patients with visceral carcinoma. *Surg., Gynecol. Obstet.*, **149**, 385–394.

Jones, H.B. (1956). Demographic consideration of the cancer problem. *Trans. N. Y. Acad. Sci., II*, **18**, 298–333.

Kaplan, E.L., and Meier, P. (1958). Nonparametric estimation from incomplete observations. *J. Am. Stat. Assoc.* **53**, 457–481.

Kraus, A.S. (1953). A review of the effectiveness of early treatment in breast cancer. *Surg., Gynecol. Obstet.*, **96**, 545–552.

Langlands, A.O., Pocock, S.J., Kerr, G.R., and Gore, S.M. (1979). Long-term survival of patients with breast cancer: a study of the curability of the disease. *Br. Med. J.*, **2**, 1247–1251.

Maetani, S., Tobe, T., Hirakawa, A., Kashiwara, S., and Kuramoto, S. (1980). Parametric survival analysis of gastric cancer patients. *Cancer*, **46**, 1709–2716.

Metcalfe, W. (1974). Analysis of cancer survival as an exponential phenomenon. *Surg., Gynecol. Obstet.* , **138**, 737–740.

McKinnon, N.E. (1954). Control of cancer mortality. *Lancet*, **i**, 251–255.

Mould, R.F., and Boag, J.W. (1975). A test of several parametric statistical models for estimating success rate in the treatment of carcinoma cervix uteri.*Br. J. Cancer*, **33**, 529–550.

Mueller, C.B., and Jeffries, W. (1975). Cancer of the breast: its outcome as measured by the rate of dying and causes of death. *Ann. Surg.*, **182**, 334–341.

Myers, M.H. (1973). Breast cancer survival over three decades. In *Recent results in cancer research: Breast cancer—A challenging problem.*(Eds: M.L. Griem,, J. V. Jensen, J. E. Ultmann and R. W. Wassler), Berlin: Springer-Verlag.

Myers, M.H., Axtell, L.M., and Zelen, M. (1966). The use of prognostic factors in predicting survival for breast cancer patients. *J. Chronic Dis.* **19**, 923–933.

Park, W.W., and Lees, J.C. (1951). The absolute curability of cancer of the breast. *Surg. Gynecol. Obstet.* **93,** 129–152.

Sorensen, B. (1958). Late results of radium therapy in cervical carcinoma. *Acta Radiol.* Suppl. 169, 65–75.

Stocks, P. (1950). Methods of measuring results in the treatment of cancer. *J. Fac. Radiol.* , **1**, 187–197.

Cancer Treatment: End Point Evaluation
Edited by B.A. Stoll
© 1983 John Wiley & Sons Ltd.

Chapter

2   IAN E. SMITH

Measuring Response in Incurable Cancer

In treating incurable cancer, the first aim is to improve, or at least preserve, the quality of remaining life as much as possible. The second is to attempt to prolong survival, with the proviso that this does not compromise quality of life unacceptably. The therapeutic dilemma is of course, that the degree of morbidity which might be tolerable in an attempt at cure could be quite unacceptable in the case of the incurable patient. The measurement of response to treatment in incurable cancer must take this morbidity into account.

This chapter discusses the main techniques currently used in measuring response to treatment in incurable cancer. It is the author's belief that some of these have serious inadequacies in assessing whether the two main aims of treatment are being achieved. Therefore, in the final section, guidelines to possible improvements in approach will be outlined.

OBJECTIVE TUMOUR RESPONSE AND ANTI-TUMOUR ACTIVITY

Objective measurement of tumour regression has become in recent years the single most widely used criterion for assessing response to therapy in the incurable patient. Its validity in terms of patient benefit therefore needs critical examination.

Tumour shrinkage has always been considered a reasonable aim for cancer treatment, whether by surgery, radiotherapy of drugs. For many years the way in which this was recorded was left largely to the clinician's individual judgment, and new forms of therapy often brought enthusiastic, but sometimes widely differing, claims from therapeutic pioneers. As an example, the response rate for advanced squamous cell carcinoma of lung treated with chemotherapy has been reported as ranging from 0 to 100% (Selawry, 1974), and for pancreatic carcinoma as ranging from 0 to 67% (Hurley and Ellison, 1960).

It therefore became clear that strict objective criteria were required both to measure the anti-tumour activity of new forms of treatment and also to enable comparisons to be made with conventional therapy. From this, the concept of strictly defined objective tumour response emerged to become the main, and often the only, yardstick in the literature for assessing anti-tumour activity. Different systems have been used, although with an increasing trend towards conformity (WHO, 1979). For some tumour types the criteria used are elaborate: for example, objective response for all likely sites of metastatic disease in breast carcinoma is usually defined by standard UICC criteria which were published originally in a seven-page document (Hayward and Rubens, 1977).

Whatever the details used in different systems of measurement, all include two main definitions: complete remission (CR) is defined as disappearance of all clinical evidence of tumour; partial response (PR) is defined as a 50% or greater reduction in measurable tumour for an arbitrary period, usually of at least one month.

Although discussed more fully in a later chapter, some technical difficulties in measurement and interpretation need to be mentioned. The achievement of a partial response will depend on whether the required 50% reduction in tumour size relates to diameter, area or volume (and these vary in the literature). The first is clearly the most rigorous, a 50% reduction in diameter being equivalent to a 75% reduction in area and an 87.5% reduction in volume (or at least roughly so, assuming tumours to be 'circles' or 'spheres'). These details must therefore be included for response data to be assessed and compared accurately.

The achievement of a complete remission will often depend upon the intensity with which residual tumour is sought. A laparotomy after treatment for Hodgkin's disease or ovarian carcinoma will reveal residual disease in some patients who might otherwise be judged as in complete remission (Wiltshaw, 1981; Schwartz and Smith, 1980). The same is true for repeat bronchoscopy after treatment for lung cancer (Ihde *et al.*, 1979) and for other examples of investigation. Such details need to be specified for accurate assessment of response data.

Another problem is that some tumours are anatomically inaccessible for careful measurement, pancreatic carcinoma being an obvious example. A bias may be inevitable from the fact that tumour response can be measured only in relatively accessible sites (Smith and Schein, 1979).

The site of metastatic involvement may present another problem, as for example in the assessment of response in bone. Recalcification of lytic lesions on x-ray is usually used as an objective measurement (Hayward and Rubens,

1977) but this process is often delayed. Furthermore, subjective relief of bone pain after treatment is not uncommonly seen without recalcification (Smith *et al.*, 1978). Recently, attempts have been made to overcome these problems using serial measurements on isotopic bone scans (Citrin *et al.*, 1981) or biochemical parameters of bone metabolism. Changes in urinary hydroxyproline excretion for example, have been claimed to provide earlier evidence of response in bone than do other parameters (Powles *et al.*, 1975).

Finally, for a few tumours the system can hardly be made to work at all in a practical way. Prostatic carcinoma with its palpable but almost unmeasurable primary site, and its radiologically little changed sclerotic bone metastases, is the most obvious example. Here, alternative methods of assessment based on weight gain, relief of symptoms, performance status and serum enzyme changes are used instead (BMJ Editorial, 1980).

Despite the difficulties described, the measurement of objective tumour response has to a considerable extent fulfilled its original function, that is to give a formal measurement of the anti-tumour activity of a specific therapy and to allow comparison with other forms of treatment.

One example is in the use of cytotoxic drugs in the treatment of advanced non-small cell lung cancer, where, in the past, 'responses' in up to 100% of patients were being reported (Selawry, 1974). Recent critical analysis by the yardstick of objective tumour response has demonstrated that conventional drugs, even when used in combination, rarely achieve response rates in excess of 20%, while complete responses are very rare (Livingston, 1977). This has relieved clinicians of any ethical 'pressure' to use conventional chemotherapy for these tumours and patients need therefore no longer be exposed to unpleasant and ineffective treatment.

Instead, either symptomatic treatment alone can be offered, or else new drugs can be tested as first-line treatment in the context of a carefully supervised clinical trial at a time in the natural history of the tumour when they have the best chance of showing anti-tumour efficacy. Based on this approach, a new drug combination using vindesine and cisplatin has been shown to have greater anti-tumour activity than conventional agents in such tumours (Gralla *et al.*, 1981), and this treatment can now be assessed for patient benefit.

A second example concerns the activity of cytotoxic drugs in advanced breast cancer. Reassessment of the early conventional drugs used against this tumour, but using strict criteria of objective response, has again shown a significantly lower response rate than was generally claimed in the past (Hoogstraten and Fabian, 1979); response rates fell from 45% to 22% for 5-fluorouracil (5–FU), from 45% to 22% for cyclophosphamide and from 40% to 17% for thiotepa. Thus, a more realistic yardstick is now available against which the anti-tumour activity of alternative forms of treatment may be compared in breast cancer.

CLINICAL SIGNIFICANCE OF OBJECTIVE TUMOUR RESPONSE

Although objective tumour response has importance in the assessment of anti-tumour activity, the real question is the extent to which this measure correlates with clinical benefit to the patient. This is vitally important because tumour response is increasingly widely used as the main, and indeed often the only criterion for assessing therapeutic benefit.

For example, a combination of vindesine and cisplatin has recently been advocated as superior to other forms of therapy for advanced malignant melanoma, on the basis of a 30% response rate (Dodion *et al.*, 1981). No survival data were given and no mention was made of effect on quality of life, although it was noted that all patients experienced severe nausea and vomiting, the majority developed alopecia, and neurotoxicity and renal impairment were noted in some. Likewise, a three-drug regimen has been advocated as having 'definite advantage' over single-drug treatment for advanced colonic cancer on the basis of a higher response rate alone; no significant difference in survival was observed, and quality of life was not assessed in any detail (Falkson and Falkson, 1976).

Again, in a much quoted trial, chemotherapy was claimed to be superior to endocrine therapy in the treatment of advanced breast carcinoma principally on the basis of a higher response rate (Priestman *et al.*, 1977). Yet in a subsequent analysis, no significant survival difference was seen for the two different treatments (Priestman *et al.*, 1978). To be fair to the authors, this was one of the few published trials in which an attempt was made to assess quality of life associated with each of the treatments.

These examples are in no way isolated. Objective tumour response is used throughout the literature not simply as the main criterion for assessing treatment benefit but often as the *only* one. In a recent review of chemotherapy for gastrointestinal malignancies, tabulated data from 45 separate studies are given for response rate alone; even in the text, survival data are only rarely discussed and quality of life not at all (Smith *et al.*, 1979).

The same is true for a review of advanced breast cance therapy tabulating 62 forms of treatment (Rubens, 1979), and for bladder and prostatic cancer tabulating 22 treatment studies (Stoter *et al.*, 1979). Many similar examples could be quoted. What, then, is the basis for the assumption that objective response alone correlates with the fundamental criteria of treatment benefit, namely quality of life and survival?

Although quality of life is dealt with in detail in a subsequent chapter, a few points need to be made here. The first is that the great majority of published studies make no attempt to record quality of life in any detail as a treatment end-point. Those that do tend to use some standard measure of patient performance status, the best known of which is probably the Karnofsky scale (Karnofsky and Burchenal, 1948). The limitations of this type of assessment are two-fold: first they give only a fairly crude measure of the degree of physical dependence or independence of the patient and take little account of possible social and psychological problems; secondly, and more importantly, they are an *objective* measure of how the clinician perceives the patient's quality of life, and not a *subjective* account by the patient himself.

One technique which attempts to allow the patient to grade his own quality of life in physical, social and emotional terms is that of linear analogue self-assessment (LASA). The technique has become a standard and reproducible tool for psychological testing (Bond and Lader, 1974) but has so far had very limited use in assessing response to cancer therapy. A pilot study suggests that the technique can be used to monitor changes in quality of life during treatment in patients with advanced breast cancer (Priestman and Baum, 1976) and perhaps also to compare the effects of different types of treatment on quality of life (Baum *et al.*, 1980).

Changes in LASA scores correlated with objective tumour responses both to endocrine therapy and to chemotherapy, but some aspects of these studies were a little surprising, in particular the finding that scores were consistently higher for patients on chemotherapy than on endocrine therapy. The work needs repeating and expanding but the LASA technique may be of potential importance in the measurement of response in incurable cancer.

TUMOUR RESPONSE AND SURVIVAL

Complete response

Complete response to therapy is a necessary prerequisite for cure, and the achievement of complete remission, even if only in a few patients at first, has come to be regarded as an important milestone in the development of curative treatment. Even for incurable patients, the achievement of a complete remission whether by surgery, radiotherapy or chemotherapy is usually associated with a better prognosis than is absence of response. Some examples are given in Tables 1 to 3.

In the case of surgery, attempts at tumour resection for incurable disease (or disease with little chance of cure) are restricted to a few tumour types. The patients with complete resection have a longer median survival than those whose tumours are unresectable; examples include gastric carcinoma (Lawrence and Lawrence, 1980), advanced intraperitoneal ovarian carcinoma (Griffiths *et al.*, 1979), and recurrent colorectal carcinoma (Holyoke and Ledesma, 1981). For some tumours, however, including pancreatic carcinoma, it is dubious whether complete resection is associated with any significant degree of prolonged survival (Shapiro, 1975).

In the case of radiotherapy for advanced cancer, a similar survival advantage for complete or near-complete responders over non-responders

Table 1 Correlation of degree of tumour 'response' with survival after surgery

Tumour	Median survival (months)			Reference
	CR	PR	NR	
Stomach	15	9	4.5	Lawrence and Lawrence (1980)
Colorectal (recurrent)	50	21	12	Holyoke and Ledesma (1981)
Pancreas	12[a]		8[b]	Shapiro (1975)
Lung	16[a]		8[b]	Sherman and Weichselbaum (1981)
Ovary	22[c]	9[d]		Griffiths *et al.* (1979)

[a] Resectable
[b] Non-resectable
[c] Residual nodules, <1.5 cm diameter
[d] Residual nodules, >1.5 cm diameter

has been demonstrated for several tumour types including deeply infiltrating bladder carcinoma (Wallace and Bloom, 1976; van der Werf-Messing, 1979), carcinoma of uterine cervix (Dische *et al.*, 1980)), and probably lung cancer, although here the difference is relatively small (White and Boles, 1981).

Finally, in the case of chemotherapy, a clear-cut survival benefit has likewise been shown for most tumours in which complete remissions can be achieved: examples include acute leukaemia, malignant teratoma (Einhorn *et al.*, 1981), Hodgkin's disease (de Vita *et al.*, 1980), and ovarian cancer Young *et al.*, 1978: de Palo *et al.* 1981). Occasional exceptions are suggested in the literature. Two studies have reported that patients with certain indolent lymphomas who achieve complete remission on chemotherapy do not survive significantly longer than non-responders (Ezdinli *et al.*, 1978; 1980).

Our own experience with the endocrine agent, aminoglutethimide, in advanced breast cancer suggests that complete responders have the same survival probability as those whose disease merely remains stable, although

Table 2 Correlation of degree of tumour response with survival after radiotherapy

Tumour	Median survival (months)			Reference
	CR	PR	NR	
Bladder	36	12[b]		Wallace and Bloom (1976)
	40[a]		15	van der Werf-Messing (1979)
Lung	17	10	7	White and Boles (1981)
	13[a]		7	Salazar *et al.* (1976)
Cervix	96	24	8	Salazar *et al.* (1976)

[a] CR + PR
[b] PR + NR

Table 3 Correlation of degree of tumour response with survival after chemotherapy

Tumour	Median survival (months)			Reference
	CR	PR	NR	
Ovary	36	16	7	Young *et al.* (1978)
	21	13[b]		de Palo *et al.* (1981)
Small cell lung	12	9	3	Maurer *et al.* (1980)
Non-small cell lung	—	22[c]	6	Gralla *et al.* (1981)
	—	10[d]	6	Gralla *et al.* (1981)
	—	6	5	Taylor *et al.* (1980)
Breast	22[a]		8	Brambilla *et al.* (1976)
	24[a]		14	Brambilla *et al.* (1976)
	16[a]		4	Creech *et al.* (1979)
	15[a]		3	Powles *et al.* (1980)
Gastric	12		3	McDonald *et al.* (1980)
Colorectal	10		5	Lavin *et al.* (1980)
Teratoma	Cure common	11	11	Einhorn *et al.* (1981)
Hodgkin's	Cure common	11	11	de Vita *et al.*
Lymphoma (diffuse histiocytic)	Cure common	5	6	Elias *et al.* (1978)

[a] CR + PR
[b] PR + NR
[c] Low dose
[d] High dose

better than those with progressive disease on treatment (Harris *et al.*, 1981). Such exceptions are rare, however, and the general statement remains true that complete response is usually associated with significantly prolonged survival.

Partial response

The relationship between partial response and survival is more tenuous and variable than for complete response (Tables 1 – 3). In surgery, the concept of partial resection of an incurable cancer is an unusual one, and this approach is not widely used except to relieve symptoms, for example in intestinal obstruction. Partial resection for gastric cancer is reported to be associated with a slightly longer median survival than non-resection (9 months versus 4.5 months) (Lawrence and Lawrence, 1980), and the same is true for recurrent colo-rectal cancer (Holyoke and Ledesma, 1981). In contrast, little survival benefit has been demonstrated for partial (in contrast to near-complete) resection for advanced ovarian cancer (Griffiths *et al.*, 1979).

For radiotherapy, the significance of achieving a partial response appears to vary for different tumours. In advanced carcinoma of cervix, it is associated with significantly prolonged survival compared with that of non-responders (Dische *et al.*, 1980). In contrast, a survival benefit of only 3 months has been reported for partial responders over non-responders with lung cancer (Salazar *et al.*, 1976). In a further study no significant difference at all in survival between partial and non-responders was reported for adenocarcinomas, small cell carcinomas and large cell carcinomas of lung (Lee *et al.*, 1976). Likewise, for squamous cell tumours of the head and neck, no significant survival difference between partial responders and non-responders is apparent. (Mantyla *et al.*, 1979).

With chemotherapy, the survival significance of partial response also varies with tumour type (Table 3). It is unusual for partial responders to survive as long as complete responders, but for some tumours partial response still carries some survival benefit over absence of response. Examples include advanced breast cancer (Brambilla *et al.*, 1976; Creech *et al.*, 1979; Powles *et al.*, 1980a), small cell lung cancer (Einhorn *et al.*, 1978; Maurer *et al.*, 1980), non-small cell lung cancer (Gralla *et al.*, 1981), gastric cancer (Levi *et al.*, 1979; McDonald *et al.*, 1980), and perhaps ovarian cancer (Young *et al.*, 1978), although for this tumour at least one study suggests no significant difference (de Palo *et al.*, 1981). However, it should be noted from Table 3 that such survival advantages are usually of a few months only.

For several tumour types it is well established that a partial response to chemotherapy confers no significant survival benefit at all over absence of response. Examples include acute leukaemia, malignant teratoma (Einhorn *et al.*, 1981), Hodgkin's disease (de Vita *et al.*, 1980), the more aggressive lymphomas including diffuse histiocytic (Elias *et al.*, 1978), and non-small cell lung cancer treated with conventional drugs (Taylor *et al.*, 1980).

To summarize, although complete response is associated with significantly prolonged survival, at least for most tumour types, the same is not necessarily true for partial response. Partial response is an unreliable prognostic criterion. For some tumour types the treatment may be worse than useless as far as patient benefit is concerned, if significant treatment-related morbidity is coupled with lack of survival advantage. The use of objective tumour response, and in particular partial response, as the main criterion for assessing treatment benefit in terms of survival for patients with incurable disease therefore appears unwarranted.

SURVIVAL IN RESPONDING AND NON-RESPONDING PATIENTS

In contrast to the difficulties inherent both in measuring and interpreting objective tumour response, survival would appear to be an easy end-point to assess in patients with incurable disease. There are, however, important pitfalls in the interpretation of survival data and these continue to be evident both in the literature and in therapeutic decision-making for the individual patient. Such pitfalls can lead to unjustified claims for the survival benefit of treatment.

It has already been shown for some but not all tumours, that patients who achieve an objective response to therapy survive longer than those who fail to respond. This is all too frequently interpreted to mean that treatment itself prolongs survival. For example, a paper describing a 9 month median survival after partial resection for advanced stomach cancer compared with 4.5 months for tumours where no resection was attempted, states that 'palliative resection ...appears to prolong survival' (Lawrence and Lawrence, 1980). Similarly, in a report on radiotherapy for inoperable lung cancer, the authors conclude that 'treatment directed at improving local control can therefore have a significant effect on survival' (White and Boles, 1981). Similar claims are regularly made for chemotherapy.

Treatment *may* of course prolong survival but such data do not allow this conclusion to be drawn. Response to therapy may simply be a feature of a tumour with an inherently good prognosis. For example, complete response to surgery implies a tumour in which excision is possible by virtue of its being sufficiently localized in the first place, perhaps because of detection at an early stage in its natural history or because of biological characteristics which lead to slow growth and absence of early metastatic spread. Likewise, clinical responsiveness to radiotherapy or chemotherapy might simply be one of many biological features of a tumour with an innately good prognosis. In other words, patients whose tumours respond to treatment might have done better than non-responders even without treatment.

Clinical evidence for this contention comes from a multicentre study comparing different chemotherapy regimens for advanced colorectal carcinoma (Lavin *et al.*, 1980). Responders survived significantly longer than non-responders, but it was also observed that the median interval between diagnosis and start of treatment was significantly longer for responders than for non-responders, suggesting that the former were a biologically different group with a longer natural history independent of therapy.

There is another facet to this argument. Patients whose tumours fail to respond to therapy might actually have survival shortened by treatment, particularly where this is followed by rapid deterioration. It is well recognized that a laparotomy for an inoperable intra-abdominal malignancy is often associated with rapid subsequent deterioration. Similarly, it seems unlikely that intensive radiotherapy or chemotherapy which fails to achieve a tumour response in an already debilitated patient would be beneficial. In fact for some tumours there is good evidence (see below) that ineffective treatment actually does shorten life.

Clear-cut evidence for survival benefit from treatment can only be obtained by comparing a treated group of patients with a matched non-treated group, ideally in a randomized trial. For a few incurable tumours, such trials have been conducted. In small cell lung cancer, clear-cut evidence for prolongation of survival by chemotherapy is well established (Bunn and Ihde, 1981). Likewise for pancreatic carcinoma, at least one such trial has suggested clear-cut survival benefit (Mallinson *et al.*, 1980). In contrast, no evidence for survival benefit following chemotherapy for advanced colorectal carcinoma has been demonstrated, despite the fact that responders live longer than non-responders (Moertel, 1975). Even more disturbing is the demonstration in at least two control trials in non-small cell lung cancer that the addition of chemotherapy shortened survival (Landgren *et al.*, 1973; Brunner *et al.*, 1973).

For many tumour types no such therapeutic trials have been conducted, sometimes because of 'clinical instinct' that treatment must be beneficial and sometimes through the mistaken belief that such evidence already exists, based on the 'responders living longer' argument described above. The fallacy inherent in such an argument is further illustrated in a recent analysis of the survival impact of chemotherapy for advanced breast carcinoma. Today in the United Kingdom, chemotherapy is more widely prescribed for this tumour than for any other; but although it is well established that responders to this treatment survive longer than non-responders (Brambilla *et al.*, 1976; Creech *et al.*, 1979; Powles *et al.*, 1980a), nevertheless no control randomized trial of chemotherapy has ever been published and indeed many would consider such a trial unethical.

In one study, survival in a group of patients treated with combination chemotherapy was compared to an earlier group who did not receive this treatment because of its lack of availability at the time (Powles *et al.*, 1980a). No significant difference in survival was seen between the two groups, despite the fact that chemotherapy responders lived significantly longer than non-responders. Despite criticism of this study based on 'the responders surviving longer than non-responders' argument (Greenspan, 1980), no contradictory data have so far been published.

It is important not to misinterpret this point. All who have treated advanced breast cancer with chemotherapy have seen critically ill patients with extensive liver metastases or pulmonary carcinomatous lymphangitis respond dramatically to chemotherapy and survive for many months or even years with a good quality of life. The fact that an *overall* benefit cannot be demonstrated may well reflect the possibility that the advantages of treatment in some patients are outweighed by the disadvantages to non-responding patients. The latter may result from morbidity of treatment, denial of potentially worthwhile hormone therapy or perhaps even the failure to recognize that some patients would have done better with symptomatic measures alone.

Whatever the reasons, there are two main conclusions to be drawn. First, the potential survival benefit from a given therapy cannot simply be inferred by comparing responders and non-responders. Secondly, appropriate selection of patients for any form of treatment with potential morbidity is essential if overall benefit is not to be outweighed by overall harm.

SURVIVAL FROM WHEN?

A further problem which can lead to misinterpretation of survival data concerns the reference point from which survival is measured. By convention, survival after treatment is nearly always measured from the time treatment was started. This is reasonable for tumours with a short natural history or where treatment is initiated as soon as the diagnosis is made; acute leukaemia, testicular teratoma and paediatric malignancies are obvious examples.

In contrast, difficulties arise for tumours with a relatively long natural history and for which tumour regressions but not cures are possible with therapy; examples would include radiotherapy for inoperable lung carcinoma, chemotherapy for the nodular or indolent lymphomas, and endocrine therapy or chemotherapy for advanced breast carcinoma. Here the problem in management is not what treatment to use, but when to use it. This question can be answered only if survival is measured from the diagnosis, irrespective of when treatment is started. All too commonly, however, no account is taken of the natural history of the disease, and in the literature survival is recorded simply from the start of treatment. This can lead to fundamental misinterpretation of true survival benefit, as the following examples illustrate.

Assume a tumour with an untreated natural history of, say, two years, during the first year of which the patient is asymptomatic.

Example 1 Consider a treatment A which in fact has no influence on survival, given either at the time of diagnosis or at the time of first symptoms. Figure 1 shows that treatment A given at diagnosis achieves a survival *from the start of treatment* twice as long as if given at the time of symptoms. By this criterion A would seem to be twice as effective if given early. This of course is nonsense, and indeed if treatment A has any morbidity whatsoever, there would be a disadvantage in early therapy.

Example 2 Consider now a comparison of the same ineffective treatment A with effective treatment B which increases survival by, say, six months even if started only at the time symptoms appear. Figure 2 shows that the true survival advantage of B over A (30 months versus 24 months) is entirely concealed if measured from the start of treatment, A appearing quite wrongly superior to B (24 months versus 18 months).

Example 3 Consider finally a more extreme case in which ineffective treatment actually shortens survival by, say, 25% (this is no mere hypothesis,

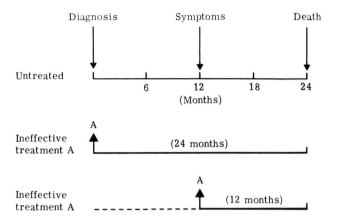

Figure 1 Survival after ineffective treatment A started either at the time of diagnosis or at the time of first symptoms. (see text for details.)

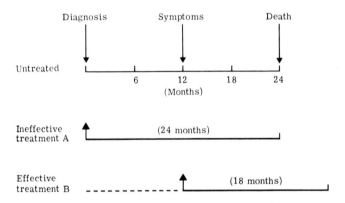

Figure 2 Survival after ineffective treatment A started at diagnosis, compared with effective treatment B started at the time of first symptoms. (See text for details.)

as studies quoted above for chemotherapy in some types of lung cancer have already shown). As Figure 3 shows, this treatment given at the time of diagnosis would lead to a greater shortening in true survival than given only when symptoms appeared (18 months versus 21 months). Yet an entirely fallacious case could still confidently be made for the advantages of starting A at once rather than delaying until symptoms developed based on survival from the start of treatment (18 months versus 9 months).

Similar examples could be given. The point they illustrate may seem obvious, yet by convention, survival after treatment is nearly always

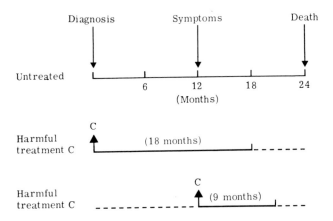

Figure 3 Survival after harmful treatment C started either at diagnosis or at the time of first symptoms. (See text for details.)

measured in the literature from the start of treatment and not from diagnosis. This applies even to indolent tumours with a long natural history.

Data from the occasional published studies where natural history is taken into account tend to emphasize the pitfalls. The study on survival after chemotherapy for breast cancer already quoted demonstrates no overall survival advantage from the diagnosis of first metastases (Powles *et al.*, 1980a). A randomized trial comparing immediate radiotherapy for advanced inoperable lung cancer in asymptomatic patients with a 'wait and see' policy in which treatment was delayed until symptoms developed showed no survival benefit (and no improved quality of life) for those given immediate treatment (Durrant *et al.*, 1971).

To summarize, the observation that responders to therapy survive longer than non-responders merely demonstrates the prognostic significance of response and does not necessarily imply that the treatment itself is the cause of prolonged survival. Likewise, for tumours with a long natural history, the real influence of treatment on survival can only be assessed if the latter is measured from the time of diagnosis and not from the start of the treatment itself.

GUIDELINES TO MANAGEMENT AND MEASURING RESPONSE IN INCURABLE CANCER

With the above limitations in mind, the following is proposed as an approach to improved management and measurement of response in the incurable patient.

Curable or incurable?

The first and most important question to be decided is whether the patient is potentially curable or incurable, since this will determine the aims and often the intensity of therapy. Too often, and particularly with combination chemotherapy, intensive and toxic treatment, which might be justified if cure were a possibility, is advocated where no such possibility exists.

Survival versus quality of life

It has already been emphasized that the main aims of treatment for the incurable patient are first to improve or maintain as good a quality of life as possible and secondly to prolong survival where possible. A dilemma may arise here in trying to balance these two aims when a treatment which prolongs survival does so only at the expense of considerable morbidity. There are no easy answers to this, and indeed different patients may opt for different priorities.

Evidence for this comes from a recent study investigating the attitudes of normal individuals (not patients) to the hypothetical decision of having to opt for surgery for laryngeal carcinoma with loss of normal speech (and hence impaired quality of life) or radiotherapy with speech preservation but shortened survival (McNeil *et al.*, 1981). It was found that different individuals opted for different priorities. Further similar studies would be of value in this important and hitherto largely neglected area of therapy, but the implication is that patients may have to be more involved in this type of decision-making than in the past.

Indications for active treatment

It cannot be emphasized too strongly that the diagnosis of incurable cancer is not in itself an indication for specific anti-cancer treatment. However satisfying the achievement of tumour regression may be to the clinician, the inadequacy of this aim (in isolation) in terms of real patient benefit, has been clearly shown.

The first consideration should be whether the patient has tumour-related symptoms. Their presence constitutes one of the main indications for starting treatment. For the asymptomatic patient, the decision is much more difficult. Sometimes the imminent risk of unpleasant or potentially irreversible symptoms would justify prophylactic therapy; examples include lytic bone metastases threatening fracture, or spinal cord compression. Occasionally some form of treatment might be necessary purely for psychological reasons, for the patient aware of the diagnosis and unhappy about 'nothing being done'.

The only indication for starting treatment in the asymptomatic patient would be clear evidence that survival in that disease could be prolonged without intolerable morbidity. The absence of such evidence for some tumours and the fallacies in interpretation of survival data for others have already been pointed out. For most tumour types, therefore, the clinician faced with the dilemma of when to treat should either attempt to participate in a trial designed to answer this question or should adopt a conservative, 'wait and see' policy. This means waiting at least until the tempo of the disease has been established, and for most patients until symptoms have developed. At present too many patients with incurable cancer are being treated simply because the tumour is there.

Age and general medical condition

Age and general medical condition must be considered in selecting potentially curable cancer patients for radical therapy. Pneumonectomy for lung cancer (Shields *et al.*, 1972) and more recently marrow transplantation for acute leukaemia (Powles *et al.*, 1980b) are two examples. The same applies to treatment for incurable cancer, and treatment which may offer a good chance of prolonged survival for the relatively young and fit patient may be inappropriate and inferior to simple palliative measures in the elderly and the medically unfit.

Measuring response to treatment

The decision as to whether to continue anti-cancer treatment is just as important as the initial decision to start, and treatment should be considered as a therapeutic trial which requires constant monitoring. All too often the main, and even the only, measurement applied to treatment effectiveness is the objective tumour response, whatever the cost in investigations and inconvenience to the patient.

For the symptomatic patient the main aim of treatment is relief of symptoms, and this should be the main criterion for assessing response. Objective evidence of tumour regression is of course also helpful in overall assessment if it can be readily obtained, but it is of secondary importance. Tumour response at the expense of decreased quality of life may in many instances not be worth having; conversely, symptomatic relief even without tumour regression is usually worth while, and an indication for continuing treatment.

Duration of treatment

For chemotherapy this can be a difficult question. The pressure to continue such treatment in the patient who has achieved benefit is strong. Most published studies advocate or imply that chemotherapy should be continued indefinitely or until relapse, for the common solid tumours including advanced breast cancer (Greenspan *et al.*, 1963; Canellos *et al.*, 1974; Jones *et al.*, 1975; Brambilla *et al.*, 1976), lung cancer (Cohen *et al.*, 1977; Israel *et al.*, 1977; Gralla *et al.*, 1981), and gastrointestinal cancer (McDonald *et al.*, 1980; Lavin *et al.*, 1980). Yet the evidence to support this approach is weak. One control trial in the treatment of small cell lung cancer has shown significantly prolonged survival for a subgroup of patients with limited disease treated with maintenance chemotherapy, but not for patients with more extensive disease (Maurer *et al.*, 1980).

Other studies, however, have suggested that treatment lasting only a few months for this tumour type may achieve as good survival results as prolonged therapy (Johnson *et al.*, 1978) and our own, as yet unpublished, data support this. In myeloma, no advantage has been shown for continuing chemotherapy once complete remission has been achieved (Alexanian *et al.*, 1975), and no benefit for maintenance chemotherapy after maximum symptomatic relief in the nodular lymphomas has been demonstrated (Portlock, 1980). Likewise, control trials have shown that maintenance chemotherapy adds no further survival benefit for potentially curable tumours including Hodgkin's disease (de Vita *et al* 1980), and malignant teratoma (Einhorn *et al.*, 1981).

Further data on this difficult question are clearly needed, particularly for the common tumours in which chemotherapy is increasingly being used, and the question is most likely to be answered by control clinical trials. The clinician faced with this problem should consider joining such a trial should one exist. Alternatively, there is little in the literature to argue against a conservative approach in which treatment should be stopped once maximum clinical benefit has been achieved if side-effects are significantly impairing quality of life.

CONCLUSION

The two main aims of treatment in patients with incurable cancer are improvement in quality of life and prolongation of survival. Measurement of response to treatment should therefore aim principally at measuring the extent to which these aims are achieved; the measurement of objective tumour response, although often useful, is of secondary importance.

The influence of treatment on survival can be properly assessed only if the latter is measured from the time of diagnosis; a false impression of survival benefit may be gained if it is measured merely from the start of treatment.

By no means all patients are likely to benefit from active therapy. The diagnosis of incurable cancer should not in itself be considered an indication to start treatment.

REFERENCES

Alexanian, R., Balcerzak, S., Bonnet, J.D., *et al.* (1975). Prognostic factors in multiple myeloma. *Cancer*, **36**, 1192–1201.

Baum, M., Priestman, T., West, R.R., *et al.* (1980). A comparison of subjective responses in a trial comparing endocrine with cytotoxic treatment in advanced carcinoma of the breast. In *Breast cancer: experimental and clinical methods* (eds H.T. Mouridsen, and T. Palshof) New York: Pergamon Press. pp. 223–226.

BMJ Editorial (1980). Prostatic cancer: the response to treatment dilemma. *Br. Med. J.*, **1**, 883–884.

Bond, A., and Lader, M.H. (1974). The use of analogue scales in rating subjective feelings. *Br. J. Med. Psychol.*, **47**, 211–218.

Brambilla, C., de Lena, M., Rossi, A., *et al.* (1976).Response and survival in advanced breast cancer after 2 non-cross resistant combinations. *Br. Med. J.*, **1**, 801–804.

Brunner, K.W., Marthaler, T., and Mullerm, W. (1973). Effects of long term adjuvant chemotherapy with cyclophosphamide for radically resected bronchogenic carcinoma. *Cancer Chemother. Rep.*, **4**, 125–132.

Bunn, P.A., and Ihde, D.C. (1981). Small cell bronchogenic carcinoma: a review of therapeutic results. In *Cancer treatment and research*, vol. 1, *Lung cancer* (ed. R.B. Livingston), The Hague: Martinus Nijhoff pp. 169–208.

Canellos, G.P., de Vita, V.T., Gold, G.L., *et al.* (1974). Cyclical combination chemotherapy for advanced breast carcinoma. *Br. Med. J.*, **1**, 218–220.

Citrin, D.L., Hougen, C., Zweibel, W., *et al.* (1981). The use of serial bone scans in assessing response of bone metastases to systemic treatment. *Cancer*, **47**, 680–685.

Cohen, M.H., Creaven, R.J., Fossieck, B.E., *et al.* (1977). Intensive chemotherapy of small cell bronchogenic carcinoma. *Cancer Treat. Rep.*, **61**, 349–354.

Creech, R.H., Catalano, R.B., Harris, D.T., *et al.* (1979). Low dose chemotherapy of metastatic breast cancer with CAMF versus sequential CMF and adriamycin. *Cancer*, **43**, 51–59.

de Palo, G., Demicheli, R., Valagussa, P., *et al.* (1981). Prospective study with HEXA-CAF combination in ovarian carcinoma. *Cancer Chem. Pharmacol.*, **5**, 157–161.

de Vita, V.T., Simon, R.M., Hubbard, S.M., *et al.* (1980). Curability of advanced Hodgkin's disease with chemotherapy. *Ann. Intern. Med.*, **92**, 587–595.

Dische, S., Bennett, M.H., Saunders, M.I., *et al.* (1980). Tumour regression as a guide to prognosis: a clinical study. *Br. J. Radiol.*, **53**, 454–461.

Dodion, P., Mulder, M., Cavalli, F., *et al.* (1981). Combination chemotherapy with *cis*-platin and vindesine in advanced malignant melanoma. *UICC Conf. on Clinical Oncology*, Lausanne. Conference Abstracts, p. 126.

Durrant, K.R., Berry, R.J., Ellis, F., *et al.* (1971). Comparison of treatment policies in inoperable bronchial carcinoma. *Lancet*, **i**, 715–719.

Einhorn, L.A., Bond, W.H., Hornback, N., *et al.* (1978). Long-term results in combined-modality treatment of small cell carcinoma of the lung. *Semin. Oncol.*, **5**, 309–313.

Einhorn, L.H., Williams, S.D., Troner, M., *et al.* (1981). The role of maintenance therapy in disseminated testicular cancer. *New Engl. J. Med.*, **305**, 727–731.

Elias, L., Portlock, C.S., and Rosenberg, S.A. (1978). Combination chemotherapy of diffuse histiocytic lymphoma with CHOP. *Cancer*, **42**, 1705–1710.

Ezdinli, E.Z., Costello, W.G., Idi, F., *et al.* (1980). Nodular mixed lymphocytic–histiocytic lymphoma. Response and survival. *Cancer*, **45**, 261–267.

Ezdinli, E.Z., Costello, W.G., Lenhard, R.E., *et al.* (1978). Survival of nodular versus diffuse pattern lymphocytic poorly differentiated lymphoma. *Cancer*, **41**, 1960–1996.

Falkson, G., and Falkson, H.C. (1976). Fluoro-uracil, methyl-CCNU and vincristine in cancer of the colon. *Cancer*, **38**, 1468–1470.

Gralla, R., Casper, E.S., Kelsen, D., *et al.* (1981). *Cis*–platin and vindesine combination chemotherapy for advanced carcinoma of the lung: a randomised trial investigating two dosage schedules. *Ann. Intern. Med.*, **95**, 414–420.

Greenspan, E.M. (1980). Chemotherapy and survival in breast cancer (Letter). *Lancet*, **i**, 983.

Greenspan, E., Fieber, M., Lesnick, G., *et al.* (1963). Response of advanced breast carcinoma to the combination of the anti-metabolite methotrexate and the alkylating agent thio-tepa. *J. Mt Sinai Hosp.* , **30**, 246–267.

Griffiths, C.T., Parker, L.M., and Fuller, A.F. (1979). Role of cytoreductive surgical treatment in the management of advanced ovarian carcinoma. *Cancer Treat. Rep.*, **63**, 235–240.

Harris, A.L., Smith, I.E., and Powles, T.J. (1981). Aminoglutethimide in the treatment of advanced breast cancer. *Cancer Res.*, **42** (Supp), 3405s–3408s.

Hayward, J.L., and Rubens, R.D. (1977). Assessment of response to therapy in advanced breast cancer. *Br. J. Cancer*, **35**, 292–298.

Holyoke, E.D., and Ledesma, E.L. (1981). Diagnosis and surgical treatment of colon and rectal cancer. *Curr. Concepts Oncol.*, **3**, 3–7.

Hoogstraten, B., and Fabian, C. (1979). A reappraisal of single drugs in advanced breast cancer. *Clin. Cancer Trials*, **2**, 101–109.

Hurley, J.D., and Ellison, E.H. (1960). Chemotherapy of solid cancer arising from the gastro-intestinal tract. *Ann. Surg.*, **152**, 568–582.

Ihde, D., Bevnath, A., Cohen, M., *et al.* (1979). Utility of fibre-optic bronchoscopy in assessing response to chemotherapy in small cell lung cancer. In *Lung cancer: progress in therapeutic research* (eds. F. Muggia, and M. Rozencweig) New York: Raven Press. pp. 543–548.

Israel, L., Depierre, A., Choffel, C., *et al.* (1977). Immunochemotherapy in 34 cases of oat cell carcinoma of the lung with 19 complete responses. *Cancer Treat. Rep.* , **61**, 343–347.

Johnson, R.E., Brereton, H.D., and Kent, C.H. (1978). 'Total' therapy for small cell carcinoma of the lung. *Ann. Thorac. Surg.*, **25**, 509–515.

Jones, S.E., Durie, B.G.M., and Salmon, S.E. (1975). Combination chemotherapy with adriamycin and cyclophosphamide for advanced breast cancer. *Cancer*, **36**, 90–97.

Karnofsky, D.A., and Burchenal, J.H. (1948). The clinical evaluation of chemo-therapeutic agents in cancer. In *Evaluation of chemotherapeutic agents* (ed. C.M. MacLeod). New York: Columbia University Press. p. 191.

Landgren, R.C., Hussey, D.H., Samuels, M.L., *et al.* (1973). A randomised study comparing irradiation alone to irradiation plus procarbazine in inoperable bronchogenic carcinoma. *Radiology*, **108**, 403–406.

Lavin, P., Mittelman, A., Douglass, H., *et al.* (1980). Survival and response to chemotherapy for advanced colorectal adenocarcinoma. *Cancer*, **46**, 1536–1543.

Lawrence, W.T., and Lawrence, W. (1980). Gastric cancer : the surgeon's view point. *Semin. Oncol.*, **7**, 400–417.

Lee, R.E., Carr, D.T., and Childs, D.S. (1976). Comparison of split-course radiation therapy and continuous radiation therapy for unresectable bronchogenic carcinoma : 5 year results. *Am. J. Roentgenol.*, **126**, 116–122.

Levi, J.A., Dalley, D.N., and Aroney, A.S. (1979). Improved combination chemotherapy in advanced gastric cancer. *Br. Med. J.*, **2**, 1471–1473.

Livingston, R.B. (1977) Combination chemotherapy of bronchogenic carcinoma. 1. Non-oat cell. *Cancer Treat. Rev.*, **4**, 153–165.

McDonald, J.S., Schein, P.S., Wooley, P.V., *et al.* (1980). 5–Fluorouracil, doxorubicin and mitomycin (FAM) combination chemotherapy for advanced gastric cancer. *Ann. Intern. Med.*, **93**, 533–536.

McNeil, B.J., Weichselbaum, R., and Parker, S.G. (1981). Speech and survival. Tradeoffs between quality and quantity of life in laryngeal cancer. *New Engl. J. Med.*, **305**, 982–987.

Mallinson, C.N., Rake, M.O., Cocking, J.B., *et al.* (1980). Chemotherapy in pancreatic cancer: results of a controlled prospective randomised multi-centre trial. *Br. Med. J.*, **281**, 1589–1591.

Mantyla, M., Kortekangas, A.E. Valavaara, R.A., *et al.* (1979). Tumour regression during radiation treatment as a guide to prognosis. *Br. J. Radiol.*, **52**, 972–977.

Maurer, L.H., Tullok, M., Weiss, R.B., *et al.* (1980). A randomised combined modality trial in small cell carcinoma of lung. *Cancer*, **45**, 30–39.

Moertel, C.G. (1975). Clinical management of advanced gastro-intestinal cancer. *Cancer*, **36**, 675–682.

Portlock, C.S. (1980). Management of indolent lymphomas *Semin. Oncol.*, **7**, 292–301.

Powles, T.J., Coombes, R.C., Smith, I.E., *et al.* (1980a). Failure of chemotherapy to prolong survival in a group of patients with metastatic breast cancer. *Lancet*, **i**, 580–582.

Powles, T.J., Leese, C.L., and Bondy, P.K. (1975). Hydroxyproline excretion in patients with breast cancer and response to treatment. *Br. Med. J.*, **2**, 164–166.

Powles, R.L., Morgenstern G., Clink, H.M., *et al.* (1980b). The place of bone marrow transplantation in acute myelogenous leukaemia. *Lancet*, **i**, 1047–1050.

Priestman, T.J., and Baum, M. (1976). Evaluation of quality of life in patients receiving treatment for advanced breast cancer. *Lancet*, **i**, 899–900.

Priestman, T., Baum, M., Jones, V., *et al.* (1977). Comparative trial of endocrine versus cytotoxic treatment in advanced breast cancer. *Br. Med. J.*, **1**, 1248–1250.

Priestman, T., Baum, M., Jones, V., *et al.* (1978). Treatment and survival in advanced breast cancer. *Br. Med. J.*, **2**, 1673–1674.

Rubens, R.D. (1979). Breast cancer. In *Cancer chemotherapy* (ed. H.M. Pinedo) Amsterdam: Excerpta Medica. Chap. 18, pp.376–411.

Salazar, O.M., Rubin, P., *et al.* (1976). Predictors of radiation response in lung cancer. *Cancer*, **37**, 2636–2650.

Schwartz, P.E., and Smith, J.P. (1980). Second look operations in ovarian cancer. *Am. J. Obstet. Gynecol.*, **138**, 1124–1130.

Selawry, O.S. (1974). The role of chemotherapy in the treatment of lung cancer. *Semin. Oncol.*, **1**, 259–272.

Shapiro, T.M. (1975). Adenocarcinoma of the pancreas: a statistical analysis of biliary by-pass vs. Whipple resection in good risk patients. *Ann. Surg.*, **182**, 715–720.

Sherman, D.M., and Weichselbaum, R.R. (1981). The use of pre-operative radiation therapy in the treatment of lung carcinoma. In *Lung cancer*, (ed. R.B. Livingston). The Hague: Martinus Nijhoff. Chap. 4, pp.63–73.

Shields, T.W., Higgins, G.A., and Keehn, R.J. (1972). Factors influencing survival after resection for bronchial carcinoma. *J. Thorac. Cardiovasc. Surg.*, **64**, 391–398.

Smith, F.P., Byrne, P.J., Cambaren, R.C., *et al.* (1979). Gastro-intestinal cancer. In

Cancer chemotherapy (ed. H.M. Pinedo). Amsterdam: Excerpta Medica. Chap. 15, pp. 292–316.

Smith, F.P., and Schein, P.S. (1979). Chemotherapy of pancreatic cancer. *Semin. Oncol.*, **6**, 368–377.

Smith, I.E., Fitzharris, B.M., McKinna, J.A., *et al.* (1978). Aminoglutethimide in treatment of metastatic breast carcinoma. *Lancet*, **ii**, 646–649.

Stoter, G., Rosencweig, M., and Pinedo, H.M. (1979). Genito-urinary tumours. In *Cancer chemotherapy* (ed. H.M. Pinedo). Amsterdam: Excerpta Medica. Chap. 16, pp.317–339.

Taylor, R.E., Smith, I.E., Ford, H.T., *et al.* (1980). Failure of intensive combination chemotherapy to control adenocarcinoma or large cell anaplastic carcinoma of lung. *Cancer Chemother. Pharmacol.*, **4**, 271–273.

van der Werf-Messing, B. (1979). Pre-operative irradiation followed by cystectomy to treat carcinoma of the urinary bladder category T3 NX, 0–4MO. *J. Radiat. Oncol., Biol. Phys.*, **5**, 395–401.

Wallace D.M., and Bloom H.J.G. (1976). The management of deeply infiltrating bladder carcinoma: control trial of radical radiotherapy versus pre-operative radiotherapy and radical cystectomy (first report). *Br. J. Urol.*, **48**, 587–594.

White, J.E., and Boles, M. (1981). The role of radiation therapy in the treatment of regional non-small cell carcinoma of the lung. In *Lung Cancer* (ed. R.B. Livingston) The Hague: Martinus Nijhoff. Chap. 6, pp. 113–156.

WHO (1979). Handbook for reporting results of cancer treatment. *WHO Offset Publication* no. 48. Geneva: World Health Organization.

Wiltshaw, E. (1981). personal communication.

Young, R.C., Chabner, B.A., Hubbard, S.P., *et al.* (1978). Advanced ovarian adenocarcinoma. A prospective clinical trial of melphalan versus combination chemotherapy. *New Engl. J. Med.*, **299**, 1261–1266.

Cancer Treatment: End Point Evaluation
Edited by B.A. Stoll
© 1983 John Wiley & Sons Ltd.

Chapter

3   A.C. BEGG

Clinical Relevance of Experimental End-points

INTRODUCTION

In experimental cancer, the end-points of growth delay and local tumour control are the ones most closely resembling the human end-points of palliation and cure respectively. In this respect they are the most clinically relevant assays, but other types of assay provide different but complementary information. It is the comparison of assays that may lead to treatment improvement, and in striving for clinical relevance, the choice of experimental tumour model, treatment dose, and regime deserves as much attention as the assay system.

Most of the techniques to be discussed can be applied to different types of treatment although most were designed with a specific treatment in mind, e.g. growth delay for radiation, and per cent increase in lifespan (%ILS) for chemotherapy. Surgical excision as a treatment cannot be assessed by most of the techniques discussed here but is generally used only as a tool in the laboratory, e.g. removing the primary tumour to allow measurement of development time for metastases.

In attempting to answer the question of how relevant an experimental assay is to the human situation, other equally important questions become apparent at the same time. Some of these are :

How relevant is the type of tumour to a human tumour (e.g. its differentiation or immunogenicity)?

Are the doses used experimentally in the range of possible doses for human use?

Are the methods of restraining animals (jig design, use of anaesthetics) introducing artefacts so that the results cannot be compared with or extended to human treatment?

This review will confine itself to the subject of tumour response and will not refer to the large subject of experimental end-points for normal tissue damage. Clinicians or experimentalists interested in assays available for studying normal tissues are referred to the reviews by Fowler and Denekamp (1977) and Field and Michalowski (1979). These deal mainly with radiation damage.

GROWTH DELAY

This end-point was developed largely by Thomlinson (1960) to investigate the potential of hyperbaric oxygen to increase the radiation response of rat tumours (Figure 1). The concept is very simple. The growth of tumours is delayed by the treatment for a given period, after which more-rapid growth is resumed. The magnitude of the delay is used as a measure of the effectiveness of the treatment. The method is simple to carry out, requiring only that the tumour be accessible for measurement. For subcutaneous, intramuscular, and intradermal tumours, vernier calipers are used routinely to measure three perpendicular diameters of each tumour at several intervals during its growth history, both before and after treatment.

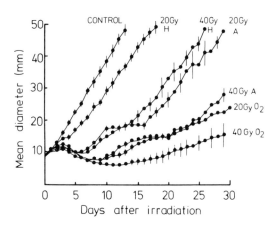

Figure 1 An example of the growth delay assay. In this experiment, groups of rats bearing subcutaneous RIB$_5$ tumours were given graded doses of x-rays on day 0. The tumours were irradiated with the animals breathing air (A) or hyperbaric oxygen (O_2), or with the tumour blood supply clamped off to render all cells hypoxic (H). The error bars are ±1 standard error of the mean. Dose–response curves can be obtained by plotting the time to reach a given size against dose (see Figure 2). (Redrawn from Thomlinson, 1960.)

The method has also been used in the clinic, employing either calipers (Thomlinson, 1979; Ashe *et al.*, 1979) or serial radiographs (Breur, 1966; Malaise *et al.*, 1972; Van Peperzeel, 1972) to assess tumour size. The time taken to reach a given size is then determined for each tumour. The end-point size is typically taken as twice or four times the treatment volume. The time for untreated tumours to reach the end-point size is then subtracted from the equivalent times for treated tumours in order to calculate the delay in growth.

The growth delay method has three main advantages to the experimentalist: (1) it can be applied to almost all transplantable solid tumours; (2) it can cover a wide range of response and therefore of dose; and (3) little or no prior knowledge of the tumour's sensitivity to treatment is required, in contrast to some of the techniques discussed below. It has been successfully used to study a wide variety of treatments, particularly when radiation is involved. Some examples of these are the effect of hyperbaric oxygen in modifying radiation response (Thomlinson, 1960; Thomlinson and Craddock, 1967), investigations into fractionated versus single doses in radiotherapy (Denekamp and Harris, 1976), comparison of x-rays with high linear energy transfer (LET) radiations such as neutrons and heavy ions (Field *et al.*, 1968; Barendsen and Broerse, 1969), and radiosensitization of hypoxic cells by electron affinic compounds (Denekamp and Harris, 1975, 1976) (see Figure 2). In addition to these radiation studies, the growth delay end-point is frequently used in studies of other treatment modalities such as cytotoxic drugs and hyperthermia.

The growth delay assay has a potential disadvantage for basic studies in that it does not directly indicate the amount of cell killing caused by the treatment. Obviously, as the delay is increased by higher treatment doses, it is highly likely that greater cell killing has occurred. However, the relationship between delay and cell killing is not a simple one and is crucially influenced by the proliferation kinetics of the cells that survive the treatment.

It has been shown, for example, that surviving tumour cells can proliferate more rapidly soon after radiation or drug treatment than before (Hermans and Barendsen, 1969; Stephens and Peacock, 1977). As there have only been a few studies of this type, it is not known how universal the phenomenon is. Where it occurs, the magnitude of growth delay would give an incorrect prediction of the surviving fraction when calculated using the *pre*-treatment growth rate.

The increased proliferation rate of the surviving tumour cells occurs in the period of no growth or even shrinkage of the tumour as a whole. However, another effect can become important as the tumour begins to regrow macroscopically, particularly after radiation treatments. This is a decreased growth rate compared with untreated tumours, resulting from damage to the stroma, or bed, of the tumour.

This effect is demonstrated by experiments in which untreated tumours

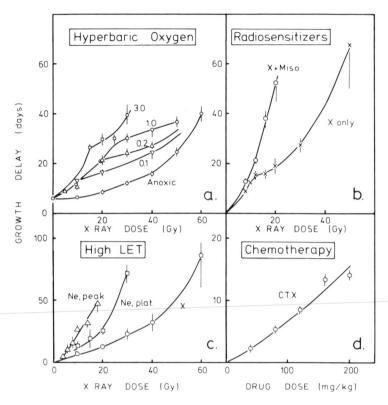

Figure 2 Four examples of the use of the growth delay assay. (a) Hyperbaric oxygen studies on the rat RIB₅ tumour. The figures against each curve are the atmospheric pressure of oxygen breathed by the rats at the time of irradiation. (Redrawn from Thomlinson and Craddock, 1967.) (b) Effect of the hypoxic cell radiosensitizer, misonidazole, on the mouse carcinoma CBA CA NT. (Redrawn from Denekamp and Harris, 1975.) (c) Comparison of x-rays with accelerated neon ions (Ne) in the plateau and peak regions of the depth–dose distribution. (Redrawn from Curtis *et al.*, 1978.) (d) The effect of cyclophosphamide (CTX) injected intraperitoneally, on the WH CA MT mouse tumour.

implanted into irradiated sites grow significantly more slowly than in unirradiated sites. This is termed the tumour bed effect (TBE) (Stenstrom *et al.*, 1955; Hewitt and Blake, 1968; Urano and Suit, 1971) and clearly shows that the overall tumour growth rate is not simply a reflection of the inherent proliferation capacity of its cells. The consequence of the TBE is that the growth delay for a given treatment will vary depending on the end-point size chosen, since the growth curves for treated and untreated tumours will no longer be parallel. The choice of a larger end-point size will result in a larger estimate of delay.

The magnitude of the TBE varies with radiation dose, but in a non-linear manner. Initially the growth rate reduction increases with increasing dose, but this is usually followed by a plateau at high doses. The non-linear dose–response relationship for growth rate reduction, or TBE, can result in a biphasic dose–response curve for tumour growth delay. Interpretation of the shape of growth delay dose–response curves after irradiation must therefore be treated with caution (Begg, 1982).

Growth rate reductions after drug treatment have also been observed (Begg *et al.*, 1980) although the magnitudes of the reductions are usually smaller than after irradiation. The shape of curves of growth delay versus dose after drug treatment will therefore suffer considerably less distortion than after x-rays. The cause of growth rate reduction after drug treatment can less easily be attributed to local stromal damage since the treatment is systemic and general animal health has also been known to affect tumour growth rate (Brown, 1979).

One further aspect of the growth delay assay that makes the correlation between cell killing and growth delay worse, particularly for drugs, is mitotic delay or cytostasis. Rowley *et al.* (1979) clearly demonstrated this with adriamycin (ADM). These workers found tumour surviving fractions which were not significantly different from 1.0 at all times tested after administration of 10 mg/kg ADM to rats bearing H–4–II–E hepatomas. This same drug dose, however, caused a large delay in growth of the tumours of approximately 10 days. In the same series of experiments, an x-ray dose of 15 Gy caused a smaller growth delay of only 7–8 days despite a large decrease in the surviving fraction down to approximately 2%.

Adriamycin was evidently more cytostatic than cytocidal, whilst irradiation was obviously markedly cytocidal but less cytostatic, the surviving cells repopulating the tumour with the short average doubling time of just over 1 day. It is therefore impossible to predict the surviving fraction from a knowledge of growth delay, and vice versa. This point will be returned to later.

With regard to clinical relevance of the growth delay assay, the difficulty of relating delay to cell killing in no way prevents results of delay experiments being relevant to the clinic. The slowed growth rate of tumours after irradiation and the prolonged cytostasis observed after some drugs would both serve in the clinic to prolong the life of the patient. They are therefore important components in their mechanisms of action. Indeed, even if other methods of tumour assay were used, these factors would require growth delay studies in addition to cell killing studies in order to determine their magnitude.

SHRINKAGE RATE

If complete regrowth curves are obtained for different doses of a particular treatment, there are several parameters in addition to growth delay that

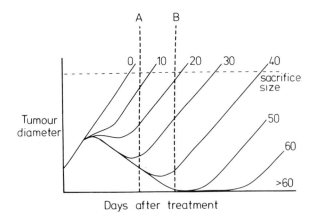

Figure 3 Schematic diagram of the changes of tumour size after treatment with graded single doses. The scales and treatment doses are arbitrary. The diagram shows (i) the common regression rate of tumours after all doses sufficiently large to induce regression and (ii) that after complete regression regrowth will occur at different times depending on the dose given. Complete regression is therefore a poor quantitative measure of response. This schema will apply to treatment with cytotoxic agents as well as to radiation therapy. (See text for discussion of the use of the different end-point times A and B.)

can be and have been used to assess the efficacy of treatment. The rate of regression is a frequently used parameter, particularly in the clinic, and has been the subject of some controversy. Thomlinson (1979), basing his conclusion on both animal and human growth studies, maintains that regression rate is a function of the individual tumour's stroma and the response of the host. It is therefore not a reflection of the treatment given.

The curve shapes depicted in Figure 3 for animal tumours treated with single doses of x-rays illustrate that there is a common regression rate after all doses sufficiently high to induce regression. Similar results have been found in other animal tumours, although each type of tumour has its own regression rate. In this case regression rate is no guide to treatment efficacy.

Thomlinson also found from many measurements in patients with carcinoma of the breast that, in individual patients given sequential chemotherapy and radiotherapy, regression rates after each treatment type were similar. These regression rates varied markedly from patient to patient given the same treatment (Thomlinson, 1979). These observations would also suggest that for this human cancer it is the biology of the tumour and not the treatment that determines the regression slope. The lack of correlation between

Table 1 Correlation of tumour regression rate after treatment with prognosis

Tumour	Schedule	Correlation	Reference
Animal studies			
C3H mammary carcinoma	Single doses	No	Suit *et al.* (1965)
C3H mammary carcinoma	Single doses	No	Denekamp (1977)
C3H mammary carcinoma	Fractionated	Yes	Denekamp (1977)
RIB$_5$	Single dose	No	Thomlinson (1960)
Clinical studies			
Breast		No	Thomlinson (1979)
Lung		No	Dische and Saunders (1980)
Cervix		Yes	Dische *et al.* (1980)
Cervix		Yes	Marcial and Bosch (1970)
Cervix		Yes	Grossman *et al.* (1973)
Oropharynx and oral cavity		No	Suit *et al.* (1965)
Oropharynx and oral cavity		Yes	Barkley and Fletcher (1977)
Head and neck		Yes	Mantylä *et al.* (1979)

regression and prognosis is also supported by other clinical studies (Suit *et al.*, 1965; Dische and Saunders, 1980)

On the other hand, Denekamp (1977) found a strong positive correlation between regression rate and ultimate tumour control in animal studies with the C3H mammary carcinoma. This was only true, however, for fractionated irradiations, with a far weaker correlation found for single doses. Some clinical trials have also found a correlation between regression rate and control. A summary of the results of these trials and the animal studies is given in Table 1. It appears that for single doses of x-rays there is no correlation between regression rate and prognosis. For fractionated doses in animals and in human cancer the situation is more complex, a correlation being observed in some sites but not in others.

Shrinkage rate has been correlated with reoxygenation rate (Denekamp, 1972) and could therefore partly explain the greater radiosensitivity of rapidly shrinking tumours. Why this dos not occur in all sites is a matter for speculation. It may be that reoxygenation is not important in these tumours or does not correlate with regression rate. Some reoxygenation can occur without shrinkage, although in the limited number of animal tumours studied reoxygenation was greatest in tumours which shrank fastest.

MINIMUM VOLUME

Another parameter that is sometimes used as an indication of treatment efficacy is the minimum volume that tumours reach before they regrow. Referring again to the regrowth curves in Figure 3, two problems with this end-point become apparent. At low doses many tumours do not shrink at all but simply show a transient slowing in growth rate. Defining a minimum volume in this case is arbitrary or impossible.

The second problem occurs at high doses which produce complete regression followed either by subsequent tumour regrowth or not (= cure). At all doses greater than the smallest required to cause complete regression, the minimum volume is the same, i.e. below the detection threshold. There is therefore no increase in response with increasing dose for this end-point at high doses. The low-dose problem may not occur with all tumours but the high-dose problem will.

A final point about the minimum volume end-point is that the range of response is necessarily limited to sizes between zero and the treatment size. The growth delay end-point encompasses a comparatively larger response range (of time instead of size) and thus it can resolve smaller dose differences.

VOLUME RATIOS

A final parameter that is extracted from growth and regrowth curves is the ratio of volumes of treated to untreated tumours at a given day after treatment. Usually many different treatments are compared in the one experiment, and only one set of measurements of tumour diameter, volume or weight is made after treatment to save work and time. The time chosen for the measurement is usually based on previous knowledge of the tumour's growth rate.

The problems with this assay can again be seen by referring to Figure 3. If the end-point time is chosen to be at A, all tumours given doses greater than or equal to 30 Gy will be at the same volume due to the fact that the regression rate is independent of dose. If end-point time B is chosen, doses less than 40 Gy will be resolved, but not doses greater than 40 Gy. It would appear, then, that the later the end-point times the better, except that animals with tumours given low doses will have been sacrificed to prevent suffering by them. The dose range covered by this end-point is therefore limited, and the end-point time needs to be carefully chosen to maximize the dose range resolved. For these reasons, growth delay is again a better choice of end-point than volume ratio at a given time.

When serial measurements of tumour size are carried out in the clinic, it is usually on patients with advanced disease, e.g. multiple metastatic nodules. The patients may therefore die of their disease before regrowth of the nodule(s) being investigated occurs. In these cases information on the efficacy of the treatments being compared may have to be obtained from a minimum volume or volume ratio end-point rather than from growth delay. These end-points may well distinguish the better treatment, but are not likely to provide quantitative information on the increase in therapeutic efficiency.

TUMOUR CONTROL (TCD$_{50}$)

The dose required to control 50% of treated tumours (TCD$_{50}$) is an end-point which is essentially an extension of the growth delay assay to high doses after which some tumours show an infinite delay, i.e. the animals are cured. Experimentally, groups of tumour-bearing animals are given a graded series of doses, and the proportion of tumours controlled (no regrowth observed by a specified time) is recorded in each group. The TCD$_{50}$ can be read off a plot of per cent tumours controlled versus treatment dose. Enough time must be allowed for all the non-cured tumours to regrow, otherwise the TCD$_{50}$ estimate will be too low (Fowler *et al.*, 1975).

This end-point has been widely used in radiation studies, particularly of factors affecting the efficacy of fractionated x-ray treatments (Fowler *et al.*,

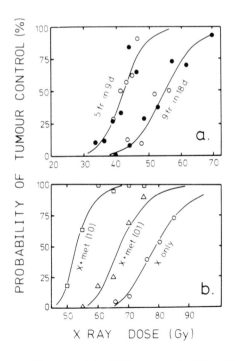

Figure 4 Two examples of the use of the TCD$_{50}$ assay. (a) The efficacy of two different x-ray fractionation schemes on C3H mouse mammary carcinomas: five fractions in 9 days versus nine fractions in 18 days. Open and closed circles are data from two separate experiments. (Redrawn from Fowler *et al.*, 1975.) (b) Radiosensitization by metronidazole in the WH CA MT tumour. Figures in brackets are the radiosensitizer doses in mg/g. (Redrawn from Sheldon and Hill, 1977.)

1974; Howes, 1969; Suit and Maeda, 1967), and in studies of radiosensitizing agents (Begg *et al.*, 1974; Sheldon and Hill, 1977) (Figure 4). The method can also be used in chemotherapy studies, although only in restricted situations. Most non-immunogenic solid tumours in animals which are treated at sizes typically used in radiobiology experiments (≥ 6 mm) are not cured by most of the available chemotherapeutic agents. If very small tumours are used, cures can be obtained and thus the TCD_{50} end-point employed.

One advantage of the method over the growth delay assay is that the rate of tumour regrowth does not influence the assay, since only a yes/no answer concerning regrowth is required. Tumour bed damage is therefore of no consequence and only the physiological state of the tumour cells at the time of treatment is important, i.e. whether oxic or hypoxic, proliferating or non-proliferating, etc.

A major disadvantage of the technique, however, pariculary with radiation treatments, is that many animal tumours have metastasized by the time of treatment. Consequently, a large proportion of the animals will die from metastatic disease before it is known whether or not their tumours will recur. This severely restricts the proportion of tumour types that can be studied by the TCD_{50} method. The tumours used with this technique therefore have a metastasis incidence usually less than 10%.

In chemotherapy studies, if relatively large primary tumours are controlled it is likely that micrometastases will be controlled as well, reducing or eliminating the problem. For radiation studies, different sites or methods of implantation of the tumour can be tried which may reduce the incidence of metastases. Two other possible solutions to the metastasis problem are either to treat when the tumours are small, before metastasis has occurred to a significant extent, or to eradicate the metastases separately, if they occur at one major site only, e.g. radiation treatment of the lungs to eradicate lung metastases.

One further disadvantage of the TCD_{50} technique is the length of time of the assay (at least 2 months for a tumour with a doubling time of 1–2 days, and 4–6 months for a tumour with a doubling time of 5 days). In addition, some knowledge of the treatment sensitivity of the tumour is needed to plan the dose range in order to avoid obtaining either cures or recurrences in all groups.

Despite these disadvantages, the TCD_{50} method can provide useful and accurate information on tumour sensitivity and its modification by various agents, fractionation schemes, etc. It requires less total measurement time than the growth delay assay, and when the two end-points have been compared over similar dose ranges they have given similar answers (Fowler *et al.*, 1980). It also appeals to clinicians and is not complicated by overall time in fractionated treatments, a problem with most other assays.

PER CENT INCREASED LIFESPAN (%ILS)

This type of experiment is widely used in the screening of new chemotherapeutic agents and almost exclusively involves the use of extremely rapidly
growing tumours in the peritoneal cavity of mice, e.g. the P388 lymphoma
and the L1210 leukaemia (Law *et al.*, 1949; Potter and Briggs, 1962). The
treatment, usually intraperitoneal injection of a cytotoxic drug, is given either
one or several days after tumour cell inoculation. The time of death of
animals in each treatment group is recorded. The mean time of death of
treated animals is compared with that of untreated animals and the per cent
increase in lifespan is calculated from the day of tumour inoculation. The
method is very easy to use and is quick due to the rapid growth rate of the
tumours used.

In other variations of the technique the tumour is implanted intracerebrally
or subcutaneously (Chirgos *et al.*, 1962). When tumours similar to the L1210
leukaemia are used, the mice succumb from generalized metastatic disease.
However, there are other brain tumour models, e.g. 9L gliosarcoma (Barker
et al., 1973), in which death, as in glioblastoma patients, is due to the primary
tumour growth. The choice of which type of tumour to use should depend on
the characteristics of the human disease that the animal tumour is meant to
model.

The three main criticisms of this end-point are that (1) it is not always clear
what the animal died of; (2) the mouse is simply used as a small incubator;
and (3) the mice suffer in dying of their tumour burden, evoking ethical
questions. Mice inoculated with tumour cells i.p. may die either of their
primary tumour, or from generalized metastatic disease, or from drug
toxicity. A change in the mode of death with dose or drug type may give
misleading results.

The second criticism applies only to experiments in which intraperitoneal
tumours are treated with intraperitoneally administered drugs. In this case
there are no drug delivery problems, but these exist and are extremely
important in treatment of solid tumours where the drug has access to the
tumour only through an often disordered and deficient vascular system. In
addition, the drug is frequently administered in the early stages of tumour
development when the proliferative fraction is high and the tumour is
consequently sensitive to cycle-specific drugs. For these reasons the system
when used in this way is a highly artificial one. These criticisms do not apply
to intracerebrally inoculated tumours.

The ethical problems with this end-point are the same as with LD_{50}
experiments (the dose of cytotoxic agent required to kill 50% of treated
animals). They are more severe than with other tumour end-points because
mice with large tumours in growth delay or TCD_{50} experiments are humanely

sacrificed before the mouse begins to suffer from its tumour burden, with no loss of relevant data from the experiment. Because of the ethical problems, and the questionable relevance of the assay to treatment of solid tumours or even leukaemias, the %ILS end-point should be avoided whenever possible.

CELL SURVIVAL ASSAYS

In these assays the tumour is treated *in situ* and some time after treatment the tumour is excised, a cell suspension made, and the clonogenic potential of the treated cells tested. The test can be made by plating the cells in petri dishes and subsequently looking for growth of colonies, or by inoculating known numbers of cells back into animals. In the latter case either the latent periods (time for the tumours to reach a given size) or the TD_{50} (the number of cells required to produce 50% tumours) (Hewitt and Wilson, 1961) can be measured after subcutaneous inoculation. Another method is to inject the cells intravenously and count the number of lung colonies produced several weeks later (Hill and Bush, 1969). In all cases an estimate of the fraction of cells surviving the treatment is obtained.

The experimental advantages of the *in vitro* assay are that it is quicker (usually taking between 1 and 3 weeks from the time of treatment) and that fewer animals are required than for other assays such as growth delay and TCD_{50}. It is also unaffected by damage to the host and produces a direct estimate of cell killing. Its main disadvantage is that it can only be used on a limited range of tumours, i.e. those that will grow readily in culture preferably with a plating efficiency of greater than 10%, or those that have been selectively adapted to grow *in vitro*.

The need for selection is becoming less of a limitation with an increase in understanding of the culture conditions most favourable for tumour growth, e.g. soft agar, lowered oxygen tension, addition of red blood cells, etc. (Courtenay and Mills, 1978). However, most tumours used in this assay are fast-growing anaplastic tumours. There are no differentiated carcinomas available for use, for example. The relevance of cell survival assay to the clinic is therefore probably less important than the relevance of the types of tumours used (Rockwell, 1980).

Another potential disadvantage of cell survival assays is that the surviving fraction is often markedly dependent on the time between treatment and tumour excision, due to such processes as repair of potentially lethal damage (PLD) (Phillips and Tolmach, 1966; Hahn *et al.*, 1973). PLD repair is simply the rise in surviving fraction observed as the time between treatment and assay is increased. Following PLD repair the surviving fraction may continue to rise due to the onset of proliferation, making the choice of assay time a difficult one (Twentyman, 1979).

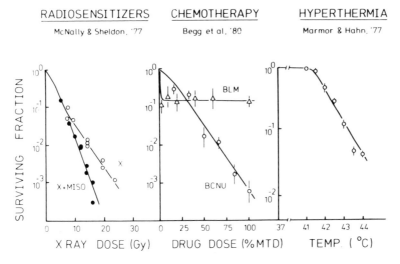

Figure 5 Three examples of the use of cell survival assays in which the tumours were treated *in vivo* and the cell survival assayed by colony formation *in vitro*. *Left*: radiosensitization by misonidazole in the WH CA MT tumour. *Middle*: chemotherapy of the EMT6/SF tumour with bleomycin (BLM) and the alkylating agent BCNU (MTD = maximum tolerated dose). *Right*: cell killing by radiofrequency heating of EMT6 tumours. (Graphs redrawn from the publications referred to in each panel.)

A factor opposing the surviving fraction increase due to PLD repair is the death of nutritionally deprived cells if left *in situ*, but rescued by tumour excisions soon after treatment (McNally, 1973; Van Putten, 1968). A further complication is that the process of disaggregating a tumour, usually with the use of enzymes, is a potentially toxic one. This was shown clearly in one series of experiments demonstrating a markedly increased sensitivity to bleomycin as a result of disaggregation (Twentyman, 1977).

Despite its potential disadvantages, the cell survival assay has been useful in elucidating such processes as PLD repair, and has been used in a variety of studies including those on radiosensitizers (McNally and Sheldon, 1977; Brown, 1975), chemotherapy (Begg *et al.*, 1980; Twentyman and Bleehen, 1976; Stephens and Peacock, 1977), and hyperthermia (Marmor *et al.*, 1977) (Figure 5). It is probably most useful when used in conjunction with other assays, since differences between assays can often lead to valuable information about the agent being tested. To be most relevant to the clinic, the assay should be made after the completion of PLD repair (greater than 6 h after treatment), since PLD repair will be able to occur if tumours are left *in situ*.

The TD$_{50}$ assay for cell survival is historically important as being the first used to define the cell survival characteristics of a tumour treated *in situ*

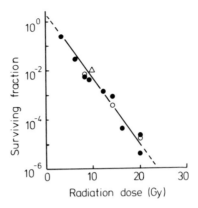

Figure 6 Cell survival curve of CBA leukaemia cells treated with ^{60}Co γ-rays *in vivo* and assayed for cell survival using the TD_{50} assay. Open circles, mice breathing 95% oxygen; closed circles, mice breathing air. (Redrawn from Hewitt and Wilson, 1961.)

(Hewitt and Wilson, 1959) (Figure 6). The assay is slower than the *in vitro* assay and requires many more animals. However, it is more widely applicable since the tumour does not have to grow *in vitro* but only in its natural habitat, the animal. It has been shown in some systems to give identical results to the *in vitro* assay (Steel and Adams, 1975) and so, if a particular tumour will grow in culture, the *in vitro* assay should be used for reasons of economy and speed, and to save animals.

The lung colony and latent period assays require fewer animals than the TD_{50} assay and are usually slightly quicker. The range of surviving fractions covered by the TD_{50} and lung colony assays is limited by the take rate and lung colony forming efficiency (CFE) respectively of untreated tumour cells. The TD_{50} can be lowered and the lung CFE raised by various procedures, the most common one being the addtion of lethally irradiated tumour cells to the test cells. (Hewitt and Wilson, 1961; Hill and Bush, 1969). This manipulation increases the dose range that the assays can cover. It also reduces the problem of selection, since a larger fraction of the tumour cells contributes to growth in the subcutaneous site or in the lung. In all these assays the most important feature is the fact that the tumour cells must be disaggregated before survival assessment. The method of assessment, whether *in vitro* or *in vivo*, appears to be of secondary or no importance to the result.

^{125}I-IODODEOXYURIDINE; RADIOACTIVITY LOSS

Iododeoxyuridine (IUdR) is an analogue of thymidine and is thus incorporated into the DNA of all cells in DNA synthesis at the time of injection.

Loss of ^{125}I radioactivity after ^{125}IUdR injection has been used to measure cell loss rates from tumours (Begg, 1977; Dethlefsen, 1971; Porschen and Feinendegen, 1973). It was found that treating ^{125}IUdR-labelled tumours with a cytocidal agent increased radioactivity loss rates from the tumours. This could therefore be used as a measure of damage. The increase in radioactivity loss after treatment cannot be related to cell killing mainly because ^{125}IUdR released from dying cells can be extensively reutilized by the surviving proliferating cells.

The advantages of the technique are that it is quick (1 to 2 weeks) and that it allows oxic and hypoxic subpopulations to be investigated separately by varying the time between ^{125}IUdR injection and treatment. The longer this interval the greater the proportion of labelled cells that will have moved into hypoxic regions (Porschen *et al.*, 1974). The disadvantage of the method is that the dose-response relationship for radioactivity loss occurs over a small dose range, or is absent in some tumours (Figure 7). As an experimental tool it is a useful and interesting assay in a limited number of animal tumours. As a general test of damage to a range of tumours, one of the other methods mentioned above offers more scope and reliability.

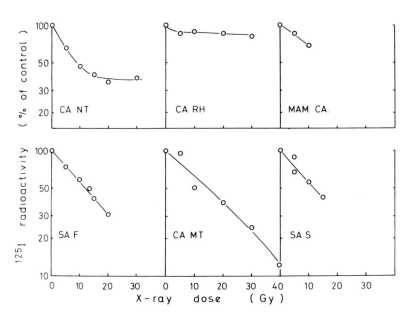

Figure 7 X-ray dose–response curves for six different solid tumours in mice using the ^{125}IUdR assay. Mice were injected intraperitoneally with 20 μCi ^{125}IUdR (a thymidine analogue) and their tumours irradiated 8 h later. The ^{125}I radioactivity remaining in the treated tumours, expressed as a percentage of that in untreated tumours, 8 days after injection is plotted as a function of x-ray dose.

Regarding its relevance to the clinic, the assay has been used to investigate such phenomena as hypoxic cell radiosensitization (Begg *et al.*, 1974), hyperthermia (Weber *et al.*, 1978), chemotherapy (Hofer, 1969), and high LET radiation (Begg and Fowler, 1974; Porschen and Feinendegen, 1973), all of which are currently being tested in the clinic. It is therefore capable of selecting potentially new forms of treatment in a limited number of tumour systems. These tumours, however, are usually anaplastic solid tumours or ascites tumours, and so the question of relevance of the tumour rather than of the assay may again be more pertinent.

DISCUSSION

The questions that a clinician might ask of an experimentalist are 'what new forms of treatment are there', 'are they likely to work in the clinic', and 'how can the present forms of treatment be improved'? The choice of assay to best answer each of these questions will vary, although all of the assays mentioned in this chapter are capable of detecting potential new forms of treatment, and to that extent they are all clinically relevant.

However, the question of whether a new treatment will work in human cancer is more complex. Hypoxic cell radiosensitizers, for example, were shown to be effective in all the assays mentioned, initially by using high doses of drug and high single doses of radiation. In the clinic, neither the levels of drug nor radiation would be tolerated. To predict their possible clinical usefulness, subsequent experiments were needed with much smaller drug doses to give plasma levels that could be achieved in humans, together with small fractionated doses of x-rays. Fractionated treatments are very difficult to interpret with the cell survival and ^{125}IUdR assays but less difficult for other assays (growth delay, TCD_{50}). The more clinically relevant experiments are therefore automatically restricted in this case to particular *in situ* end-points.

In addition, the experimentalist can be more certain of a treatment's potential clinical application if they have tested it against a variety of animal tumours which vary in growth rate and histology. This too is a limitation on the choice of assay. The correlation of treatment efficacy with one or both of these parameters can point to possible mechanisms of action and indicate in which type of human tumour the treatment may be most effective. Human tumour xenografts may be valuable as one of the test systems in order to show that the treatment is effective against human as well as rodent cells. Again, it is the tumour and the dose levels used, in addition to the type of assay, which brings the experiment closer to the clinical situation.

In order to compare treatments, it is vital to understand the biological mechanisms behind their effect and to understand fully the assay system used. The use of more than one assay system concurrently is often invaluable for this. For example a comparison of the TCD_{50} and cell survival assays in the WH CA MT tumour indicated that the chronically hypoxic cells but not the aerobic cells or the aerobic cells made acutely hypoxic could repair potentially lethal damage. This led to incorrect estimates of hypoxic fraction by the TCD_{50} method (McNally and Sheldon, 1977) since it was assumed that acutely and chronically hypoxic cells had the same radiosensitivity.

In the same tumour it was found that in the cell survival assay the radiation sensitivity ($1/D_o$) was less if the cells were plated in agar rather than on plastic, and only this lower radiosensitivity estimate (agar) could account for the high TCD_{50} (Stephens *et al.*, 1980). The agar method is obviously the more relevant to *in situ* treatments. In other examples, in which growth delay and cell survival were compared (Begg, 1980; Twentyman, 1980; Stephens and Peacock, 1977; Rowley *et al.*, 1979), it became clear that the rates of proliferation after different cytotoxic treatments could be vastly different, a highly important point in determining the overall effect of treatment. Two drugs which produce equal cell killing can therefore give markedly different growth delays. The drug giving the slower post-treatment proliferation rate would therefore be more beneficial to the patient if cure were not achieved.

It is worth pointing out again that recognizing the problems with these assays does not necessarily make them less useful. In the process of finding the problems, useful information on treatment mechanisms often emerges, and knowing the problems also allows the assay to be used more intelligently.

It is always necessary to return to more basic studies than the *in situ* treatment studies mentioned here, in order to understand how the treatment works at a more fundamental level. New drugs are often tested at the subcellular level, then at the cellular level (*in vitro*), and finally in the whole animal. *In vitro* studies will often demonstrate a drug to be an effective cytotoxic agent, but the gap from there to the clinic is huge. There is no information from these studies whether the drug will be toxic to the animal, or whether it will reach the tumour in adequate concentrations. Consequently, although variables such as proliferation rate, oxygenation, pH, etc., can be finely controlled in *in vitro* studies, for clinical relevance animal studies ultimately have to be done. To be more certain about the clinical application of a treatment, tumours in at least one species other than a mouse should also be investigated, such as spontaneous dog tumours (Owen, 1980).

Finally, the clinician may wish to know not merely the end-points to take notice of in experimental animals, but which end-points can also be used on the cancer patient. Of the techniques mentioned in this chapter, the ones most suited to human application are growth delay and complete and partial regression. The latter is used commonly, particularly in chemotherapy studies. As discussed above, growth delay is the better, more quantitative, assay and has been used successfully to measure the effects of both radiotherapy and chemotherapy, usually on patients with multiple metastatic nodules.

These studies will undoubtedly be helped by advances in the imaging technologies of computed assisted tomography (CAT scanning) and ultrasound (see *Br. J. Cancer*, **41**, Suppl. IV, 1980, for reviews).

Another new technology that may contribute to the testing of treatment sensitivity in humans is that of flow cytometry. By fluorescence of DNA-bound dyes and light scatter measurements, this technique can often distinguish normal cells from cancerous cells. In addition, it can then determine the proliferative state of the cancer cells before and after treatment. This can sometimes provide an early guide to prognosis (see Melamed *et al.*, 1979). Flow cytometry methodology is still being developed and therefore its full potential is as yet unknown.

It may be possible to carry out cell survival studies in human tumours if biopsies were taken before, during, and after treatment, followed by successfully growing the tumour cells *in vitro* or in immune-suppressed animals. A variation of this technique now being tested is to first take a tumour sample from an untreated patient and subsequently to treat the tumour cells *in vitro*, or as a xenograft in immune-suppressed mice. Both these methods are one step removed from direct clinical relevance compared with a clonogenic assay of tumour cells treated in the patient. Growth *in vitro* or as a xenograft can introduce artefacts in estimates of sensitivity to treatment (for reviews see Dendy, 1980; Steel and Peckam, 1980).

It may also be possible to use the [125]IUdR assay in the patient, but in addition to the radiotoxicity problem this would provide no benefit over the growth delay assay. Consequently, growth delay appears to be the best choice for experimental human treatment studies, with cell survival studies possibly complementing these in future.

CONCLUSION

There is often a difference between experimentalists and clinicians in the information that they require from an assay. The experimentalist is used to asking how many cells survived a given treatment, and so will think in terms of cell survival curve parameters such as mean lethal dose (D_o) and extrapolation number (n). The clinician usually has no way of knowing the surviving fraction and will assess treatment efficacy on such parameters as percentage cures or tumour-free interval before recurrence. These parameters for *in situ* assays, however, can also be used in the laboratory and there have been many attempts to relate tham to the amount of cell kill.

I have described these correlations, or lack of them, but do not wish to leave the impression that an assay is of little value without a one-to-one correlation of its parameters with surviving fraction. Cell kill is by no means the only criterion in judging the merits of a treatment, as I have demonstrated, but it is very useful in understanding mechanisms of action, particularly in studies of interaction between two or more agents.

It is inevitable in assessing these end-points that a considerable part of the discussion has centred on the problems which all end-points have. It therefore needs to be emphasized that the problems associated with an assay should not automatically be either a deterrent to its use, or lead to discounting of the results as wrong or irrelevant. Knowing the problems should lead to better use of an assay, and allow clinicians and experimentalists to make a more informed assessment of the results, and to make a more informed choice of end-point for their own use.

Acknowledgments

I would like to thank Drs Julie Denekamp, Jack Fowler, Nicolas McNally and Fiona Stewart for helpful criticism of the manuscript. My thanks also to Dr Stewart for her help with the diagrams and collation of the references and to Mrs Eileen Marriott for typing the manuscript.

REFERENCES

Ashe, D.V., Peckham, M.J., and Steel, G.G. (1979). The quantitative response of human tumours to radiation and misonidazole. *Br. J. Cancer*, **40**, 883.

Barendsen, G.W., and Broerse, J.J. (1969). Experimental radiotherapy of a rat rhabdomyosarcoma with 15 MeV neutrons and 300 kV X-rays: I. Effects of single exposures. *Eur. J. Cancer,* **5**, 373.

Barker, M., Hoshino, T., Gurcay, O., Wilson, C.B., Nielson, S., and Downie, R. (1973). Development of an animal brain tumour and its response to therapy. *Cancer Res.,* **33**, 976.

Barkley, H.T., and Fletcher, G.H. (1977). The significance of residual disease after external irradiation of squamous cell carcinoma of the oropharynx. *Radiology*, **124**, 493.

Begg, A.C. (1977). Cell loss from several types of solid murine tumour: comparison of ^{125}I-iododeoxyuridine and tritiated thymidine methods. *Cell Tissue Kinet.*, **10**, 409.

Begg, A.C. (1980). Analysis of growth delay data: potential pitfalls. *Br. J. Cancer*, **41**, Suppl. IV, 93.

Begg, A.C. (1982). The influence of rate of tumour regrowth on the shape of dose response curves in growth delay experiments. (in preparation).

Begg, A.C., and Fowler, J.F. (1974). A rapid method for the determination of tumour RBE. *Br. J. Radiol.*, **47**, 154.

Begg, A.C., Fu, K.K., Kane, L.J., and Phillips, T.L. (1980). Single agent chemotherapy of a solid murine tumor assayed by growth delay and cell survival. *Cancer Res.*, **40**, 145.

Begg, A.C., Sheldon, P.W. and Foster, J.L. (1974). Demonstration of radiosensitization of hypoxic cells in solid tumours by metronidazole. *Br. J. Radiol.*, **47**, 399.

Breur, K. (1966). Growth rate and radiosensitivity of human tumours I. *Eur. J. Cancer*, **2**, 157.

Brown, J.M. (1975). Selective radiosensitization of the hypoxic cells of mouse tumours with the nitroimidazoles metronidazole and Ro 07–0582. *Radiat. Res.*, **64**, 633.

Brown, J.M. (1979). Drug or radiation changes to the host which could affect the out-come of combined modality therapy. *Int. J. Radiat. Oncol., Biol. Phys.*, **5**, 1151.

Chirgos, M.A., Humphreys, S.R., and Goldin, A. (1962). Effectiveness of Cytoxan against intracerebrally and subcutaneously inoculated mouse lymphoid leukaemia L1210. *Cancer Res.*, **22**, 187.

Courtenay, V.D., and Mills, J. (1978). An *in vitro* colony assay for human tumours grown in immune suppressed mice and treated *in vivo* with cytotoxic agents. *Br. J. Cancer*, **37**, 261.

Curtis, S.B., Tenforde, T.S., Parks, D., Schilling, W.A., and Lyman, J.T. (1978). Response of a rat rhabdomyosarcoma to neon- and helium-ion irradiation. *Radiat. Res.*, **74**, 274.

Dendy, P.P. (1980). The use of *in vitro* methods to predict tumour response to chemotherapy. *Br. J. Cancer*. **41**, Suppl. IV, 195.

Denekamp, J. (1972). The relationship between the 'cell loss factor' and the immediate response to radiation in animal tumours. *Eur. J. Cancer*, **8**, 335.

Denekamp, J. (1977). Tumour regression as a guide to prognosis: a study with experimental animals *Br. J. Radial.*, **50**, 271.

Denekamp, J., and Harris, S.R. (1975). Tests of two electron-affinic radiosensitizers *in vivo* using regrowth of an experimental carcinoma. *Radiat Res.*, **61**, 191.

Denekamp, J., and Harris, S.R. (1976). The response of a transplantable tumor to fractionated irradiation. I. X-rays and the hypoxic cell radiosensitizer Ro 07–0582. *Radiat. Res.*, **66**, 66.

Dethlefsen, L.A. (1971). An evaluation of radioiodine-labelled 5–iodo–2′–deoxy-uridine as a tracer for measuring cell loss from solid tumours. *Cell Tissue Kinet.*, **4**, 123.

Dische, S., Bennett, M.H., Saunders, M.I., and Anderson, P. (1980). Tumour regression as a guide to prognosis : a clinical study. *Br. J. Radiol.*, **53**, 454.

Dische, S., and Saunders, M.I. (1980). Tumour regression and prognosis : a clinical study. *Br. J. Cancer*, **41**, Suppl. IV, 11.

Field, S.B., Jones, T., and Thomlinson, R.H. (1968). The relative effects of fast neutrons and X-rays on tumour and normal tissue in the rat. *Br. J. Radiol.*, **41**, 597.

Field, S.B., and Michalowski, A. (1979). Endpoints for damage to normal tissues. *Int. J. Radiat. Oncol., Biol. Phys.*, **5**, 1185.

Fowler, J.F., and Denekamp, J. (1977). Radiation effects on normal tissues. In *Cancer: a comprehensive treatise*, vol. 6 (ed. F.F. Becker). New York: Plenum. p.139.

Fowler, J.F., Denekamp, J., Sheldon, P.W., Smith, A.M., Begg, A.C., Harris, S.R., and Page, A.L. (1974). Optimum fractionation in X-ray treatment of C3H mouse mammary tumours. *Br. J. Radiol.*, **47**, 781.

Fowler, J.F., Hill, S.A., and Sheldon, P.W. (1980). Comparison of tumour cure (local control) with regrowth delay in mice. *Br. J. Cancer*, **41**, Suppl. IV, 102.

Fowler, J.F., Sheldon, P.W., Begg, A.C., Hill, S.A., and Smith, A.M. (1975). Biological properties and response to X-rays of first generation transplants of spontaneous mammary carcinomas in C3H mice. *Int. J. Radiat. Biol.*, **27**, 463.

Grossman, I., Kurohara, S.S., Webster, J.H., and George, F.W. (1973). The prognostic significance of tumour response during radiotherapy in cervical carcinoma. *Radiology*, **107**, 411.

Hahn, G.M., Ray, G.R., Gordon, L.F., and Kallman, R.F. (1973). Response of solid tumour cells to chemotherapeutic agents *in vivo*. Cell survival after 2 and 24 hours exposure. *J. Natl Cancer Inst.*, **50**, 529.

Hermans, A.F., and Barendsen, G.W. (1969). Changes of cell proliferation characteristics in a rat rhabdomyosarcoma before and after X-irradiation. *Eur. J. Cancer*, **5**, 173.

Hewitt, H.B., and Blake, E.R. (1968). The growth of transplanted murine tumours in pre-irradiated sites. *Br. J. Cancer*, **12**, 808.

Hewitt, H.B., and Wilson, C.W. (1959). A survival curve for mammalian leukaemia cells irradiated *in vivo* (implications for the treatment of mouse leukaemia by whole-body irradiation). *Br. J. Cancer*, **13**, 69.

Hewitt, H.B. and Wilson, C.W. (1961). Survival curves for tumour cells irradiated *in vivo*. *Ann. N.Y. Acad. Sci.*, **95**, 818.

Hill, R.P., and Bush, R.S. (1969). A lung-colony assay to determine the radiosensitivity of the cells of a solid tumour. *Int. J. Radiat. Biol.*, **15**, 435.

Hofer, K.G. (1969). Tumor cell death *in vivo* after administration of chemotherapeutic drugs. *Cancer Chemother. Rep. 1*, **53**, 273.

Howes, A.E. (1969). An estimation of changes in the proportion of hypoxic cells after irradiation of transplanted C3H mouse mammary carcinomas. *Br. J. Radiol.*, **42**, 441.

Law, L.W., Dunn, T.B., Boyle, P.J., and Miller, J.H. (1949). Observations on the effect of a folic acid antagonist on transplantable lymphoid leukaemias in mice. *J. Natl Cancer Inst.*, **10**, 179.

McNally, N.J. (1973). A comparison of the effects of radiation on tumour growth delay and cell survival. *Br. J. Radiol.*, **46**, 450.

McNally, N.J., and Sheldon, P.W. (1977). The effect of radiation on tumour growth delay cell survival and cure of the animal using a single tumour system. *Br. J. Radiol.*, **50**, 321.

Malaise, E.P., Charbit, A., Chavaudra, N., Combes, P.F., Douchez, J., and Tubiana, M. (1972). Change in volume of irradiated human metastases. Investigation of repair of sublethal damage and tumour repopulation. *Br. J. Cancer* **26**, 43.

Mantyla, M., Kortekangas, A.E., Valavaara, R.A., and Nordman, E.M. (1979). Tumour regression during radiation treatment as a guide to prognosis. *Br. J. Radiol.*, **52**, 972.

Marcial, V.A., and Bosch, A. (1970). Radiation induced tumour regression in carcinoma of the uterine cervix: prognostic significance. *Am. J. Roentgenol., Radiat. Ther. Nucl. Med.*, **108**, 113.

Marmor, J.B., Hahn, N., and Hahn, G.M. (1977). Tumour cure and cell survival after localized radiofrequency heating. *Cancer Res.*, **37**, 879.

Melamed, J.N., Mullaney, T., and Mendelsohn, G. (eds) (1979). *Flow cytometry and cell sorting*. New York: John Wiley & Sons.

Owen, L.N. (1980). Canine osteosarcoma and canine mammary carcinoma. In *Developments in oncology*, vol. 4, *Metastasis: clinical and experimental aspects* (Ed. K. Hellmann). The Hague: Martinus Nijhoff. p. 75.

Phillips, R.A., and Tolmach, L.J., (1966). Repair of potentially lethal damage in X-irradiated HeLa cells. *Radiat. Res.*, **29**, 413.

Porschen, W., and Feinendegen, L.E. (1973). Biologische In-vivo-dosimetrie von 15-MeV Neutronen bei normalem und tumorzellen-zellmarkierung mit jod–125–desoxyuridin. *Strahlentherapie*, **145**, 27.

Porschen, W., Feinendegen, L.E., Muhlensiepen, H., Piepenbring, W., and

Bosiljanoff, P. (1974). *In vivo* measurements of radiosensitivity of different cell populations within sarcoma-180 in mice. *Radiat. Res.*, **59**, 307.

Potter, M., and Briggs, G.M. (1962). Inhibition of growth of an amethopterin sensitive and amethopterin resistant pair of lymphocytic neoplasms by dietry folic acid deficiencies in mice. *J. Natl Cancer Inst.*, **28**, 341.

Rockwell, S. (1980). *In vivo–in vitro* tumour cell lines: characteristics and limitations as models for human cancer. *Br. J. Cancer*, **41**, Suppl. IV, 118.

Rowley, R., Bacharach, M., Hopkins, H.A., Macleod, M., Rittenour, R., Moore, J.V., and Looney, W.B. (1979). Adriamycin and X-radiation effects upon an experimental solid tumor resistant to therapy. *Int. J. Radiat. Oncol., Biol. Phys.*, **5**, 1291.

Sheldon, P.W., and Hill, S.A. (1977). Hypoxic cell radiosensitizers and local control by X-rays of a transplanted tumor in mice. *Br. J. Cancer*, **35**, 795.

Steel, G.G., and Adams, K. (1975). Stem-cell survival and tumor control in the Lewis lung carcinoma. *Cancer Res.*, **35**, 1530.

Steel, G.G., and Peckam, M.J. (1980). Human tumour xenografts: a critical appraisal. *Br. J. Cancer*, **41**, Suppl. IV, 133.

Stenstrom, K.W., Vermund, H., Mosser, D.G., and Marvin, J.F. (1955). Effects of röntgen irradiation on the tumor bed. 1. The inhibiting action of local pre-transplantation röntgen irradiation (1500 r_a) on the growth of mouse mammary carcinoma. *Radiat. Res.*, **2**, 180.

Stephens, T.C., and Peacock, J.H. (1977). Tumour volume response, initial cell kill and cellular repopulation in B16 melanoma treated with cyclophosphamide and 1-(2-chloroethyl)-3-cyclohexyl-1-nitrosourea. *Br. J. Cancer*, **36**, 313.

Stephens, T.C., Peacock, J.H., and Sheldon, P.W. (1980). Influence of *in vitro* assay conditions on the assessment of radiobiological parameters of the MT tumour. *Br. J. Radiol.*, **53**, 1182.

Suit, H.D., and Maeda, M. (1967). Hyperbaric oxygen and radiobiology of a C3H mouse mammary carcinoma. *J. Natl Cancer Inst.*, **39**, 639.

Suit, H.D., Lindberg, R., and Fletcher, G.H. (1965). Prognostic significance of extent of tumour regression at completion of radiation therapy. *Radiology*, **84**, 1110.

Thomlinson, R.H. (1960). An experimental method for comparing treatments of intact malignant tumours in animals and its application to the use of oxygen in radiotherapy. *Br. J. Cancer*, **14**, 555.

Thomlinson, R.H. (1979). Measurement of the response of primary carcinoma of the breast to treatment. *Br. J. Radiol.*, **52**, 341 (abstract).

Thomlinson, R.H., and Craddock, E.A. (1967). The gross response of an experimental tumour to single doses of X-rays *Br. J. Cancer*, **21**, 108.

Twentyman, P.R. (1977). Artefact introduced into clonogenic assays of bleomycin toxicity. *Br. J. Cancer*, **36**, 642.

Twentyman, P.R. (1979). Timing of assays: an important consideration in the determination of clonogenic cell survival both *in vitro* and *in vivo*. *Int. J. Radiat. Oncol., Biol. Phys.*, **5**, 1213.

Twentyman, P.R. (1980). Experimental chemotherapy studies: intercomparison of assays. *Br. J. Cancer*, **41**, Suppl. IV, 279.

Twentyman, P.R., and Bleehen, N.M. (1976). The sensitivity to cytotoxic agents of the EMT6 tumour *in vivo*. Comparative response of lung nodules in rapid expoential growth and of the solid flank tumour. *Br. J. Cancer*, **33**, 320.

Urano, M., and Suit, H.D. (1971). Experimental evaluation of the tumor bed effect in C3H mouse mammary carcinoma and for C3H mouse fibrosarcoma. *Radiat. Res.*, **45**, 41.

Van Peperzeel, H.A. (1972). Effects of single doses of radiation on lung metastases in man and experimental animals. *Eur. J. Cancer,* **8**, 665.

Van Putten, L.M. (1968). Oxygenation and cell kinetics after irradiation in a transplantable osteosarcoma. In *Effects of radiation on cellular proliferation and differentiation.* Vienna: IAEA. p.493.

Weber, H.J., Porschen, W., Dietzel, F., Muhlensiepen, H., and Feinendegen, L.E. (1978). *In vivo* analysis of the influence of combined hyperthermia and gamma irradiation on euoxic and hypoxic tumour cells. In *Cancer therapy by hyperthermia and radiation* (eds C. Streffer, S. Seeber, K.R. Trott, and J.E. Robinson). Baltimore: Urban and Schwarzenberg.

Chapter

4   LUCIEN ISRAËL

Evaluating Response in Soft Tissue Tumour

In order to evaluate the efficacy of a given treatment and to compare different types of cancer therapy, we need to define 'response' to treatment. The definition should permit reproducible evaluation from one situation to another and from one investigator to another.

CRITERIA OF RESPONSE

It has come to be widely accepted that the response of a soft tissue tumour to therapy can be defined as a *partial response* when there is a decrease of at least 50% of the product of two perpendicular diameters of a measurable tumour (corresponding to a two-thirds decrease in spherical tumour volume). In the case of multiple tumours, there must be no increase in size of any of the tumours for a response to be designated as partial.

The reason for choosing this criterion was the difficulty in measuring tumour dimensions accurately, and the variability of measurements from one individual observer to another. Only a reduction by more than 50% in tumour size can be considered to indicate, with any degree of reliability, that effective tumour reduction has taken place. Consequently, only responses that meet this requirement are worth considering in evaluating a therapeutic modality.

Complete response is defined as complete disappearance of all tumour, as assessed by the same methods that were used to determine tumour size before treatment. *Progression* is defined as an increase in the product of two perpendicular diameters of a tumour by 25%, over the smallest volume recorded at any time, either before or during treatment. Progression of tumour growth shows inefficacy of the treatment on which progression occurs and, accordingly, calls for discontinuation of that treatment. Standards for defining progression are rightly less stringent than those for defining regression. A situation is classified as *no change* when variation in tumour size falls between a partial response and progression, i.e. between a 50% decrease and a 25% increase in size.

In addition to the magnitude of a response, it is important to define the *duration of the response*. This is the time that elapses between the date that partial response is first documented and the date that progression is recorded.

Definition of 'soft tissue' includes muscle, skin, fat, connective tissue, hematopoietic and lymphatic tissue, blood vessels, and peripheral nerves. Bone is excluded and so are viscera such as lung, liver, kidney and pancreas. Some superficial palpable tumours, such as intra-abdominal metastases from ovarian carcinoma, are also classified as soft tissue tumours.

TECHNICAL ASPECTS OF EVALUATING RESPONSE IN SOFT TISSUE TUMOUR

For *deep-seated tumours* (e.g. intra-abdominal or pelvic masses) the concept of evaluable, as opposed to measurable, disease was introduced. This distinction arose from the inaccuracy of measuring deep-seated tumours and the indirect methods used to make the measurements. It has become somewhat outdated since the introduction of CT scanning which can be used to measure a pelvic or retroperitoneal mass with a high degree of accuracy, thus making such tumours assessable in a therapeutic trial. Other methods used to measure deep-seated tumours and to assess their response to therapy include plain roentgenograms, lymphangiography, arteriography, and ultrasonograms.

For *palpable tumours*, such as skin nodules, superficial lymphadenopathy, chest or abdominal wall tumours, and soft tissue tumours of the limbs, measurement is generally easy and can be made either directly across the skin or by means of a caliper. One must exert the same pressure on the tissue covering the tumour from one measurement to the next, otherwise the thickness of the subcutaneous tissue will inevitably distort the results. Superficial palpable tumours may also be measured radiologically (e.g. by xerography of a muscle tumour in a limb).

Some *skin tumours*, such as superficial melanoma metastases, mycosis fungoides or basal cell carcinomas, tend to spread superficially without perceptibly extending into the subcutaneous tissue. For such tumours, only the area can be measured. Since this type of superficial tumour may be irregularly shaped or may consist of multiple small tumours, serial photographs are essential for measuring response.

It may be useful to mention the possible use of *biochemical markers* as indicators of response to therapy in soft tissue tumour, e.g. β-HCG in testicular choriocarcinoma, or carcinoembryonic antigen in peritoneal metastases from breast or colon carcinomas. In the author's opinion, decrease by more than 50% in the level of an abnormal secretion should be taken into account in assessing the response of tumours to therapy. Clinical studies need to investigate the correlation between changes in the volume of tumours and their ability to secrete biochemical markers.

SPECIAL PROBLEMS IN EVALUATING RESPONSE

The treatment of tumours by local hyperthermia has been reported to induce fibrotic changes rather than shrinkage of the tumour mass (Storm *et al.*, 1979). The implication is that measurement of volume, whether by clinical or roentgenographic methods, does not accurately reflect the response of malignant tumours to this treatment modality. In our experience (Israël and Besenval, 1981) the response of liver metastases to such treatment is best monitored by ultrasonograms. Responding liver metastases undergo liquefaction (necrosis), followed a few weeks later by calcification and a hyperdensity state that is readily distinguishable from active tumour.

Another situation in which response may be difficult to assess is that of skin metastases treated by intralesional immunotherapy. Such lesions generally exhibit an intense inflammatory reaction with an increase in volume, followed by suppuration and necrosis. When the lesion heals it may leave a fibrotic scar and only biopsy can ascertain that tumour has been eradicated.

The efficacy of chemotherapy for recurrence in previously irradiated areas is difficult to evaluate owing to radiation-induced tissue fibrosis. Radiotherapy also causes fibrotic vascular changes within the tumour, thus reducing the accessibility to chemotherapeutic agents. For these reasons, tumours recurring in previously irradiated areas are unreliable situations in which to evaluate the efficacy of chemotherapy.

CELLULAR ASPECTS OF EVALUATING RESPONSE

Not all the cells in a tumour mass are tumour cells. Macrophages, lymphocytes, fibroblasts, and normal cells of the tissue in which the tumour develops contribute to the 'tumour volume'. It is widely held that tumour volume regression or progression involves the same proportion of normal and tumour cells, but in fact this has never been clearly shown. Tumours of different sizes may behave differently with regard to the proportion of normal and tumour cells that contribute to the reduction in mass that we record as the response.

In addition, necrosis is more marked in larger tumours, and results in a diminished blood supply, and hence poorer accessibility to drugs. Investigational protocols should ensure that tumours being compared for response have an equal chance of responding. In practice this would mean stratifying for small tumours (less than 2 cm in diameter), medium-sized tumours (2 to 5 cm) and large tumours (greater than 5 cm).

Chemotherapy may produce changes in the degree of differentiation of a tumour by selectively killing more undifferentiated cells, thus leaving a higher proportion of differentiated cells within the tumour. The usual cytostatic agents more readily kill undifferentiated cells, that is stem cells or clonogenic cells responsible for rapid growth of a tumour mass. In contrast, most hormonal agents are more active against differentiated cells (more likely to have oestrogen receptors) than against undifferentiated cells.

The degree of cell differentiation may not be critical in all situations, but the efficacy of new agents may depend on this criterion. Hence it may be of the utmost importance to evaluate the response of a tumour as a function of its degree of differentiation.

Tumour cell kinetics play an integral part in evaluating response to therapy. Some drugs are able to increase cell loss, thus interfering with tumour growth, without actually killing proliferating tumour cells. Drugs which interfere with coagulation and/or the adhesion process could also reduce tumour recurrence rates without direct cell killing. It would be useful to measure the growth fraction of the tumours we treat so that tumours with different growth fractions could be studied separately for their response to therapy. This point will be discussed later under the heading of tumour doubling time.

The clinician observing tumour response to treatment must have some idea of the number of cells involved if he is to form a realistic picture of the biological significance of the response. A tumour 1 cm in diameter contains approximately 10^9 cells, a tumour 10 cm in diameter contains 10^{12} cells, and a tumour just too small to be detected clinically can contain 10^8 or even 5×10^8 cells. The implication is that a clinically spectacular response which produces 'disappearance' of a tumour 10 cm in diameter has in fact reduced the number of cells from 10^{12} to less than 10^8, i.e. four logs. Although this is a significant result and beneficial to the patient, up to 10^8 cells remain to be killed in order to achieve eradication of the tumour.

In this regard, clinical investigators note that partial responses are generally of much shorter duration than complete responses for comparable tumours, a finding consistent with cell kinetic considerations. In terms of survival prolongation, a partial response is of practically no benefit in the case of rapidly growing tumours. Clinical trials looking to improve existing therapy should aim at complete response as the goal.

TUMOUR DOUBLING TIME AND EVALUATION OF RESPONSE TO THERAPY

The observed tumour doubling time is the overall result of a number of factors including the growth fraction, extent of cell loss, the grade of differentiation, and the mean tumour cell cycle time. Although it is generally impossible to determine all these factors individually for a given tumour, assessment of their net result (doubling time) provides useful information about the biology of tumours. Unpublished data from our Institute indicates that there is some relationship between doubling time and immune status. Doubling time may be influenced by the tumour's ability to synthesize growth factors and may also be related to differentiation (Chahinian and Israël, 1976) and cell loss (Israël and Chahinian, 1969).

Doubling time and treatment trials

An immediate advantage of determining doubling time would be to ensure comparability of the groups being treated in a trial. It has been shown that the doubling time of solid tumours may vary from 10 to 400 days (Israël *et al.*, 1971). These extremes obviously represent different diseases in terms of biological behaviour, even though they may be pathologically indistinguishable. About half of all measurable solid tumours have a doubling time of less than 100 days, with a very broad distribution for the other half. It is claimed that the doubling time of a tumour may be related to its tendency to metastasize, both in terms of the number of metastases and their time of appearance. If this is true, prognosis may depend, at least in part, on the doubling time of the tumour.

Investigational protocols should include stratification for doubling time so as to compare that which is comparable (Israël, 1972). The fact that stratification for doubling time is not performed accounts, at least in part, for the non-reproducibility of treatment results from one centre to another in studies with relatively small numbers of patients (e.g. a few hundred). Very large numbers of patients would be required to ensure homogeneous distribution of doubling times by chance alone.

Doubling time is a crucial factor for determining optimal cytotoxic treatment schedules (Israël and Duchatellier, 1971). We have shown that a treatment can potentially eradicate a tumour only if at least four courses are administered *per doubling time*. It is clear then that, if the treatment schedule is not tailored to tumour doubling time, some tumours in a given study will be treated optimally whereas others will not.

Doubling time and progression

The doubling time of a tumour remains constant within its clinically detectable phase (Collins *et al.*, 1956). This means that the course of a tumour is relatively predictable on the basis of its doubling time. Another implication of a constant doubling time is that, as soon as treatment is discontinued or as soon as all the sensitive cells have been killed, the tumour resumes its previous spontaneous growth rate. We have shown (Israël *et al.*, 1972) that it is resumed immediately after maximum regression is achieved, without a 'plateau' phase.

If progression is viewed in this light, then it appears that the definition of progression in current protocols is unsatisfactory. For tumours of short doubling time, the time that elapses between maximum regression and progression, as currently defined, will be short and hence of no major consequence. For tumours of relatively long doubling time, however, several weeks of useless and even harmful treatment may be wasted before a patient is finally acknowledged to be 'progressing' and taken off treatment. Obviously, it is mandatory to evaluate response duration but this must not run counter to the best interests of the patient. Determination of a tumour's doubling time provides a way of reconciling the two.

Doubling time and the significance of a response

Evaluating a clinical response, and assessing its clinical significance in terms of benefit to the patient, are two entirely different things. Here again, tumour doubling time is a critical factor. For example, a decrease in tumour cell mass by say 10^4 cells in a tumour of very short doubling time may last only a short time and produce minimal prolongation of survival. In contrast, for tumours of long doubling time, a 'no change' or even therapy-induced slowing down of the growth rate may imply significant prolongation of survival. We have calculated survival gain in relation to the response of tumours to therapy and their spontaneous doubling times (Chahinian and Israël, 1969). This illustrates how relative the concept of response is, and how carefully it must be interpreted if one hopes to improve upon current results and to assess this improvement realistically.

CONCLUSION

In evaluating response in soft tissue deposits of cancer, we have stressed the difficulty of defining end-points. Response to treatment is a biological phenomenon intimately associated with the tumour's 'biological behaviour' in a broad sense of the term. Attempts to compare response rates and median durations of response in tumours that belong to different subgroups in terms of biological behaviour will lead to meaningless results. Stratifying tumours according to their doubling times would be a step in the right direction in ensuring that we compare that which is comparable.

REFERENCES

Chahinian, P., and Israël, L. (1969). Survival gain and volume gain. Mathematical tools in evaluating treatments. *Eur. J. Cancer*, **5**, 625.

Chahinian, P., and Israël, L. (1976). Rates and patterns of growth of lung cancer. In *Lung cancer: Natural history, prognosis, and therapy* (eds L. Israël, and P. Chahinian). New York: Academic Press. p.63.

Collins, F.P., Loeffler, R.K., and Tivey, H. (1956). Observations on growth rates of human tumours. *Am. J. Roentgenol.*, **76**, 988.

Israël, L. (1972). L'évaluation des traitements anticancéreux dans les tumeurs mesurables. In *The design of clincial trials in cancer therapy* (ed. M. Staquet). Bruxelles: Editions Scientifiques Européennes. p. 190.

Israël, L., and Besenval, M. (1981). Essai phase I, phase II d'une hyperthermie localisée par radiofréquence dans 49 cas de cancers profonds. *Bull. Cancer*, **68**, 296.

Israël, L., and Chahinian, P. (1969). Le temps de doublement des cancers bronchiques. *Rev. Fr. Etudes Clin. Biol.*, **14**, 703.

Israël, L., and Duchatellier, M. (1971). Growth fraction, resistance, schedule-doubling time relationship sequential versus simultaneous combinations, as evaluated by a mathematical model of response to chemotherapy. *Eur. J. Cancer*, **7**, 545.

Israël, L., Duchatellier, M., and Chahinian, P. (1972). Predictability models for drug resistance. In *Advances in antimicrobial and antineoplastic chemotherapy*. München, Berlin, Wien: Urban and Schwarzenberg. p. 775.

Israël, L., Soucquet, R., Combes, P.F., Douchez, J., and Chahinian, P. (1971). Le temps de doublement spontané et thérapeutique des cancers broncho-pulmonaires. *J. Fr. Méd. Chir. Thorac.*, **25**, 115.

Storm, F.K., Harrison, W.H., Elliot, R.S., and Morton, D.L. (1979). Normal tissue and solid tumor effects of hyperthermia in animal models and clinical trials. *Cancer Res.*, **39**, 2245.

Cancer Treatment: End Point Evaluation
Edited by B.A. Stoll
© 1983 John Wiley & Sons Ltd

Chapter

5 SANTILAL PARBHOO AND AYAD WAHBA

Evaluating Response in Lesions of Lung, Liver, and Central Nervous System

This chapter will review traditional and developing forms of assessment in lesions of the lungs, liver, and central nervous system. Few reports of serial examination using newer techniques are available. Critical assessment of the newer techniques is also required as application of these is often invasive, and expensive both in their financial and morbidity aspects.

One of the great benefits of properly conducted clinical trials is the insight it gives us into the usefulness of the investigations we commonly request almost as a matter of routine. External review of trial data should sharpen the criteria indicating the frequency and need for special investigations.

It is essential for the clinician to establish initially the pathological extent of the disease being treated, as all future assessment of reponse or deterioration will depend on it. A single follow-up investigation is of limited value because, if it shows a dramatic change, it is very likely that the benefit will be obvious on clinical assessment. But the less detectable clinical improvements (which are much more common) are more likely to be identified by serial investigations.

DEFINITION AND DURATION OF RESPONSE

Clinical observation is the corner-stone of assessment of response to treatment, and the development of controlled clinical trials has dictated the use of strict objective criteria to assess response. These still present problems. For example, new lesions may appear while others regress, when the tumour is heterogeneous (Parbhoo, 1981). In addition, many lesions are not easy to measure, including pulmonary infiltration, pleural effusion, and diffuse liver metastases.

Objective response is usually taken as a decrease in size of measurable lesions, usually a decrease of 50% or more in the product of the diameters of the individual lesions. Where multiple lesions are present, up to eight lesions are measured at each examination. The measurement is either two-dimensional or three-dimensional depending on the facility available, e.g. a plain radiograph of the chest compared to three-dimensional information available from a CAT scan of the brain. Measurement in other areas is becoming possible, such as the introduction of electronic cursors to measure discrete lesions in ultrasonic pictures of the liver.

Where lesions are evaluable but non-measurable, such as pulmonary infiltration, pleural effusion, and diffuse infiltration of the liver, serial changes may be appreciable on plain x-ray, scintiscan or ultrasound examinations. Attempts are being made to quantify these changes by computer and, if successful, this will be a major advance in assessing such lesions, which are at present subject to a great deal of observer bias. The UICC has introduced standardized criteria for the assessment of response (Hayward *et al*, 1977) and the Karnofsky–Burchenal (1948) assessment of the patient's performance status is important in the general assessment of the patient's response to treatment.

Definition of response duration is controversial and the overall response duration should be taken as the period from the start of treatment to the date of first observation of progressive disease. The period of complete response should be from the date that complete response was first recorded to the date of first observation of progressive disease.

The survival period may be too crude a measure to assess response when drug regimes are relatively ineffective. It is also important to stress that objective response of the lesion may not give a clue to the ultimate survival of the patient. It is probably more accurate to record the period of survival in clinical studies from the date of diagnosis of the primary or metastatic disease to death, rather than from the commencement of treatment to death (see Chapter 2).

PULMONARY NEOPLASMS

Evaluation of the response of primary and secondary lung neoplasms to different modalities of treatment is complicated by the fact that the variety of histological tumour types respond differently to any particular treatment. The histopathology and biology of primary lung cancer is tabulated in Table 1.

Pulmonary metastases occur in about 30% of patients with malignant disease coming to autopsy and as seen from Table 2, the incidence of pulmonary secondaries varies according to the primary tumour. Occasionally patients present with metastatic lesions without any evidence of primary disease, despite extensive search.

Measurement of the response to treatment in plain radiographs depends on the pattern of pulmonary metastases (Table 3). It may be difficult if there are

Table 1   Primary lung cancer

	Types	Incidence (%)	Biology
A	Squamous cell	50	Well differentiated; slowly growing
B	Oat cell (small cell anaplastic)	18	Highly malignant; metastasize early
C	Large cell anaplastic	18	Intermediate behaviour
D	Adenocarcinoma	11	Often peripheral; no sex difference; not related to smoking

Table 2   Frequency of pulmonary metastases at autopsy (after Willis, 1973)

Site of primary tumour	Frequency (%) in autopsy series
Oral and pharyngeal	30
Oesophagus	20
Stomach	20
Intestines	15
Liver	20
Pancreas	20
Breast	55
Uterus	15
Ovary	10
Prostate	40
Thyroid	65
Kidney	75
Malignant melanoma	60
Osteosarcoma	75
Chorionepithelioma	75
Overall incidence in all malignant disease	30

Table 3   Patterns of pulmonary metastases

Number	Single, multiple, or miliary
Size	Similar or dissimilar (? due to repeated showers of tumour emboli)
Distribution	Bilateral (commoner in basal than in apical areas), peripheral and subpleural, or diffuse (miliary)
Shape	Discrete rounded 'cannon ball' metastases (e.g. hypernephroma), fuzzy poorly defined areas (e.g. breast cancer), plaques in subpleural position, or diffuse sheet of tumour encasing lung

Table 4   Complications of lung neoplasms (after Riordan, 1979)

Intrathoracic spread beyond the lung
Pleural effusion
Superior vena caval obstruction
Recurrent laryngeal paralysis
Phrenic paralysis
Oesophageal obstruction
Chest wall involvement
Pericarditis
Brachial plexus involvement ⎫
Horner's syndrome   ⎬ Pancoast tumour

Non-metastatic manifestations
Clubbing
Hypertrophic pulmonary osteoarthropathy
Inappropriate vasopressin secretion
Ectopic ACTH secretion
Ectopic parathormone secretion
Carcinoid syndrome
Gynaecomastia
Thyrotoxicosis
Hypoglycaemia
Dementia
Cerebellar ataxia
Myelopathy
Peripheral neuropathy
Myopathy
Myasthenia

diffuse changes compounded by underlying chronic respiratory disease, lymphatic permeation, pleural effusion, bronchial occlusion, and supervening bronchopneumonia. Lymphatic permeation by tumour is a particular problem in that it excites the formation of dense stroma with compression of air sacs as in other fibrotic disease.

Clinical assessment will include simple measurement of respiratory function, assessment of improvement or progression of extrapulmonary manifestations, or changes in the non-metastatic manifestations as shown in Table 4.

Radiology

The plain PA and lateral chest views are still the mainstay of assessment. A major problem in assessing the x-rays is the site of the tumour, e.g. a central tumour produces hilar enlargement whereas a peripheral one presents as a nodule, an irregular density or rarely as a cavitating mass (Figure 1(a)–(c)). Some tumours tend to produce rounded metastases which are easily measured (such as hypernephroma or sarcoma) whereas in carcinoma of the breast the lesions are often less suitable for measurement. Metastases require to have a relatively sharp outline and to be spherical, to be measured serially.

Difficulties in assessing response are encountered when several crops of metastases appear over the period of evaluation or when the tumour is in a

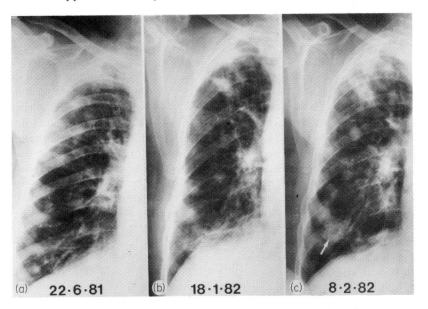

(a) 22·6·81   (b) 18·1·82   (c) 8·2·82

Figure 1 Serial radiographs of a patient with lung metastases from breast cancer showing cavitation of deposits following cytotoxic therapy.

site where it is partly obscured by other shadows, associated collapse or consolidation. Pleural effusions are difficult to evaluate as their assessment in terms of volume is extremely inaccurate (Davis *et al.*, 1963). Lung compression due to a large effusion will also make assessment difficult, as will also lung fibrosis after radiotherapy to the chest.

To help overcome some of these problems, it is important to deal with pleural effusions adequately and to be constantly on the look out for infection which may pass unnoticed in an immunocompromised patient on cytotoxic and corticosteroid treatment. It has recently been suggested that comparison of radiographs may be helped by placing plastic strips with radio-opaque markers on the patient's chest prior to examinations taken on the same machine with the same settings (Watson, 1981).

Tomography is often used to identify a lung lesion but is seldom used for follow-up. However, in the case of cavitation which may occur following necrosis, particularly in squamous carcinoma, follow-up tomography may be of some help. Differentiation from a lung abscess distal to bronchial obstruction or from tuberculous cavitation is important.

Bronchography

This is sometimes used for diagnosis but rarely to assess reponse in primary carcinoma of the lung.

Computerized Axial Tomography

The major use of CAT scans in pulmonary neoplastic disease has been in the detection of disease not discovered by radiographic means, especially in staging patients with primary disease elsewhere, and in the recognition of bronchogenic metastases. It is a much more sensitive technique than other available radiological procedures and, in addition, lymph nodal enlargement can be seen.

Plain film tomography (PFT) is said to be more accurate for the detection of nodular calcification than is a CAT scan. The former technique, in the AP and posterior oblique views, is also better than the CAT scan in determining hilar abnormality and whether the abnormality is due to an enlarged lymph node, enlarged pulmonary artery or hilar mass (Muhm, 1980).

The more widespread use of CAT scans and their greater availability will probably lead to fewer 'curative' operations for primary disease since multiple small pulmonary metastases will be recognized. It may also lead to a better evaluation of response to treatment in pulmonary metastases than has hitherto been possible. With the CAT scan, the data are stored electronically and, by manipulation of the contrast, either the thoracic cage or the lung parenchyma can be seen. The difference in density between the lesion and the surrounding tissue is important, and where the difference is great, the resolution is better, allowing small lesions to be seen. Thus, in the lung parenchyma 2–3 mm lesions can be recognized whereas in solid organs, such as the liver, lesions smaller than 1.5–2 cm in diameter are rarely seen.

Because of its ability to visualize mediastinal nodes and distortion of the mediastinum clearly, this technique has a great advantage over traditional techniques. It can also monitor the response to treatment, and determine changes in the tumour size or changes in density, such as when the tumour undergoes necrosis with little change in size (Husband, 1980). Unfortunately, the radiation exposure to the skin for 10 consecutive slices is approximately 3.5 r which is similar to the exposure during a barium meal examination.

Ultrasound examination

The sonographic evaluation of lung disease has not been widely explored. It is certainly a technique which will recognize a small pleural effusion with blunting of the costophrenic angles, at little extra cost in time during examination of the liver.

Scintiscanning

Pulmonary scintiscanning has been used to assess ventilation perfusion defects in the lung due to tumour or associated infection. Certain isotopes seem to have a predilection for tumour types such as the anaplastic small cell carcinoma, and gallium-67 has been used to predict the efficacy of radiation therapy in reducing tumour size (Higashi *et al.*, 1980). Possible use of this isotope has been suggested in assessing the response to treatment also, but there is little information available. Moreover, gallium-67 is expensive and not readily available.

Nuclear magnetic resonance

Although nuclear magnetic resonance (NMR) is still very much in the experimental stage, preliminary investigations have been carried out and clinical studies are very promising. NMR combines a high degree of sensitivity with some indication of the underlying pathology. As it does not carry the risks of radiation, it should allow frequent examinations to assess response, but the cost of this facility is however still formidable.

Cytology

The accuracy of the results of cytology depends on the expertise of the cytologist, and is also related to a close collaboration between the clinician and cytologist. Apart from its diagnostic advantages it is also useful when a lung lesion is near the surface and a needle can be guided into it under ultrasound control. Little is known about the usefulness of cytology in monitoring response to treatment in pulmonary neoplasms, since difficulties confront the cytologist when looking at changes caused by radiation and chemotherapy.

Good cytological facilities can provide a positive diagnosis in over 80% of central and in up to 50% of peripheral lung tumours (Riordan, 1979). Three or four fresh early-morning sputa are required. It is generally recognized that sputum cytology in patients suspected of having a carcinoma is more effective than either bronchial washings or bronchial biopsies in making a diagnosis. However, serial examination of sputa during the course of treatment may be difficult to interpret because of the changes due to treatment and it is important that the cytologist knows of previous and current treatment. Bronchoscopic material is equally suitable.

The cytological exmination of pleural effusions in patients with malignant disease is essential because there may be other reasons for these patients to develop pleural effusions. Even in patients who develop recurrent effusions, cytological assessment should be repeated before treatment is given.

Fine-needle percutaneous aspiration of a pulmonary lesion under x-ray control is used extensively to provide a cytological diagnosis. The theoretical risk of implantation secondaries in the needle tract does not appear to be a practical problem (Robbins *et al.*, 1954; Berg and Robbins, 1962). Repeated percutaneous biopsies are rarely done but this technique may provide valuable objective data regarding response in treated tumours that apparently show no change in size. Complications such as pneumothorax and haemothorax are fortunately rare, but stringent criteria require to be applied before repeat fine-needle aspiration is carried out in lung lesions.

Endoscopy

Bronchoscopy

The development of the small-calibre fibre-optic bronchoscope allows apical and more peripheral lesions to be reached in a high proportion of cases and bronchoscopy plays a great part in the initial diagnosis of the underlying tumour. It is also valuable in the assessment of patients who have had irradiation therapy to the lungs, when radiographs of the chest may be difficult to interpret due to factors such as atelectasis, underlying chronic lung disease, pneumonitis, and radiation fibrosis. The routine use of bronchoscopy in lieu of, or in addition to, chest radiographs is not warranted if the chest x-rays show measurable lesions.

Mediastinoscopy

This has been used to assist in the diagnosis and to assess whether the patient is fit for thoracotomy. While it plays an important part in the initial management of patients, it clearly has very little place in the follow-up period.

Tumour markers

Despite the continuing enthusiasm for biological markers, there are few clinical indications for their use in evaluating lung cancer response to therapy.

Carcinoembryonic antigen (CEA)

This antigen may be present in all types of primary lung cancer. While all histologic types of lung cancer produce CEA, adenocarcinoma characteristically produces the highest values. Whenever measurable amounts of CEA are found at presentation, it is possible that serial measurement of this antigen may be useful following treatment either by surgery or radiotherapy. It may indicate the extent of eradication of the tumour as well as warning of early recurrence (Vincent *et al.*, 1979).

Calcitonin

This polypeptide hormone was initially thought to be exclusively produced in excess by medullary thyroid carcinoma, a tumour of C cells. In 1973, Silva *et al.* reported that small cell carcinoma (oat cell) of the lung also produced calcitonin. The picture is however somewhat confused since hypercalcitonaemia of thyroidal origin can also occur in patients with lung cancer, perhaps as a response to bone resorption and impending hypercalcaemia. As in the case of many other tumour markers, calcitonin is also found in patients with tuberculosis, pneumonia, chronic obstructive pulmonary disease, breast cancer, pregnancy, chronic renal failure, Zollinger–Ellison syndrome, pancreatitis, and pernicious anaemia. More recent developments indicate that calcitonin is an heterogenuous marker and one could therefore differentiate hypercalcitonaemia of bronchogenic cancer from that of medullary thyroid cancer.

LIVER CANCER

Metastatic deposits in the liver are almost never single and indeed there may be a series of showers of emboli. Overall, 50% of all tumours in the portal system spread to the liver and approximately one-third of all dissemi-

Table 5   Frequency of hepatic metastases at autopsy (after
Willis, 1973)

Site of primary tumour	Average of collected series (%)	Willis (%)
Stomach	33	46
Colon	33	53
Pancreas	60	73
Breast	41	49
Uterus	12	20
Oesophagus	27	41
Overall incidence in all malignant disease		36

Table 6   Complications of hepatic cancer

Jaundice	Calcification
Liver failure	Liver abscess
Portal vein thrombosis	
Portal hypertension	Budd Chiari
Necrosis	syndrome
Haemorrhage	(hepatic outflow block)
Rupture	Hypoglycaemia

Table 7   Local problems affecting evaluation of hepatic metastases

1. Diffuse as against discrete change
2. Underlying chronic liver disease, e.g. cirrhosis, cholangitis.
3. Liver congestion (outflow obstruction, cardiac failure, pericardial effusion)
4. Distortion of liver due to drug toxicity, tumour necrosis, surgery, radiotherapy, invasion of major vessels or bile ducts
5. Density of tumour:
    solid
    necrotic centre
    calcification
    high mucus content
    vascularity of tumour
6. Omental masses attached to liver
7. Co-existent ascites

nated tumours finally involve the liver (Table 5). Slowly growing tumours may virtually replace the liver, but liver function remains reasonably good, since the liver reserve is great. In general, metastatic deposits tend to be less differentiated than the primary tumour.

A host of complications may occur as a result of the extension of primary or secondary hepatic cancer and will affect the assessment of response (Table 6). In addition, various local and regional factors will affect the evaluation of tumour extent in the liver (Table 7). The therapeutic modality used may itself distort liver architecture markedly, due to extensive localized or diffuse necrosis with or without subsequent fibrosis.

The diagnostic need to confirm liver metastases cannot be overemphasized. While primary liver cancer either of the liver cells or biliary tree will be confirmed histologically in the majority of cases, this is rare in the case of liver secondaries. The clinical signs and symptoms, biochemistry or other special investigations may be suggestive of liver metastases, yet the changes may be due to underlying liver disease, alcoholism, and gallstones. Apart from obtaining histological or cytological material wherever possible, it is vital that we should be able to measure the effect of treatment on liver metastases directly. Prolongation of survival time in these patients may reflect response of lesions other than those in the liver. Hence, estimation of liver-specific enzymes and isoenzymes, ultrasound examination, and scintiscans are valuable in separating improvement in liver function and tumour regression from response at other sites of tumour.

Toxicity from drug therapy may interfere with assessment of response, and various forms of hepatotoxicity have been observed after prolonged courses of cytotoxic drugs. Most information is available on methotrexate (Colsky *et al.*, 1955; Menard *et al.*, 1980; Podurgiel *et al.*, 1973). Recent studies by the Milan group in patients receiving adjuvant cytotoxic chemotherapy for breast cancer (cyclophosphamide, methotrexate, and 5-fluorouracil) have ruled out significant chronic liver damage over a five-year follow-up (Bajetta *et al.*, 1981). However, liver function tests do alter during treatment and may interfere with proper assessment of response in liver metastases.

Clinical assessment of reponse

The general well-being of the patient is best assessed by a standard performance index such as the Karnofsky–Burchenal index or the UICC performance status as outlined by Hayward (1980). The extent of clinical hepatomegaly should be clearly marked pictorially in follow-up forms, and measurements should be taken in the mid-clavicular line and in the epigastrium. Careful note should be made of pain and areas of tenderness over the liver. The presence of a hepatic rub will indicate extension to the capsule of the liver.

In primary or metastatic liver cancer, jaundice is not a constant feature unless extensive involvement has occurred. The depth of jaundice has little relation to the extent of hepatic involvement during the early stages of invasion. Deep jaundice usually implies invasion of the biliary tree, or compression of the primary bile duct by tumour. Ascites is a common accompaniment especially late in the disease, and is present in about 50% of patients with primary liver cell cancer.

In large tumours, whether primary or secondary, the relief of pain and tenderness following either hepatic artery ligation or cytotoxic chemotherapy is a good guide to response, and may occur some time before clinical shrinkage of the liver is apparent. However, the development of pain and tenderness over the liver in a patient previously without local symptoms, may also signify response to treatment if the tumour has undergone necrosis and causes stretching of the hepatic capsule due to oedema.

While the liver is the most frequent site of blood-borne metastases at autopsy (Table 5), the much lower incidence recorded during life indicates the low sensitivity of the various imaging devices currently available. The high incidence of blood-borne metastases from outside the portal system, as well as the equal incidence in the cirrhotic as opposed to the non-cirrhotic liver, suggests the importance both of hepatic artery tumour emboli and local liver factors conducive to the growth of secondaries.

Many reports have shown that the right lobe has a higher incidence of secondaries from the portal system but there is no evidence that the right lobe receives a segregated blood supply. Instead, it appears that the high incidence in the right lobe is merely because this lobe forms the major part of the liver and therefore will have a greater number of secondary deposits (Willis, 1973). Liver metastases are almost always multiple and form well shaped spheres, except when they impinge on the hepatic capsule or are traversed by major vessels or bile ducts.

Metastatic deposits can reach enormous sizes, particularly in secondaries from melanoma, carcinoids, and colonic carcinoma where enlarged livers up to 12 500 g have been recorded. Even with this colossal enlargement, the shape is usually retained and the capsule is intact. The probable reason is that most of the tumours are slowly growing, and attain the enormous size by allowing the capsule and blood supply to stretch. In contrast, rapid growth results in loss of blood supply, haemorrhage, and capsular rupture as seen in hepatocellular carcinoma. Even with gross enlargement of the liver, if the multiple deposits are small, hepatic scan may merely show an enlarged liver without showing any focal defects.

The major complications which interfere with the initial and subsequent assessment of response of these tumours to treatment have been summarized in Table 6. The degenerative changes of central necrosis, haemorrhagic liquefaction, and cystic change have an important bearing on the images obtained by ultrasound examination, scintiscanning, and computerized tomography or angiography.

While most metastatic growths in the liver appear as circumscribed tumours, diffuse tumour infiltrations are also seen. The tumours most frequently responsible are breast carcinoma and melanoma. If the tumour is scirrhous, a cirrhosis-like picture may emerge (Willis, 1973). Hence a nodular liver resembling cirrhosis in a patient with cancer requires biopsy at the time of laparoscopy if this is being carried out.

A further factor which has a bearing on assessing response is that secondary deposits in the liver appear to grow at a faster rate than metastatic deposits elsewhere. Many hepatic metastases show mitosis greatly in excess of the mitotic activity seen in the primary tumour or its metastases elsewhere. Hence recognition of hepatic metastases by our crude imaging techniques probably means that these deposits will grow very much more quickly and therefore may not have the same degree of response to treatment as shown by other sites. A number of other local problems which affect the evaluation of response have been summarized in Table 7.

The small number of patients who have successful surgical resection of a primary hepatocellular carcinoma or the rare solitary liver secondary, appear to show little abnormality in their biochemical and imaging patterns after the immediate post-operative period. This is due to the fact that, as the tumour grows, the rest of the liver has compensated, and usually liver function is in fact normal. Therefore, abnormalities appearing at a later date indicate possible recurrence of the tumour or the further development of previously unnoticed secondary deposits.

Biochemical assessment of response

These tests may be divided into those usually considered as liver function tests, and others which are labelled 'tumour markers' (shown in Table 8). The

Table 8   Biochemical assessment of response in hepatic cancer

---

'Liver function' tests
Serum enzymes
    alkaline phosphatase
    5'–nucleotidase
    alkaline phosphatase (hepatic)
    aspartate transaminase
    gamma-glutamyl transferase

Serum bilirubin
Serum proteins (total)
Serum albumin
Prothrombin ratio/index

Tumour marker assessment
Alpha-fetoprotein
Carcinoembryonic antigen
Human chorionic gonadotrophin
Serotonin and its products

enzymes in common usage as liver function tests are markers of liver damage or membrane leakage rather than measures of synthetic function. Gamma-glutamyl transferase is the most sensitive enzyme test, but the results may be vitiated by alcohol intake prior to blood sampling. Wiener and Sachs (1978), Winchester *et al.* (1978), and White *et al.* (1979) have highlighted the usefulness of liver function tests, especially alkaline phosphatase, in relation

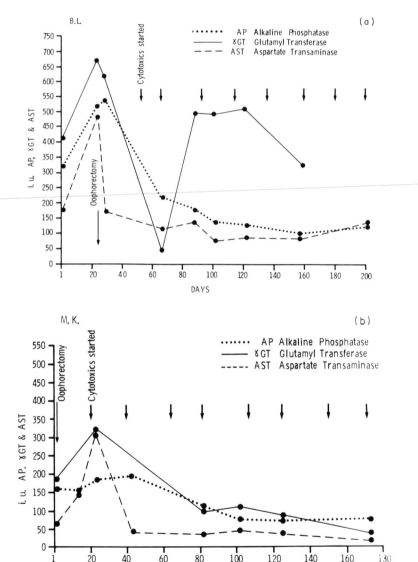

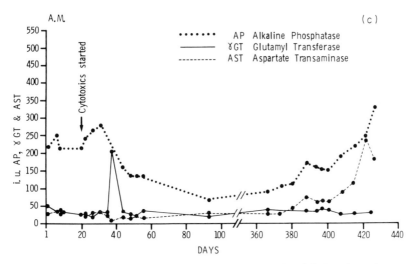

Figure 2 Changes in serum levels of alkaline phosphatase (AP) (*N*0–65), and aspartate transaminase (AST) (*N*=5–40) in three patients with hepatic metastases from breast cancer, following treatment by oophorectomy combined with a low-dose adriamycin, cyclophosphamide, prednisolone (ACP) regime (Parbhoo *et al.*, 1982b). (a) Initial rise in enzyme levels after oophorectomy followed by gradual fall in AP and AST levels. This patient had a visible 12 cm hepatomegaly, which has become impalpable over the 11 month period of therapy. (b) Dramatic response to treatment in enzyme levels correlated with clinical improvement. Patient also showed response in lung and bone deposits. (c) Complete response in liver secondaries as assessed clinically, biochemically, and on CAT scan after 12 cycles of treatment. AP and AST levels began to rise again after 12 months, associated with recurrence of hepatic metastases but with little change in the γGT levels.

to the economic use of scintiscanning. The burden of their message is that isotopic liver scans are unlikely to provide additional useful information either in initial staging or follow-up, in patients in whom the alkaline phosphatase levels are normal.

Most clinicians use a battery of hepatic enzyme tests to assess response to treatment. The usefulness of a combination of alkaline phosphatase, aspartate transaminase, and gamma-glutamyl transferase is shown in Figure 2 (a–c) and explained in the legend. Both primary and secondary tumours of the liver may cause a disproportionate elevation of the plasma alkaline phosphatase compared to the rise in bilirubin, but the reason for this is not entirely clear. In patients with bone and hepatic secondaries, isoenzymes, especially quantitative values of alkaline phosphatase isoenzymes, have proved to be invaluable in assessing a response by metastases at these two sites (Parbhoo *et al.*, 1982a). Since deposits in one organ may respond to treatment while metastases in another site may show no change or progress, prospective studies of serial assays of multiple enzymes are essential.

Ligation of the hepatic artery or angiographic embolization results in transient elevation of the enzyme levels and this may be marked when extensive necrosis occurs in livers virtually replaced by tumour. The gross disturbance in liver enzymology usually returns to normal after 7–10 days following hepatic artery ligation. Large rises in enzyme levels may indicate that infusion therapy either via the portal vein or the hepatic artery should be temporarily stopped.

In contrast to the enzyme tests, serum albumin and the prothrombin ratio/index provide a measure of hepatic synthetic function. The former has a long half-life of approximately 3 weeks while the latter test represents the measurement of a short half-life protein of approximately 6 h. These two estimations therefore provide a good index of the functional capacity of the liver and serve two purposes. First, they indicate the probable tolerance of the liver to cytotoxic therapy and, secondly, their return to normal indicates improvement in hepatic function.

The tumour markers of greatest use in primary hepatocellular carcinoma and metastatic disease are shown in Table 8. High levels of alpha-fetoprotein (AFP) are found in 70% of patients with primary hepatocellular carcinoma. Marked regional differences are apparent, e.g. primary hepatocellular carcinoma in South African and West African blacks and Eastern European patients carries at 90% positivity for AFP, whereas the majority of patients in Britain are negative. If detected, it may be useful for assessment of residual disease after surgery, or during and after chemotherapy. In the presence of shadows on x-rays or defects on scans, serial tumour markers may be a guide as to the institution of further therapy. Residual lesions seen on x-ray or scanning may be due to differentiation of the tumour or, more commonly, to extensive necrosis. AFP is not found in patients with cholangiocarcinoma.

While 80–100% of colorectal cancer patients with liver metastases have raised levels of carcinoembryonic antigen (CEA), its role in management is unclear. This is because CEA is cleared mainly by the liver, and patients with chronic liver disease, obstructive biliary disease, and liver abscess will all have raised levels (Loewenstein and Zamcheck, 1978). Falling CEA levels suggest (but are not diagnostic of) response to therapy while rising levels are incompatible with tumour regression. However, CEA levels do not appear to be related to tumour bulk and *in vitro* observations suggest that raised levels of CEA are related to tumour anoxia and increased doubling time (Ellison *et al.*, 1976; Bronstein *et al.*, 1980).

The urinary level of 5-hydroxyindole acetic acid (5HIAA) in the carcinoid syndrome is a good guide to the activity of metastatic deposits and therefore measures response to treatment, whether by chemotherapy, percutaneous embolization of the hepatic artery, resection or enucleation of the tumour.

Following successful treatment of hepatic carcinoid, the 5HIAA urinary level falls to normal with complete symptomatic relief. Recurrent tumour may be recognized by serial 5HIAA estimations.

Several rare manifestations of primary hepatocellular carcinoma may provide good tumour markers when present. They include hypoglycaemia, hypercalcaemia due to parathormone or parathormone-like hormones, and porphyrin-producing tumours.

Radiology

The plain abdominal radiograph will show elevation and distortion of the diaphragm due to an enlarged liver. Occasionally, calcification may be seen in both primary and secondary tumours of the liver (Khilnani, 1961; Saghatoeslami *et al.*, 1962; Campbell and Greenberg, 1981).

Selective coeliac and superior mesenteric angiography is invaluable in the initial assessment of primary and secondary tumour by allowing precise evaluation of the anatomy of the arterial tree and vascularity of the tumour. Cholangiocarcinoma and metastatic tumours are relatively avascular, but show distortion and displacement of the vascular pattern (Boijsen and Abrams, 1965; Bosniak and Phanthumachinda, 1966).

The advantages of arteriography are that it will show the site of the primary tumour and whether it is multicentric. It will also show the site and size of secondaries, and the degree of vascularity may suggest the possible diagnosis. Against this, one must balance the disadvantages. It is a painful and expensive procedure involving a large radiation dose. Therefore, one cannot repeat arteriography unless a hepatic artery catheter is left *in situ* for serial studies during chemotherapy infusion treatment. Occasionally repeat angiography is carried out to assess the success of embolization of tumours such as carcinoids or when these have produced further symptoms. (Such a follow-up study is shown in Figure 3 (a)–(d).

Hepatic artery ligation or percutaneous selective embolization during arteriography may produce worthwhile palliation in metastatic liver disease, especially in metastatic carcinoid. The pain and tenderness usually disappear and patients show improvement in general well-being for months and sometimes years. For extensive hepatic replacement, repeated embolization can be carried out over several days to reduce the sudden massive volume of necrosis that occurs after total hepatic artery ligation, and so prevents severe toxicity or hepatic failure. For long-term serial studies and hepatic artery infusion therapy, the catheter is best inserted at laparotomy as it is easily displaced from the vessel if inserted by the percutaneous route.

The conventional hyperosmolar contrast media produce vasodilatation and hence pain. Newer contrast media such as meglumine and sodium ioxaglate (Hexabrix 320, May & Baker) have considerably lower osmolality and cause

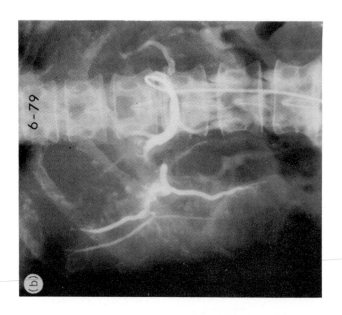

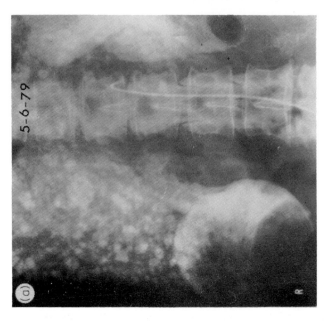

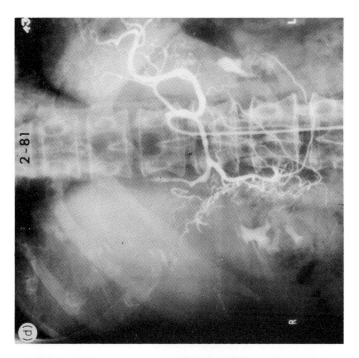

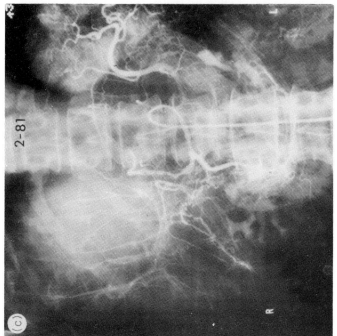

Figure 3 Selective hepatic angiography in a patient with extensive hepatic carcinoid metastases: (a) and (b) before and after embolization of tumour (June 1979); (c) and (d) before and after second embolization for recurrent tumour (February 1981).

markedly less pain. These more physiological contrast media should allow repeated studies to be carried out to assess the progress of tumours following treatment, but the catheter angiographic technique may be replaced by the development of equipment to carry out intravenous angiography.

Scintiscanning

Isotopic liver scanning is relatively simple and relatively non-invasive. It has a high degree of sensitivity in the detection of focal abnormalities greater than 2 cm in size, but a low specificity, since chronic underlying disease such as cirrhosis and abnormal blood flow patterns affect distribution of the isotope. Furthermore, the minimal size of lesions detected deep within the liver is probably of the order of 4 cm.

Most reports on liver metastases indicate that the sensitivity is of the order of 80% but emphasize the non-specificity of the investigation (Leyton *et al.*, 1973). In a *post-mortem* study of patients who had a liver scan within 28 days of death, the accuracy of the scan was 81%, the false positive rate 15%, and the false negative rate 21% (Ostfeld and Meyer, 1981). The predictive value of a positive test in these patients was very high but it may not apply to early cancer. Standardization of the images presented to the observer may help, but it is unlikely that a more critical or standardized assessment of interpreting the scans will improve the accuracy greatly since the basic problem appears to be the variable uptake of the isotope.

The most widely used isotope is ^{99m}Tc sulphur colloid, which is taken up by the Kupffer cells. Any area in the liver where Kupffer cells are absent, such as tumour, cyst, abscess, fatty infiltration or fibrosis or an area devoid of vascularity, will show up as a defect. The region of the porta hepatis often shows decreased activity (Sample *et al.*, 1977) and this abnormal pattern may be due to the vascular anatomy, dilatation of the biliary tree or tumour.

Other isotopes such as rose bengal, selenomethionine and gallium have been used to identify the tumour itself. These isotopes are not widely used and have been superseded by other investigations. Gallium is also avidly taken up by inflammatory lesions such as hepatic or subhepatic abscess.

Ultrasonography or computerized tomography of a defect seen on the scrintiscan may be used to resolve the nature of the scintiscan filling defect and in this respect the investigations are complementary. The use of both scintiscan and ultrasound examination increases the diagnostic accuracy to over 95%. In our hands, serial scintiscans of the liver with technetium-99 sulphur colloid in patients with metastatic breast cancer have been less rewarding than ultrasound examination, especially in early diagnosis of metastases and in assessing response to treatment at a late stage. Once focal deposits are clearly seen, scintiscan is a simple technique of follow-up to assess the size of the lesions (Parbhoo *et al.*, 1982c) but it will not indicate the degree of necrosis in a tumour which is responding without changing much in size.

Refinements in the technique of scintigraphy, such as emission tomography, have been reported (Granowska and Britton, 1981). To overcome the problems of isotope uptake surrounding the defect to be examined, transverse sections through areas that are equivocal on the standard liver scan are compared quantitatively with a normal area. Conventional radiopharmaceuticals available to any medical physics department can be used (single photon emission tomography). Positron emission tomography using a radionucleide with a short half-life, (< 25 min) will allow greater definition but has the disadvantage that it requires a cyclotron locally as well as a team to operate it in close proximity to the clinical scanning room. Emission tomography will detect lesions either seen as equivocal areas or missed on conventional scans but it remains to be seen whether it will prove useful in the detection and follow-up of diffuse infiltrating lesions.

Ultrasound examination

The rapid technical advances in ultrasound equipment have improved both the definition and contrast of the pictures as well as the recording and storage of the data. Some of the current limitations of naked-eye examination (subject to observer bias) may be eliminated in the future by computer analysis of the ultrasonic signals (Barnett and Morely, 1980). Ultrasound examination is a non-invasive, relatively cheap, repeatable technique, and is now available in most general hospitals.

The major drawback of ultrasound examination is that it is highly dependent upon the skill and expertise of the individual operator. In experienced hands it is probably the best method currently available for the detection and follow-up of hepatic metastases, but it is virtually useless in unskilled hands. Good assessment of the parenchyma as well as the vasculature, vena cava, portal vein, and surrounding structures is obtained. One also obtains information on the density of the mass, and one can use ultrasound for guiding a needle to obtain specimens using either the conventional B scanner or a specifically designed aspiration biopsy transducer probe.

Factors which affect echo formation in adjacent soft tissues with varying acoustic impedance are not well understood, but are thought to be due mainly to tissue density. The velocity of sound in soft tissue also varies and appears to be influenced by collagen content. The latter is thought to be the main source of internal echoes on grey-scale ultrasound scans (Fields and Dunn, 1973; Calderon *et al.*, 1976). Factors which limit the usefulness of ultrasound examination are marked obesity, bowel gas, and difficulty in visualizing structures under the rib cage.

Sonography has become the investigation of choice in the initial management of the jaundiced patient suspected of having bile duct obstruction and, if dilated ducts are seen, they can be further examined by percutaneous cholegraphy or retrograde endoscopic cannulation of the common duct.

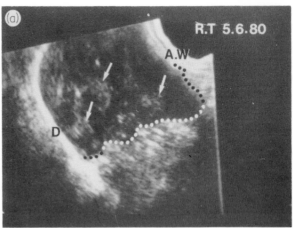

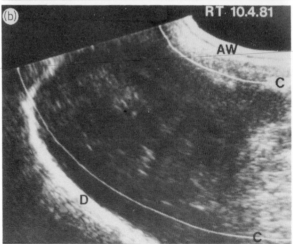

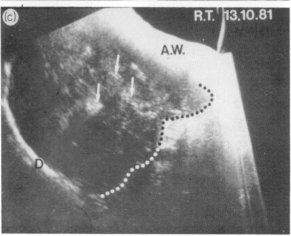

Simple enlargements, or distortions such as Riedel's lobe, are easily excluded on ultrasound examination. If a malignant deposit is discrete but exhibits little difference in echo characteristics from the adjacent tissue it will be missed, but the technique will detect liver metastases greater than 1 cm with reasonable accuracy depending on the number of deposits and the ultrasound features.

Reports claim a 90% accuracy in the detection of liver deposits greater than 1 cm (Taylor and Grade, 1980; Smith *et al.*, 1976). The liver deposits may be echo-dense, contain low-level echoes or present a target appearance with an echo-dense zone surrounded by a ring of low-level echoes (Barnett and Morely, 1980). Less commonly, the lesion may present a cystic appearance due to necrosis. Gravity layering of necrotic material within a secondary deposit has also been recorded (Baker and Morin, 1977). A number of authors have suggested that the sonographic appearances of metastatic disease depends on the type of tumour. Dense lesions have been found especially with adenocarcinoma arising from the colon (Scheible *et al.*, 1977). Similarly Cosgrove and McCready (1978) have indicated that in some cases it may be possible to suggest the tissue of origin of the deposits, as they noted that approximately one-third of gastrointestinal and urogenital metastases were brightly reflecting, whereas other carcinomas and all sarcomas and lymphomas were always poorly reflecting. In contrast, Green *et al.* (1977) reported less correlation between the sonographic patterns of metastases and the primary tissue of origin or histologic type of neoplasm. Tumours of the same primary origin or those with a very similar histologic pattern often had different ultrasonic appearances.

In general, adenocarcinomas of the colon tend to produce more dense echo-reflecting secondaries and are therefore easier to assess on follow-up than are other tumours such as metastatic breast cancer. Diffuse infiltration of the liver without discernible discrete deposits (as in lymphoma or miliary metastases) is difficult to evaluate on sonography. Ultrasound examination is of special value in resolving abnormalities seen in the porta hepatis on the scintiscan, since it has a greater specificity in evaluating the *nature* of the lesion found on scintiscanning.

Responding tumour masses may show necrosis, a decrease in size or change in echo reflectivity. Initial reports suggested that, if the deposits were

---

Figure 4 Serial ultrasound examination in a 76-year-old patient with liver metastases and ascites from breast cancer, treated with a low-dose adriamycin, cyclophosphamide, prednisolone regime. (a) Irregular liver with multiple focal metastases. (b) Diffusely mottled liver with no focal lesions, but liver is enlarged and irregular. Cursors for measurement (C) are shown. (c) Irregular liver with bright areas (? healed areas following necrosis). The dark areas posterior to the bright areas are due to a combination of signal weakness (loss of acoustic penetration) and reflection of signal by dense tissue (? scarring). Key: Dotted line indicates edge of liver; AW=abdominal wall; D=diaphragm; K=kidney; bd=bile duct; P.ef= pleural effusion.

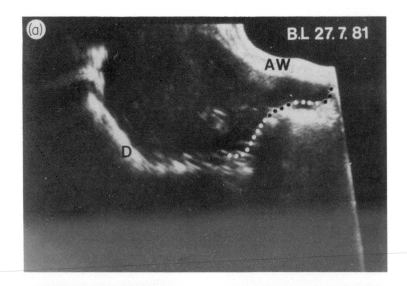

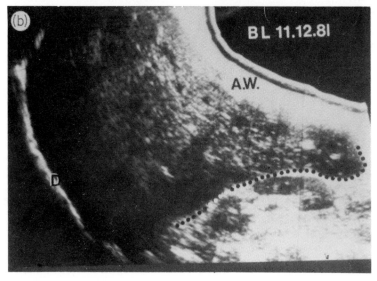

Figure 5 Same patient as in Figure 2 (a); serial ultrasound examination of liver. (a) Patient presented with visible liver enlargement, and the protrusion of the abdominal mass is clearly seen. (b) After oophorectomy and ACP regime, abdominal mass has receded and sonograph shows bright areas in anterior portion of the liver while the posterior part of the liver is thrown into darkness as in Figure 4(c).

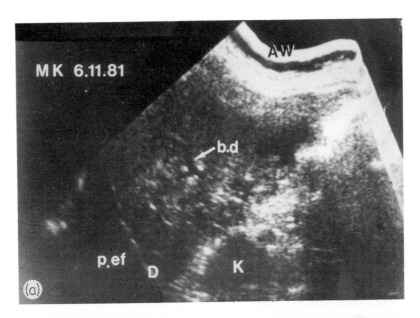

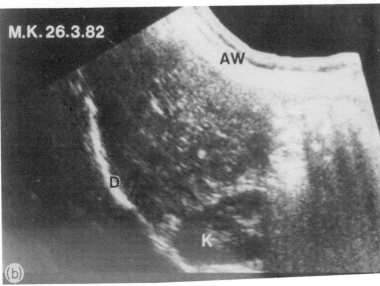

Figure 6 Same patient as Figure 2(b); Serial ultrasound examination of liver. (a) Irregular enlarged liver with metastases and dilated bile duct (bd). Note pleural effusion (p.ef). (b) Improvement at 4 months after beginning therapy. Pleural effusion and dilated ducts no longer seen.

responding, a tumour mass becomes smaller and brighter but, to date, few long-term serial studies have been carried out. Our own experience with examination at three-monthly intervals in patients with hepatic metastases from breast cancer has revealed a variety of patterns. The change may be subtle, especially in the diffusely infiltrated liver (Hinton and Parbhoo, 1982), and metastases in different parts of the liver respond differently and seldom show necrosis, although this is easily recognized (Figures 4–6). Replacement of diffuse infiltration of the liver following a complete response leaves a relatively normal liver, whereas a response in a liver grossly distorted by large metastases will result in a deformed liver although metastases are no longer seen.

Sonography will rapidly assess dilatation of ducts in patients who have been treated for major bile duct cancer, and may also reveal segmental obstruction at follow-up in patients where extension of the tumour has occurred, causing elevation of the alkaline phosphatase but no jaundice. Use of electronic calipers or cursors (Figure 4(b)) on the ultrasound picture provides a means of easy measurement of response or progression of focal lesions.

Computerized axial tomography

In expert hands and with proper selection of patients, there is no doubt that this is probably the best method of assessing secondary deposits once the liver function tests become abnormal. Most workers agree that the accuracy is less dependent on the expertise of the observer than with ultrasound examination. The problem of lack of contrast between the structure to be examined and the normal tissue, causing non-visualization of the lesion, has been partly overcome by contrast enhancement for low-attenuation areas in the liver. Using this technique, lesions down to 0.5 cm in diameter have been detected. In early or diffuse infiltrative metastatic disease, CAT scans have only a minor role in documenting and assessing response, e.g. lymphoma involving the liver (Best and Blackledge, 1980). Thus, in expert hands ultrasound examination yields similar quality information to that from CAT scans, but like CAT scans, ultrasound examination is poor in assessing diffuse disease.

In the jaundiced patient the combination of sonography followed by percutaneous transhepatic cholegraphy in a patient with dilated ducts is as accurate as CAT scans, cheaper and yields much more useful information for the surgeon prior to operation. CAT scans will however provide highly accurate visualization of the abnormal biliary tree in patients with intra-hepatic duct carcinoma who have had surgery or radiotherapy, without recourse to invasive techniques when these patients develop recurrent jaundice.

Histology and cytology

Needle biopsy is the commonest method of establishing a tissue diagnosis in primary hepatocellular cancer but is less frequently used in the assessment of metastatic hepatic disease. Blind percutaneous biopsy has a false negative rate which approaches 50% in malignant disease (Conn, 1972). The ability to select the site accurately by reference to hepatic scans, through an ultrasound probe or during laparoscopy, should increase the practice of liver biopsy so that treatment and assessment of response may be based on a histological diagnosis of metastatic cancer. Multiple defects seen by the scintiscan or ultrasound examination, as well as nodules seen at laparoscopy, may be misleading.

Where cytological expertise is available, it is suggested that fine-needle aspiration cytology be carried out with ultrasound control in serial studies. There are so far no reports on the use of serial biopsies in patients undergoing long-term treatment for hepatic metastases. Biopsy techniques are contra-indicated in highly anaplastic tumours such as hepatoblastoma, in patients with hepatic outflow obstruction or congestion, and those with biliary obstruction in whom surgical intervention is not intended.

Laparoscopy

The wider use of laparoscopy has allowed confirmation of the findings seen on ultrasound examination or scintiscans when these have been equivocal. Tumour deposits varying from a few seedlings under the capsule to large nodules may be seen. The large ones may show umbilication as a result of tumour necrosis or cicatricial contraction. Nodules from a pigmented melanoma are easily recognized.

In those patients with malignant disease associated with chronic liver disease such as cirrhosis, laparoscopy may be the only way of assessing the liver status and taking guided biopsies other than at laparotomy. Laparoscopy will probably play an increasing role in the selection of patients for treatment of liver metastases when the diagnosis of liver involvement is equivocal. At the same time one can assess extrahepatic spread, biopsy peritoneal seedlings, and aspirate peritoneal fluid for cytology.

INTRACRANIAL NEOPLASMS

In assessing response to treatment in intracranial neoplasms, clinical evalua-tion is often difficult as the sensorium may be affected by tumour, effects of drugs, raised intracranial pressure or cerebral oedema. If the primary tumour is operable it is usually removed and few follow-up studies are carried out to evaluate change. The management of brain metastases and inoperable primary tumours is usually palliative. If submitted to radiotherapy or chemotherapy, the assessment of response is usually based on symptoms and signs. Survival periods even with treatment are short, improvement in neurological function is limited, and little effort is made to carry out further investigations.

The recently improved management of advanced malignant disease, and particularly of its metastases in bone and liver, has led to prolongation of survival. Since most of the drugs used in cytotoxic chemotherapy do not cross the blood–brain barrier in sufficient concentration, the central nervous system is an unprotected reservoir for metastatic seeding. CNS metastases are likely to become an increasingly important therapeutic problem as a result of the improved management of cancer. Greater efforts are now being made to provide some degree of protection to the brain during and after adjuvant or intensive cancer chemotherapy for certain tumours.

There has been almost no effort made to evaluate critically the response of intracranial neoplasms to different treatment modalities such as chemotherapy, radiation, surgery or a combination of these. Patients in controlled trials will obviously require some form of objective measurement and those currently available need to be evaluated.

Clinical assessment

One needs to be as objective as possible in assessing general performance status (Karnofsky–Burchenal index) as well as specific mental functions, because 50% of patients with metastases in the brain do not show clinical signs capable of measurement. The major symptoms which can be assessed are, first, those of raised intracranial pressure (headache, vomiting, papilloedema, and occasionally hydrocephalus) and, secondly, the function based on the site of the tumour itself and its resultant compression of the surrounding brain which may impair cognitive function and cause hemiparesis, the two most important symptoms.

Recovery of function following extirpation of the tumour may be incomplete due to permanent damage caused by the tumour. In these patients the response will be measured in terms of further deterioration and survival. In the majority of patients who have received radiotherapy for metastatic disease in the brain, any improvement seen is short-lived, the mean survival time being 6.5 months (Bloom, 1979). The presence of extensive disease elsewhere will affect the assessment of response and often make it impossible to determine whether treatment to the cerebral metastases has made any difference at all to survival.

Scintiscanning

Since most neurosurgical centres in the western world now have CAT scan facilities, the usefulness of brain scintiscans has been questioned. Standard scintiscans offer only a 75% accuracy in identifying cerebral metastatic lesions (Brooks, 1974) but, although CAT scans may have replaced isotope scans in tumour diagnosis, the latter may be used more often in the future for assessing reponse. The technique of emission tomographic imaging increases the accuracy, sensitivity, and specificity compared with standard isotope scans (Ell, 1980).

Computerized tomography

This technique has been established as the most valuable single diagnostic tool for the investigation of intracranial tumours. It is much more sensitive and specific than the scintiscan, with the ability to detect lesions 6–10 mm in diameter and therefore excellent for the detection of multiple metastases (Black, 1979a). Additional advantages of this technique are that it will show the ventricular system and extent of oedema around the tumour.

Positive identification of metastases may not always be possible, as the scan configuration and enhancement with intravenous dyes are not specific for tumours. Some 40% of small cerebral metastases are missed by the CAT scan. The major problems of evaluating lesions even with enhancement by contrast media, are the vascularity of the tumour and the surrounding stroma, cerebral oedema, brain displacement, obstructive hydrocephalus, and destruction or sclerosis of the overlying skull.

Few follow-up CAT scan studies are available but the difficulties in interpretation noted in diagnosis will probably be magnified following treatment with radiotherapy or chemotherapy. Occasional studies after radiotherapy are available to assess response as shown in Figure 7 (a)–(c).

Tumour markers

In contrast to the excellent physical techniques now available to assess the intracranial tumour mass, no good technique is available to assess its biological activity and cell population. The measurement of tumour markers in the cerebrospinal fluid (CSF) may offer a method of assessing response to treatment serially but the dangers of obtaining CSF (in terms of the serious complication of brain herniation and meningitis) cannot be overemphasized. A large number of tumour markers have been studied in CSF (Kaye and Bagshawe, 1979) but the only marker of clinical value is the CSF human chorionic gonadotrophin in gestational choriocarcinoma.

(a)

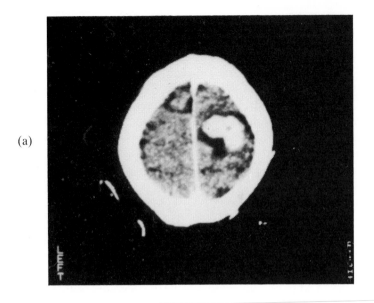

(b)

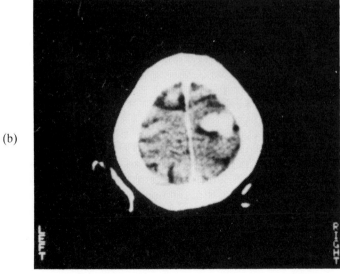

(c)

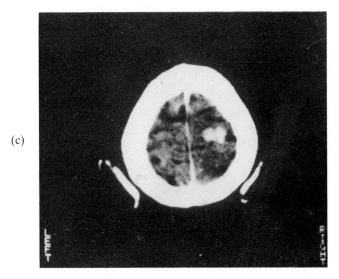

Figure 7 Inoperable cerebral tumour treated with radiotherapy. Serial CAT scans show response of tumour. After 5 weeks there is marked reduction in oedema around tumour and 5 weeks later there is marked reduction in tumour size. By courtesy of Dr A. Valentine.

SPINAL CORD NEOPLASMS

As with cerebral metastases, recent advances in the treatment of cancer may lead to a higher proportion of patients developing spinal cord compression due to tumour, because of the high incidence of bone metastases in the vertebral column. The mechanism of cord dysfunction may involve direct compression of the spinal cord by epidural tumour or tumour within the cord itself, ischaemic dysfunction due to interruption of blood supply by tumour, vasculitis following radiotherapy, or vertebral collapse.

In some patients, several of these mechanisms may co-exist and it may be difficult to disentangle the various changes which have occurred in the spine and cord due to the tumour, decompressive surgery, radiotherapy, and invasive radiology. Residual oily contrast media may themselves cause arachnoiditis and contribute to the patient's symptoms.

Clinical assessment

Ambulation is the best criterion of response to treatment for paraplegia or paraparesis. Although receovery from paraplegia due to spinal cord compression is uncommon, Livingston and Perrin (1978) report that a series of 20 patients, five were ambulant and continent of urine 6 months following surgery. Apart from the degree of ambulation, evaluation of bladder function and anal sphincteric tone is an essential part of the clinical assessment of response.

The response may be graded as follows: (a) complete — patient fully ambulant with no neurological abnormalities; (b) good partial response — patient walking with residual neurological signs; (c) poor partial response — considerable residual disability with minor relief of symptoms or signs; (d) no response — failed therapy with no objective improvement in either signs or symptoms. In each of these grades, detailed criteria would require to be laid down so that minor changes woud be properly evaluated. Black (1979b) has summarized the results of treatment for spinal cord or cauda equina compression by metastatic tumour in the literature. He found that improvement occurs in 51% following surgical decompression plus radiotherapy, compared to 30% with decompression alone and 46% with radiotherapy alone.

Special investigations

There is little detailed information on the follow-up assessment of spinal cord compression by special investigations. Radiological tomography will show osteolytic and sclerotic areas as well as the extent of collapse of the vertebral column. Microfocal radiology will help define the bone lesion more clearly. Good definition of the vertebrae is obtained on CAT scans but residual myelographic material may interfere with the interpretation. The use of new non-irritating myelographic opaque media should help in repeat examinations in those patients with recurrent symptoms.

Isotopic bone scans are helpful in that they show areas of greatest activity, and examination of serial scans with quantitation will be helpful in difficult cases (Parbhoo *et al.*, 1980). This is of particular use in patients where x-ray changes are still extensive, but isotopic bone scan shows that the disease is only locally active in one or two vertebrae. Both surgery and radiotherapy will clearly alter local isotopic uptake, and this has to be borne in mind when assessment is made of quantitative studies of isotopic uptake.

BEST USE OF CURRENT INVESTIGATIONS IN EVALUATING RESPONSE

(1) The clinician has to match the frequency of the plethora of tests available to their usefulness in management, to patient comfort and compliance, and to their cost-effectiveness. Well designed trials, especially controlled ones,

dictate the use of objective criteria, even though many are poorly understood and non-specific. Better and more stringent criteria of assessment require to be applied both in trials and in our day-to-day management of patients.

(2) It is important to discuss the clinical problems with the radiological or medical physics team and decide as to which test would be the most suitable in a particular situation. Similarly, every effort should be made to standardize methods of evaluation when trials are being carried out in national or international studies with external assessors. To obtain the maximum benefit from specialized tests, one should provide the service departments not only with adequate clinical information but also with subsequent feedback as to the usefulness of the tests carried out.

(3) Whenever regular monitoring is to be carried out, a *planned* programme of serial investigation for the particular type and site of tumour should apply to routine work as well as to clinical trials. Enthusiastic individuals in the various service departments should collaborate with clinicians to provide an efficient, cohesive, cost-effective service.

(4) The following schedule of tests is recommended for monitoring reponse.

Lungs

Once lesions are seen on plain x-rays, simple radiology is adequate at three-monthly intervals unless complications such as infection intervene. Investigations will include PA and lateral chest views, tomography of single lesions, and oblique views of the hilar area.

Liver

The following 'liver function' tests need to be carried out at monthly intervals: plasma alkaline phosphate, plasma γ-glutamyl transferase, plasma aspartate transaminase, serum albumin, plasma bilirubin, and prothrombin index/ratio.

Ultrasound examination of the liver, biliary tree, and costophrenic angles should be done at three-monthly intervals. Clearly, these tests have to be repeated earlier if there is no response to therapy and treatment has to be altered.

Central nervous system

In the absence of critical published reports, no clear guidelines as to assessment of response can be suggested at this stage. They will have to await the outcome of studies critically correlating clinical improvement with information obtained from CAT scans and other objective evidence of response. The pooling of data from multiple centres is essential in the development of a databank, especially in the uncommon types of tumour.

FUTURE DEVELOPMENTS IN EVALUATION OF RESPONSE

(1) Computerization is certain to be used to analyse data from angiograms, scintiscans, and ultrasound examination. Although the cost is still high, this will be compensated for by the reduction in the total number of investigations and the decrease in invasive procedures.

(2) Computerization of the data from ultrasound examination should remove some of the subjective errors inherent in its interpretation, and should be particularly valuable in assessing response in follow-up examination. Rapid access to data of the patient's previous ultrasound examination will allow the operator to carry out a similar probing, and will lead to a greater standardization in the individual patient's pictures.

(3) Availability and wider application of electronic manipulation of isotopic scan data (as in emission tomography) will allow greater definition of lesions hitherto not seen on the standard scan.

(4) Isotopes which are excreted by the hepatic cells into biliary tree (such as ^{99}mTc HIDA) are used in the diagnosis of biliary tract disease. They have recently been applied to the detection and assessment of intrahepatic lesions (Schulze *et al.*, 1981) and the pictures seen with this technique appear to be superior to the standard gamma camera pictures of Tc sulphur colloid scans.

(5) The development of intravenous angiography using small doses of radio-opaque medium will allow repeated examinations without catheterization.

(6) Nuclear magnetic resonance (NMR) is now being assessed in the detection of clinical disease (Koeze, 1982) and the images produced by NMR are already being compared with CAT scans in many research centres. In addition to providing better definition, NMR has the advantage that there is no danger from ionizing radiation. Furthermore, the NMR machine is able to produce projections or slices in any plane, simply by orientating the magnetic field gradient into the desired plane.

(7) Nuclear magnetic resonance can also be used to scan the metabolism of specific elements such as phosphorus. This may well give us some insight into the biological behaviour of tumours before, during, and after treatment.

(8) Advances will be made in the quantitation of isoenzymes which are specific for the tumour stroma and for the type of cells surrounding the lesion.

There is a need to develop better methods of assessing hepatic function as opposed to hepatocellular damage, and to separate the toxic effect of chemotherapy on normal liver cells from damage to the tumour cells.

(9) The development of specific tumour markers by the use of monoclonal antibodies will allow for greater precision in the serial evaluation of specific tumours.

Notwithstanding all the major developments in electronic gadgetry and sophisticated micro-biochemistry, there will continue to be a need for critical clinical assessment of the patient using the feedback from detailed clinical, biochemical, and physical investigations. The quality of life and patient well-being must always remain our paramount objective during the evaluation of response to treatment for cancer.

Acknowledgments

I thank my colleagues (Les Berger, David Bernstein, Robert Dick, Chandra Grubb, Sidney Rosalki, Basil Stoll, and Alan Valentine) in various disciplines for helpful discussions during the preparation of this review and the loan of illustrative material. I thank my secretary Denise Young for the preparation of the manuscript and Julie Phipps and Mollie Graneek for the artwork.

REFERENCES

Bajetta, E., Buzzoni, R., Giardini, R., and Bonnadonna, G. (1981). Liver assessment in women receiving adjuvant CMF chemotherapy. *Tumori*, **67**, 27–30.

Baker, D.A., and Morin, M.E. (1977). Gravity dependent layering in necrotic metastatic carcinoma to the liver. *J. Clin. Ultrasound*, **5**, 282–283.

Barnett, E., and Morely, P. (1980). Ultrasound in cancer assessment. In *Cancer: assessment and monitoring* (eds T. Symington, A.E. Williams, and J.G. McVie. Edinburgh: Churchill–Livingstone. p.p. 221–239.

Berg, J.W., and Robbins, G.F. (1962). A late look at the safety of aspiration biopsy. *Cancer*, **15**, 826–827.

Best, J.J.K., and Blackledge, G. (1980). The use of computed tomography of the abdomen in the initial assessment and monitoring of patients with lymphoma. In *Cancer: assessment and monitoring* (eds T. Symington, A.E. Williams, and J.G. McVie). Edinburgh: Churchill–Livingstone. pp. 188–203.

Black, P. (1979a). Metastatic tumours of the central nervous system: cerebral metastases. In *Complications of Cancer* (ed. M.D. Abeloff). Baltimore: Johns Hopkins University Press. Chap. 12, pp. 283–312.

Black, P. (1979b). Metastatic tumours of the central nervous system: spinal metastases. In *Complications of cancer* (ed. M.D. Abeloff). Baltimore: Johns Hopkins University Press. Chap. 13, pp313–356.

Bloom, H.J.G. (1979). Intracranial secondary carcinomas and disseminating gliomas: treatment and prognosis. In *CNS complications of malignant disease* (eds J.M.A. Whitehouse, and H.E.M. Kay). London: Macmillan. pp. 306–323.

Boijsen, E., and Abrams, S.H.L. (1965). Roentgenologic diagnosis of primary carcinoma of the liver. *Acta Radiol. (Diag.)*, **3**, 257–277.

Bosniak, M.A., and Phanthumachinda, P. (1966). Value of arteriography in the study of hepatic disease. *Am. J. Surg.*, **112**, 348–355.

Bronstein, B.R., Steele, Jr, G.D., Ensminger, W., Kaplan, W.D. Lowenstein, M.S., Wilson, R.E. Forman, J., and Zamcheck, N. (1980). The use and limitations of serial plasma carcinoembryonic antigen (CEA) levels as a monitor of changing metastatic liver tumour volume in patients receiving chemotherapy. *Cancer*, **46**, 266–272.

Brooks, W. (1974). Clinical limitations of brain scanning in metastatic disease. *J. Nucl. Biol. Med.*, **15**, 620–621.

Calderon, C., Vilkomerson, D., and Mezrich, R. (1976). Differences in attentuation of ultrasound by normal, benign and malignant breast tissue. *J. Clin. Ultrasound*, **4**, 249–254.

Campbell, G.D., and Greenberg, S.D. (1981). Pleural mesothelioma with calcified liver metastases. *Chest*, **79**, 229–230.

Colsky, J., Greenspan, E.M., and Warren, T.N. (1955). Hepatic fibrosis in children with acute leukaemia treated with folic acid antagonists. *Arch. Pathol.*, **59**, 198–206.

Conn, H. (1972). Rational use of liver biopsy in the diagnosis of hepatic cancer. *Gastroenterology*, **62**, 142–146.

Cosgrove, D.0., and McCready, V.R. (1978). Diagnosis of liver metastases using ultrasound and isotope scanning techniques. *J. R. Soc. Med.*, **71**, 652–657.

Davis, S., Gardner, F., and Qvist, G. (1963). The shape of a pleural effusion. *Br. Med. J.*, **1**, 436–437.

Ell, P.J. (1980). Emission tomography. In *Cancer: assessment and monitoring*, (eds T. Symington, A.E. Williams, and J.G. McVie. Edinburgh: Churchill–Livingstone. pp. 291–306.

Ellison, M.L., Lamb, D., Rivett, J., and Neville, A.M. (1976). Quantitative aspects of CEA output by a human lung carcinoma cell line. *J. Nat Cancer Inst.*, **59**, 309–312.

Fields, S., and Dunn, F. (1973). Correlation of echographic visualizability of tissues with biological composition and physiological state. *J. Acoust. Soc. Am.*, **54**, 809–812.

Granowska, M., and Britton, K. (1981). Annual review : nuclear medicine. *Hosp. Update*, **7**, 1239–1250.

Green, B., Bree, R.L., Goldstein, H.M., and Stanley, C. (1977). Gray scale ultrasound evaluation of hepatic neoplasms: patterns and correlations. *Radiology*, **124**, 203–208.

Hayward, J.L., Carbone, P.P., Heuson, J.C., Kumaoka, S., Seagaloff, A., and Rubens, R.D. (1977). Assessment of response to therapy in advanced breast cancer. *Cancer*, **39**, 1289–1294.

Hayward, J.L. (1980). Cancer assessment and monitoring. In *Cancer : assessment and monitoring* (eds T. Symington, A.E. Williams, and J.G. McVie). Edinburgh: Churchill–Livingstone. pp. 34–39.

Higashi, T., Wakao, H., Nakamura, K., Shimura, A., Yokohama, T., Suzuki, S., Watanabe, K., and Kruglik, G.D. (1980). Quantitative gallium 67 scanning for predictive value in primary lung carcinoma. *J. Nucl. Med.*, **21**, 628–632.

Hinton, J., and Parbhoo, S.P. (1982). unpublished data.

Husband, J. (1980). Computed tomography. In *Oncology supplement: Scientific foundations of oncology* (eds T. Symington, and R.L. Carter). London: Heinemann. pp. 131-142.

Karnofsky, D.A., and Burchenal, H.J. (1948). Evaluation of chemotherapeutic agents. In *Evaluation of chemotherapeutic agents* (ed. C.M. MacLeod). New York: Columbia University Press. pp. 191–205.

Kaye, S.B., and Bagshawe, K.D. (1979). Chemical markers in spinal fluid for tumours of the central nervous system. In *CNS complications of malignant disease* (eds J.M.A. Whitehouse, and H.E.M. Kay). London: Macmillan. pp. 306–323.

Khilnani, M.T. (1961). Calcified liver metastases from carcinoma of the colon. *Am. J. Dig. Dis.*, **6**, 229–232.

Koeze, T.H. (1982). Applications of nuclear magnetic resonance in medicine. *Br. J. Hosp. Med.*, **27**, 402–407.

Leyton, R.A., Halpern, S., and Leopold, G. (1973). Correlation of ultrasound and colloid scintiscan studies of the normal and diseased liver. *J. Nucl. Med.*, **14**, 27–33.

Livingston, K.E., and Perrin, R.G. (1978). The neurosurgical management of spinal metastases causing cord and cauda equina compression. *J. Neurosurg.*, **49**, 839–843.

Loewenstein, M.S., and Zamcheck, N. (1978). Carcinoembryonic antigen (CEA) levels in benign gastrointestinal disease. *Cancer*, **42**, 1412–1418.

Menard, D.B., Gisselbrecht, C., Marty, M., Reyes, F., and Dhumeaux, D. (1980). Antineoplastic agents and the liver. *Gastroenterology*, **78**, 142–164.

Muhm, J.R. (1980). Role of computed tomography in evaluation of intrathoracic lesions. *J. Thorac. Cardiovasc. Surg.*, **79**, 469–470.

Ostfeld, D.A., and Meyer, J.E. (1981). Liver scanning in cancer patients with short interval autopsy correlation. *Radiology*, **138**, 671–673.

Parbhoo, S.P. (1981). Heterogeneity in human mammary cancer. In *Systemic control of breast cancer*, vol.4, *New aspects of breast cancer* (ed. B.A. Stoll). London: William Heinemann. pp. 55–77.

Parbhoo, S.P., Alani, H., Agnew, J.E., and Stoll, B.A. (1980). Serial quantitative skeletal scintigraphy in breast cancer. In *Metastases—clinical and experimental aspects* (eds K. Hellman, P. Hilgard, and S. Eccles). The Hague: Martinus Nijhoff. pp. 326–330.

Parbhoo, S.P., Rosalki, S., Wahba, A., Stoll, B.A., Hinton, J., Alani, H., Jacob, G., and Graneek, M. (1982a). Value of quantitative alkaline phosphatase isoenzymes in assessing response in patients with bone and hepatic metastases from breast cancer. (in preparation).

Parbhoo, S.P., Stoll, B.A. Hinton, J., Wahba, A., Walker, A., and Bell, A. (1982b). An effective low dose adriamycin, cyclophosphamide, prednisolone combination for hepatic metastases in breast cancer?. *Proc. 1st Nat. Congr. on Senology*, Athens, 4–7 April 1982.

Parbhoo, S.P., Woods, J., Hinton, J., Stoll, B.A., and Wahba, A. (1982c). Role of serial technetium 99m sulphur colloid scans in patients with liver metastases from breast cancer receiving chemotherapy. (In preparation).

Podurgiel, B.J., McGill, D.B., Ludwig, J., Taylor, W.F., and Muller, S.A. (1973). Liver injury associated with methotrexate therapy for psoriasis. *Mayo Clinic Proc.*, **48**, 787–792.

Riordan, J.F. (1979). Chronic lung diseases. Carcinoma of the bronchus. *Br. J. Hosp. Med.*, **22**, 120–127.

Robbins, G.F., Brothers, III, H.J., Eberhart, W.F., and Quan, S. (1954). Is aspiration biopsy of breast cancer dangerous to the patient? *Cancer*, **7**, 774–778.

Saghatoeslami, M., Khodarami, K., and Epstein, B.S. (1962). Calcified intrahepatic metastases from carcinoma of the breast. *J. Am. Med. Assoc.*, **181**, 1139–1140.

Sample, W.F., Gray, R.K., Poe, N.D., Graham, L.S., and Bennett, L.R. (1977).

Nuclear staging, tomographic nuclear imaging and gray scale ultrasound in the evaluation of the porta hepatis. *Radiology*, **122**, 773–779.

Scheible, W., Gosink, B.B., and Leopold, G.R. (1977). Gray scale echographic patterns of hepatic metastatic disease. *Am. J. Roentgenol.*, **129**, 983–987.

Schulze, P.J., Stritzke, P., and Stolzenbach, G. (1981). Liver imaging and detection of liver metastases with 99m Tc–HIDA. *Nuklearmedizin*, **20**, 214–219.

Smith, I.E., Taylor, K.J., McCready, V.R. Powles T.J., and Bondy P.K. (1976). A comparison of grey-scale ultrasound with other methods for the detection of liver metastases from breast carcinoma. *Clin. Oncol.*, **2**, 47–53.

Taylor, K.J.W., and Grade, M. (1980). Abdominal ultrasound for general surgeons. *Recent advances in surgery* no. 10 (ed. S. Taylor). Edinburgh: Churchill–Livingstone. pp. 135–159.

Vincent, R.G., Chu, T.M., and Lane, W.W. (1979). The value of carcinoembryonic antigen in patients with carcinoma of lung. *Cancer*, **44**, 685–691.

Watson, J.V. (1981). What does 'response' in cancer chemotherapy really mean? *Br. Med. J.*, **283**, 34–37.

White, D.R., Maloney, J.J., Muss, H.B., Vance, R.P. Barnes, P., Howard, V., Rhyne, L., and Cowan, R.J. (1979). Serum alkaline phosphatase determination. Value in the staging of advanced breast cancer. *J. Am. Med. Assoc.*, **242**, 1147–1149.

Wiener, S.N., and Sachs, S.H. (1978). An assessment of routine liver scanning in patients with breast cancer. *Arch. Surg.*, **113**, 126–127.

Willis, R.A. (1973). *The spread of tumours in the human body*, 3rd ed. London: Butterworths.

Winchester, D.P., Sener, S.F., Khandekar, J.D., Oviedo, M.A., Cunningham, M.P., Caprini, J.A., Burkett, F.E., and Scanlon, E.F. (1978). Symptomatology as indicator of recurrent or metastatic breast cancer. *Cancer*, **43**, 956–960.

Chapter

6 BASIL A. STOLL

Quality of Life as an Objective in Cancer Treatment

INTRODUCTION

The best interests of the cancer patient are not always served by aggressive investigation and treatment. Yet, particularly in the USA, these procedures are often continued almost until the terminal stage, mainly 'to show the patient that a positive attempt is being made to retard the progress of the disease' (Stehlin and Beach, 1966). This attitude has been stimulated especially by increased 'awareness' among cancer patients and their families, and by the proliferation of new treatment agents which tend to raise unrealistic hopes both among physicians and their patients.

In conflict with this trend is the physician's humanistic training that treatment at any price is not justifiable. One may be forced to compromise the cancer patient's quality of life for a high likelihood of prolonging survival but, as stressed in preceding chapters, this cannot be justified for conjectural or minimal gain in survival (see Chapter 2). Pressure by relatives for active treatment is often maintained right up to the bitter end, but only the physician can have the knowledge to balance profit and loss on behalf of the patient.

In such a decision, the patient himself should be given an informed choice wherever possible; his decision may well differ from that of the family. It will obviously depend on his age, and his attitude to risk-taking and to the side-effects and stress which usually result from active treatment (Palmer et al., 1980). In advanced disease, the patient should rarely be confronted for a decision (Schnaper, 1982), but instead, the patient's wishes can often be deduced by compassionate listening rather than by scientific discussion. To make such difficult judgments obviously needs meaningful communication between physician and patient.

Patients develop a wide variety of emotional reactions to having cancer — usually anxiety and depression, but sometimes denial or anger (Derogatis *et al.*, 1979; Leigh *et al.*, 1980). Cancer patients stress that their peace of mind depends a great deal on the confidence and understanding that they build up with the physician directing their management (Fiore, 1979; Cousins, 1979). While confidence in some patients can be inspired by a confident appearance and reassuring noises from the physician, other patients need to discuss their anxieties. Therefore, to provide support for each patient as an individual must involve the physician in getting to know him. Anticipating the patient's emotional reactions is the art of medicine as contrasted with the science of medicine (Reisner, 1980).

On the basis of these principles, the topic of this chapter will be discussed under the following headings:

How patients cope with cancer.
Quality of life — balancing profit and loss.
Incurable cancer — management stage by stage.
Communicating with the patient.
Doctors are only human.

HOW PATIENTS COPE WITH CANCER

In the patient with an apparently curable cancer, the quality of life after treatment will depend on his ability to cope emotionally both with the implied threat to life and also with the physical problems associated with the disease and its treatment. Every patient requires reassurance and explanations from all members of the medical team at this stage. Subsequently, the patient's mental reaction will depend mostly on his own emotional resources and on the amount of moral support available from relatives (Peck, 1972; Green, 1979; Mages *et al.*, 1981).

Apart from the anxieties of short-term loss of health and earning capacity, the patient also faces possible long-term effects of treatment, mutilation, fear of relapse, and death. It is therefore surprising that complaints of anxiety or depression are recorded by physicians in only a very small proportion of case histories (Derogatis *et al.*, 1979; Silberfarb *et al.*, 1980). One factor is that most patients believe that symptoms of anxiety will be regarded as a sign of inadequacy or weakness. Their major psychological complaints tend to refer to more socially acceptable reasons for loss of self-confidence, such as mutilation from surgery, amputation, mastectomy, laryngectomy or colostomy.

A possible second reason why cancer patients rarely mention psychological problems to their doctors is that they regard them as too busy, and involved only with their physical well-being (Levine *et al.*, 1978; Maguire *et al.*, 1978).

It is said that most patients do not like to upset their medical attendants; patients most popular with doctors and nurses are the ones who always appear to be cheerful and grateful and obey orders without question.

A third reason is that doctors, on their part, do not enquire too specifically about the patient's peace of mind. It is said that less than 1% of communication between doctor and patient is concerned with the patient's emotional reaction to the diagnosis of cancer or its complications (Maguire *et al.*, 1974). Yet it has been stressed that cancer patients need to work through their anxiety, just as bereaved people need to work through their mourning (Gyllenskold, 1982). This involves the need to think and talk about the experience, and also to give open expression to emotions such as tears or anger.

It is probably unnecessary to go as far as Maguire *et al.* (1974) who suggest that the patient needs to be asked specifically his view of the illness, about symptoms suggestive of anxiety or depression, and about the effect of the illness on the patient's job, marriage, sexual adjustment, social life, and leisure activities. Nevertheless, some 'conversational' therapy is essential so that the clinician can *listen* to the patient in an unhurried manner. This type of communication can provide considerable insight into the patient's personality and attitude to his disease, without an appearance of probing (Stehlin and Beach, 1966).

Doctors who do not favour the conversational approach argue that a light-hearted, jollying, and casual attitude gives the patient confidence, whereas too much discussion increases anxiety. There are indeed some highly anxious patients who prefer their doctors to be omniscient. In other patients, however, the anxiety or depression associated with the diagnosis is not dispelled by ignoring it — it merely discourages the patient from revealing it. It is often found that the patient's spouse appears more anxious than the patient himself. Wives often become overprotective in an effort to relieve their own anxiety, and in this way may actually hinder the patient's readjustment — both physical and mental.

During active treatment, most patients are usually absorbed (or even overwhelmed) by the day-to-day, or hour-to-hour activity involved. Subsequently, reaction commonly sets in with complaints of tiredness, weakness, and loss of self-confidence. At this stage especially, more prolonged discusssions with the physician may help to build up the patient's confidence in recovery and prospects of near-normal life. By listening rather than by talking, the physician may also be able to assess the ability of the patient to accept the diagnosis, disfigurement or disability, and this may provide early warning of the likelihood of the patient breaking down under stress.

Not all patients cope mentally by adjusting to and accepting the diagnosis. Denial attitudes are more common than was previously thought, and are said to persist in up to 20% of cases (Simpson, 1982). Denial is not an all-or-none phenomenon nor should it be regarded as abormal. It is part of the psychological defences of each individual, and under normal circumstances should be supported by the physician. Seemingly intelligent people insist on denying that they are suffering from cancer even after having been told the diagnosis, and such denial should not be discouraged (Stehlin and Beach, 1966; Simpson, 1982). Denial is of course unhealthy if it leads to deliberate delay in reporting the manifestations of cancer by ignoring them.

It is said that cancer patients go through five consecutive phases in their emotional reaction to cancer (Kubler-Ross, 1969), from the initial shock through denial, anger, and dependence to final acceptance. In practice, however, many patients appear to remain held up at one stage for a prolonged period, or may miss a stage, or may keep returning to the same stage (O'Neill, 1975). The initial shock proceeds to denial in some cases ('Not me, surely?') but an alternative reaction is overt anger ('Why me?'). As a result, hostility may be expressed to relatives or medical staff, and this anger reaction is often behind the bitter blame one sometimes hears from patients against a previous doctor or hospital. Sometimes a feeling of guilt may predominate and the patient believes that his own actions have precipitated the disease as a judgment. Such emotions often have a religious colouring.

Most patients tend to develop a feeling of dependence on their major medical advisor so that they can identify with the physician's fight against the disease and thus overcome their sense of helplessness. The reaction of physicians varies. While some feel unhappy at a patient's continued dependence, others enjoy the exalted position and assume so much authority that it delays the patient from coming to terms with his disease (Luce, 1979).

Patients need to proceed to acceptance, the stage at which they adjust emotionally to the diagnosis (Senescu, 1963). It has been suggested (Mages *et al.*, 1981) that the patient's pattern of adaptation to the diagnosis can be clearly recognized by three or four months after the primary treatment, and is unlikely to change much after that unless there is a change in the medical condition. This applies both to good and to poor psychosocial adaptation.

Emotional breakdown may occur in some patients before the acceptance stage is reached, and the most likely times for breakdown, apart from the time of diagnosis, are at the first appearance of recurrence or metastasis, or at the onset of the terminal phase. It is claimed that the patient at high risk to emotional breakdown may be recognized by certain psychosocial characteristics (Worden and Weisman, 1977): a history of failure to cope in the presence of stress; evidence of psychological instability or a history of a multiproblem background; low socio-economic status or little moral support from those around.

In the majority of patients, anxiety tends to decrease after a year or two without any sign of recurrence (Surawicz *et al.*, 1976; Holland and Mastrovito, 1980). By the time five or more years without recurrence have passed, the vast majority of patients are said to show few signs of psychosocial disability (Craig *et al.*, 1974). A study among breast cancer patients showed that, even two years after mastectomy, more than 80% of patients had resumed their preoperative responsibilities (Eisenberg and Goldenberg, 1966).

In summary, therefore, the majority of cancer patients know that the disease may be lethal, but most maintain the hope that they will overcome it. Most patients cope unaided or with the help of their families but usually develop some degree of dependency on the physician. Denial is more common than is realized, and should not be discouraged.

QUALITY OF LIFE — BALANCING PROFIT AND LOSS

Every form of cancer treatment must have a price in terms of morbidity. In the case of treatment aiming at cure, a high degree of morbidity or disfigurement may be acceptable to the patient as the price to be paid. In the case of advanced cancer, however, it is axiomatic that palliative treatment must not cause morbidity more distressing than the symptoms it seeks to relieve.

When palliation of local symptoms by radiotherapy is considered on this basis, the balance sheet is relatively simple. One can usually promise that pain will be eased and a tumour reduced and that, in the case of brain or mediastinal metastases, survival will almost certainly be prolonged as a result of relieving pressure by the tumour. The price to be paid is occasional radiation sickness which is usually transient, predictable, and easily countered.

On the other hand, palliation by systemic therapy (whether endocrine or cytotoxic) has a second aim in addition to that of local palliation. Its goal is to arrest all foci of cancer in the body and thereby prolong life. The latter has been demonstrated only in the case of leukaemia and lymphoma, testicular teratoma and kidney embryoma, and possibly for small cell lung cancer and pancreatic cancer (see Chapter 2). In the case of the vast majority of solid cancers, it may *possibly* be achieved in individual cases, but cannot be predicted. Yet, the pursuit of cancer arrest by the use of systemic therapy is widespread. Since its value is conjectural in the majority of cases, any resulting vitiation in the patient's quality of life needs to be justified and the patient must be given an informed choice (Shingleton and Shingleton, 1980). The problem is that, while the cost in morbidity can usually be predicted, the benefit to the patient is quite unpredictable.

Because of our inadequate knowledge, patients with advanced cancer may be treated very differently between one clinic and another and between one physician and another. These differences in treatment practice result from differences in aim, and they can be summed up as follows:

(a) Using the minimum of treatment needed for palliation, as and when symptoms appear. The various treatments are used sequentially and are saved up as far as possible.

(b) Using aggressive combination treatments in pursuit of cancer remission and prolongation of life, either in the context of a clinical trial or empirically.

(c) Treating mainly for 'supportive' reasons in order to maintain hope in the patient and relatives.

The differences between the first and second approaches are summed up in a recent discussion on the management of advanced breast cancer (Tormey, 1981): 'For a physician in private practice, the concept of using minimal sequential therapy has some advantage in the sense of decreased overall toxicity and simplicity of administration. On the other hand, the physician in research (sic) is looking for a regression which is going to produce complete remission rates in excess of 50%, because that is the point at which we see an occasional cure in other cancer.' Tormey is presumably referring to the patient's participation with informed consent in a controlled clinical trial.

Before presenting the balance sheet to the patient who is to receive systemic therapy for advanced cancer, we must be clear about our aims. In doing this, how do we measure the degree of benefit to the patient; how do we compare different types of morbidity with each other; how we do balance benefit against morbidity from the point of view of the patient?

Measuring the benefit

Chapter 2 provides a full discussion of the problems involved in measuring response in incurable cancer. It has been pointed out that because we are unable to measure accurately the response to treatment in late cancer, we are not clear as to which objectives are worth pursuing and which are not (Watson, 1981). As an example, UICC criteria of response to systemic therapy in soft tissue lesions of breast cancer specify a minimum 50% decrease in the area of a lesion (Hayward *et al.*, 1977). This is equivalent to a mean decrease in diameter of about 30%. There are few patients to whom a reduction in a lump's diameter by one-third has anything but psychological value, particularly if its duration is a matter of a few months only.

It is obvious that alopecia and intermittent gastrointestinal upset (common complications of nearly all cytotoxic therapy) are a high price to pay for a 50—60% chance of tumour shrinkage (or partial relief of pain) for a median duration of a few months. Even a possible prolongation of life by a month or two could hardly justify vitiating the quality of the patient's last few months of life. It is clear therefore that, in the majority of cases, the price is being paid by the patient for the privilege of maintaining hope. The patient is being shown 'that a positive attempt is being made to retard the progress of his disease' (Stehlin and Beach, 1966).

Most patients with advanced cancer (and also their relatives) do indeed expect active treatment, and become depressed (or resentful) if told that nothing further can be done to prolong life. Some may go to quacks in their despair. To avoid such despair, many patients are treated for 'supportive' reasons. An example of this is a series of patients with gastrointestinal cancer who were treated by a 'low toxicity' combination of cytotoxic agents (Gough *et al.*, 1981). Objective evidence of tumour regression was noted in only one out of the 25 cases treated, yet 23 of the patients and their relatives expressed their satisfaction with the treatment after completing three months of chemotherapy. The authors of the report conclude that 'general care and support are important determinants of the patient's subjective response to a chemotherapy program'.

But what degree of toxicity or unpleasantness is justifiable if treatment is being given mainly for 'supportive' reasons? In some countries, we are told, patients expect cancer treatment to be nasty and certainly given at the point of a needle rather than by mouth. If there are no such expectations, might it not be kinder to give the patient a course of multivitamin therapy instead? One often hears a relative say of the chemotherapy treatment after a patient's death, 'If I had known beforehand what unnecessary misery it would cause, I would not have agreed to it.' Or is this being wise after the event?

Some part may be played in the choice of unsuitably aggressive treatment by the unrealistic hopes of many clinicians. It has been said that success with combination therapy in leukaemia, lymphoma, and testicular teratoma has encouraged many oncologists to practise aggressive treatment in patients with advanced solid cancer where cure is not a reasonable objective (Tobias and Harper, 1981). In our present state of knowledge, quality of life must suffer if an attempt is made to cure the incurable.

Combination chemotherapy has doubled the response rates in cancer which were previously achieved by single-agent therapy. Yet a recent report shows that the mean length of survival in patients treated by combinaton chemo-therapy at a major UK cancer centre was no longer than in previous years when patients had not received this treatment (Powles *et al.*, 1980). Combinations of cytotoxic agents certainly increase the potential for a wider spectrum of complications.

Comparing different types of morbidity

The second problem in palliation is to compare different types of morbidity. Most treatments have unpleasant side-effects and the difficulty is to compare different degrees of unpleasantness *to the individual concerned*. For example, assuming that the two treatments are equally palliative, for a woman with breast cancer would one choose loss of scalp hair from cytotoxic therapy as against stimulation of facial and body hair growth from androgen therapy? Or choose intermittent cytotoxic injections, nausea, and malaise for months as against the short-term morbidity of transnasal hypophysectomy?

McNeil *et al.* (1978) have shown that a proportion of patients with lung cancer, when given a choice between radical surgery (carrying a higher chance of cure but also a high risk of operative mortality) or radiation therapy (carrying a lower risk of cure but little risk of immediate death) will reject the surgical method. These patients are averse to taking risks, and life in the next few months is more important to them than possible survival in the distance future. The same group (McNeil *et al.*, 1981) report that when people were asked to select between laryngectomy for laryngeal cancer (carrying a higher chance of cure but loss of speaking ability) and radiation therapy (carrying a possibly lower chance of cure but retaining speech), many said they would reject surgery.

Alopecia is one of the more unpleasant side-effects of cytotoxic therapy. Although it is associated with only about 20% of the agents currently used in palliative therapy, these happen to be the most effective and most widely used of the agents (bleomycin, cyclophosphamide, doxorubicin, and vinca alkaloids). These agents are commonly used also in the adjuvant treatment of high-risk cancer patients after surgery, when the alopecia together with the stresses, investigations, and anxieties of the periodic visits entailed lead many patients in apparent remission to decide to discontinue treatment.

Such decisions are of course a function of age and personal attitudes, but it is above all the *patient's* attitude which must prevail — it is he or she who takes the risk or suffers damage to the quality of life. Yet, in the majority of cases, the doctor makes the choice of palliative treatment for the patient on the basis of his particular training, his familiarity with a technique, and his own personal attitudes to the side-effects. In the process, he may tend to minimize the disadvantages of the method which he advocates.

There may be other reasons why the physician may minimize the morbidity of treatment he uses. One report notes that trained interviewers recognized toxicity following cytotoxic therapy in 90% of a group of patients, when clinicians recognized it in only 60% of cases (Maguire *et al.*, 1980). In the same group, disclosure of toxic symptoms to a surgeon was found to be considerably less than to an oncologist, the conclusion being that patients avoid complaining to some of their medical attendants, either for fear of losing their sympathy or because communication barriers are greater.

The problem is that quality of life is almost impossible to measure. It is commonly assessed as the proportion of his time the patient spends in pain-free activity. The most widely used measure of subjective response to treatment in patients with advanced cancer is based on the so-called 'performance status' (Karnofsky and Burchenal, 1948). This is the observer's assessment of the patient's status of daily activity and return to independence at intervals after treatment. Gough *et al.* (1981) found that a structured and detailed questionnaire used at intervals to assess subjective response to treatment gave no more information than the physical performance status as an index of improvement or deterioration.

Self-rating questionnaires have also been tried in such cases, but their disadvantage is that they are liable to be influenced by the image which the patient may wish to project, or thinks is expected. One investigation of this type (Craig *et al.*, 1974) reported that in 134 patients who had been submitted to mastectomy for cancer nine months or more previously, the quality of life, as measured by physical and psychosocial criteria, was not significantly different from that in 260 control women. How much meaning can we ascribe to such a finding in view of the well known physical and psychological consequences of a diagnosis of breast cancer, the subsequent mastectomy, and other associated treatments?

To try to achieve a more complete picture of the patient's symptoms, feelings, and performance, linear analogue self-assessment has been suggested (Priestman and Baum, 1976). The patient marks along a series of scales the point most appropriate to each sympton or activity, and the scores are added together to give an index. Serial assessments are again possible and can be compared. A major criticism is that all factors are given equal weighting in such an assessment. For example, a woman may suffer complete alopecia following treatment, but a fall in score on this account would be compensated in the final tally by an improved ability to do housework. How important is the latter compared to the former in assessing a patient's quality of life?

Balancing benefit against morbidity

In selecting a palliative treatment, the clinician must assess not only the likelihood of a response but also its possible duration, promptness, and degree of remission. These must then be judged in the context of the estimated life expectation of the patient. Against these conjectural benefits must be set the more predictable factors, such as the side-effects of treatment, their effect on the patient's activity, and their possible effects on the patient's mood. Travelling to and from hospital, repeated investigations, and vene-puncture must also be taken into account.

A decision based on so many imponderables is easier to make when the patient has a severe symptom such as pain, which requires urgent palliation. The decision is much more difficult if, for example, the patient has small or non-symptomatic metastases in skin, nodes, lung or liver. 'Anticipatory' palliative treatment may have a place under these conditions, as has also treatment on a psychological supportive basis. Aggressive systemic therapy with a doubtful chance of prolonging life has little place in these cases.

Adjuvant chemotherapy after surgery is widely used in the treatment of patients at high risk to recurrence. Some publications tend to minimize its morbidity, and it may be instructive to compare in this respect reports from the USA and from the UK on patients' psychosocial reactions to a course of such treatment in breast cancer. A report on 50 women from the University of California Medical Center (Meyerowitz *et al.*, 1979) concluded that, although their family and social life had been disrupted, the majority of the patients reported that the side-effects were acceptable for the sake of their health.

Yet, from the Royal Marsden Hospital in London a report on a similar regime showed that nausea, vomiting, malaise, and alopecia in the treated group had interfered to such an extent with the patients' lifestyles that 30% of the group said that the treatment had been 'unbearable' or 'could never be gone through again' (Palmer *et al.*, 1980). Another report from the UK using trained interviewers found that, whereas 50% of patients receiving mastectomy displayed an anxiety state or other psychiatric problems subsequently, these occurred in 80% of patients receiving adjuvant chemotherapy in addition (Maquire *et al.*, 1980).

Motivation is obviously the major factor determining the 'acceptability' of side-effects in such cases. In the USA, the patients assumed that the treatment was likely to help them as individuals, while in the UK report, the patients knew they were taking part in a clinical trial. In fact, the results of the study contributed to the decision of the UK group to stop the trials. They felt that such morbidity was justifiable only if it could be proved to result in a considerable improvement in prognosis.

INCURABLE CANCER — MANAGEMENT STAGE BY STAGE

It was pointed out above that the intensity of treatment carried out on patients with incurable cancer often differs grossly between one clinic and another. There is wide variation also in (a) the amount of investigation carried out before treatment, (b) the relative use of radiotherapy and chemo-endocrine treatment, and (c) the degree of follow-up investigation after the initial treatment. These differences are of course related to the different aims and aspirations of treatment, i.e. localized palliation of cancer *or* an attempt to achieve a remission (and so increase the duration of survival) *or* treatment given mainly to maintain hope in the patient.

While palliation by radiation therapy aims to alleviate the symptoms of advanced cancer in order to maintain the quality of life, local treatment of this type can also prolong life under specific circumstances. These include relief of pressure from the tumour at vital sites such as brain, spinal cord or mediastinum; healing of an ulcerated tumour in a viscus or externally; or reduction in the quantity of opiates required by the patient.

The writer's approach to palliative therapy is based on two principles established in the previous section. The first is that the management of the patient must at all times balance conjectural benefits against the likely effect of the proposed treatment on the patient's quality of life. The second principle is the acknowledgment that, in the vast majority of solid cancers, life is unlikely to be prolonged either by more aggressive or by earlier therapy (see Chapter 2). This means that sequential treatment is preferred, starting with the most simple, and keeping alternative treatments in reserve as long as possible.

Management of incurable cancer will be considered under the following categories:

The asymptomatic patient.
The symptomatic patient.
The terminal patient

The asymptomatic patient

If the above principles of therapy are accepted, there is no advantage to be gained by repeated time-consuming and expensive searches for occult metastases in the asymptomatic patient. Investigations not only cause the patient inconvenience and distress, but also lead to anxiety as to the results of the tests. As far as the clinician is concerned, evidence of blood-borne metastasis at one site presumes the presence of widespread systemic disease. Apart from occasions when the clinical extent of the disease needs to be known (e.g. when treatment policy is being changed), proof of occult metastases elsewhere merely converts a guarded prognosis into a gloomy one. It is far more likely to harm the quality of life than to help it (Brewin, 1981).

Having established that a patient has asymptomatic metastases from solid cancer, there is no clinical evidence to support the *theoretical* argument that early systemic treatment must prolong life because (a) a smaller tumour burden is easier to eradicate and (b) it may stop secondary tumours from throwing off 'tertiary' metastases. If aggressive systemic therapy is added to local radiation therapy when the first metastasis becomes manifest clinically, it may delay the clinical appearance of the next metastasis. But there is no firm evidence in the vast majority of solid cancers that the total length of survival is any different than if one delayed the same systemic therapy until the next metastasis became clinically overt.

The value of delaying treatment as long as possible is that the tempo of cancer growth varies enormously between one patient and another. Even in the same patient, cancer does not always advance irrevocably at the same rate (Stoll, 1982a). Although the future course can sometimes be predicted on the basis of variables such as microscopic type of tumour, stage of disease at presentation, and sites of metastatic involvement, wide variations exist between one patient and another in the tempo and pattern of metastasis.

Recognition of the tempo of asymptomatic disease permits selection of a suitable form of management out of the following:

1. No treatment at all is advised for slowly growing tumour (often manifested by a long recurrence-free interval) in the absence of symptoms from metastases and no danger of serious complications.
2. Localized radiotherapy and conservative management is usually adequate to control localized recurrence or metastasis.
3. Aggressive treatment associated with morbidity is justified only for aggressive spread of disease, and then only if the physical and mental condition of the patient justifies it.

For relatively small metastases not causing symptoms, there is usually no advantage to be gained by early therapy unless it is for anticipatory or supportive reasons. It is usually far better for the patient to continue as normal a life as possible, until symptoms do appear. Activity should be restricted only if there is a danger that it may cause symptoms or cause complications such as a pathological fracture. If asymptomatic metastases are to be treated because of anxiety in the patient or relatives, they must clearly understand that there is no firm evidence that such treatment will prolong survival.

Anticipatory treatment of asymptomatic metastases is usually given by radiation therapy. It implies that symptoms are expected to arise from these lesions in the near future, but such treatment must in all cases be based on informed clinical experience, and not given indiscriminately on a 'prophylactic' basis. It may be indicated in the case of relatively small mediastinal or cerebral metastases where their further growth may threaten life, or for lytic deposits in long bones where a pathological fracture might subsequently incapacitate the patient. It is quite unnecessary for asymptomatic slowly growing metastases in skin or regional nodes in elderly patients, or for symptomless sclerotic metastases, or for one or two small x-ray opacities in the lung fields or for defects found in a routine scintiscan of the liver.

The use of aggressive treatment associated with morbidity can be justified in the asymptomatic patient only under clearly specified conditions. First, in those *few* tumour types where the evidence is clear that survival may be prolonged by such therapy (see Chapter 2). Even in such a case, the patient must be given the opportunity to balance any morbidity from the proposed treatment against the possible advantages. Secondly, a patient whose tumour type is not in the above category can be entered with informed consent into a controlled clinical trial of a new regime, either if the disease shows a rapid tempo of growth or if it is requested for psychological reasons. If these conditions are not fulfilled, only systemic therapy carrying little or no morbidity is justified. On the whole, systemic therapy, whether cytotoxic or endocrine, is better saved until its use is demanded by the patient's symptoms.

Treatment of symptomatic metastases

Only in the case of locally recurrent solid cancer can one justify aggressive therapy aiming at eradicating the disease. The applies equally whether the treatment to be selected is surgery, radiotherapy or systemic chemotherapy. The decision must depend on the site and histopathological characteristics of the tumour and on the patient's age, mental attitude, and physical fitness to withstand aggressive treatment. In the case of blood-borne metastases from the vast majority of solid cancers, intensive treatment is called for only if they fail to respond to simpler palliative measures.

We noted above that there is no firm evidence to justify aggressive local treatment of a distant metastasis by surgery or radiation therapy on the basis that it may be solitary or that it may prevent spread of 'tertiary' metastases from the secondary deposit. There are, of course, recorded cases where surgical removal or high-dose irradiation of an apparently solitary secondary deposit in lungs, bone or liver has been followed by prolonged survival, but this almost certainly reflects the type of slowly growing disease which produces an apparently solitary metastasis. Aggressive treatment of so-called metastases is not justified either by pathological concepts or by the results of treatment.

If there are multiple symptomatic metastases, the most troublesome or the most life-endangering ones should be the first to be treated. A sequential plan of treatments is projected from the outset, progressing from the most simple to the most complex, each step using the minimum treatment necessary for palliation. One starts with the best-tolerated treatment, taking into account first that measurable shrinkage of a local tumour is by no means synonymous with improved quality of life, and secondly that the burden to the patient must be commensurate with possible benefits from such a treatment.

Palliative surgery may be necessary for intractable pain, fluid drainage, obstruction, pathological fracture or ulcerated tumour. However, the practice of 'second look' (re-exploring the abdomen after a resection in the hope of dealing with recurrence) has little justification. Positive findings almost certainly indicate the need for radiation or systemic therapy, and second look presents no proven advantage over waiting for recurrence to manifest clinically.

Radiation therapy is most commonly used for palliation of localized disease. In the case of a relatively small tumour, it may be worth a short course of radiation therapy even if the tumour is presumed to be only moderately radiosensitive, because localized radiation therapy is associated with minimal morbidity. As an alternative to radiation therapy, systemic therapy by combination cytotoxic agents may also achieve regression of local disease. If, however, its duration is only a matter of a few months and the disease is again recrudescent by the time the morbidity of systemic therapy has settled, one must question whether palliation has been achieved.

Systemic therapy is, however, clearly indicated in symptomatic disease where the tumour type is clearly known to have prolongation of survival associated with objective evidence of tumour regression. As always, the patient must be informed of any morbidity involved, so that he can balance it against the potential benefit. Systemic therapy may be used also in the case of tumours not in the above category, if the patient's tumour is too disseminate to be controlled by localized therapy, or is growing at a rapid tempo, or if such treatment is requested by the patient. Treatment is by entry with informed consent into a controlled trial or alternatively by a regime known to be effective in that disease.

When a decision has been made to use systemic therapy for breast or prostatic cancer, some clinicians start with a combination of endocrine and cytotoxic methods. This is, in my opinion, an example of *overkill* except in the case of rapidly advancing disease. Wherever possible, treatment should be selected according to specific host/tumour characteristics (e.g. oestrogen receptor characteristics of the tumour or age group of the host) and should be the minimum necessary for palliation. Such a policy has the advantage that it does not exhaust all possible modalities but leaves alternative methods for later use. In the case of breast cancer, there is no evidence that by using two such modalities together, concurrently, there results a longer overall survival than by using them separately (Carter, 1981).

The management of advanced local disease by a combination of localized radiation therapy and systemic therapy is also, in our present state of knowledge, an example of overkill. Regression of the local disease following such combined treatment is common, but often leads to the systemic therapy being continued for long periods without any evidence that it has been involved in the tumour control. As mentioned earlier, such a combination may lead to greater delay before recurrence but the price paid in additional morbidity is often high, and there is no firm evidence that total survival is any longer than if the same systemic therapy was delayed until recurrence took place.

In the practice of sequential therapy, one does not progress to a second type of therapy until adequate time has been allowed to assess the results of the first treatment. Whereas relief of pain following radiotherapy to bone metastases may take only two weeks, that from endocrine therapy or cytotoxic therapy may be delayed four to six weeks. As far as tumour regression is concerned, the latter methods usually take about two months before it manifests in soft tissue masses, or even longer in the case of endocrine therapy (Glick *et al.*, 1980).

When systemic therapy has shown itself capable of controlling tumour growth, we are still uncertain whether it should be persisted with (either continuously or intermittently) until the tumour reappears or whether it should be stopped when maximum regression is obtained (see Chapter 2). A mixed response to therapy does not preclude its continued use. For example, if localized soft tissue tumours have regressed on systemic therapy, yet in the meanwhile a new metastasis has appeared in bone, the systemic therapy can be continued and radiation therapy used to control the bone metastasis.

There is no indication to plague the patient with frequent and repeated follow-up investigations after treatment. In 90% of cases, the development of new metastases is heralded by symptoms, and while chest x-rays or liver function tests may occasionally uncover occult disease, serial bone scans as a routine are not justified (Winchester *et al.*, 1979). Serial liver and brain scans are certainly not justified.

The terminal stage

The patient with advanced cancer not only has to contend with physical symptoms but also has to cope emotionally with the threat of dying. The degree of this additional anxiety is often related to the tempo at which the disease is progressing. As patients' dependence on treatment increases, so their anxiety tends to focus on possible ways in which they may die (e.g. choking, suffocating, pain, paralysis, etc.). It is at this stage, especially, that the physician has to extend himself to provide hopefulness and compassionate care. Even if he cannot prolong survival, he can offer physical comfort, and his reassurance can play as crucial a role as the physical treatment which be provides.

When terminal care is the goal, investigations must be restricted to those which will improve symptom control. When attempts to prolong life are still appropriate, active treatment is justified only after discussing the probable morbidity and possible duration of response with the family and patient. Unproven treatments should be used only as part of a carefully controlled clinical trial and, even then, only at the request of the patient and relatives. Cytotoxic therapy should, in general, be withheld from elderly patients with widely disseminate disease and in poor condition. 'Suffering in the patient is intensified if treatment, used in a last ditch attempt to save the patient, causes unpleasant side effects' (Maguire, 1982).

The duration of a palliative treatment must be commensurate with the patient's life expectation. It is not justifiable to occupy the last few weeks or months of a patient's life with a prolonged course of activity therapy in a hospital. Death of a cancer patient in the middle of a course of treatment (whether radiotherapy or cytotoxic agents) can be justified if the treatment is an attempt at cure and a calculated risk is being taken. If, however, a patient dies in the middle of a palliative course of treatmemt, it may indicate poor clinical judgment on the part of the physician.

In extenuation, it is sometimes suggested that a decision to treat has been forced by the patient or relatives demanding that no stone be left unturned. But it is the physician's responsibility to provide time for discussion and balanced explanation, while at the same time showing compassionate understanding of the anxiety of patient and relatives. The hopes of the latter are often unrealistic and it is clear that our duty is to the patient and not to assuage relatives. We should not feel guilty if we do not offer technically complex treatments in this highly scientific age, but it often takes more time to explain why we do not advise it than it takes to arrange such treatment.

There comes a time when aggressive treatment is no longer appropriate: the physician's need to treat and the family's need to treat are unacceptable reasons for active therapy (Mount, 1978). It is important to explain to the family that the stage is *not* one where 'nothing more can be done', even if therapy can no longer control the disease progress. The goal is now to alleviate suffering because nothing can be done to prolong life *without too great a cost in side-effects*. The control of symptoms then becomes the priority.

In summary, therefore, all treatment for metastatic solid cancer is palliative and, when several types of effective treatment are available, the less unpleasant methods should be offered first. Because such decisions are based on many imponderables, it may be useful to give some prime examples of *inappropriate* palliation (Stoll, 1982b):

Aggressive treatment of asymptomatic metastases.
The use of two methods in combination where one would be adequate.
Prolonged duration of a palliative treatment in relation to the patient's life expectation.
Severe morbidity from a treatment in relation to the degree of palliation which can be hoped for.

COMMUNICATING WITH THE PATIENT

Not being told what is wrong with them is probably the most common complaint levelled by patients against their doctors. But, certainly in the UK, it is likely that the cancer patient who complains that he is not told enough is expressing a sense of insecurity, rather than a lack of information (Brewin, 1977). Such insecurity may result from what the patient believes is a lack of interest by the doctor in his symptoms, or from the doctor's failure to have gained the patient's confidence.

Some information is of course commonly withheld from the cancer patient, although recent years have seen pressures to permit patients more participation in decisions affecting the management of their disease (Schain, 1980). In the past, the physician was the ultimate authority and it was enough for him to show such respect for the cancer patient's point of view as would a reasonable parent for that of his adolescent child. No-one really questioned this attitude, as the physician's code of ethics requires him to provide the patient with hope at all times, and, logically, he avoided information which might cause despair.

In 1961, a survey in the USA (Oken, 1961) showed that almost 90% of physicians withheld knowledge of the diagnosis of cancer from their patients unless it was necessary for getting the patient to accept treatment, or was essential for the patient to plan his future. The same questionnaire was issued a few years ago, and this time 98% of USA physicians stressed the importance of being totally frank with their cancer patients (Novack *et al.*, 1979). It is said that most patients now prefer the doctor to act as a technical advisor while the patient weighs the evidence and makes the ultimate decision as to treatment.

It is claimed by proponents of this attitude that increasing the patient's participation in decision-making helps to prevent a feeling of helplessness and has few disadvantages, because improvements in cancer treatment have now changed its previously sinister reputation. In fact, the change in attitude in the USA is probably due more to alterations in social opinion on the rights of patients, to changes in legal requirements, and to malpractice suits. These factors are gradually assuming greater importance in European medicine as doctors begin to retreat into the practice of defensive medicine.

But does this change in attitude also indicate an erosion of the traditional doctor–patient relationship? On the subject of this relationship, a patient has written that 'the most potent medicine available to the physician is the confidence placed in him by the patient' (Cousins, 1979). This confidence imples not that cure is at his fingertips nor even that he is a leading expert in his field, but that the physician can be trusted and relied on always to serve the patient's best interests.

On this basis, should the cancer patient be told the worst? It is clear that information should be withheld if it might damage the patient and cause despair. But evasion of the truth is usually detected, and blank denial of the diagnosis may increase the patient's fears and lose his trust in the physician, because most patients suspect the diagnosis in any case. But equally, there is no place for the naked truth. An 'escape window' must be provided so that optimism can be maintained.

It is clear also that the method of informing the patient and its timing is crucial. In all cases, it must take note of cues from the patient in setting the pace of disclosure. Unfortunately 'much of medical education is devoted to learning how to gather and evaluate facts, but little on how to divulge them' (Reisner, 1980). It is unfortunate too that such explanations are very time-consuming. Because of these difficulties, many physicians prefer to talk in approximate half-truths.

Wherever possible, unspoken communication is certain to have a greater impact than words. A smile, a touch of the hand or an arm around the shoulder may show that the physician wants to help and knows how to help. On the other hand, unconscious cues such as a worried facial expression and awkward gaps of silence in the discussion will tend to suggest to the patient that the physician may be avoiding an honest relationship.

How much should the cancer patient be told? It is obviously unnecessary to inform him of every possible complication of treatment, of conjectural benefit of one treatment as against another or of all the controversies in medical opinion. Above all, any statistical commitment as to prognosis should be avoided—published figures are merely averages taken from wide extremes. Although it is currently popular for physicians to be honest with cancer patients, a question such as 'When am I going to die?' should not be answered literally. It is an expression of the patient's fears rather than a desire for knowledge (Luce, 1979).

Complex and technical explanations will confuse even an intelligent patient and leave him anxious, so it is important that excessive information is not given to the uncomprehending patient or to the one who is emotionally unstable. In general, it is unnecessary, and even harmful, to discuss the more complex aspects of the disease and it is essential always to encourage optimism and hope of overcoming the disease.

A recent study of 256 cancer patients in the USA concluded that knowledge of their condition helps many patients to preserve hope (Cassileth *et al.*, 1980). But what about the patients who do not want such information? How does one distinguish patients who want to have a hand in decision-making from those who prefer others to decide. Information-seekers can sometimes be recognized by their mention of similar cases and their outcome, questions on treatment and sometimes a request for 'time to think things over'. Information-avoiders usually ask no questions except 'When do you want me in?' and are obviously looking for authoritarian, confident, decision-making.

The most difficult problem is posed by the patient who asks searching questions yet appears to the physician to be emotionally unsuited to receive blunt answers (Stoll, 1979). Most of the patients who 'want to know the worst, so that I can be prepared' or who say 'I haven't got cancer, have I?' are not asking for information but for reassurance. In deciding what to say to such patients, the doctor may have little to go on. He may have some information from the family doctor, but, especially in hospital practice, he has little knowledge of the patient's emotional resources or of his psychological history. He gets little help from relatives who usually try to exact a promise that the patient shall not be told the true situation.

Usually the physician has to make up his own mind. It is important therefore to have adequate time for unpressured discussion with the patient alone. Hope and confidence must be stimulated at all costs, whether the patient is an information-seeker or an information-avoider. While most physicians agree that the patient should be told no more than he asks, there are some who suggest that the doctor should always enquire specifically if there is any more information that the patient desires (Reynolds *et al.*, 1981; Spencer-Jones, 1981).

What do most cancer patients wish to know about their disease? There is obviously gross variation among patients according to social and cultural settings, and also according to individual attitudes of denial. It is even suggested that people vary from time to time in what they want to admit to themselves about their disease (Simpson, 1982; Gyllenskold, 1982). On this basis one cannot divide information-seekers from information-avoiders, but information must be given according to the patient's needs at any particular time. As a general rule, one should give the patient only *as much information as he asks for, can comprehend, and can emotionally accept.* Fortunately, the patient who does not want to know is generally unlikely to ask.

In a study of hospital patients in the UK, it was found that, of those who suspected that they had cancer, only one-third wanted confirmation of the diagnosis (McIntosh, 1976). Again, of those patients who suspected that they had cancer, only one-seventh wanted to know the prognosis. No patient wanted to know if the disease was likely to prove fatal. What most wanted was a progress report from time to time — whether cancer was absent or whether it had recurred.

A recent report from the USA (Cassileth *et al.*, 1980) suggests that 87% of younger cancer patients want full participation in the doctor's decision compared to 51% of older patients. Only about 10% of all patients wanted no information at all, and another 10% wanted only minimal or optimistic information. Yet, in another series in the USA (Leigh *et al.*, 1980), it was found that, in a group of 100 patients who were all told of their diagnosis of cancer before being treated, subsequent questioning showed that 48% of men and 16% of women claimed that they were not aware of the diagnosis. In addition, 81% of the men and 63% of the women regarded their illness as not being severe in spite of the information they had received.

This might appear to be evidence of denial in about one-third of cases. Yet it is possible that some of the patients did not 'take in' what the physician had said originally, or it may possibly have been a shock of which the patient did not wish to be reminded (Aitken-Swan and Easson, 1959).

In summary, it is obvious that the psychological reaction of the patient may impede free communication between doctor and patient. The majority of patients are realistic and moderately optimistic, but there are also extremes—patients who deny and those who are deeply depressed and anxious.

DOCTORS ARE ONLY HUMAN

In the preceding section we have stressed the variability in personality among cancer patients. There is often a bland assumption that physicians are uniformly caring and understanding. Even if this were not their reason for joining the medical profession, it is assumed that they learn to establish empathy with the sick (Gyllenskold, 1982), whom they then treat with understanding, patience, and compassion. Is this really so?

Doctors have to fulfil a double role in their treatment of the cancer patient. First, they need an objective and detached attitude to put the patient through unpleasant tests or treatments. Secondly, they need an understanding of each patient's anxieties which will then lead to empathy—a feeling for the patient without loss of identity. Many doctors, unfortunately, find it difficult to alternate between the two roles (Gyllenskold, 1982). They find it difficult to put themselves in the patient's place and, when it comes to the psychological problems of the cancer patient, many clinicians are unhappy and out of their depth.

To gain the patient's confidence, physicians need psychological resources and supportive qualities which are quite different from those derived from a study of the latest medical literature. While some doctors are adept at sensing their patient's emotional needs, others tend to ignore them and busy themselves in non-essential investigations or in vigorous trials of new treatment.

What are the specific fears of the cancer patient? The term 'cancer' is linked with the idea of death in the minds of most laymen. They have practically all known people die from cancer, while those patients who recover from cancer treatment rarely talk about it. The current fear of cancer is said to be greater than the fear of death itself—it is popularly believed to involve gradual wasting away, loss of control, constant pain, and suffering. It is associated with the fear of being a burden to all around or of being abandoned.

As a result, the clinician who has to inform a patient that cancer is advancing may appear in the position of a judge delivering a death sentence. This is even more so if the physician's experience in the management of cancer has engendered a feeling of ineffectual hoplessness. He says little to the patient and this in turn leads to absence of empathy. Subsequent discussions are often limited to technical medical problems.

Young people take up the profession of medicine for a variety of reasons. The clinician's task involves not only problem-solving, decision-making, and technical knowledge but also sensitivity to the emotional state of the patient and providing moral support. Doctors are obviously not equal in their capacity to demonstrate compassion, understanding, and support in a tangible form. Sometimes, too, the 'chemistry' between doctor and patient may not be right; doctors and patients rarely choose each other.

The medical student sees little of the team care necessary in the management of the cancer patient—particularly of the late cancer patient. He is barely trained in the psychological management of severe illness, and often feels helpless when faced with the psychological, family, and social problems of the cancer patient. He may try to ignore them, or else compensate for a feeling of inadequacy by showing professional overactivity. Such busy behaviour often satisfies the family members who wish to be reassured that no stone had been left unturned. It usually fails to meet the needs of the patient.

Medical training is generally successful in one objective—it teaches that death is the enemy and that the doctor stands somewhat in the position of St George. As a result, most clinicians (and indeed, most medical personnel including nurses) become paternalistic in their behaviour to the patient. Paternalism associated with superior knowledge inspires confidence in most patients. But unhappily, paternalism can be of two types—a benevolent caring variety associated with empathy, or an arrogant or patronizing variety associated with vanity. It depends on the personality of the individual.

The arrogant-type doctor may feel threatened when his mastery is called into question. This may occur for example when a promised 'cure' in cancer ends with manifestations of recurrence. Because of the doctor's sense of failure, he may pass the patient on to an assistant or to a colleague, just when the patient's need is greatest. The paternalistic attitude may be used to fend off too many questions and often prevents the patient giving essential information about his physical or psychological reaction to treatment. The patient does not wish to appear ungrateful, or risk losing the doctor's sympathy by complaining.

The arrogant-type doctor tends to be highly critical of any suggestion that ancillary personnel may be useful in identifying the psychological needs of his patients or even that doctors need training in this skill. It is a generalization that, because of their technical training in prompt decision-making, most doctors find it difficult to work in with members of other disciplines. Having been trained to make rapid decisions in what he thinks are the best interests of the patient, the physician tends to assume that he knows best.

On the other hand, most physicians show a paternalism which is clearly associated with empathy. Many argue that it is cruel to ask the patient to take difficult medical decisions and that, in any case, the patient is not qualified to judge the situation objectively (Gillon, 1981). They believe that the majority of patients expect their physicians to take full responsibility and that paternalism and domination are essential for the physician's effectiveness. They may list alternatives to the patient but recommend a specific choice. They think it unethical to say 'Go ahead and choose, it's your life' (Ingelfinger, 1980).

In general, doctors tend to defend entrenched and conservative attitudes in medicine and are slow to accept changing social attitudes around them. There is, however, an increasing realization that physicians should recognize and accept the variety of psychological reactions and needs among cancer patients (Blanchard *et al.*, 1981; Sanson-Fisher and Maguire, 1980). While one patient may choose to be dependent and maintain a child-like faith in the physician, another may prefer a skilled advisor to a father figure. The doctor's attitude must above all be flexible.

In Western materialist society, emphasis tends to be placed on quantity— more is better. Longer life is unquestionably regarded as better than shorter life, and the technical training of doctors lays increasing stress on machine-controlled survival and spare-part surgery. But should we fight incessantly to add months to the cancer patient's life or should we fight for good-quality life only? It depends on whether the patient is a risk-taker by nature, and only the patient can make the decision. The clinician needs not only wide experience of the disease and considerable clinical judgment, but also a sense of compassion to steer the course best suited to the individual patient and his disease.

To all patients with advanced cancer the physician must offer *hope* and this often involves support of the patient's denial defence mechanisms. Patients should be given to understand that cancers behave differently in different people and that many patients with incurable cancer undergo remissions which may last for many years. Physical methods of treatment are used, but they should *not be given as a substitute for psychological support*.

Finally, there is a need to discuss physicians' personal attitudes to death. Few people have enough insight to evaluate their own prejudices, and, in the case of the physician, this may present problems in the management of the pre-terminal cancer patient. One of the symptoms of our modern detribalized society is that we are unable to cope confidently with death. Mere discussion of the process of dying and interment makes most laymen feel awkward and inadequate. It has been said that physicians can help patients face their fears only if they are able to recognize their own.

Up to the beginning of this century, death among young and old was common from tuberculosis and the complications of the specific fevers. Most patients died in the presence of relatives at home, and only about 5% of deaths occurred in hospitals. In the last 80 years, however, death has become institutionalized and about 65% of all people now die in hospital, often with tubes attached to every orifice. (It is possible to compensate for this gross indignity that the patient is encouraged to float away with a clouded mind.)

Death is hardly mentioned in our medical institutions, yet a recent report (Hinton, 1980) suggests that a majority of pre-terminal cancer patients are aware of their condition. Over one-third experience distressing symptoms of anxiety or depression, and the figure is even higher in patients under 50 who feel themselves also angry and cheated. About three-quarters of late cancer patients are said to recognize that they might die soon and speak of this to their spouses or to medical personnel, and it appears to be rare for patients to maintain denial to the end (Kubler-Ross, 1969).

Hinton (1980) stresses that terminal patients are less likely to experience anxiety or depression if they can discuss their problems. But the patient's willingness to talk about death depends on whether the attendants are prepared to listen and help in this awareness. They rarely are.

CONCLUSION

(1) Two recent developments in medical practice threaten the quality of life in the cancer patient. First, increased anxiety among patients who are aware of their diagnosis, and inevitably of the progress of the disease. Secondly, attempts to assuage this anxiety by agents which offer the hope (if not the substance) of delaying the growth of solid cancer.

(2) The emotional reaction of the cancer patient to his disease needs constant support and understanding from the physician. While patients respond to the paternalistic approach, most require some empathy with the medical attendants which will establish hope and confidence in the patient. Conversational therapy will help most patients work through their fears. Enthusiastic investigation and aggressive treatment are no substitute.

(3) There is no firm evidence that aggressive systemic therapy prolongs life in the vast majority of patients with advanced solid cancer. Yet it is capable of vitiating the patient's quality of survival. Palliative therapy should therefore proceed sequentially, the less unpleasant methods being offered first. Some prime examples of inappropriate palliation are aggressive treatment of asymptomatic metastases; the use of two methods of treatment in combination where one would be adequate; prolonged duration of a palliative treatment in relation to the patient's life expectation; severe morbidity from a treatment in relation to the degree of palliation which can be hoped for.

(4) The training of physicians should include an insight into their own emotional reaction to the cancer patient, to failure of their treatment, and to death. As a result, the patient's quality of life should benefit.

REFERENCES

Aitken-Swan, J., and Easson, E.C. (1959). Reactions of cancer patients on being told their diagnosis. *Br. Med. J.*, **1**,779.

Blanchard, C.G., Ruckdeschel, J.C., Cohen, R.L.E., *et al*. (1981). Attitudes towards cancer; the impact of a comprehensive oncology course on second year medical students. *Cancer*, **47**, 2756.

Brewin, T.B. (1977). The cancer patient; communication and morale. *Br. Med. J.*, **11**, 1623.

Brewin, T.B. (1981). The cancer patient—too many scans and X-rays? *Lancet*, **ii**, 1098.

Carter, S.K. (1981). The interpretation of trials; combined hormonal therapy and chemotherapy in disseminated breast cancer. *Breast Cancer Res. Treat.*, **1**,43.

Cassileth, B.R. Zupkis, R.V., Sutton Smith, K., *et al.* (1980). Information and participation preferences among cancer patients. *Ann. Intern. Med.*, **92**, 832.

Cousins, N. (1979). Medical ethics; is there a broader view? *J. Am. Med. Assoc.*, **241**, 2711.

Craig, T.J., Comstock, G.W., and Geiser, P.B. (1974). Quality of survival in breast cancer; a case control comparison. *Cancer*, **33**,1451.

Derogatis, L.R., Feldstein, M., Morrow, G., *et al.* (1979). A survey of psychotropic drug prescriptions in an oncology population. *Cancer*, **44**, 1919.

Eisenberg, H.S., and Goldenberg, I.S. (1966). Measurement of quality of survival of breast cancer patients. In *Clinical evaluation of breast cancer* (eds, J.L. Hayward, and R.D. Bulbrook). New York: Academic Press. p. 93.

Fiore, N. (1979). Fighting cancer—one patient's perspective. *New Eng. J. Med.*, **301**,284.

Gillon, R. (1981). The function of criticism. *Br. Med. J.*, **283**,1633.

Glick, J.H., Creech, R.H., Torri, S., *et al.* (1980). Tamoxifen plus sequential CMF chemotherapy versus tamoxifen alone in postmenopausal breast cancer. *Cancer*, **45**,735.

Gough, I.R., Furnival, C.M., and Burnett, W. (1981). Patient attitudes to chemotherapy for advanced gastro-intestinal cancer. *Clin. Oncol.*, **7**,5.

Green, S. (1979). Psychological consequences of cancer. *Practitioner*, **222**, 173.

Gyllenskold, K. (1982). *Breast cancer. The psychological effect of the disease and its treatment*. London: Tavistock Publications. p.84.

Hayward, J.L., Carbone, P.P., Heuson, J.C., *et al.* (1977). Assessment of response to therapy in advanced breast cancer. *Cancer*, **39**,1289.

Hinton, J. (1980). Whom do dying patients tell? *Br. Med. J.*,**281**,1328.

Holland, J.C., and Mastrovito, R. (1980). Psychologic adaptation to breast cancer. *Cancer*, **46**,1045.

Ingelfinger, F. (1980). Arrogance. *New Engl. J. Med.*, **303**,1507.

Karnofsky, D.A., and Burchenal, J.H. (1948). In *Evaluation of chemotherapeutic agents* (ed. C.M. MacLeod) New York: Columbia University Press. p.101.

Kubler-Ross, E. (1969). *On death and dying*. New York: Macmillan.

Leigh, H., Ungerer, J., and Percarpio, B. (1980). Denial and helplessness in cancer patients undergoing radiation therapy. *Cancer*, **45**,3086.

Levine, M.P., Silberfarb, P.M., and Lipowski, Z.J. (1978). Mental disorders in cancer patients. *Cancer*, **42**,1385.

Luce, J.K. (1979). Selecting patients for supportive therapy. In *Mind and cancer prognosis* (ed. B.A. Stoll). Chichester: John Wiley & Sons. p.127.

McIntosh, J. (1976). Patients' awareness and desire for information about diagnosed but undisclosed malignant disease. *Lancet*, **11**,300.

McNeil, B.J., Weichselbaum, R., and Pauker, S.G. (1978). Fallacy of the five year survival in lung cancer. *New Engl. J. Med.*, **299**,1397.

McNeil, B.J., Weichselbaum, R., and Pauker, S.G. (1981). Speech and survival. Tradeoffs between quality and quantity of life in laryngeal cancer. *New Engl. J. Med.*, **305,982.**

Mages, N.L., Castro, J.R., Fobair, P., *et al.* (1981). Patterns of psychosocial response to cancer; can effective adaptation be predicted? *Int. J. Radiat. Oncol., Biol. Phys.*, **7**,385.

Maguire, G.P. (1982). The personal impact of dying. In *The dying patient* (ed. E. Wilkes). Lancaster: MTP Press. p.233.

Maguire, G.P., Julier, D.L., Kawton, K.E., and Bancroft, J.H.J. (1974). Psychiatric morbidity and referral on two general medical wards. *Br. Med. J.*, **1**,268.

Maguire, G.P., Lee, E.G., Bevington, D.J., *et al.* (1978). Psychiatric problems in the first year after mastectomy. *Br. Med. J.*, **2**,963.

Maguire, G.P., Tait, A., Brooke, M., *et al.* (1980). Psychiatric morbidity and physical toxicity associated with adjuvant chemotherapy after mastectomy. *Br. Med. J.*, **281**,1179.

Meyerowitz, B.E., Sparks, F.C., and Spears, I.K. (1979). Adjuvant chemotherapy for breast carcinoma; psychosocial implications. *Cancer*, **43**, 1613.

Mount, B.M. (1978). Palliative care of the patient with terminal care. In *Genito-urinary cancer* (eds D.G. Skinner, and J.B. de Kernion). Philadelphia: W.B. Saunders. p.535.

Novack, D.H., Plumer, R., Smith, R.L., *et al.* (1979). Changes in the physician's attitude towards telling the cancer patient. *J. Am. Med. Assoc.*, **241**,897.

Oken, D. (1961). What to tell cancer patients. *J. Am. Med. Assoc.*, **175**,1120.

O'Neill, M.P. (1975). Psychological aspects of cancer recovery. *Cancer*, **36**,271.

Palmer, B.V., Walsh, G.A., McKinna, J.A., *et al.* (1980). Adjuvant chemotherapy for breast cancer; side effects and quality of life. *Br. Med. J.*, **281**,1594.

Peck, A. (1972). Emotional reactions to having cancer. *Radiology*, **114**,591.

Powles, T.J., Coombes, R.C., Smith, I.E., *et al.* (1980). Failure of chemotherapy to prolong survival in a group of patients with metastatic breast cancer, *Lancet*, **i**,580.

Priestman, T.J., and Baum, M. (1976). Evaluation of quality of life for patients receiving treatment for advanced breast cancer. *Lancet*, **i**,899.

Reisner, S.J. (1980). Words as scalpels. Transmitting evidence in the clinical dialogue. *Ann. Intern. Med.*, **82**,837.

Reynolds, P.M., Sanson-Fisher, R.W., Poole, A.D., *et al.* (1981). Cancer and communication; information giving in an oncology clinic. *Br. Med. J.*, **282**,1449.

Sanson-Fisher, R., and Maguire, P. (1980). Should skills in communicating with patients be taught in medical schools? *Lancet*, **ii**,523.

Schain, W.S. (1980). Patients' rights in decision making. *Cancer*, **46**,1035.

Schnaper, N. (1982). The age old question of euthanasia. In *Controversies in oncology* (ed. P.H. Wiernik). New York: John Wiley & Sons. p.279.

Senescu, R.A. (1963), The development of emotional complications in the patient with cancer. *J. Chronic Dis.*, **16**,813.

Shingleton, W.W., and Shingleton, A.B. (1980). Ethical considerations in the treatment of breast cancer. *Cancer*, **46**,1031.

Silberfarb, P.M., Maurer, L.H., and Crouthamel, C.S. (1980). Psychosocial aspects of breast cancer patients during different treatment regimes. *Am. J. Psychiatr.*, **137**,450.

Simpson, M.A. (1982). Therapeutic uses of truth. In *The dying patient* (ed. E. Wilkes). Lancaster: MTP Press. p.255.

Spencer-Jones, J. (1981). Telling the right patient. *Br. Med. J.*, **283**,291.

Stehlin, J.S., and Beach, K.H. (1966). Psychological aspects of cancer therapy. *J. Am. Med. Assoc.*, **197**,140.

Stoll, B.A. (1979). Is hope a factor in survival? In *Mind and cancer prognosis* (ed. B.A. Stoll). Chichester: John Wiley & Sons. p.183.

Stoll, B.A. (1982a). Prolonged survival in breast cancer. In *Prolonged arrest of cancer* (ed. B.A. Stoll). Chichester: John Wiley & Sons. p.59.

Stoll, B.A. (1982b). Management of disseminated breast cancer. In *The dying patient* (ed. E. Wilkes). Lancaster: MTP Press. p.111.

Surawicz, F.G., Brightwell, D.R., Weitzel, W.D., *et al.* (1976). Cancer, emotions and mental illness; the present state of understanding. *Am. J. Psychiatr.*, **133**,1306.

Tobias, J.S., and Harper, P.G. (1981). Who should treat cancer? *Lancet*, **i**,884.

Tormey, D.C. (1981) Discussion on presentation by Engelsman, E. *Rev. Endocr. Relat. Cancer*, Suppl. 8, 48.

Watson, J.V. (1981). What does response in cancer chemotherapy really mean? *Br. Med. J.*, **283**,34.

Winchester, D.P., Sener, S.F., Khandekar, J.D., *et al.* (1979). Symptomatology as an indicator of recurrent or metastatic breast cancer. *Cancer*, **43**,956.

Worden, J.W., and Weisman, A.D. (1977). Coping behavior and suicide in cancer. *Am. J. Med. Sci.*, **273**,169.

Cancer Treatment: End Point Evaluation
Edited by B.A. Stoll
© 1983 John Wiley & Sons Ltd.

Chapter

7 M.H. CULLEN

Acceptable Damage to Normal Tissue

INTRODUCTION

The starting point for judgments concerning the acceptability of normal tissue damage from cancer treatment should always be a realistic expectation of the beneficial effects of that treatment. Clearly, patients and doctors are prepared to accept a high level of toxicity where cure is a reasonable objective. Palliation, on the other hand, requires non-toxic treatments, almost by definition.

At the present time surgeons, radiotherapists, and chemotherapists also administer therapies which fall between these extremes. That is, they are neither *curative* (where a significant proportion of patients achieve normal survival) nor are they merely *palliative* (where symptom relief or prevention are the only objectives). The middle group may be called *retardative* and applies to those therapies which, as well as relieving or preventing symptoms, slow or temporarily reverse the progression of the disease, thus offering a prolongation of survival but not amounting to cure, in the vast majority of patients.

For this group in particular, judgments about the acceptability of undesired effects become more difficult as they become more important. This is especially so since the same treatment may be used in all three settings. The problem is compounded by wide differences between patients in what they will accept and also by often undeclared discrepancies between doctor and patient on this point.

As a baseline, it would be most helpful to have reliable quantitative data on the normal tissue damage caused by tumours themselves, and then compare

139

the altered patterns of injury resulting from treatment. Data of this sort are not available. We are also limited in our judgments by inadequate figures demonstrating unequivocal prolongation of survival resulting from many apparently retardative cancer treatments. The literature of cancer chemotherapy, in particular, contains numerous survival curves demonstrating that responders to a given therapy live longer than those who fail to respond. This is not conclusive evidence that prolonged survival results from treatment (discussed in Chapter 3). It implies that the therapist was convinced of his treatment's value and saw no need to compare it in a randomized trial, either with the best currently available treatment or with no treatment at all.

If one is sometimes uncertain about survival benefit with cancer treatment, how much more often is there doubt concerning the precise chance of symptomatic benefit? With these difficulties in mind, this chapter reviews, system by system, the damaging effects of chemotherapy and radiotherapy.

GASTROINTESTINAL TRACT

Nausea and vomiting are major causes of morbidity from cancer chemotherapy. They cause nutritional or electrolyte disturbances and may be indirectly fatal in patients with chemosensitive tumours who refuse treatment. The mechanisms are not known, but the onset is often delayed for several hours, arguing against a direct action on the chemoreceptor trigger zone or vomiting centre. The drugs particularly associated with this problem are mustine, dacarbazine, doxorubicin, cisplatin, lomustine, and cylcophosphamide.

Phenothiazines such as prochlorperazine are the most widely used antiemetic agents, and although they have generally been superior to placebo in controlled studies the benefit is marginal to most patients (Frytak and Moertel, 1981). For this reason a number of other agents have been studied with particular reference to the vomiting associated with cisplatin which is resistant to conventional drugs. The cannabinoids, δ-9-tetrahydrocannabinol and nabilone, have antiemetic activity in these circumstances but the side-effects of ataxia, sedation, and dysphoria have been common and they are not reliably effective with high-dose cisplatin (Lucas and Laszlo, 1980; Steele *et al.*, 1980).

The butyrophenones, haloperidol and droperidol, have both demonstrated efficacy in controlling chemotherapy-induced vomiting when other agents have failed (Neidhart *et al.*, 1980; Grossman *et al.*, 1979). An interesting recent report from Gralla *et al* (1981) shows that high-dose intravenous metoclopramide (i.e. a total of 10 mg/kg given in five divided doses from 30 min before to 8½ h after therapy) was more effective than placebo or prochlorpazine in randomized double-blind trials in patients receiving cisplatin.

Side-effects were minor and infrequent. Further studies of these agents are necessary to evaluate fully their clinical role.

Anticipatory nausea and vomiting is an even more difficult problem in a minority of patients and is very resistant to treatment. In a small number of patients Morrow (1981) has found some success using behavioural techniques.

Radiotherapy, particularly wide-field irradiation involving the abdomen, also causes nausea and vomiting which is generally alleviated using conventional agents (prochlorperazine, metoclopramide).

By analogy with other kinetically active normal tissues, one might expect that the intestinal mucosa would be a potential site of damage from anti-proliferative agents. There is evidence in animal studies that this is indeed the case. Malabsorption and histological abnormalities have been demonstrated with a number of antineoplastic drugs, but the clinical relevance of these findings is as yet undefined.

Shaw *et al.* (1979), as well as reviewing the animal work, report a small but well controlled study of their own in ten patients receiving combination chemotherapy for various solid tumours not involving the small intestine. Using Crosby capsule biopsy before and following chemotherapy, they showed villous blunting in the second biopsies in three patients, and using a battery of tests for malabsorption showed some impairment of fat, xylose, and vitamin A absorption after chemotherapy in some of their patients.

Slavin *et al* (1978) have reported findings in 33 adults dying from acute leukaemia treated with cytosine arabinoside as well as other drugs. However, they implicate the cytosine arabinoside in the production of widespread mucosal abnormalities including surface and glandular epithelial atypia, immaturity, and necrosis. The resulting breakdown of the mucosal barrier was thought to contribute to the serious infections caused by endogenous bacteria and fungae seen in these patients. There is a clear need for further studies of intestinal function during and after chemotherapy.

Radiotherapy at doses above 3000 rad to the abdomen can cause partial or subtotal villous atrophy, microvillous atrophy, reduced mucosal enzyme activity, and malabsorption. In general these acute effects of radiation injury are transient and the resulting diarrhoea settles rapidly. The late effects of intestinal irradiation can be more serious but are uncommon. Deital and Vasic (1979) described 35 patients who required hospitalization for late intestinal injuries presenting from two months to several years following radiation to the abdomen, pelvis or perineum. This was less than 3% of all patients who had received such radiotherapy. The problems encountered included continuing enteritis, proctocolitis, stricture, perforation, and fistulae.

There is evidence that combined modality treatment (particulary irradiation plus doxorubicin and actinomycin D) can in some circumstances cause quite unacceptable gastrointestinal damage (Ransom *et al.*, 1979).

MUCOCUTANEOUS REACTIONS

The spectrum of mucocutaneous toxicity from antitumour agents includes the stigma of alopecia, the unpleasantness of stomatitis, and the pain of local extravasation. The damaging effects of these agents on hair, mucous membranes, and skin will be discussed separately.

Hair

Temporary hair loss is an inevitable effect of agents which interfere with cell proliferation and it is not surprising that alopecia is a common dose-related side-effect of doxorubicin, cyclophosphamide, vincristine, methotrexate, bleomycin, daunomycin, 5–fluorouracil, and cranial irradiation (Levin and Greenwald, 1978). Following the cessation of therapy, normal hair growth resumes; indeed regrowth may commence during continued treatment.

An important part of minimising the distress caused by alopecia is to warn the patient before commencing treatment so that a wig may be ordered if desired. However, scalp tourniquets can delay hair loss and more recently, scalp cooling during administration of rapidly tissue-fixed drugs such as doxorubicin may significantly reduce the degree of hair loss (Dean et al., 1981). There is as yet little evidence to refute the theoretical objection that these methods of reducing scalp blood flow during chemotherapy administration may result in a protected sanctuary for future recurrent disease.

Mucous membrances

Oral mucositis is a common and important acute toxic reaction to a number of antineoplastic drugs. Not only is oral ulceration painful and unpleasant, but it may lead to impairment of nutrition. The agents most frequently responsible are methotrexate, 5-fluorouracil, cytosine arabinoside, doxorubicin, actinomycin D, daunorubicin, and bleomycin (Spiegel, 1981). Stomatitis and ulceration may result directly from inhibition of cell proliferation in the oral mucosa or indirectly as a result of drug-induced neutropenia with consequent local infection. Treatment is primarily aimed at alleviating symptoms with topical anaesthetics and cleansing mouthwashes, while maintaining adequate fluid and food intake. In the minority of cases where candida species are isolated, antifungal mouth washes and lozenges may speed recovery.

Radiotherapy may also have severely damaging effects on the oral mucosa and related tissues, some of which may persist long after the cancer has been eradicated (Dreizen et al., 1977). Radiation-induced xerostomia secondary to salivary gland damage is rapid in onset, and irreversible after high doses. Management is purely palliative. Xerostomia contributes to dental decay which can be rampant unless stringent protective steps are taken. Mucositis and loss of taste are common side-effects of oral radiotherapy which are usually reversible, but recovery may take several weeks after the end of treatment.

Skin

(a) Local extravasation reactions

A severe local extravasation reaction with prolonged pain, necrosis, ulceration, and ultimately contracture is among the most devastating unwanted effects of intravenous chemotherapy. The agent most commonly implicated is doxorubicin but actinomycin D, daunorubicin, mitomycin, mustine, vinblastine, vincristine, and dacarbazine are sometimes involved. Agents such as these should be administered only by experienced individuals carefully following the guidelines suggested by Ignoffo and Friedman (1980) and by Spiegel (1981).

Apart from stopping the injection immediately extravasation is suspected, there is little agreement as to the best immediate management of this problem. Ignoffo and Friedman (1980) advocate aspirating the subcutaneous bleb and instilling an antidote of which they list several for different situations and then warming the site of extravasation. Larson (1981), on the other hand, deplores the use of such antidotes and suggests a conservative approach with alternate cooling and warming. Barlock *et al.* (1977) prefer multiple intradermal and subcutaneous injections of hydrocortisone in and around the site of extravasation and a film of 1% hydrocortisone cream applied topically.

Once ulceration has occurred, Zweig and Wallach (1980) use sodium hypochlorite solution (which rapidly decomposes doxorubicin *in vitro*) applied to the ulcer base as a wet dressing with a thin film of petroleum jelly around the edge. There is more agreement on the proper management of cases which fail to settle rapidly. Early wide local excision with skin grafting is indicated in cases where necrosis, ulceration, and pain are not obviously resolving. Recent reports that topical dimethylsulphoxide can prevent doxorubicin-induced skin ulcers in animals need confirmation (Desai *et al.*, 1981).

(b)Generalized reactions

A number of antineoplastic drugs can produce cutaneous pigmentation. With busulfan, the syndrome resembles Addison's disease clinically with weakness, weight loss, nausea, anorexia, and hypotension as well as hyperpigmentation. Biochemical evidence of adrenal insufficiency has not been reported. Hyperpigmentation is not uncommon following bleomycin therapy. Skin folds, scars, scratch marks and injection sites may all be involved. More rarely, doxorubicin causes pigmentation of variable distribution including skin, nails, and mucous membranes. Other drugs have occasionally been associated with hyperpigmentation including 5-fluorouracil, cyclophosphamide, methotrexate, and mithramycin (Levine and Greenwald, 1978).

Reactivation of a radiation dermatitis ('radiation recall') in a previously irradiated field is sometimes seen following doxorubicin and actinomycin D and more rarely with other drugs (Adrian *et al.*, 1980). Other deeper tissues may also be involved in this process, including previously irradiated areas of oesophagus, lung, and bladder.

A wide variety of other skin reactions are recorded with antineoplastic drugs (Levine and Greenwald, 1978) but there are few agents which cause eruptions with any frequency. Cutaneous side-effects occur in the majority of patients who have received more than 200 mg of bleomycin (Cohen *et al.*, 1973). In addition to alopecia, pigment changes, and oral ulceration already discussed, cutaneous ulcers, morbilliform eruptions, a scleroderma-like reaction with infiltrated plaques, nodules, and linear bands on the hands histologically showing dermal sclerosis have all been reported. These changes are reversible on stopping the drug.

With increasing use of megavoltage irradiation, skin reactions are generally mild since maximum doses fall in subcutaneous tissues. The key pathological change is endarteritis obliterans associated with dense fibrous tissue producing the woody feel of heavily irradiated soft tissue. The principal risk in this situation is infection which can rapidly lead to massive tissue breakdown and ulceration.

BONE MARROW

The major cause of mortality from antitumour agents is granulocytopenia leading to overwhelming infection. For only a few drugs, for example vincristine, L-asparaginase, bleomycin, and the hormones, is myelosuppression not the dose-limiting toxicity. With the effectiveness and increasing availability of platelet transfusions, isolated secondary thrombocytopenia (i.e. less than 20 000/mm^3) should not be a cause of death from cancer treatment although HL-A matching may be required in circumstances where allo-immunization is a problem (Mittal *et al.*, 1976).

Precise indications and protocols for giving platelet transfusions are discussed in an excellent review by Higby and Henderson (1981). The prevention and management of infections in granulocytopenic patients, on the other hand, is much less straightforward. The number of episodes of severe infection rises steeply with neutrophil counts below 1000 (Bodey, 1975) and mortality is related, amongst other factors, to the duration of neutropenia. The prompt diagnosis and treatment of such infections with parenteral antibiotics and, in certain circumstances, granulocyte transfusions can be life-saving but not invariably so. This topic is the subject of a number of recent review articles (Rodrigues and Ketchel, 1981; Higby and Henderson, 1981).

There is some evidence supporting the use of protected environments and prophylactic antimicrobial agents in the management of patients who are severely neutropenic. These rather complex data together with the practicalities of infection prevention during granulocytopenia are discussed by Schimpff (1980) and by Young (1981). It is clearly vital that clinicians using these agents have a thorough understanding of the severity and duration of myelosuppression that may be expected from any particular regime and be prepared to justify the risks involved and vigorously manage these complications should they arise.

The time course of neutropenia varies widely from the brief and rapidly occurring nadir of vinblastine to the very delayed nadir associated with the nitrosoureas. The latter may also exhibit a rather unpredictable cumulative myelotoxicity.

Other important variables in determining myelotoxicity include the schedule of drug administration (e.g. bolus injection versus continuous infusion—for cell-cycle stage-specific agents), bone marrow involvement by the malignant process, and concurrent or prior irradiation of haemopoietic marrow. Total nodal irradiation in Hodgkin's disease, for example, involves treatment of approximately 60–70% of the active adult bone marrow and both acute and late effects are observed. The peripheral blood counts decline after the first 2–3 weeks of treatment, recovering within 2–4 weeks of interrupting therapy (Kaplan, 1972). Following completion of therapy it may then take several months for peripheral counts to return to normal.

Rubin and Scarantino (1978) have studied bone marrow recovery with isotope scanning in Hodgkin's disease patients treated with total nodal irradiation. They found no evidence of in-field regeneration six months to one year after irradiation. At 1–2 years 54% of patients showed evidence of regeneration within the irradiated fields; at 2–3 years, 66%; at 4–5 years, 75%. It is thus not surprising that antineoplastic chemotherapy given in extensively irradiated patients can produce severe and sometimes precipitous myelosuppression. Close cooperation between medical oncologist and radiotherapist is necessary for successful treatment with combined modalities.

There is increasing evidence that some cytotoxic drugs can cause a long-lasting proliferative defect in the haemopoietic stem cell compartment as well as the better known acute effects. Botnick *et al.* (1979) have compared the effects of various drugs on self-renewal potential of the stem cell compartment (CFU-S) in mice. Busulphan was found to be the most damaging since it killed the most primitive stem cells preferentially. 5-Fluorouracil was the least damaging to the proliferative capacity of the stem cell compartment, while carmustine and cyclophosphamide damaged it in an intermediate way. The authors suggest that this may relate to the late marrow failure sometimes seen following busulphan and carmustine.

NERVOUS SYSTEM

Neurotoxicity from cancer therapy can take many forms and a wide range of individual antineoplastic agents may exert very damaging and long-lasting effects on both peripheral and central nervous systems. Cancer drugs and radiotherapy have been the subject of comprehensive reviews of this topic (Weiss *et al.*, 1974; Sheline *et al.*, 1980).

The vinca alkaloid, vincristine, is unique in its dose-limiting effect of neurotoxicity. The related drug, vinblastine, has a similar spectrum of unwanted effects on the nervous system, but its bone marrow depressing activity limits the doses given such that neurotoxicity is rarely a problem. The newer vinca alkaloid, vindesine, is both neurotoxic and myelotoxic but possibly to a rather lesser extent than vincristine and vinblastine, respectively.

Loss of the ankle deep tendon reflex is virtually universal in patients receiving therapeutic doses of vincristine (Holland *et al.*, 1973). Numbness of fingertips and toes and paraesthesiae are extremely common and rarely serious enough to discontinue effective treatment. Severe pains in the jaw or throat occasionally follow the first or second dose of vincristine but rarely continue with further treatment. The most disabling manifestation of vincristine neurotoxicity is motor involvement, the symptoms of which are dose-related and are preceded by areflexia. Typically the dorsiflexors of toes and ankle and extensors of wrists and fingers are affected symmetrically. Recovery following discontinuation of treatment is slow and may be incomplete.

Cranial and autonomic nerves may both be the prominent site of involvement (Sandler *et al.*, 1969), presenting, for instance, with ptosis or diplopia; or with constipation which may progress to severe ileus and faecal impaction or orthostatic hypotension. The key to preventing the severe neurological side-effects of vincristine is regular and careful review of patients receiving the drug and discontinuing its administration at the earliest sign of potentially serious damage.

Peripheral neuropathy has been observed during treatment with cisplatin (Hadley and Herr, 1979). It is primarily axonal and sensory, resembling that seen with other heavy metals, and may be irreversible. A more common problem is ototoxicity consisting of high-frequency hearing loss.

Procarbazine is associated with a mild peripheral neuropathy and disorder of conscious level in a small (around 10%) proportion of patients receiving daily oral therapy (Weiss *et al.* 1974). 5-Fluorouracil can rarely cause an acute cerebellar syndrome which although not total-dose-related is seen more frequently with intensive regimes. It is completely reversible on discontinuation of therapy and may also remit on lowering the dose or increasing the interval between courses (Moertel *et al.*, 1964).

The psychiatric complications of cancer therapy have been poorly studied. A recent review by Peterson and Popkin (1980) discusses affective and organic mental disorders associated with agents such as vinblastine, L-asparaginase, mitomycin, and hexamethylmelamine, and the well known psychotic reactions occasionally observed with prednisone. These all seem reversible on stopping the offending drug. The more important effects of methotrexate are discussed below.

Neurotoxicity of leukaemia therapy

In assessing the unwanted effects of central nervous system prophylaxis as part of the treatment of acute lymphocytic leukaemia (ALL), it is important to remember that long-term survival has undoubtedly increased as a result. The treatment and prevention of overt CNS leukaemia commonly involves the combination of irradiation and intrathecal methotexate, and toxicity may be acute, subacute or delayed.

Most patients receiving CNS radiotherapy experience mild nausea, vomiting, headache, and anorexia, which is usually self-limiting. Within 1 to 2 months after completing prophylactic cranial radiation, 40% of patients with ALL develop somnolence, lethargy, and anorexia, which is again generally transient but in severe cases may be treated successfully with adrenocorticosteroids (Freeman *et al.*, 1973). The most common type of intrathecal methotrexate neurotoxocity is acute arachnoiditis. Usually occurring within 12 h of administration, it is characterized by headache, nausea, vomiting, nuchal rigidity, and fever with a CSF granulocytic pleocytosis. It too will usually disappear spontaneously within 72 h (Haghbin, 1977). The mechanism underlying this reaction is not known but it seems to be related to the drug itself rather than to the diluent (Pizzo *et al.*, 1979).

A myelopathy or encephalopathy may develop within days to weeks after starting intrathecal methotrexate therapy. This subacute toxic reaction, manifested as para- or quadriparesis, cranial nerve palsies, seizures or cerebellar dysfunction, appears to be related to the dose and duration of methotrexate therapy and has been observed following high-dose intravenous therapy. Neurological sequelae are minimal. Pizzo *et al.* (1979) have suggested that careful monitoring of the CSF methotrexate concentration, and adjusting the dose in those patients with abnormally high levels, reduces the incidence of acute and subacute neurotoxicity.

A delayed form of methotrexate neurotoxicity developing after months or years presents clinically with dementia, personality change, ataxia, spasticity, and occasionally seizures. The pathological appearances, consisting of discrete areas of coagulative necrosis, axonal damage, and reactive astrocytosis, have been observed in 6% of cases with ALL at autopsy (Price and Jamieson, 1975). The risk of developing this syndrome appears to be increased by cranial irradiation and is related to the cumulative dose of methotrexate. There are some recent data suggesting an adverse effect of CNS prophylaxis on intellectual function in children with ALL (Moss *et al.*, 1981).

HEART

The principal total-dose-limiting effect of the anthracycline antibiotics, doxorubicin and daunorubicin, is congestive cardiomyopathy. This may be insidious in onset, the first symptoms being tachycardia and cough, or it may come on abruptly, presenting as typical congestive cardiac failure (CCF). This may develop during treatment but there are recorded instances of heart failure developing six months to almost a year from the last dose (Minow *et al.*, 1975; Von Hoff *et al.*, 1977). Presentations with fatal pulmonary infarction and with cerebral emboli from mural thrombi have also been reported.

The incidence (and probably the severity) of CCF is directly related to the cumulative dose of the drug, being 3.5% after 400 mg/m^2, 7% at 550 mg/m^2, and 18% at 700 mg/m^2 for doxorubicin (Von Hoff *et al.*, 1979). For daunorubicin, the figures are 1.5% incidence of CCF at a total dose of 600 mg/m^2 and 12% at 1000 mg/m^2 (Von Hoff *et al.*, 1977). For both drugs there is a continuum of increasing risk with increasing total dose. For doxorubicin the slope increases at around 450–500 mg/m^2 and it is recommended that the drug be stopped when this total cumulative dose is reached, except in the infrequent patient in whom the threat of disease and the benefit of further doxorubicin therapy clearly outweigh the risk of heart failure.

Patients who receive mediastinal or left chest wall radiotherapy before, with or after doxorubicin therapy appear to be at increased risk of cardiomyopathy (Bristow *et al.*, 1978), but although an arbitrary cut-off dosage of 400 mg/m^2 has been recommended there are inadequate data available at the present time to support this (Von Hoff, 1980). Furthermore, it is not clear whether prior heart disease predisposes to doxorubicin cardiomyopathy, although patients over 70 are at increased risk (Bristow *et al.*, 1978).

The most frequent histological abnormalities are myofibrillar lysis and cytoplasmic vacuolization — features not distinctly different from those associated with many other cardiomyopathies (Billingham *et al.*, 1978). Probably all patients have some cardiac damage when treated with these drugs and will become symptomatic if a sufficient total dose is given (Henderson and Frei, 1980). A number of agents (e.g. digoxin, α -tocopherol) have been suggested as possibly reducing the risk of cardiotoxocity based upon unproven hypotheses concerning the pathogenesis of the disorder. As yet there is no convincing evidence to support their use.

It has recently been reported that prolonged intravenous infusion of doxorubicin (compared with intravenous bolus injection) significantly reduces the risk of damage without compromising antitumour activity (Benjamin *et al.*, 1981). If this finding is confirmed in larger studies, the inconvenience and expense of hospitalization for 48–96 h infusions will need to be weighed against the risk of cardiomyopathy. There is no serial, non-invasive test of left ventricular function of proven value in decreasing the incidence of doxorubicin–induced cardiomyopathy (Henderson and Frei, 1980). Acute cardiac toxicity is much less of a clinical problem although ECG changes are reported during or shortly after doxorubicin administration.

A serious, although uncommon, problem is an acute fatal myopericarditis following very high-dose cyclophosphamide administration, e.g. 144–270 mg/kg prior to bone marrow transplantation (Mills and Roberts, 1979). 5-Fluorouracil can rarely cause acute cardiotoxicity, ranging from mild angina without persisting electrocardiographic changes to frank myocardial infarction (Villani *et al.*, 1979). Administration of this drug should be discontinued immediately if precordial pain occurs.

As well as increasing the risk of doxorubicin-induced cardiomyopathy, ionizing radiation in the therapeutic dose range can damage the human heart in its own right (Stewart and Fajardo, 1971). An exudative pericarditis is the most common lesion, occurring usually within a year of initiation of radiation therapy. This generally follows a benign course, but can progress to tamponade and pericardial constriction. Large volume irradiation to the heart may also result in diffuse myocardial fibrosis. The risk of both lesions is dose-dependent.

LUNG

Interstitial pneumonitis is the principal dose-limiting toxic effect of bleomycin. The clinical features include non-productive cough, dyspnoea, sometimes fever with diffuse râles on physical examination (Willson, 1978). Radiographically bilateral basal infiltrates may progress to a diffuse interstitial pneumonitis. Hilar adenopathy or pleural effusion due to bleomycin toxicity have not been reported. Progressive arterial hypoxaemia, restrictive ventilatory defect, and decreased diffusion capacity for carbon monoxide are found on lung function testing and may pre-date symptoms or x-ray abnormalities (Pascual *et al.*, 1973).

The histological changes have been recently reviewed by Sostman *et al.* (1977) and include diffuse alveolar damage, organizing interstitial pneumonia, and interstitial pulmonary fibrosis. The incidence of bleomycin-induced pulmonary damage is related to the total dose of drug administered

(Blum *et al.*, 1973) and increases with the age of the patient. Review of over 1000 bleomycin-treated patients demonstrated no life-threatening pulmonary disease at a total dose of below 150 mg (Sostman *et al.* 1977). However, in one series the incidence reached 66% in patients who received 359 mg/m^2 and a mortality of 10% is reported among patients receiving more than 550 mg/m^2 (Schein and Winokur, 1975).

Thoracic irradiation appears to enhance bleomycin-induced lung damage both when given at the same time as the drug (Catane *et al.*, 1979) and when radiation precedes drug therapy (Samuels *et al.*, 1976). The latter authors accepted an *overall* bleomycin-related mortality of 5% in view of the 75% response rate and substantially improved survival achieved with bleomycin combination chemotherapy in metastatic testicular cancer. However, in patients who have received thoracic irradiation, careful consideration must be given to the toxicity-risk:benefit ratio whenever bleomycin is used. There is also evidence of synergism between prior bleomycin therapy and a high concentration of inspired oxygen at operation. Goldiner *et al.* (1978) recommend low concentrations of inspired oxygen during and after surgery in patients who have received bleomycin treatment.

Bleomycin should be withdrawn as soon as symptoms, x-ray abnormalities or significant changes in pulmonary function appear and, if no infective cause is found, lung biopsy should be performed. Should this indicate toxicity, permanent withdrawal of bleomycin is mandatory. The process frequently progresses but may be reversible. There are insufficient data to assess the role, if any, for corticosteroids in the treatment of bleomycin pulmonary toxicity (Sostman *et al.*, 1977).

Busulfan is the drug of choice in the treatment of chronic myelogenous leukaemia. Long-term therapy is a prerequisite for the appearance of busulfan lung—the average interval being more than four years from starting treatment (Sostman *et al.*, 1977). Respiratory symptoms, abnormal chest x-ray findings and pulmonary function tests develop in 2.5–11.5% of patients who receive the drug. Clinically it usually resembles the picture described for bleomycin, although an acute onset has been described. The process usually, although not invariably, progresses despite withdrawal of the drug and a fatal outcome is common (Schein and Winokur, 1975).

The nitrosoureas, particularly carmustine, have been reported to cause pulmonary fibrosis, albeit rarely, following cumulative doses in the range 580–2100 mg/m^2. This problem has recently been reviewed by Weiss and Muggia (1980). These authors also discuss the more transient, non-dose-related pneumonitis occasionally associated with methotrexate, as well as the fibrotic reactions (resembling those due to bleomycin and busulfan) seen rarely with mitomycin, cyclophosphamide, and chlorambucil. Procarbazine is occasionally associated with a hypersensitivity pneumonitis.

The pulmonary effects of radiation therapy have been comprehensively reviewed by Gross (1977). The clinical syndrome can be divided into two consecutive phases: an acute pneumonitis occurring within 2 to 6 months after therapy and later a fibrotic phase. Cough and dyspnoea are the principal features of radiation pneumonitis. They may last for as little as a week and subside without sequelae or persist for a month or more subsiding gradually. Despite symptomatic improvement, the majority of patients with pneumonitis will eventually develop radiological pulmonary fibrosis. In a few severely affected patients the distorted pulmonary architecture may result in chronic respiratory insufficiency.

The incidence and severity of radiation damage are related to the volume of lung irradiated, the total dose, the rate of its delivery, and the quality of the radiation. Concomitant chemotherapy, previous radiation therapy, and steroid withdrawal potentiate the damaging effects of radiation. As for treatment, most centres commence high-dose cortiscosteroid therapy as soon as pneumonitis is diagnosed, gradually reducing the dose over several weeks.

KIDNEY AND BLADDER

Cisplatin has been the major recent addition to the medical oncologist's armamentarium, made possible only since the irreversible nephrotoxicity which characterized its early use has been avoidable. Autopsy and animal experimental data suggest that this renal toxicity is analogous to the acute tubular necrosis of heavy-metal poisoning (Gonzales-Vitale *et al.*, 1977), manifest as a fall in glomerular filtration rate (GFR) causing a rising creatinine. Forced hydration and diuresis have dramatically reduced the risk of nephrotoxicity.

Examining this phenomenon in depth, Stark and Howell (1978) have reported a careful study of both glomerular and tubular function in 15 patients having 49 courses of cisplatin (20 mg/m^2/day for 5 days with 1000 ml saline prehydration). With this regime there was no immediate or cumulative increase in serum creatinine and only a small transient fall in GFR. No tubular dysfunction was demonstrable. Four patients with pre-existing renal insufficiency (GFR 17–44 ml/min/m^2) experienced no significant additional nephrotoxicity. With a more vigorous hydration and diuretic programme, it has been possible to administer safely 50 mg/m^2 of cisplatin in a 2 h outpatient regimen (Vogl *et al.*, 1981).

Nephrotoxicity has become a significant problem with methotrexate only since the introduction of very high-dose therapy with folinic acid rescue. In one study the serum creatinine increased by more than 50% in over half the patients (Pitman *et al.*, 1975). Since the methotrexate is eliminated largely unchanged, any reduction of its renal clearance will greatly enhance its myelotoxicity. Forced hydration and alkalinization of the urine have been recommended to reduce the risk of nephrotoxicity and lower doses with more prolonged courses of folinic acid rescue are mandatory in patients with lowered GFR.

Nephrotoxicity is the principal dose-limiting toxic effect of streptozotocin. The kidney is also a very radiosensitive organ and the whole of both organs should be excluded from radiation fields if possible. Irradiation of only part of one kidney can result in hypertension months or years later. If kidney irradiation cannot be avoided, an upper dose limit of 2000 rad has been recommended (Strickland, 1980).

Acrolein is a degradation product of cyclophosphamide which contributes little to the antitumour effects of the drug. However, its release in the bladder is known to be the cause of haemorrhagic cystitis which can complicate high-dose cyclophosphamide therapy and, more rarely low-dose treatment given for long periods (Bischel, 1979). Maintaining a forced diuresis during and shortly after intravenous administration of high doses significantly reduces the risk of this complication.

In addition, 2-mercaptoethane sulphonate sodium (mesnum) has been shown to prevent cyclophosphamide-induced cystitis by reacting with and inactivating acrolein *in vivo* (Scheef *et al.*, 1979). Ifosfamide is also metabolized to acrolein and mesnum is effective in preventing the urothelial toxicity which has hitherto been a major dose-limiting factor with this drug (Bryant *et al.*, 1980).

LIVER AND METABOLIC EFFECTS

Abnormal liver function test (LFT) results are common in patients with disseminated malignant disease and it is often impossible to assess their significance. However, a number of antineoplastic drugs have been frequently associated with mild hepatotoxicity and a few, only rarely, with severe toxicity. With methotrexate, for instance, there is a slight but definite risk of hepatic fibrosis and cirrhosis which is said to be commoner with the now little used continuous oral regime (Weinstein, 1977). Liver function test abnormalities are not reliable indicators of this problem. L-Asparaginase produced LFT abnormalities in 76 of 123 patient trials reported by Land *et al.* (1972), but only eight cases were taken off the study because of hepatotoxicity. Fatty change was the prominent histological abnormality.

6-Mercaptopurine hepatotoxicity is heralded by elevations in serum transaminase levels, at times accompanied by increases in serum alkaline phosphatase and bilirubin (Schein and Winokur, 1975). Histologically, hepatocellular necrosis and biliary stasis are the most specific findings. In general, the LFT abnormalities return to normal after discontinuing therapy. Hepatotoxicity is also reported with a number of other drugs including the nitrosoureas, streptozotocin, chlorambucil, dacarbazine, mustine, and 6-thioguanine, but is very rarely dose-limiting (Creaven and Mihich, 1977).

There are a number of rather poorly understood metabolic complications of cancer chemotherapy which will be discussed briefly. Vincristine administration is occasionally associated with the syndrome of inappropriate ADH secretion occurring several days after single or multiple doses, usually in association with other signs of neurotoxicity (Stuart, *et al.* 1975), as well as elevated ADH levels. Cyclophosphamide (and ifosfamide) in high dosage is also associated with brief, self-limiting water retention which may result from a direct effect of cyclophosphamide on the renal tubule (Bode *et al.*, 1980).

Hyperuricaemia leading to renal failure is a potentially fatal complication of rapid tumour lysis following chemotherapy for leukaemia and lymphoma in particular (Pochedly, 1974). Prophylactic allopurinol given with or before chemotherapy plus adequate hydration has greatly reduced the risk of this occurrence. Patients who are hyperuricaemic before treatment should be given allopurinol to lower the uric acid level to normal before chemotherapy is commenced. Should acute renal failure develop, urgent rehydration and alkalinization of the urine is recommended; however, in oliguric patients the former must be carefully judged and the latter may be impossible. In the absence of volume depletion, the only effective treatment is haemodialysis (Lancet Editorial, 1974).

Chemotherapy may contribute to several other metabolic disturbances seen in acute leukaemia (Afzal Mir and Delamore, 1978; O'Regan *et al.*, 1977); in particular, hyponatraemia and hypokalaemia (secondary to an increased osmolal clearance caused by a release of electrolytes, urea, urate, etc., during chemotherapy) and aminoaciduria and hyperphosphaturia (resulting from proximal tubular dysfunction). Rapid cell lysis with chemotherapy for acute promyelocytic leukaemia can exacerbate the bleeding diathesis characteristic of this disease (Jones and Saleem, 1978).

Mithramycin, rarely used as an antitumour drug, causes hypocalcaemia (possibly by inhibiting the action of parathyroid hormone on the osteoclast) and is now regularly used to treat hypercalcaemia due to malignant disease. The finding that streptozotocin caused hyperglycaemia through an effect on the pancreatic islets led to its use against islet cell tumours. L-Asparaginase can quite commonly cause a reversible diabetic state requiring short-term insulin therapy, and cisplatin is known to cause hypomagnesaemia secondary to inappropriate renal tubular loss which is occasionally symptomatic (Schilsky and Anderson, 1979).

Metabolic complications of cancer therapy are rarely dose-limiting when the clinician is aware of, and prepared for, their occurrence.

IMMUNITY AND HYPERSENSITIVITY REACTIONS

There exists a considerable literature describing the immunosuppressive properties of antineoplastic drugs in experimental animals (reviewed by

Haskell, 1977). There is much less information on which to evaluate these immunosuppressive effects in man in the clinical setting. However, it would appear that most antineoplastic drugs inhibit antigen recognition or processing, or depress clonal amplification of lymphocytes. In general, maximum depression of the primary humoral immune response is observed when antiproliferative drugs are given close to the time of antigenic stimulation. Pre-existing humoral immunity (the secondary response) is less commonly affected at the doses ordinarily used in cancer chemotherapy (Markoe and Saluk, 1979).

For both single-agent and combination chemotherapy, phytohaemagglutinin responses, macrophage migration as well as primary antibody responses are reduced but recover almost completely within 2–3 days of stopping therapy (Haskell, 1977). It seems likely that these demonstrable abnormalities are related to the opportunist (protozoal, viral, and fungal) infections occurring in patients, particularly those with leukaemia and lymphoma, treated with antineoplastic drugs. The immunosuppression of malignant disease itself as well as the use of broad-spectrum antibacterial antibiotics may also contribute.

Irradiation of the immune system (which may include treatment of large volumes of blood in transit in the irradiated field) has also been shown to interfere with normal immune responses. Furthermore, the abnormalities can persist for much longer periods after exposure than is the case with chemotherapy. For instance, radiation suppresses primary antibody formation even if given several weeks prior to immunization. As with chemotherapy, secondary antibody responses are more resistant. Reduction in cell-mediated immunity is also demonstrable following radiotherapy which in some cases may persist for periods in excess of 10 years (reviewed by Markoe and Saluk, 1979).

Hypersensitivity reactions are uncommon with the vast majority of cancer chemotherapeutic agents but are occasionally serious and life-threatening (Weiss and Bruno, 1981). L-Asparaginase from *Escherichia coli* has the highest incidence of hypersensitivity reactions of all anticancer agents ranging from 6 to 43% of patients reported. The higher figures have occurred in series where the drug was used as a single agent. In combination with vincristine, prednisone, and 6-mercaptopurine (which may act as immunosuppressants), the incidence is 10% or less.

Intramuscular administration is as effective as intravenous but much less commonly associated with hypersensitivity problems. The clinical picture is variable but may include urticaria, dyspnoea, agitation, hypotension, facial oedema, abdominal cramps, laryngo-spasm and stridor, rash, pruritus, and loss of consciousness. Treatment is with antihistamines, corticosteroid, and adrenaline if necessary. Following the development of hypersensitivity, an antigenically distinct L-asparaginase from *Erwinia carotovora* should be substituted. Similar reactions are seen much less commonly following cisplatin, daunorubicin, and doxorubicin administration.

Doxorubicin can cause a localized urticaria at the site of drug injection— the so-called 'flare'. This does not preclude further treatment with the drug and probably does not involve antibodies or sensitized lymphocytes. Bleomycin quite commonly (20–25% of patients) causes pyrexia 1 to 4 h after injection and rarely this is associated with marked hypotension. Very occasionally intravenous cyclophosphamide and methotrexate can cause anaphylactic reactions. Vincristine, vinblastine, 5-fluorouracil, the nitro-soureas, hydroxyurea, 6-thioguanine, 6-mercaptopurine, mithramycin, acti-nomycin D, and dacarbazine have *not* as yet been recorded as causing verified hypersensitivity reactions (Weiss and Bruno, 1981).

SECOND MALIGNANCIES

Most oncologists can recall at least one patient developing a second malignant disease as a result of successful treatment of an earlier tumour. Before reviewing the evidence available on induced second malignancies, it is worth remembering that most studies show an increased risk of second tumours with minimal or no therapy in patients with malignant disease (Bender and Young, 1978). Nevertheless, radiotherapy and chemotherapy, and in particular the two combined, are associated with an expanding literature on second malignancies.

Radiotherapy

Arsenau *et al.* (1972), reporting 149 patients who received intensive radio-therapy for Hodgkin's disease, described three patients with second tumours—an incidence 3.8 times that expected. Senyszyn *et al.* (1970) reviewed 13 cases of sarcoma occurring within the irradiated field in patients with breast cancer having had post-operative radiotherapy. The authors estimate the relative risk in these circumstances as substantially less than 0.22%.

Boice and Hutchison (1980) have made an extensive study of leukaemia risk in women who have been treated with radiotherapy for cervical cancer. Among 28 490 women followed up between 1960 and 1970, 13 cases of leukaemia were observed. On the basis of general population rates, 15.5 cases would have been expected. In summary, the risk following therapeutic doses of radiation are very small and, in general, related to dose and time since the initial treatment (Hutchison, 1976).

Chemotherapy

Despite rather heterogeneous treatment groups in the literature, it is becoming clear that long-term single-alkylating-agent therapy is associated with an increased risk of acute non-lymphocytic leukaemia. Reimer *et al.* (1977) reviewed 5455 patients treated for advanced ovarian cancer. Thirteen cases of acute leukaemia were recorded compared to 0.62 cases expected (relative risk = 21.0). All 13 had received alkylating agents but nine also received radiotherapy. The relative risk was calculated as 171.4 for patients followed for two years or more. Of nine patients autopsied, six had no evidence of residual ovarian cancer.

This risk rate represents an incidence of only 0.3% of all patients treated and the authors stressed that the benefits of treatment clearly outweighed the risks in such a tumour with a poor prognosis. Other reports of acute leukaemia following long-term chemotherapy with alkylating agents alone or in combination stress the high incidence of refractory anaemia preceding the leukaemia by several months, and the extreme resistance to treatment and short survival characteristic of the induced leukaemias (Kapadia *et al.*, 1980; Auclerc *et al.*, 1979).

Chemotherapy with radiotherapy

The study of Arsenau *et al.* (1972) cited above was the first to highlight convincingly the synergistic carcinogenic potential of the two treatment modalities. Patients who received intensive chemotherapy and radiotherapy (generally total nodal irradiation) had a 29-fold increased incidence of a second tumour compared to a three- to four-fold increase for either modality alone. This group went on to investigate the sequencing of the two forms of treatment and found that by far the highest-risk group were those patients who had received intensive radiotherapy, then relapsed and received intensive chemotherapy (Canellos *et al.*, 1975).

The Stanford experience of patients with Hodgkin's disease treated electively with irradiation followed immediately by adjuvant combination chemotherapy is reported by Coleman *et al.* (1977). They report an actuarial risk of leukaemia of 3.2% at seven years compared with a risk of 4.7% where chemotherapy was used to 'salvage' radiotherapy relapses. There were no cases in patients having radiotherapy or chemotherapy alone but the number at risk in the latter group was small. The now extensive and complicated literature on multiple primary cancers in Hodgkin's disease has been well reviewed recently along with a discussion of statistical methods of analysis by Brody and Schottenfeld (1980).

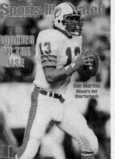
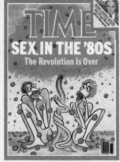
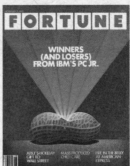
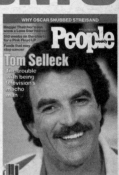
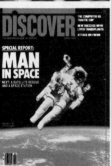
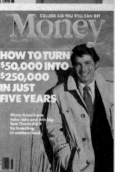

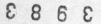

ENDOCRINE EFFECTS

Gonadal effects

The reproductive potential of patients receiving cancer chemotherapy has only recently been the subject of concern and hence detailed study. The emergence of long-term survivors following treatment for Hodgkin's disease, lymphoblastic leukaemia, and choriocarcinoma has allowed retrospective and more recently prospective studies of gonadal function. The effects of chemotherapy vary with the sex of the patient and the age at which treatment occurred (Schilsky *et al.*, 1980).

(a) Effects in adult man

Total-dose-dependent depletion of the germinal epithelium lining the seminiferous tubules is the primary testicular lesion seen following alkylating-agent therapy (Miller, 1971). Complete aplasia of germinal cells but sparing Sertoli cells and the interstitial Leydig cells are the typical testicular biopsy appearances, and are associated with high serum follicle-stimulating hormone (FSH) levels.

In a prospective study of patients with Hodgkin's disease, Chapman *et al.* (1981) report azoospermia and elevated FSH levels in all of 14 men after completion of only two cycles of chemotherapy. However, even before therapy 12 of 37 patients had inadequate sperm counts, and histological abnormalities (predominantly tubular hyalinization and thickening of the basement membrane) were noted in eight of nine pretreatment testicular biopsies. During therapy, 17 of 21 men had mild or absent libido which did not correlate with changes in testosterone level.

Reversibility of testicular damage is unpredictable but there is no doubt that spermatogenesis may recover with increasing time off chemotherapy—15 to 49 months in one study following cyclophosphamide (Buchanan *et al.*, 1975). Combination chemotherapy may also be followed by recovery of tubular function although there is some evidence that procarbazine-containing regimes produce particularly long-lasting azoospermia, more than 52 months in five of six patients studied by Roeser *et al.* (1978).

The radiation tolerance of the normal testis is well worked out but the dose received during an inverted 'Y' field for Hodgkin's disease for instance varies considerably with technique and method of testicular shielding. Slanina *et al.* (1977) report a very high incidence of azoospermia and oligospermia in patients studied up to nine years following treatment which included the use of a testicular capsule. Thar and Million (1980), however, claim that, with careful shielding, the total dose can be kept below 100 rad and that complete recovery will occur in the majority of patients by two years.

Notwithstanding the findings of Chapman *et al.* (1981) discussed above, sperm banking should be offered to all patients facing the high probability of induced sterility although conception rates using preserved semen remain around 50% (Ansbacher, 1978) for healthy donors and almost certainly less for cancer patients.

(b) Effects in adult women

Ovarian fibrosis with follicle destruction, elevation of serum FSH, luteinizing hormone (LH), and reduction in serum oestradiol are the characteristics of chemotherapy-induced ovarian failure. Symptoms of oestrogen deficiency and premature menopause may result. The greater the total dose of alkylating agent (the most frequently studied group of drugs) and the older the woman, the more likely it is to be irreversible.

The latter observation also holds for combination chemotherapy. Chapman *et al.* (1979) studied the effects of mustine, vinblastine, procarbazine, and prednisolone (MVPP) in 41 women aged 20 to 51 with advanced Hodgkin's disease. Five (12%) had normal ovarian function (as assessed by hormone and menstrual status) after a minimum follow-up of 10 months. However, 69% of women under 30 continued to have regular or irregular menses. Schilsky *et al.* (1981) note similar findings in 27 women treated with MOPP alone or plus radiation excluding the pelvis. Forty-six per cent had ovarian failure when studied (median, nine years after treatment). Eighty-nine per cent of these were older than 25 at the time of treatment in contrast to 80% of patients under 25 who continued to menstruate regularly.

Horning *et al.* (1981) have recently reported data on young women (median age at treatment, 23 years) showing return of regular menstruation in 56% of 34 patients at a median follow-up period of 45 months from combination chemotherapy for Hodgkin's disease. This study also demonstrates an apparent additive effect of total lymphoid irradiation (after midline oophoropexy) with chemotherapy. Forty-seven per cent of women treated with irradiation alone retained regular menstruation compared with 20% receiving combined treatment. Pregnancies occurred in all three groups of patients with no foetal wastage or birth defects.

Examining the effects of irradiation alone following oophoropexy in Hodgkin's disease, Thomas *et al.* (1976) reported that the operation itself had little effect on fertility in that successful pregnancies occurred in four of six young women in whom the ovaries had received little or no irradiation. Four patients who received an ovarian dose of 150 rad over four weeks showed normal menstrual function and gonadotrophin levels. One subsequently became pregnant. Of the ten patients who received 500–3500 rad to the ovaries, eight had persisting amenorrhoea and two had resumed menstrual cycles following 6 to 24 months amenorrhoea, one of these having become pregnant. Age, as well as dose, is an important variable influencing the effects of radiation on fertility in women. For example, over 40 years of age, 400 rad results in 100% sterility, whereas in younger women the figure is around 30% (Ash, 1980).

(c) Effects in boys

The effects of alkylating-agent therapy on the pre-pubertal testis again seem to be total-dose-related. In one study, boys receiving total cyclophosphamide doses of 6.2 to 14.3 g between 6½ and 10 years previously had normal sperm counts, gonadotrophin levels, and testicular histology, whereas those receiving 11.8 to 39.3 g were azoospermic and had germinal aplasia (Etteldorf *et al.* 1976).

The effects of chemotherapy avoiding alkylating agents and methylhydrazines may be a great deal less damaging on the pre-pubertal testis as reported by Blatt *et al.* (1981). Fourteen boys with acute lymphoblastic leukaemia were followed for a median 5½ years. All had normal testicular function as determined by serum gonadotrophin and testosterone levels and by pubertal development on examination throughout the follow-up period. Semen samples from all six of the patients tested were essentially normal. The authors conclude that the administration of antileukaemic chemotherapy can be compatible with normal gonadal development.

There is a suggestion that MVPP chemotherapy *during* puberty may affect both germ cell and Leydig cell function (Sherins *et al.*, 1978). In 10 pubertal boys treated for Hodgkin's disease, elevated FSH and LH levels with low normal serum testosterone levels were recorded in nine who developed gynaecomastia.

(d) Effects in girls

There are very few well-documented reports of ovarian function in girls receiving antineoplastic chemotherapy before the menarche. In one study in acute leukaemia (Siris *et al.*, 1976), the vast majority of patients demonstrated normal ovarian function although the chemotherapy consisted primarily of antimetabolites and, as has been seen in the other patient groups, it is alkylating agents and methylhydrazines which produce the most damaging effects. Irradiation in childhood for abdominal malignancy invariably results in permanent ovarian failure even when the field extends no further than the sacral promontory (Shalet *et al.*, 1976).

In the curative therapy group, which is the main concern in this section, even a high probability of sterility may well be acceptable if it is unavoidable. Nevertheless, there is a clear need for more detailed prospective studies of gonadal function following cancer chemotherapy including newer agents like cisplatin so that accurate advice, support and, if necessary, replacement therapy may be given to patients. At the same time, efforts must continue to find treatments of equal effectiveness with less damaging late effects.

In patients whose reproductive capacity is preserved following cancer treatment, the question of the outcome of pregnancy is clearly important. The more recent but still largely anecdotal data available suggest no increased incidence of spontaneous abortion or foetal abnormality following chemotherapy given to the father at or prior to the time of conception or to the mother prior to gestation or after the first trimester (Blatt *et al.*, 1980). However, there is some evidence of an increased incidence of spontaneous abortion and foetal abnormality in women previously treated with both chemotherapy and irradiation (Holmes and Holmes, 1978) and considerable anecdotal evidence showing increased risk from chemotherapy and irradiation alone in the first trimester (Stewart and Kneale, 1970; Nicholson, 1968).

Hypothalamus pituitary

There is no convincing evidence that chemotherapy impairs hypothalamic–pituitary function in man. However, cranial radiotherapy can cause abnormalities of pituitary hormone production particularly in children. Those who have been studied following successful treatment for intracranial tumours demonstrate a tendency to short stature and impaired growth hormone response to insulin hypoglycaemia (Shalet and Beardwell, 1979). These authors recommend regular measurements of growth rate in children who have received cranial irradiation and test of growth hormone secretion if growth is impaired.

Abnormalities of TSH and ACTH production may also result from high-dose irradiation to the hypothalamic–pituitary axis, the incidence gradually increasing with time.

Thyroid

Radiation-related thyroid dysfunction has recently been studied by Schimpff *et al.* (1980) in patients treated for Hodgkin's disease. Among 169 patients treated with mantle irradiation, 112 (66%) had evidence of thyroid dysfunction. In 69 (41%) elevated TSH was the sole abnormality, and in 43 (25%) a high TSH was accompanied by a low serum T4 level. Thyroid dysfunction developed slowly with the maximum incidence being reached at six years. Adjuvant chemotherapy did not significantly affect either the incidence or severity of thyroid dysfunction. These authors recommend six-monthly TSH estimations in these patients as well as in patients with head and neck cancer who have received thyroid irradiation, with thyroxine replacement given to those with an elevated level.

TISSUE DAMAGE FROM HORMONAL AGENTS

These agents have patterns of adverse effects which differ in many ways from those resulting from cytotoxic therapy and are therefore discussed separately.

Diethylstilboestrol in prostatic cancer

Following the demonstration of an increased cardiovascular mortality in patients with prostatic cancer treated with 5 mg of diethylstilboestrol daily, a dose of 1 mg was shown to be safe and effective. Many centres now use 3 mg daily since this more reliably suppresses plasma testosterone, although there is recent evidence that cardiovascular complications and mortality at this dose may be unacceptable in patients with localized disease (Glashan and Robinson, 1981). In addition, the majority of patients experience gynaeco-mastia and nipple soreness which generally improves with time despite continued therapy, and fluid retention requiring diuretic therapy is not uncommon. Nausea and vomiting are relatively rare in the male and can usually be prevented by gradually building up the dose which should be taken at night, if necessary with an antiemetic.

Estramustine

This combination of an oestrogen moiety with an alkylating agent shows promise in the management of prostatic cancer. Its principal toxic effect is gastric irritation with nausea, occasionally vomiting and diarrhoea. Taylor (personal communication) has experience in over 100 patients teated with estramustine, and although gynaecomastia, nipple soreness, and fluid reten-tion occur commonly, they are less of a problem than with stilboestrol. As with oestrogens, cardiovascular complications may prove troublesome (Glashan and Robinson, 1981).

Tamoxifen

The anti-oestrogen tamoxifen is now used extensively in advanced breast cancer and the unwanted effects have been well documented. Heel *et al* (1978) have reviewed the side-effects described in 16 studies in a total of 825 patients treated with daily dosages usually of 20–40 mg. The problems were rarely serious, causing a drop-out rate due to side-effects of less than 5%. Hot flushes (15.5%), gastrointestinal symptoms (11.4%), leukopenia (15.5%), thrombocytopenia (9.3%), hypercalcaemia (17%), and headache (8.5%) were the most frequent complaints. The haematological abnormalities were not life-threatening and returned towards normal in all patients within a few weeks despite continued treatment.

Aminoglutethimide

This inhibitor of adrenal steroid synthesis is under evaluation in the treatment of breast cancer. In one recent study 58% of patients had appreciable side-effects including lethargy and drowsiness (37%), rash (30%), nausea (8%), and depression (4%) (Smith *et al.*, 1981). The rash, which is erythematous, maculopapular, and sometimes associated with malaise and fever, occurs early in treatment and resolves within about a week despite continued therapy. Seven out of 97 patients treated in the above-mentioned study had side-effects severe enough to warrant stopping treatment.

Androgens and oestrogens in breast cancer

Facial hirsutism and deepening of the voice are common side-effects of androgen therapy, affecting about one-third of patients taking 25–40 mg fluoxymesterone daily for longer than three months (Stoll, 1972). Fluid retention, gastrointestinal intolerance, and hepatotoxicity are rarely severe enough to necessitate interruption of therapy.

Nausea and vomiting are the commonest side-effects of oestrogen administration in women but may be minimized by a gradual dose escalation to the required level and by taking the oestrogen at night with an antiemetic. Fluid retention, breakthrough bleeding, and stress incontinence of urine are not uncommon (Stoll, 1977).

Corticosteroids

Adrenocorticosteroids are widely used in cancer treatment both as primary therapy (e.g. breast cancer and lymphomas) and in the management of complications (e.g. hypercalcaemia, cerebral oedema). Generally they are used for short periods and therefore the familiar long-term complications of steroid therapy are rarely seen. However, more acute problems do occur (e.g. fluid retention, dyspepsia, hypokalaemia, mental disturbances, infection, impaired glucose tolerance, and acne) which can often be circumvented by dose reductions. Appetite stimulation and a feeling of well-being are often useful side-effects of corticosteroid therapy in cancer patients.

CONCLUSION

This review is by no means an exhaustive account of the effects of antineoplastic agents. New or investigational drugs have been largely ignored through lack of space but are the subject of review articles to which interested readers are referred (Carter *et al.*, 1981; Wierzba *et al.*, 1981; Young *et al.*, 1981).

It is apparent from the discussion of antiproliferative drugs that their use is more commonly accompanied by seriously damaging adverse effects than is that of any other class of drug. In general, their therapeutic index is low and in many circumstances a certain degree of toxicity must be accepted if any therapeutic advantage is to be achieved. Because of this, medical oncologists quickly become accustomed to observing toxicity problems in their patients. These problems can become as much a part of cancer chemotherapy as post-operative pain is a part of cancer surgery. Once toxicity has been accepted as inevitable by the oncologists, then their patients will often do likewise and fail to report very unpleasant treatment-related symptoms. An even more serious result of the toxicity of such cancer therapy is the refusal by patients or by the parents of paediatric patients to accept treatment even of the curative category because of fear of side-effects.

While the search for new and better treatments for cancer goes on, it is vital that we look harder for ways of ameliorating (or better still, avoiding) the undesired effects of those we use at present. In Hodgkin's disease, for example, alternative regimes with less immediate toxicity than MOPP have been advocated (McElwain *et al.*, 1977) as well as still other combinations which may carry a lower risk of second malignancies (Valagussa *et al.*, 1980). Clearly the question of equal effectiveness needs to be clearly answered before such major changes in treatment policy are widely applied.

Using the same agents but in different ways is another approach to toxicity reduction. The apparently lower incidence of cardiac damage from doxorubicin when given as a constant infusion rather than by bolus injection has already been discussed. The use of folinic acid to abolish the myelotoxicity of methotrexate and thus allow very high doses to be given is now an established part of the oncologist's repertoire. Unfortunately, clear evidence of enhanced efficacy of these high doses is often sparse.

Two novel approaches to reducing myelotoxicity have been recently tested. Hedley *et al.* (1978) showed that a small intravenous dose of cyclophosphamide given seven days before high-dose melphalan appeared to result in more rapid recovery of white cell counts than when the 'priming' agent was omitted. Treating small cell anaplastic carcinoma of the bronchus, Lyman *et al.* (1980) found that lithium carbonate (which is known to produce leukocytosis in psychiatric patients) significantly reduced chemotherapy-related neutropenia and infections. However, their control group may have experienced more infectious complications than most other workers observe with similar regimes. Furthermore, the clear superiority of severely myelotoxic regimes in this disease is yet to be established. Others addressing this question in lung cancer and other tumours are using autologous bone marrow rescue techniques to bypass myelotoxicity.

Dose rate is clearly of crucial importance in considerations of toxicity in cancer chemotherapy. Frei and Canellos (1980) argue that it is only in highly sensitive tumours that a steep and generally linear dose-response curve is observed. For relatively resistant tumours, increasing the dose may have little effect on response, but will often increase the toxicity in sensitive normal tissues. The lack of similarly quantitative data on the adverse effects of cancer treatments has been discussed by Young (1979). In place of the list of organs or tissues affected which appear in most reports, Young argues for dose-response and time–response curves of toxic effects as a more meaningful and appropriate guide to therapists administering these drugs.

The normal tissue damage resulting from radiotherapy has been well documented over the years. However, it is becoming increasingly apparent that major interactions between radiotherapy and chemotherapy can seriously complicate the management of cancer patients (Vaeth, 1979). In this chapter, combined effects on the lungs, heart, bone marrow, gonads, gastrointestinal tract, and effects on the incidence of second malignancies have been discussed. Close collaboration between the radiotherapist and medical oncologist is clearly more important than ever.

In summary, radiotherapy and chemotherapy with the drugs discussed in this review are used with palliative, retardative or curative intent in different malignant diseases or at different stages in the treatment of a single disease. Outside the clinical trial setting, oncologists should have a clear idea in which category any particular treatment falls and a thorough understanding of the probable and possible unwanted effects which he should be able to justify. He must continually adjust the risk–benefit equation as treatment progresses, and be prepared to stop that treatment as soon as the risks outweigh the benefits. Within trials, the clinical investigator should in addition maintain a constantly vigilant attitude towards side-effects which should be recorded, and where possible quantified, and reported in full.

REFERENCES

Adrian, R.M., Hood, A.F., and Skarin, A.T. (1980). Mucocutaneous reactions to antineoplastic agents. *CA*, **30**, 143.

Afzal Mir, M., and Delamore, I.W. (1978). Metabolic disturbances in acute myeloid leukaemia. *Br. J. Haematol.*, **40**, 79.

Ansbacher, R. (1978). Artificial insemination with frozen spermatozoa. *Fertil. Steril.*, **29**, 375.

Arsenau, J.C., Sponso, R.W., Levin, D.L., Schnipper, L.E., Bonner, H., Young, R.C., Canellos, G.P., Johnson, R.E., and DeVita, V.T. (1972). Nonlymphomatous malignant tumours complicating Hodgkin's disease. *New Engl. J. Med.*, **287**, 1119.

Ash, P. (1980). The influence of radiation on fertility in man. *Br. J. Radiol.*, **53**, 271.

Auclerc, G., Jacquillat, C., Auclerc, M.F., Weil, M., and Bernard, J. (1979). Post-therapeutic acute leukemia. *Cancer*, **44**, 2017.

Barlock, A.L., Howser, D.M., and Hubbard, S.M. (1977). Nursing management of adriamycin extravasation. *Am. J. Nursing*, **79**, 94.

Bender, R.A. and Young, R.C. (1978). Effects of cancer treatment on individual and generational genetics. *Semin. Oncol.*, **5**, 47.

Benjamin, R., Legha, S., MacKay, B., Ewer, M., Wallace, S., Valdivieso, M., Rasmussen, S., Blumenschein, G., and Freireich, E. (1981). Reduction of adriamycin cardiac toxicity using a prolonged continuous intravenous infusion. *Proc. Am. Assoc. Cancer Res.*, **22**, 179.

Billingham, M.E., Mason, J.W. Bristow, M.R., and Daniels, J.R. (1978). Anthracycline cardiomyopathy monitored by morphologic changes. *Cancer Treat. Rep.*, **62**, 865

Bischel, M.D. (1979). Cyclophosphamide—hemorrhagic cystitis following prolonged low dose therapy. *J. Am. Med. Assoc.*, **242**, 238.

Blatt, J., Mulvihill, J.T., Ziegler, J.L., Young, R.C., and Poplack, D.G. (1980). Pregnancy outcome following cancer chemotherapy. *Am. J. Med.*, **69**, 828.

Blatt, J., Poplack, D.G., and Sherins, R.J. (1981). Testicular function in boys after chemotherapy for acute lymphoblastic leukemia. *New Engl. J. Med.*, **304**, 1121.

Blum, R.H., Carter, S.K., and Agre, K. (1973). A clinical review of bleomycin—a new antineoplastic agent. *Cancer*, **31**, 903.

Bode, U., Seif, S.M., and Levine, A.S. (1980). Studies on the antidiuretic effect of cyclophosphamide—vasopressin release and sodium excretion. *Med. Pediatr. Oncol.*, **8**, 295.

Bodey, G.P. (1975). Infections in cancer patients. *Cancer Treat. Rev.*, **2**, 89.

Boice, J.D., and Hutchison, G.B. (1980). Leukemia in women following radiotherapy for cervical cancer: ten year follow up of an international study. *J. Nat. Cancer Inst.*, **65**, 115.

Botnick, L.E., Hannon, E.C., and Hellman, S. (1979). A long lasting proliferative defect in the hematopoietic stem cell compartment following cytotoxic agents. *Int. J. Radiat. Oncol., Biol. Phys.*, **5**, 1621.

Bristow, M.R., Mason, J.W., Billingham, M.E., and Daniels, J.R. (1978). Doxorubicin cardiomyopathy: evaluation by phonocardiography, endomyocardial biopsy and cardiac catheterization. *Ann. Intern. Med.*, **88**, 168.

Brody, R.S., and Schottenfeld, D. (1980). Multiple primary cancers in Hodgkin's disease. *Semin. Oncol.*, **7**, 187.

Bryant, B.M., Jarman, M., Ford, H.T., and Smith, I.E. (1980). Prevention of isophosphamide-induced urothelial toxicity with 2-mercaptoethane sulphonate sodium (mesnum) in patients with advanced carcinoma. *Lancet*,**ii**, 657.

Buchanan, J.D., Fairley, K.F., and Barrie, J.U. (1975). Return of spermatogenesis after stopping cyclophosphamide therapy. *Lancet*, **ii**, 156.

Canellos, G.P., DeVita, V.T., Arsenau, J.C., Whang-Peng, J., and Johnson, R.E.C. (1975). Second malignancies complicating Hodgkin's disease in remission. *Lancet*, **i**, 947.

Catane, R., Schwade, J.G., Turrisi, A.T., Webber, B.L., and Muggia, F.M. (1979). Pulmonary toxicity after radiation and bleomycin—a review. *Int. J. Radiat. Oncol., Biol. Phys.*, **5**, 1513.

Carter, S.K., Sakurai, Y., and Umezawa, H. (1981). New drugs in cancer chemotherapy. *Recent results in cancer research*, vol. 76. Berlin: Springer-Verlag.

Chapman, R.M., Sutcliffe, S.B., and Malpas, J.S. (1979). Cyotoxic induced ovarian failure in women with Hodgkin's disease. 1. Hormone function. *J. Am. Med. Assoc.*, **242**, 1877.

Chapman, R.M., Sutcliffe, S.B., and Malpas, J.S. (1981). Male gonadal dysfunction in Hodgkin's disease: a prospective study. *J. Am. Med. Assoc.*, **245**, 1323.

Cohen, I.S., Mosher, M.B., O'Keefe, E.J., Klaus, S.N., and De Conti, R.C. (1973). Cutaneous toxicity of bleomycin therapy. *Arch. Dermatol.*, **107**, 553.

Coleman, N.C., Williams, C.J., Flint, A., Glatstein, E.J., Rosenberg, S.A., and Kaplan, H.S. (1977). Haematologic neoplasia in patients treated for Hodgkins Disease. *New Engl. J. Med.*, **297**, 1249.

Creaven, P.J., and Mihich, E. (1977). The clinical toxicity of anti cancer drugs and its prediction. *Semin. Oncol.*, **4**, 147.

Dean, J.C., Salmon, S.E., Griffith, K.S., Cetas, T.C., and Mackel, C. (1981). Scalp hypothermia: a comparison of ice packs and Kold Kap® in the prevention of adriamycin induced alopecia. *Proc. Am. Soc. Clin. Oncol.*, **22**, 415.

Deital, M., and Vasic, V. (1979). Major intestinal complications of radiotherapy. *Am. J. Gastroenterol.*, **72**, 65.

Desai, M.H., Loring, L., and Tenes, D. (1981). Prevention of adriamycin induced skin ulcers in Yorkshire pigs with dimethyl sulfoxide (DMSO). *Proc. Am. Soc. Clin. Oncol.*, **22**, 362.

Dreizen, S., Daly, T.E., Drane, J.B., and Brown, L.R. (1977). Oral complications of cancer radiotherapy. *Postgrad. Med.*, **61**, 85.

Etteldorf, J.N., West, C.D., Pitcock, J.A., and Williams, D.L. (1976). Gonadal function, testicular histology, and meiosis following cyclophosphamide therapy in patients with nephrotic syndrome. *J. Pediatr.*, **88**, 206.

Freeman, J.E., Johnson, P.G.B., and Voke, J.M. (1973). Somnolence ater prophylactic cranial irradiation in children with acute lymphoblastic leukaemia. *Br. Med. J.*, **4**, 523.

Frei, E., and Canellos, G.P. (1980). Dose: a critical factor in cancer chemotherapy. *Am. J. Med.*, **69**, 585.

Frytak, S., and Moertel, C.G. (1981). Management of nausea and vomiting in the cancer patient. *J. Am. Med. Assoc.*, **245**, 393.

Glashan, R.W., and Robinson, M.R.G. (1981). Cardiovascular complications in the treatment of prostatic carcinoma. *Br. J. Urol.*, **53**, 624.

Goldiner, P.L., Carlon, G.C., Cvitkovic, E., Schweizer, O., and Howland, W.S. (1978). Factors influencing postoperative morbidity and mortality in patients treated with bleomycin. *Br. Med. J.*, **1**, 1664.

Gonzales-Vitale, J.C., Hayes, D.M., Cvitkovic, E., and Sternberg, S.S. (1977). The renal pathology in clinical trials of cis-platin um (II) diamminedichloride. *Cancer*, **39**, 1362.

Gralla, R.J., Itri, L.M., Pisko, S.E., Squillante, A.E., Kelsen, D.P., Braun, D.W., Bordin, L.A., Braun, T.J., and Young, C.W. (1981). Anti-emetic efficacy of high-dose metoclopramide: randomized trials with placebo and prochlorperazine in patients with chemotherapy induced nausea and vomiting. *New Engl. J. Med.*, **305**, 905.

Gross, N.J. (1977). Pulmonary effects of radiation therapy. *Ann. Intern. Med.*, **86**, 81.

Grossman, B., Lessin, L.S., and Cohen, P. (1979). Droperidol prevents nausea and vomiting from cis-platinum. *New Engl. J. Med.*, **301**, 47.

Hadley, D., and Herr, H.W. (1979). Peripheral neuropathy associated with cis-dichloro-diammineplatinum (II) treatment. *Cancer*, **44**, 2026.

Haghbin, M. (1977). Antimetabolites in the prophylaxis and treatment of CNS leukemia. *Cancer Treat. Rep.*, **61**, 661.

Haskell, C.M. (1977). Immunologic aspects of cancer chemotherapy. *Ann. Rev. Pharmacol. Toxicol.*, **17**, 179.

Hedley, D.W., McElwain, T.J., Millar, J.L., and Gordon, M.Y. (1978). Acceleration of bone-marrow recovery by pre-treatment with cyclophosphamide in patients receiving high-dose melphalan. *Lancet*, **ii**, 966.

Heel, R.C., Brogden, R.N., Speight, T.M., and Avery, G.S. (1978). Tamoxifen: a review of its pharmacological properties and therapeutic use in the treatment of breast cancer. *Drugs*, **16**, 1.

Henderson, I.C., and Frei, III, E. (1980). Adriamycin cardiotoxicity. *Am. Heart J.*, **99**, 671.

Higby, D.J., and Henderson, E.S. (1981). Supportive care of the seriously ill cancer patient: platelet and granulocyte transfusion therapy. In *Oncologic emergencies* (eds J.W. Yarbro, and R.S. Bornstein). New York: Grune and Stratton. p. 323.

Holland, J.F., Scharlau, C., Gailani, S., Krant, M.J., Olson, K.B., Horton, J., Schnider, B.I., Lynch, J.J., Owens, A., Carbone, P.P., Colsky, J., Grob, D., Miller, S.P., and Hall, T.C. (1973). Vincristine treatment of advanced cancer: a cooperative study of 392 cases. *Cancer Res.*, **33**, 1258.

Holmes, G.E., and Holmes, F.F. (1978). Pregnancy outcome of patients treated for Hodgkin's disease. *Cancer*, **41**, 1317.

Horning, S.J., Hoppe, R.T., Kaplan, H.S., and Rosenberg, S.A. (1981). Female reproductive potential after treatment for Hodgkin's disease. *New Engl. J. Med.*, **304**, 1377.

Hutchison, G.B. (1976). Late neoplastic changes following medical irradiation. *Cancer*, **37**, 1102.

Ignoffo, R.J., and Friedman, M.A. (1980) Therapy of local toxicities caused by extravasation of cancer chemotherapeutic drugs. *Cancer Treat. Rev.*, **7**, 17.

Jones, M.E., and Saleem, A. (1978) Acute promyelocytic leukemia: a review of the literature. *Am. J. Med.*, **65**, 673.

Kapadia, S.B., Krause, J.R., Ellis, L.D., Pan, S.F., and Wald, N. (1980). Induced acute non-lymphocytic leukemia following long-term chemotherapy. *Cancer*, **45**, 1315.

Kaplan, H.S. (1972). *Hodgkin's disease*. Cambridge MA: Harvard University Press. pp.318–326, 339.

Lancet Editorial (1974). Hyperuricaemic acute renal failure. *Lancet*, **ii**, 1266.

Land, V.J., Sutow, W.W., Fernbach, D.J., Lane, D.M., and Williams, T.E. (1972). Toxicity of L-asparaginase in children with advanced leukemia. *Cancer*, **30**, 339.

Larson, D. (1981). Management of tissue extravasation of antitumour agents. *Proc. Am. Soc. Clin. Oncol.*, **22**, 416.

Levine, N., and Greenwald, E.S. (1978). Mucocutaneous side effects of cancer chemotherapy. *Cancer Treat. Rev.*, **5**, 67.

Lucas, V.S., and Laszlo, J. (1980) Delta-9-tetrahydrocannabinol for refractory vomiting induced by cancer chemotherapy. *J. Am. Med. Assoc.*, **243**, 1241.

Lyman, G.H., Williams, C.C., and Preston, D. (1980). The use of lithium carbonate to reduce infection and leukopenia during systemic chemotherapy. *New Engl. J. Med.*, **302**, 257.

McElwain, T.J., Toy, J., Smith, I.E., Peckham, M.J., and Austin, D.E. (1977). A combination of chlorambucil, vinblastine, procarbazine, and prednisolone for treatment of Hodgkin's disease. *Br. J. Cancer*, **36**, 276.

Markoe, A.M., and Saluk, P.H. (1979). Combined effects of radiation and chemotherapy on the lymphohemopoietic system with special reference to the immune response. In *Frontiers of radiation therapy and oncology,* vol. 13, *Combined effects of chemotherapy and radiotherapy on normal tissue tolerance* (ed. J. M. Vaeth). Basel: Karger. p. 175.

Miller, D.G. (1971). Alkylating agents and human spermatogenesis. *J. Am. Med. Assoc.*, **217**, 1662.

Mills, B.A., and Roberts, R.W. (1979). Cyclophosphamide-induced cardiomyopathy. *Cancer*, **43**, 2223.

Minow, R.A., Benjamin, R.S., and Gottlieb, J.A. (1975). Adriamycin (NSC123127) cardiomyopathy—an overview with determination of risk factors. *Cancer Chemother. Rep.,* **6**, 195.

Mittal, K.K., Ruder, E.A., and Green, D. (1976) Matching of histocompatibility (HL-A) antigens for platelet transfusion. *Blood,* **47**, 31.

Moertel, C.G., Reitemeier, R.J., Bolton, C.F., *et al.* (1964). Cerebellar ataxia associated with fluorinated pyrimidine therapy. *Cancer Chemother. Rep.,* **41**, 15.

Morrow, G.R. (1981). Behavioural treatment of anticipatory nausea and vomiting during chemotherapy. *Proc. Am. Soc. Clin. Oncol.,* **22**, 396.

Moss, H.A., Nannis, E.D., and Poplack, D.G. (1981). The effects of prophylactic treatment of the central nervous system on the intellectual functioning of children with acute lymphocytic leukemia. *Am. J. Med.,* **71**, 47.

Neidhart, J., Gagen, M., and Metz, E. (1980). Haldol as an effective anti-emetic for platinum and mustard induced vomiting when other agents fail. *Proc. Am. Soc. Clin. Oncol.,* **21**, 365.

Nicholson, H.D. (1968). Cytotoxic drugs in pregnancy. *J. Obstetr. Gynaecol. Br. Commonw.,* **75**, 307.

O'Regan, S., Carson, S., Chesney, R.W., and Drummond, K. N. (1977). Electrolyte and acid-base disturbances in the management of leukemia. *Blood,* **49**, 345.

Pascual, R.S., Mosher, M.B., Sikand, R.S., De Conti, R.C., and Bouhuys, A. (1973). Effects of bleomycin on pulmonary function in man. *Am. Rev. Respir. Dis.,* **108**, 211.

Peterson, L.G., and Popkin, M.K. (1980). Neuropsychiatric effects of chemo-therapeutic agents for cancer. *Psychosomatics,* **21**, 141.

Pitman, S.W., Parker, L.M., Tattersall, M.H.N., *et al.* (1975). Clinical trial of high dose methotrexate (NSC–740) with citrovorum factor (NSC–3590)—Toxicologic and therapeutic observations. Proc. High-Dose Methotrexate Therapy. *Cancer Chemother. Rep.,* **6**, 43.

Pizzo, P.A., Poplack, D.G., and Bleyer, W.A. (1979). Neurotoxicities of current leukemia therapy. *Am. J. Pediatr. Hematol. Oncol.,* **1**, 127.

Pochedly, C. (1974). Hyperuricemia in leukemia and lymphoma. *Postgrad. Med.,* **55**, 93.

Price, R.A., and Jamieson, A.J. (1975). The central nervous system in childhood leukemia. II Sub-acute leukoencephalopathy. *Cancer,* **35**, 306.

Ransom, J.L., Novak, R.W., Mahesh Kumar, A.P., Omar Hustu, H., and Pratt, C.B. (1979). Delayed gastrointestinal complications after combined modality therapy of childhood rhabdomyosarcoma. *Int. J. Radiat. Oncol. Biol. Phys.,* **5**,1275.

Reimer, R.R., Hoover, R., Fraumeri, J.F., and Young, R.C. (1977) Acute leukemia after alkylating agent therapy of ovarian cancer. *New Engl. J. Med.* **297**, 177.

Rodrigues, V., and Ketchel, S.J. (1981). Acute infection in patients with malignant disease. In *Oncologic emergencies* (eds J.W. Yarbro, and R.S. Bornstein). New York: Grune and Stratton, p.273.

Roeser, H.P. Stocks, A.E., and Smith, A.J. (1978). Testicular damage due to cytotoxic drugs and recovery after cessation of therapy. *Aust. N. Z. J. Med.,* **8**, 250.

Rubin, P., and Scarantino, C.W. (1978). The bone marrow organ: the critical structure in radiation drug interaction. *Int. J. Radiat. Oncol. Biol. Phys.,* **4**, 3.

Samuels, M.L., Johnson, D.E., Holoye, P.Y., and Lanzoth, V.J. (1976). Large-dose bleomycin therapy and pulmonary toxicity: a possible role of prior radiotherapy. *J. Am. Med. Assoc.,* **235**, 1117.

Sandler, S.G., Tobin, W., and Henderson, E.S. (1969). Vincristine induced neuro-pathy: a clinical study of fifty leukemic patients. *Neurology* (Minneapolis), **19**, 367.

Scheef, W., Klein, H.O., Brock, N., Barkert, H., Gunther, U., Hoefer-Janker, H., Mitrenga, D., Schnitker, J., and Voigtmann, R. (1979). Controlled clinical studies with an antidote against the urotoxicity of oxazaphosphorines: preliminary results. *Cancer Treat. Rep.*, **63**, 501.

Schein, P.S., and Winokur, S.H. (1975). Immunosuppressive and cytotoxic chemotherapy: long term complications. *Ann. Intern. Med.*, **82**, 84.

Schilsky, R.L., and Anderson, T. (1979). Hypomagnesemia and renal magnesium wasting in patients receiving cisplatin. *Ann. Intern. Med.*, **90**, 929.

Schilsky, R.L., Lewis, B.J., Sherins, R.J., and Young, R.C. (1980). Gonadal dysfunction in patients receiving chemotherapy for cancer. *Ann. Intern. Med.*, **93**, 109.

Schilsky, R.L., Sherins, R.J., Hubbard, S.M., Wesley, M.N., Young, R.C., and DeVita, V.T. (1981). Long-term follow-up of ovarian function in women treated with MOPP chemotherapy for Hodgkin's disease. *Am. J. Med.* **71**, 552.

Schimpff, S.C. (1980). Infection prevention during granulocytopenia. In *Current clinical topics in infectious diseases* (eds J.S. Remington, and M.N. Schwartz). New York: McGraw-Hill. p.85.

Schimpff, S.C., Diggs, C.H., Wismell, J.G., Salvatone, P.C., and Wiernik, P.H. (1980). Radiation-related thyroid dysfunction: implications for the treatment of Hodgkin's disease. *Ann. Intern. Med.* **92**, 91.

Senyszyn, J.J., Johnston, A.D., Jacox, H.W., and Chu, F.C.H. (1970). Radiation induced sarcoma after treatment of breast cancer. *Cancer*, **26**, 394.

Shalet, S.M., and Beardwell, C.G. (1979). Hypothalamic—pituitary function following cranial irradiation. In *CNS complications of malignant disease* (eds J.M.A. Whitehouse, and H.E.N. Kay). London: Macmillan. p.202.

Shalet, S.M., and Beardwell, C.G. , Morris Jones, P.H., Pearson, D., and Orrell, D.H. (1976). Ovarian failure following abdominal irradiation in childhood. *Br. J. Cancer*, **33**, 655.

Shaw, M.T., Spector, M.H., and Ladman, A.J. (1979). Effects of cancer, radiotherapy and cytotoxic drugs on intestinal structure and function. *Cancer Treat. Rev.*, **6**, 141.

Sheline, G.E., Wara, W.M., and Smith, V. (1980). Therapeutic irradiation and brain injury. *Int. J. Radiat. Oncol., Biol. Phys.*, **6**, 1215.

Sherins, R.J., Olweny, C.L.M., and Ziegler, J.L. (1978). Gynecomastia and gonadal dysfunction in adolescent boys treated with combination chemotherapy for Hodgkin's disease. *New Engl. J. Med.*, **299**, 12.

Siris, E.S., Leventhal, B.G., and Vartukaitis, J.L. (1976). Effects of childhood leukemia and chemotherapy on puberty and reproductive function in girls. *New Engl. J. Med.*, **294**, 1143.

Slanina, J., Musshoff, K., Rahner, T., and Stiasny, R. (1977). Long-term side effects in irradiated patients with Hodgkin's disease. *Int. J. Radiat. Oncol., Biol. Phys.*, **2**, 1.

Slavin, R.E., Dias, M.A., and Saral, R. (1978). Cytosine arabinoside induced gastrointestinal toxic alterations in sequential chemotherapeutic protocols. A clinical pathologic study of 33 patients. *Cancer*, **42**, 1747.

Smith, I.E., Harris, A.L., Morgan, M., Ford, H.T., Gazet, J-C., Harmer, C.L., White, H., Parsons, C.A., Villardo, A., Walsh, G., and McKinna, J.A. (1981). Tamoxifen versus aminoglutethimide in advanced breast carcinoma: a randomised cross-over trial. *Br. Med. J.*, **2**, 1432.

Sostman, H.D., Matthay, R.A., and Putman, C.E. (1977). Cytotoxic drug-induced lung disease. *Am. J. Med.*, **62**, 608.

Spiegel, R.J. (1981). The acute toxicities of chemotherapy. *Cancer Treat. Rev.*, **8**, 197.

Stark, J.J., and Howell, S.B. (1978). Nephrotoxicity of cis-platinum (II) dichloro-diammine. *Clin. Pharmacol. Ther.*, **23**, 461.

Steele, N., Gralla, R.J., Braun, D.W., and Young, C.W. (1980). Double-blind comparison of the anti-emetic effects of nabilone and prochlorperazine on chemotherapy-induced emesis. *Cancer Treat. Rep.*, **64**, 219.

Stewart, A., and Kneale, G.W. (1970). Radiation dose effects in relation to obstetric x-rays and childhood cancers. *Lancet*, **i**, 1185.

Stewart, J.R., and Fajardo, L.F. (1971). Radiation-induced heart disease. *Radiol. Clin. N. Am.*, **9**, 511.

Stoll, B.A. (1972). Androgen, corticosteroid and progestin therapy. In *Endocrine therapy in malignant disease* (ed B.A. Stoll). London: W.B. Saunders. p. 165.

Stoll, B.A. (1977). Palliation by castration or by hormone administration. In *Breast cancer management—early and late* (ed B.A. Stoll). London: Heinemann Medical. p.133.

Strickland, P. (1980). Complications of radiotherapy. *Br. J. Hosp. Med.*, **23**, 552.

Stuart, M.J., Cuaso, G., Miller, M., and Oski, F.A. (1975). Syndrome of recurrent increased secretion of antidiuretic hormone following mutliple doses of vincristine. *Blood*, **45**, 315.

Thar, T., and Million, R.R. (1980). Complications of radiation treatment of Hodgkin's disease. *Semin. Oncol.*, **7**, 174.

Thomas, P.R.M., Winstanly, D., Peckham, M.J., Austin, C.D.E., Murrary, M.A.F., and Jacobs, H.S. (1976). Reproductive and endocrine function in patients with Hodgkin's disease: effects of oophoropexy and irradiation. *Br. J. Cancer*, **33**, 226.

Vaeth, J.M. (1979). Combined effects of chemotherapy and radiotherapy on normal tissue tolerance. *Frontiers of radiation therapy and oncology*, vol. 13. Basel: Karger.

Valagussa, P., Santoro, A., Kenda, R., Fossati Bellani, F., Franchi, F., Banfi, A., Rilke, F., and Bonadonna, G. (1980). Second malignancies in Hodgkin's disease: a complication of certain forms of treatment. *Br. Med. J.*, **1**, 216.

Villani, F., Guindari, A., and Pagnoni, A. (1979) 5-Fluorouracil cardiotoxicity. *Tumori*, **65**, 487.

Vogl, S.E., Zaravinos, T., Kaplan, B.H., and Wollner, D. (1981). Safe and effective 2 hour outpatient regimen of hydration and diuresis for the administration of cis-diamminedichloro-platinum II. *Eur. J. Cancer*, **17**, 345.

Von Hoff, D.D. (1980). The cardiotoxicity of commonly used antineoplastic agents. Columbus, Ohio: Adria Laboratories. p.7.

Von Hoff, D.D., Layard, M.W., Basa, P., Davis, H.L., Von Hoff, A.L. Rozencweig, M., and Muggia, F.M. (1979). Risk factors for doxorubicin-induced congestive heart failure. *Ann. Intern. Med.*, **91**, 710.

Von Hoff, D.D., Rosencweig, M., Layard, M., Slavik, M., and Muggia, F.M. (1977). Daunomycin-induced cardiotoxicity in children and adults: a review of 110 cases. *Am. J. Med.*, **62**, 200.

Weinstein, G.D. (1977). Methotrexate. *Ann. Intern. Med.*, **86**, 199.

Weiss, H.D., Walker, M.D., and Wiernik, P.H. (1974). Neurotoxicity of commonly used antineoplastic drugs. *New Engl. J. Med.*, **291**, 75–81, 127–133.

Weiss, R.B., and Bruno, S. (1981). Hypersensitivity reactions to cancer chemotherapeutic agents. *Ann. Intern. Med.*, **94**, 66.

Weiss, R.B., and Muggia, F.M. (1980). Cytotoxic drug-induced pulmonary disease: Update 1980. *Am. J. Med.*, **68**, 259.

Wierzba, K., Danysz, A., and Hamid, M.R. (1981). Cytostatic and immuno-suppressive drugs. In *Side effects of drugs annual*, vol.5 (ed. M.N.G. Dukes). Amsterdam: Excerpta Medica. p.407.

Willson, J.K.V. (1978). Pulmonary toxicity of antineoplastic drugs. *Cancer Treat. Rep.*, **62**, 2003.

Young, L.S. (1981). Trimethoprim-sulfamethoxazole and bacterial infections during leukemia therapy. *Ann. Intern. Med.*, **95**, 508.

Young, R.C., Ozols, R.F., and Myers, C.E. (1981). The anthracycline antineoplastic drugs. *New Engl. J. Med.*, **305**, 139.

Young, R.S.K. (1979). Problems of toxicity of anticancer drugs. *Fed. Proc.*, **38**, 113.

Zweig, J.I., and Wallach, R. (1980). Effective medical management of the adriamycin ulcer. *Proc. Am. Assoc. Cancer Res.*, **21**, 140.

Part 2

Predictive variables and measurements

Chapter

8

EDWIN R. FISHER

Histopathology and Survival Time

INTRODUCTION

It has become increasingly evident that the clinical behavior of a solid cancer is related to its biologic properties and the host response. This is in contrast with the conventional time-oriented view concerning the progression of such neoplasms which regards a cancer as growing and spreading with time. Although this latter view would attribute successful management of cancer to its early detection, it still remains to be proved that this approach can effectively alter survival rates in cancer.

The time-oriented model also fails to take into account many biological and clinical observations related to tumour biology. Kinetic studies of tumor growth clearly show that early *clinical* detection is not synonymous with early *biologic* recognition of cancer. Indeed, most recent studies of such solid cancers as those of the breast, colon, and rectum fail to corroborate any significant relationship between survival rate and duration of symptoms, i.e. period of delay before treatment (Fisher *et al.*, 1977; McDermott *et al.*, 1980; Eker, 1963). Noteworthy too is the failure to find a consistent relationship between survival rate and tumor size. These observations lead one to doubt that the clinical or pathologic staging of cancer is related to the length of time the disease has existed in the body.

A decade of experimental studies, together with considerable clinical investigations on the biology of breast cancer and the results of treatment, support an alternative hypothesis of tumor biology (Fisher, 1980). This hypothesis suggests that there is no orderly pattern of tumor spread as previously visualized, but it is the biological properties of the neoplasm and the host reaction to it that will determine the prognosis.

Yet the value of grading cancers histopathologically—a traditional index of a tumor's biologic potential—has not been universally accepted, and even Willis (1967) noted it to represent 'an arbitrary process conferring an entirely spurious impression of precision'. One reason for the doubt as to its value is the uniformly dismal prognosis of cancer at certain sites, whatever the histology. For example, while undifferentiated small and large cell cancers of the lung exhibit a more rapid clinical course than does squamous cell cancer, and this in turn appears to be more ominous than adenocarcinoma, the prognosis with all types is uniformly poor. In this disease a very large series of cases would be necessary to identify grading factors which might be of prognostic significance. The same difficulty applies to subsets of patients with cancer in whom the prognosis is highly favorable, e.g. breast cancer patients with uninvolved nodes.

Another reason for the lack of enthusiasm for histologic appraisal of a tumor's biologic properties may be related to the difficulty in establishing reproducible criteria, whether arbitrary or based upon well recognized cytologic and structural characteristics. Also, there may not be sufficient variation in the histopathologic structure of cancers at certain sites to permit such evaluation. Despite these limitations, assessment of histopathologic characteristics appears to be valuable in predicting clinical behavior for some solid cancers, especially in the case of breast cancer. This chapter will discuss also the prognostic value of pathologic characteristics for cancers of the colon, rectum, prostate, and stomach, although they do not appear to be as well established as for cancer of the breast.

BREAST CANCER

The following identification of pathologic parameters of prognostic significance in invasive breast cancer is based on a personal pathological evaluation of 1603 invasive breast cancers entered into protocol no.4 of the National Surgical Adjuvant Breast Project (NSABP). The patients were prospectively randomized depending upon clinical assessment of nodal status. Those with clinically positive regional nodes were further randomized to be treated by either radical mastectomy or total mastectomy and irradiation, and those whose nodal status was considered to be clinically negative received either radical mastectomy, total mastectomy alone, or total mastectomy with irradiation. The randomization process afforded an equal distribution of histopathologic as well as other characteristics in all of the treatment arms. Survival and treatment failure rates were found to be comparable in the various treatment arms of the clinically negative group (25% at 5 years) as well as in those with clinically positive nodes (41% at 5 years). This finding eliminates any suggestion that variation in survival or treatment failure might be attributable to different treatments.

All of the pathologic material from these patients was examined without knowledge of the clinical course of the patients involved. Thirty-six pathologic features were systematically evaluated in an attempt to discern characteristics which might influence survival or treatment failure. Details concerning these have been presented elsewhere (Fisher *et al.*, 1975, 1976a, b). Exploratory contingency table analysis of this material disclosed 18 pathologic discriminants of prognostic significance.

Treatment failure in the whole group of patients with breast cancer taken collectively (unstratified) was associated with the following: nodal metastases demonstrated pathologically; a tumor size greater than 4.0 cm, a stellate gross and microscopic appearance of the tumor border; proliferative fibrocystic disease in quadrants remote from the dominant mass; perineural space extension of the neoplasm; and the presence of lymphatic extension of tumor in quadrants remote from the dominant mass. Likelihood of treatment failure was influenced by microscopic skin and nipple involvement and tumor type. Highly favorable types were mucinous, papillary, and tubular; moderately favorable were lobular invasive and medullary; of poor prognosis was the infiltrating ductal carcinoma without special features (NOS type). The NOS in pure form was more unfavorable than that found in combination with other histologic types.

There was no prognostic difference between so-called atypical medullary cancer (Fisher *et al.*, 1975; Ridolfi *et al.*, 1977) and its classical form. Patients with tumors of high nuclear and histologic grades did worse than those whose tumors were of low nuclear or histologic grade. Note that our designation of nuclear grade is the converse of that proposed by Black and associates (Black *et al.*, 1955; Black and Speer, 1957), and more customarily employed. Tumor necrosis, lymphoid reaction to the tumor, and a comedo or solid intraductal component were all associated with increased treatment failure rates; whereas the presence of stromal elastica and tumour cell mucin production were associated with the converse. Extranodal extension of axillary metastases was more ominous than when such metastases were confined by the nodal capsule.

Preliminary attempts to rank the significance of these various discriminants by logistic regression analysis showed the pathologic nodal status to be the most dominant influence on treatment failure rates. Further, the number of involved nodes was prognostically discriminating; patients without pathologic evidence of metastases in their regional nodes exhibited a five-year treatment failure rate of only 13%, as opposed to 39% in patients with 1–3 nodal metastases and 69% in those in whom four or more nodes were involved. Because of this finding, it was decided to stratify the material according to the nodal status, viz. absent, 1–3, or four or more nodal metastases (Fisher *et al.*, 1980b).

Contingency table analysis was again performed with the 36 pathologic characteristics of breast cancer being investigated, in the three subsets identified by nodal status. Variables used for further analyses were selected on the basis of the magnitude of difference in the proportion of treatment failures as well as in the relative frequency of their occurrence. This allowed for a reasonable subset of variables for multivariate life-table analyses.

One would expect prognostic factors to apply in all subsets but the results indicated that the presence of tumor necrosis, a high histologic grade (poorly differentiated tumor), and tumors larger than 4 cm did not totally satisfy this criterion. All were observed to influence the treatment failure rates of patients whose cancers were unaccompanied by nodal metastases and, when examined by multivariate analysis, they appeared to discriminate success from failure in those patients with four or more nodal metastases. The inconsistency encountered was their failure to delineate the clinical behavior of patients with 1–3 axillary nodal metastases, a subsect of patients whose clinical behavior lies between that of patients without nodal involvement and those in whom four or more positive nodes are detected.

This inconsistency may be related, at least in part, to the size of the metastases encountered when 1–3 nodes are found to be positive. A significant number of such nodal deposits measure less than 2 mm, and, of these, most are 1.3 mm or less. The observation has been made by us (Fisher *et al.*, 1978b) as well as by others (Huvos *et al.*, 1971; Attiyeh *et al.*, 1977) that metastases of such size are associated with a treatment failure and survival rate which is indistinguishable from that of the negative node patient. Indeed, it has been demonstrated (Fisher *et al.*, 1978c) that approximately one-fourth of all cases of breast cancer whose nodal status has been assessed as being negative by routine pathologic techniques will exhibit small ($\leqslant$ 1.3 mm) occult micrometastases after more extensive sectioning. Yet, in that study, survival in those with such occult micrometastases was not found to be different from that observed in patients whose nodes remained pathologically negative after a similarly extended examination.

Histologic grading

Our scheme of histological grading of breast cancers has been presented in detail elsewhere (Fisher *et al.*, 1975, 1980a). It depends upon the estimation of nuclear grade and the presence of tubule formation, and it should be emphasized that grading is based only upon the invasive components of the cancer. Only 3% of the breast cancers in this material were found to be of low or most favorable grade, 30% were of intermediate grade, and 67% of high or most unfavorable grade.

Because of the importance of nuclear grade in assessing histologic grade, it might be suggested that the estimation of nuclear grade alone could be a sufficient discriminant of tumor differentiation. In fact, plots of survival rates according to nuclear grade closely mimic those of histologic grade, but significant differences in survival according to histologic grade may be found in patients with the same nuclear grade (Fisher *et al.*, 1980a), indicating the former to be a more refined factor of discrimination than nuclear grade alone. It is notable that the reproducibility of nuclear grading has been found by us to be 90% among three reviewers, and 94% with the same reviewer performing assessments at different times (Fisher *et al.*, 1975).

There are no unequivocal data on whether a change in histologic grade or degree of differentiation may occur during the natural history of a breast cancer, but several observations may be relevant. First, we have noted the presence of fewer poorly differentiated carcinomas among patients with the longest duration of symptoms, even though such neoplasms are larger or associated with other characteristics which might suggest a later stage in the development of their disease (Fisher *et al.*, 1977). Secondly, our material has revealed an almost unanimous agreement between the nuclear grade of nodal metastases and that of the primary breast cancer in the same patient. Also, the histologic pattern of growth noted in the primary in the vast majority of instances can be predicted from the appearance of its nodal metastasis.

Linnell *et al.* (1980) have recently suggested that so-called scar cancers may progress from well differentiated tubular to poorly differentiated tumor types. However, investigation of our own material in regard to the histo-genesis of breast cancer from radial scars indicates little difference between peripheral and central portions of such tumours, the latter site being regarded as the initial growth center of the neoplasm. This suggests that the biologic properties of breast cancer follow a predetermined course and do not change with time. There is evidence that a similar situation obtains with rectal cancer (*vide infra*).

The identification of tumor necrosis in the histologic specimen predicts a poor prognosis and the latter appears to be related to the type of necrosis as well as to its degree (Fisher *et al.*, 1978a). The mechanism whereby necrosis is related to survival is unclear. It might be expected that the net growth rate of tumors with necrotic foci would be relatively low, yet we have demonstrated the presence of necrosis to be associated with poor tumor differentiation and also with large tumors (Fisher *et al.*, 1975), 1978b).

Tumor size represents an important prognostic discriminant, but this finding was not totally consistent. Patients with tumors less than 2 cm in greatest diameter fared better than those in whom the cancer measured greater than 4 cm. Yet, the outcome of patients whose tumors measured between 2 and 4 cm was less predictable. Although there is a strong association between tumor size, histologic grade, and tumor necrosis, multivariate analyses have disclosed that all of these tumor characteristics have a somewhat independent adverse effect upon survival. Patients whose neoplasms exhibit all three adverse characteristics have a worse prognosis than those in whom only one was present.

Except for the ominous prognostic relationship of the infiltrating ductal carcinoma without special features (NOS histologic type), no other tumor types were found to be significantly related to treatment failure. However, it should be emphasized that the failure to detect a significant prognostic relationship for mucinous, tubular or papillary forms of breast cancer when the cases were stratified according to nodal status may be due to the relative rarity of these types; as noted earlier, analyses of our data without stratification as to nodal status indicate their highly favorable prognostic significance.

We have not observed a more favorable prognosis with the medullary form of breast cancer although this latter has been regarded as a favorable tumor type. Also, we have failed to discern any significant relationship between blood or lymphatic vessel invasion on the one hand and treatment failure or survival on the other. Again, this finding may be related to the relatively few cases exhibiting such changes when stratified according to nodal status. Indeed, these ominous changes are only rarely found in tumors from patients with negative nodes.

Evidence of host responsiveness

Tsakraklides *et al.* (1974) have called attention to a relationship between survival and certain histologic patterns which may possibly reflect immunologic function in the axillary nodes of patients with breast cancer. Their retrospective studies suggested that a lymphocyte-depleted appearance indicated a poor prognosis, whereas the converse applied in cases with a lymphocyte predominance pattern. An unstimulated nodal appearance or the presence of germinal center predominance suggested intermediate survival rates.

Although in an earlier study (Fisher *et al.*, 1976a) we could not find such an association, subsequent studies indicated an adverse effect of the germinal center predominance pattern on prognosis in patients without nodal metastases (Fisher *et al.*, 1980b). A similar relationship has been noted by Hunter *et al.* (1975) in a smaller series of patients. The relationship between treatment failure and germinal center hyperplasia of lymph nodes suggests that humoral antibody formation (the functional state purported to be reflected by such an appearance) may have an adverse effect upon the natural history of breast cancer. Such a view would be consonant with the proposed action of 'blocking' humoral antibodies.

There are other histopathologic characteristics reflecting host responsiveness which have received much attention as prognostic discriminants, but were not found by us to be significantly related to treatment failure. Black and associates (Black *et al.*, 1955; Black and Speer, 1958) have directed attention to the prognostic significance of a histiocyte response in axillary node sinuses, which they designated as sinus histiocytosis. They, as well as others, have observed a more or less direct relationship between the intensity of this response and survival rates. Although we previously observed a relationship between early treatment failure (12 months) and the absence of this response (Fisher *et al.*, 1975), examination of five-year treatment failure rates have failed to substantiate this relationship (Fisher *et al.*, 1980b). Black and Kwon (1978) have suggested that discrepancies in findings among investigators might be due to a failure to differentiate between so-called active and degenerative forms of this phenomenon, as only the former represents 'true' sinus histiocytosis. However, even delineation of these forms of sinus histiocytosis in our material failed to establish a significant relationship to treatment failure.

Contrary to the findings of Black *et al.* (1955), we have not observed that an intense cell reaction within a breast cancer indicates a favorable prognosis. Indeed, such infiltrates are more frequently observed in poorly differentiated tumors and are associated with a greater incidence of treatment failure when all cases of breast cancer are considered collectively. Further, we have been unable to discern any significant difference in prognosis, whether this cell reaction is principally perivenous in distribution, or diffuse without predilection for the blood vessels. Lastly, we have not observed any relationship between treatment failure and/or survival and the site of the primary cancer within the breast (Fisher *et al.*, 1980b, 1981), and the conventional belief of a poorer prognosis with medial than with lateral breast cancers is not supported.

It may be concluded that the biologic properties of a breast cancer appear to play a significant role in determining its clinical behavior, in regard to both patient survival and treatment failure. Pathologically, these properties are reflected by the degree of tumor differentiation, the tumor size and the presence of tumor necrosis. The histologic tumor type may also play a role, although this may be more closely related to the histologic grade of the tumor rather than to the pattern *per se*. Adverse host responsiveness may manifest as germinal center hyperplasia of regional lymph nodes, particularly in patients without regional nodal metastases.

COLORECTAL CANCER

There is a striking parallelism in the search and identification of pathologic prognostic discriminants for breast and colorectal carcinomas, although the information on the latter has been almost exclusively based upon retrospective enquiry. Investigations concerning prognostic pathologic discriminants for colorectal carcinoma have focused upon the stage of the disease at the time of operation and also on data reflecting the biologic properties of the cancer and the host responsiveness.

Although the stage at presentation and the biologic properties of the tumour may be related, it appears that, as in the case of breast cancer, the biologic properties of colorectal cancers (and to a lesser degree the host responsiveness) may supersede chronological considerations. Several studies have found no relationship (or surprisingly, even a converse relationship) between duration of symptoms and survival (McDermott *et al.*, 1980; Rankin and Broders, 1928; Rankin, 1933; Eker, 1963). Most studies have failed to find a significant relationship between tumor size and survival rate. Further, those investigators exploring pathologic characteristics of biologic significance note the presence of better differentiated tumors in patients with more favorable stages, and the converse in those with more advanced tumors (Dukes, 1936, 1940; Grinnell, 1939; Simpson and Mayo, 1939).

As with breast cancer, the presence of regional nodal metastases as well as the number of such involved nodes appear to represent the most significant prognostic discriminants. The influence of the number of involved nodes is aptly expressed by Dukes (1949), who noted that individuals with five or more such metastases rarely celebrate the fifth anniversary of their disease.

The histologic grading of colorectal cancer has been based mainly on a modification of the scheme first proposed by Broders (1925). Dukes (1936), although indicating that he used Broders' grading methods, emphasized that colorectal carcinomas were either adenocarcinoma or colloid in type. He recognized four grades of differentiation of adenocarcinomas on the basis of structural configuration, and emphasized that this aspect was more important than the relative number of undifferentiated cells—a departure from traditional grading techniques.

So-called colloid, gelatinous and mucoid (more properly mucinous) forms were treated as a separate group, and much debate in the past centered about the nosologic position of those carcinomas with preponderant mucin secretion (Karsner and Clarke, 1932). In fact, the quantity of mucin varies widely between tumors and, subsequently, Grinnell (1939) graded mucinous varieties with the other forms of colorectal cancer.

Grinnell analyzed these histologic characteristics of colorectal carcinomas which might be most useful for prognostic purposes and concluded that the arrangement of the glands, nuclear polarity, frequency of mitoses, and invasive tendency of the neoplasms were the most important. From this information, he formulated combined structural and cellular criteria for three grades and observed a clear relationship between grade and survival, a relationship that obtained whether lymph nodes were, or were not, involved by metastases.

His data also revealed a correlation between the stage of the disease (Dukes) and the histologic grade, and indicated that, although stage was an important consideration in prognosis, it was likely to be related to the degree of differentiation of the tumor as shown in the histologic grade. He found that histologic grading might also be useful with biopsy material since approximately 80% of the biopsies exhibited a comparable grade to that recognised in the resected tumor. This view had also been expressed previously by Stewart and Spies (1929) who also made the important biologic observation from studying serial biopsies that there was no change in the histologic grade with time.

Mention should be made of Qualheim and Gall (1953) who minimized the value of histologic grading of colorectal cancers after observing variations in the same tumor in approximately three-fourths of the cases they studied by the 'giant section' technique. However, some of the areas they considered to show such heterogeneity were actually of benign papillomatous change. More recently, Syrjanen and Hjelt (1978) found a close correlation between nuclear grade and five-year survival in colorectal cancer, apparently discarding structural configurations from consideration.

This brief account of the role of histologic grading in colorectal cancers reflects that, for the most part, the criteria for such schemes have not been carefully or consistently defined, nor is there unanimity as to what characteristics of the tumors may be important for such an approach. As a result, many pathologists merely describe whether a particular cancer is well, moderately well or poorly differentiated. It is interesting that Dukes (1950) suggested that there were three (not two, as previously cited) forms of colorectal cancer: adenocarcinoma, colloid carcinoma, and simplex varieties. However, this last appears to the writer to conform to his grade IV adenocarcinoma described previously in 1940. In addition, the descriptions and pictorial presentations of grade I cancers in many of the grading systems utilized appear to be more consistent with adenomatous or papillomatous polyps than with cancer.

Elucidation of the biologic properties of colorectal neoplasms and their prognostic significance will require detailed examination of pathologic material from *prospective* clinical trials, and large numbers of patients will be necessary to accomplish this because of the limited natural variation among these cancers. Indeed, 82% of cancers studied by Dukes (1940) were characterized as histologic grades II and III.

Other pathologic factors might reflect the biologic nature of colorectal cancers and thus be related to prognosis. These include the appearance of the neoplasm, i.e. whether it is infiltrative or pushing, or whether the tumor exhibits an intraluminal as opposed to an infiltrating macroscopic appearance (Spratt, 1974; Buckwalter and Kent, 1973; Montessori and Donald, 1978). Venous and lymphatic extension have also received attention as prognostic indices, although there is some debate as to the value of the former (Khankanian *et al.*, 1977; Talbot *et al.*, 1980).

Lastly, recent attention has been directed to assessment of the so-called transitional mucosal zone, i.e. the normal bowel adjacent to the cancer. A relationship has been noted between an increase in sialomucins and decrease in sulfomucins in this area and the extent of invasion of the bowel according to Dukes classification. (Filipe and Branfoot, 1974), as well as an inverse relationship between survival rate and the length of the transitional zone (Greaves *et al.*, 1980). Whether this represents an independent variable related to survival has not as yet been clarified.

Factors related to host responsiveness that are claimed to relate to a favorable prognosis are the presence of lymphoid or mast cell stromal response, and paracortical hyperplasia of regional lymph nodes (Pihl *et al.*, 1977). Indeed, Syrjanen and Hjelt (1978) contended that paracortical nodal hyperplasia is incompatible with nodal metastases. This finding is hypothetically consistent with the association of this nodal change with the activity of T cells, mediators of cellular immunity.

PROSTATIC CANCER

Although several systems for histopathologic grading of prostatic cancer have been utilized, their accuracy and consistency have been questioned (Mostofi, 1976). Gleason *et al.* (1974) have recently proposed a scheme based upon a prospective clinical trial, which they found to have significant prognostic value and subsequent experience with this method by others (Kramer *et al.*, 1980) has confirmed its utility. In the Gleason system, patterns of growth of prostatic cancer are assessed histologically by relatively low-power observation (40 to 100 magnifications). To account for variations in histologic pattern in a particular tumor, two patterns are recorded in each sample. Five patterns are recognized and ascribed a number which ascends with increasing malignancy. Thus, each case receives two numbers with the primary pattern indicated by the first digit.

For example, a cancer with a very well differentiated primary pattern but lesser areas that are more poorly differentiated would be scored as 1–5. The sum of the two patterns was found to be strongly related to survival rate and when combined with stage, it was even more discriminating. However, the data revealed similar favorable survival rates in patients with low histopathological scores even if they were in a more advanced stage of the disease. Combined staging and grading identified a group of patients of intermediate risk who showed improved survival following the administration of diethylstilbestrol.

In a conventional sense one might regard the Gleason scheme as a form of histological typing rather than grading. Nevertheless, it may possess therapeutic implications, and, most importantly, it signifies the importance of the biologic characteristics of prostatic cancer (as reflected by its histological appearance) in relation to prognosis. For example, it may predict a favorable natural history for the disease, when staging may suggest the reverse.

STOMACH CANCER

Numerous attempts have been made to identify histopathologic characteristics of gastric cancers which could be used as prognostic discriminants. Unfortunately, the vast majority of these studies have been concerned with the identification of the various histologic types of gastric cancer. Indeed, the literature is replete with descriptions of a host of tumor types, including adenocarcinoma, scirrhous, papillary, small cell, signet ring cell, blue cell, medullary, etc., but little prognostic information has been obtained from such an exercise. In some instances, complex schema incorporating features of both stage and histologic type have been utilized for this purpose but have not been widely adopted.

A more simplified approach was proposed by Lauren (1963) who considered only two main tumor types which he designated as intestinal and diffuse. The former represented localized or circumscribed tumors with preponderant glandular features, whereas the latter were represented by those tumors with infiltrative microscopic characteristics and decidely less gland formation. Some investigators prefer to distinguish these types of gastric cancer as either expanding and infiltrative, or pushing and infiltrative (Ming, 1977; Martin and Kay, 1964). The prognosis of the intestinal (expanding or pushing) type was better than in those with an infiltrative appearance.

The studies of Kubo (1971) are of interest in that his classification, which exhibited some relationship to survival, recognized three main types of gastric cancer: adenocarcinoma, mucoid, and diffuse. The former was divided into four subtypes stratified according to features of differentiation. Two classes of differentiation characterized the mucoid tumors, whereas the diffuse varieties were represented by signet cell, desmoplastic, and a more anaplastic variety. This classification represents a congeries of features encompassing structural characteristics as well as features of differentiation.

Black *et al.* (1954) attempted to utilize characteristics which they had recognized in other cancers, particularly those of the breast, to be useful prognostic indicators. Certainly, estimation of nuclear grade, one of their principal discriminants, is directly related to differentiation and the criteria for the various grades of differentiation are well defined by these authors. Host responses were assessed by changes in the regional lymph nodes and by the lymphoid infiltrate in the primary tumor.

They noted in a relatively small series of cases that sinus histiocytosis of regional nodes and lymphoid infiltrate of the tumor were more important discriminants than the age or sex of the patient, period of delay in treatment, and, surprisingly, even the metastatic status of the regional nodes. However, in a subsequent report (Black *et al.*, 1971), based upon a larger number of patients from the Norwegian Cancer Registry, they recognized the rarity of sinus histiocytosis in regional nodes of patients with gastric cancer, and emphasized instead nodal follicular hyperplasia as an index of host responsiveness with a favorable outcome—a situation which is the converse of that found by us (Fisher *et al.*, 1980a) in patients with breast cancer.

Favorable nuclear grade and a lymphoid response within the primary tumor were also encountered more frequently in survivors with gastric cancer than in those dying of the disease. Assessment of histologic grade according to a modification of the Broders' method performed by the Norwegian collaborators in that study revealed similar findings to that from assessing nuclear grade, although it was noted that histologic grade might supersede estimation of nuclear grade.

It might be concluded that studies attempting to relate certain histopathologic characteristics of gastric cancer to survival rate exhibit the defects of retrospective analyses as outlined previously; they lack important information which might be obtained from multivariate analyses (e.g. does the relationship of survival rate to nuclear grade or other histologic parameters still obtain in patients with positive nodes?) and have not been demonstrated to be reproducible. Nevertheless, despite these shortcomings, the findings do suggest the potential prognostic value of pathologic characteristics which may reflect the biologic properties of gastric cancer and host responsiveness.

CONCLUSION

Pathologic characteristics which reflect the biologic properties of the tumor and also the host responsiveness have been shown to be useful as prognostic discriminants. There is strong evidence of their value in the case of cancer of the breast and prostate, and, while the evidence for colorectal and gastric cancers is less convincing, it still suggests that such a practice might be useful.

The lack of confidence in, or wide acceptance of, pathologic prognostic discriminants for cancers of these sites is probably not as much a reflection of a 'failure of fit' as it is the failure of a 'true test'. Prospective randomized studies performed on large numbers of patients are necessary to resolve this problem satisfactorily.

Despite limitations, the results of almost all studies strongly imply that the biologic characteristics of the cancer and host responsiveness supersede simple mechanistic and strictly time-oriented considerations in influencing survival. Further, it seems likely that the degree of differentiation of cancers is not changed with time, at least during the portion of their life history which is available for pathologic examination.

REFERENCES

Attiyeh, F.F., Jensen, M., Huvos, A.G., and Fracchia, A. (1977). Axillary micro-metastases and macrometastases in carcinoma of the breast. *Surg., Gynecol. Obstet.*, **144**, 839.

Black, M.M., Freeman, C., Mork, T., Harvei, S., and Cutler, S.J. (1971). Prognostic significance of microscopic structure of gastric carcinomas and their regional lymph nodes. *Cancer*, **27**, 703.

Black, M.M., and Kwon, C.S. (1978). Prognostic factors. In *The breast* (eds H.S. Gallagher, H.P. Lewis, R.K. Snyderman, and J.A. Urban). St. Louis: C.V. Mosby.

Black, M.M., Opler, S.R., and Speer, F.D. (1954). Microscopic studies of gastric carcinomas and their regional lymph nodes in relation to survival. *Surg., Gynecol. Obstet.*, **98**, 725.

Black, M.M., Opler, S.R., and Speer, F.D. (1955). Survival in breast cancer cases in relation to the structure of the primary tumor and regional lymph nodes. *Surg., Gynecol. Obstet.*, **100**, 543.

Black, M.M., and Speer, F.D. (1958). Sinus histiocytosis of lymph nodes in cancer. *Surg., Gynecol. Obstet.*, **106**, 163.

Broders, A.C. (1925). The grading of carcinoma. *Minnesota Med. J.*, **8**, 726.

Buckwalter, J.A., and Kent, T.H. (1973). Colonic cancer. *Arch. Pathol.*, **95**, 366.

Dukes, C.E. (1936). Histological grading of rectal cancer. *Proc. R. Soc. Med.*, **30**, 25.

Dukes, C.E. (1940). Cancer of the rectum: an analysis of 1000 cases. *J. Pathol. Bacteriol.*, **50**, 527.

Dukes, C.E. (1949). The surgical pathology of rectal cancer. *J. Clin. Pathol.*, **2**, 95.

Dukes, C.E. (1950). The relation of histology to spread in intestinal cancer. *Br. J. Cancer*, **4**, 59.

Eker, R. (1963). Some prognostic factors for carcinoma of the colon and rectum. *Acta Chir. Scand.*, **126**, 636.

Filipe, M.I., and Branfoot, A.C. (1974). Abnormal patterns of mucus secretion in apparently normal mucosa of large intestine with carcinoma. *Cancer*, **34**, 282.

Fisher, B. (1980). Laboratory and clinical research in breast cancer—a personal adventure: The David A. Karnofsky Memorial Lecture. *Cancer Res.*, **40**, 3874.

Fisher, B., Wolmark, N., Redmond, C., Deutsch, M., and Fisher, E.R. (1981). Findings from NSABP protocol no. B–04; Comparison of radical mastectomy with alternative treatments. II. The clinical and biological significance of medial–central breast cancers. *Cancer*, **48**, 1863.

Fisher, E.R., Gregorio, R.M., and Fisher, B. (1975). The pathology of invasive breast cancer. A syllabus derived from the findings of the National Surgical Adjuvant Breast Project (protocol no.4). *Cancer*, **36**, 1.

Fisher, E.R., Gregorio, R.M., Redmond, C., Dekker, A., and Fisher, B. (1967a). Pathologic findings from the National Surgical Adjuvant Breast Project (protocol no. 4).II. The significance of regional node histology other than sinus histiocytosis in invasive mammary cancer. *Am. J. Clin. Pathol.*, **65**, 21.

Fisher, E.R., Gregorio, R.M., Redmond, C., Kim, W.S., and Fisher, B. (1976b). Pathologic findings from the National Surgical Adjuvant Breast Project (protocol no. 4). III. The significance of extranodal extension of axillary metastases. *Am. J. Clin. Pathol.*, **65**, 439.

Fisher, E.R., Palekar, A.S., Gregorio, R.M., Redmond C., and Fisher, B. (1978a). Pathologic findings from the National Surgical Adjuvant Breast Project (protocol no. 4). IV. Significance of tumor necrosis. *Human Pathol.*, **9**, 523.

Fisher, E.R., Palekar, A.S., Rockette, H., Redmond, C., and Fisher, B. (1978b). Pathologic findings from the National Surgical Adjuvant Breast Project (protocol no.4). V. Significance of axillary nodal micro and macrometastases. *Cancer*, **42**, 2032.

Fisher, E.R., Redmond, C., and Fisher, B. (1980a): Histologic grading of breast cancer. *Pathol. Annu.*, **15**, 239.

Fisher, E.R., Redmond, C., and Fisher, B. (1980b). Pathologic findings from the National Surgical Adjuvant Breast Project (protocol no.4). VI. Discriminants for five-year treatment failure. *Cancer*, **46**, 908.

Fisher, E.R., Swamidoss, S., Lee, C.H., Rockette, H., Redmond, C., and Fisher, B. (1978c). Detection and significance of occult axillary node metastases in patients with invasive breast cancer. *Cancer*, **42**, 2025.

Gleason, D.F., Mellinger, G.T., and the Veterans Administration Cooperative Urological Research Group (1974). Prediction of prognosis for prostatic adeno-carcinoma by combined histological grading and clinical staging. *J. Urol.*, **111**, 58.

Greaves, P., Filipe, M.I., and Branfoot, A.C. (1980). Transitional mucosa and survival in the human colorectal cancer. *Cancer*, **46**, 764.

Grinnell, R.S. (1939). The grading and prognosis of carcinoma of the colon and rectum. *Ann. Surg.*, **109**, 500.

Hunter, R.L., Ferguson, D.J., and Coppleson, L.W. (1975). Survival with mammary cancer related to the interaction of germinal center hyperplasia and sinus histiocytosis in axillary and internal mammary lymph nodes. *Cancer*, **36**, 528.

Huvos, A.G., Hutter, R.V.P., and Berg, J.W. (1971). Significance of axillary macrometastases and micrometastases in mammary cancer. *Ann. Surg.*, **173**, 44.

Karsner, H.T., and Clarke, B. (1932). Analysis of 104 cases of carcinoma of the large intestine. *Am. J. Cancer*, **16**, 933.

Khankanian, N., Maglivit, G.M., Russell, W.O., and Schimer, M. (1977). Prognostic significance of vascular invasion in colorectal cancer of Dukes B class. *Cancer*, **39**, 1195.

Kramer, S.A., Spahr, J., Brendler, C.B., Glenn, J.F., and Paulson, J. (1980). Experience with Gleason's histopathological grading in prostatic cancer. *J. Urol.*, **124**, 223.

Kubo, T. (1971). Histological appearance of gastric carcinoma in high and low mortality countries: comparison between Kyushu, Japan and Minnesota, USA. *Cancer*, **28**, 1971.

Lauren, P. (1963). The two histological main types of gastric carcinoma: diffuse and so-called intestinal-type carcinoma. *Acta Pathol. Microbiol. Scand.*, **64**, 31.

Linnell, F., Ljunberg, O., and Anderson, I. (1980). Breast carcinoma. Aspects of early stages, progression and related problems. *Acta Pathol. Microbiol. Scand.* Suppl. 272

McDermott, F.T., Hughes, E.S.R., Pihl, E.A., and Milne, B.J. (1980). Changing survival prospects in carcinoma of the rectum. *Br. J. Surg.*, **67**, 775.

Martin, C., and Kay, S. (1964). The prognosis of gastric carcinoma as related to its morphologic characteristics. *Surg., Gynecol. Obstet.*, **119**, 319.

Ming, S. (1977). Gastric carcinoma. A pathobiological classification. *Cancer*, **39**, 2475.

Montessori, G.A., and Donald, J.D. (1978). Invasion profile of colorectal carcinoma. *Dis. Colon Rectum*, **21**, 26.

Mostofi, F.K. (1976). Problems of grading carcinoma of prostate. *Semin. Oncol.*, **3**, 161.

Pihl, E., Malahy, M.A., Khankhanian, N., Hersh, E.M., and Maglivit, G.M. (1977). Immunomorphological features of prognostic significance in Dukes class B colorectal carcinoma. *Cancer Res.*, **37**, 4145.

Qualheim, R.E., and Gall, E.A. (1953). Is histologic grading of colon carcinoma a valid procedure? *Arch. Pathol.*, **56**, 466.

Rankin, F.W. (1933). The curability of cancer of the colon, rectosigmoid and rectum. *J. Am. Med. Assoc.*, **101**, 491.

Rankin, F.W., and Broders, A.C. (1928). Factors influencing prognosis in carcinoma of the rectum. *Surg., Gynecol. Obstet.*, **46**, 660.

Ridolfi, R.L., Rosen, P.P., Port, A., Kinne, D., and Mike, V. (1977). Medullary carcinoma of the breast. A clinicopathologic study with 10 year follow up. *Cancer*, **40**, 1365.

Simpson, W.C., and Mayo, C.W. (1939). The mural penetration of the carcinoma cell in the colon: anatomic and clinical study. *Surg., Gynecol. Obstet.*, **68**, 872.

Spratt, J.S. (1974). Carcinoma of the rectum: biologic characteristics. *Dis. Colon Rectum*, **17**, 591.

Stewart, F.W., and Spies, J.W. (1929). Biopsy histology in the grading of rectal carcinoma. *J. Pathol.*, **5**, 109.

Syrjanen, K.J., and Hjelt, L.H. (1978). Tumor-host relationships in colorectal carcinoma. *Dis. Colon Rectum*, **21**, 29.

Talbot, I.C., Ritchie, S., Leighton, M.H., Hughes, A.O., Bussey, H.J.R., and Morson, B.C. (1980). The clinical significance of invasion of veins by rectal cancer. *Br. J. Surg.*, **67**, 439.

Tsakraklides, V., Olson, P., Kersey, J.H., and Good, R.A. (1974). Prognostic significance of the regional lymph node histology in cancer of the breast. *Cancer*, **34**, 1259.

Willis, R.A. (1967). *Pathology of tumours*, 4th edn. London: Butterworths.

Cancer Treatment: End Point Evaluation
Edited by B.A. Stoll
© 1983 John Wiley & Sons Ltd.

Chapter

9 J.E. DEVITT

Lymph Node Invasion and its Significance

INTRODUCTION

The traditional view of the distant spread of carcinomas assumes that the lymphatic system is the main pathway, and that the pattern of lymph node involvement follows the natural routes of drainage (Robbins and Cotran, 1979). The afferent lymphatics of the lymph gland enter the peripheral sinus and it is here that metastatic growths due to lymphatic emboli are initially situated (Willis, 1973). These channels are often to be seen distended by the proliferating tumor cells, which extend from there into the substance of the lymph gland along the interfollicular sinuses toward the medulla.

It is postulated that the regional nodes serve as an effective barrier to further dissemination in many cases, but that more distant spread eventually occurs when excessive numbers of tumor cells and proliferation of the tumor within the lymph node itself overwhelm the filtration function. Once a node has been obstructed by tumor, spread may occur because of the diversion of lymph flow from the obstructed node into collateral channels passing to unaffected neighboring nodes. These now become the sites of arrested emboli from the original source as well as from the affected nodes.

This concept implies that there is a time when the neoplastic process has not yet spread beyond the primary site and regional lymph nodes, and provides a theoretical basis for radical surgical and radiotherapy treatment. It is justified by numerous reports of patients with lymph node metastases, whether malignant melanoma (Cohen *et al.*, 1977), breast cancer (Brinkley and Haybittle, 1977) or bronchial carcinoma (Shields, 1980), who remain clinically free of disease following local–regional treatment. Even patients with extensive regional nodal metastases may have a long survival and be apparently cured, whether with rectal carcinoma (Bacon *et al.*, 1958), breast cancer (Adair *et al.*, 1974) or malignant melanoma (Cohen *et al.*, 1977).

However, an alternative explanation for these apparent cures is that the tumor cells may have passed the 'lymph node barrier' but that the tumor–host relationship has not allowed the development of actively growing distant metastases.

Copher *et al.* (1962) observed that patients with inner quadrant breast cancer (and a higher likelihood of untreated internal mammary node metastases), did as well as patients with outer quadrant lesions. In the same year, Devitt (1962) noted that breast cancer patients treated by conservative axillary surgery did as well as those with radical axillary surgery, and observed that other reports had found that regional radiotherapy failed to improve survival rates. Both authors suggested that metastatic regional lymph nodes were not the cause of the poor outcome with which they were associated, but rather were signposts of the unfavorable tumor–host relationship that was responsible for the poor prognosis.

This chapter deals with the overwhelming statistical and biological evidence that now supports this concept in the case of breast cancer, and to a lesser extent in other types of cancer. The topic will be explored under three headings:

Statistical correlations.
Biological correlations
Therapeutic implications.

STATISTICAL CORRELATIONS

Natural history and node metastases

In all types of carcinoma the presence of regional lymph node metastases is associated with poorer survival rates. For breast cancer patients, axillary lymph node metastases reduce the survival rates by half or more at each follow-up period for 25 years (Brinkley and Haybittle, 1977). Devitt (1967) reported that axillary lymph node metastases doubled the annual mortality rates of breast cancer patients. Morson and Dawson (1974) reported that five-year survival rates of patients with carcinoma of the colon or rectum was lowered from 80% to 30% in the presence of lymph node metastases.

Karakousis *et al.* (1980) reported that the median survival rate of malignant melanoma patients without lymph node metastases was 85 months, whereas it was 26 months in those with metastases in regional nodes. Shields (1980) reported that the metastatic involvement of lobar or hilar lymph nodes reduced the survival of patients with bronchial carcinoma by one-half at both five- and ten-year follow-up periods. Prout *et al.* (1980) reported a probability of survival without progressive disease of 84% in patients with carcinoma of the prostate without nodal involvement compared to 34% for those with metastatic nodes.

Lymph node metastases have a greater prognostic significance than any other primary tumor characteristics. Cohen *et al.* (1977) found that, in malignant melanoma patients, lymph node status was more strongly correlated with survival time than was the level or thickness of the primary tumor. Clarke and Spangler (1980) found that the survival rate in breast cancer patients with negative nodes and large primary tumors was better than in those with positive nodes and primary lesions less than 2 cm in diameter. Fracchia *et al.* (1980) found that, in breast cancer, 'grave' signs in the primary lesion did not have the same effect on survival rates in patients with negative nodes as they did in patients with positive nodes. Similarly, they did not adversely affect recurrence rates in patients with no nodal involvement.

Not only are survival rates worse, but local–regional recurrence rates also are worse, in patients with regional lymph node metastases. Devitt (1967) reported that, in spite of their worse survival rates, breast cancer patients with axillary node metastases had a 17% five-year local skin recurrence rate compared to 10% for those without axillary metastases. Enker *et al.* (1979) reported that the presence of regional lymph nodes in colorectal cancers more than doubled the local recurrence rate. Karakousis *et al.* (1980) reported that 14% of malignant melanoma patients with negative lymph nodes developed regional recurrences compared to 49% of patients with histologically positive nodes. Further, in breast cancer patients at least, those with regional lymph node metastases develop recurrences earlier and survive their recurrence or metastatic disease for shorter periods of time (Shimkin *et al.*, 1954; Devitt, 1967, 1971).

Thus, when the tumor–host relationship is unfavorable, the cancer patient is more likely to have metastases in the regional nodes. In addition, local or regional recurrence will be more common, as will also be a lethal outcome. Recurrence or metastasis will appear earlier and the patient's survival of the metastases will be shorter. These last observations cannot be explained on a step-by-step, node-by-node, concept of tumor spread.

Delay before treatment and regional lymph node metastases

One would expect that a longer period of delay before seeking treatment would give the cancer more time to spread to the regional lymph nodes. While there is in breast cancer patients a suggestion that increasing delay before treatment increases the likelihood of regional lymph node metastases, the correlation is a very weak one. Bloom (1965) found that 59% of his patients with a history of less than a month had pathological involvement of the lymph nodes. It only increased to 68% of those patients who admitted to having had their tumor for three or more years.

Devitt (1967) found no significant difference in the distribution of the time delay before treatment in patients with or without axillary node metastases. Fisher *et al.* (1977) found that 52% of their patients with a duration of symptoms of one month or less had axillary lymph node metastases compared to 57% of those with a symptom duration of nine or more months. Handley (1972) reported that, when the duration of symptoms was one month or less, 52% of patients had axillary node metastases and 21% had internal mammary node metastases. When the duration of symptoms was 10 months or longer, 55% of patients had axillary lymph node metastases and 39% had internal mammary node metastases.

McDermott *et al.* (1981) reported that increasing duration of symptoms in patients with carcinoma of the rectum was not associated with an increase in the proportion with lymph node metastases.

In studying the level of axillary node involvement in breast cancer patients, Robbins and Bross (1957) observed that 28% of patients with a history of less than two months delay had Level III metastases, 30% of those with 2–6 months delay in treatment had such involvement, and 41% of those with more than 6 months delay. Proportions with only Level I involvement were respectively 13%, 10%, and 13%. In examining the effect of duration of symptoms on the number of lymph node metastases, Fisher *et al.* (1977) found that 30% of patients with a duration of symptoms of less than one month had four or more axillary lymph nodes invaded compared to 33% of patients with a duration of nine or more months.

Thus, there is a very weak relationship between the duration of symptoms in breast cancer and the presence or extent of regional lymph node metastases. While it may be logical to expect that 'older' tumors would have more time to develop lymph node metastases than 'younger' tumors, time does not in fact seem to be the major determinant; rather, it is likely to be the tumor–host relationship, as shown by the common observation of tumors with a very short history which nevertheless show extensive regional lymph node metastases.

Primary lesion characteristics and node metastases

In general, the larger the size of the primary tumor, the greater the likelihood of lymph node metastases. Fisher *et al.* (1969) reported that whereas 22% of patients with breast cancers less than 1 cm in greatest diameter had axillary lymph node metastases, there was a progressive increase in risk with increasing size, so that 63% of patients with tumors 6 cm or more in diameter had axillary lymphatic involvement. Handley (1972) observed that breast cancer patients with lesions smaller than 2.5 cm had internal mammary node metastases in 15% of cases and this increased to 45% when the lesion was greater than 5 cm in diameter. Robbins and Bross (1957) have reported greater likelihood of Level III involvement of the axillary lymph nodes with increasing size of primary tumor in the breast.

Local extension of the primary tumor also influences the likelihood of nodal metastases. Balch *et al.* (1978) have reported that patients with increasing thickness of malignant melanomas had increasing risk of lymph node involvement. Dukes (1940) reported that carcinoma of the rectum was rarely associated with lymph node metastases until it had spread by direct continuity into the perirectal fat. Prout *et al.* (1980) reported that prostatic cancers with positive nodes were more often associated with extracapsular spread and increasing T stage.

While this could be interpreted as meaning that small (young) tumors have not had time to spread to regional lymph nodes, an alternative explanation is that an unfavorable tumor–host relationship will result in larger primary tumors, greater local invasion, and a greater likelihood of regional lymph node metastases.

The degree of differentiation of the primary tumor has an important relationship to the likelihood of lymph node metastases. Dukes (1940), using a four-grade classification of carcinoma of the rectum, found that the incidence of lymph node involvement increased from 24% in those patients with the most differentiated tumors to 93% in those with the least differentiated. Dukes (1940) also observed a relationship between differentiation and the number of lymph nodes involved in rectal carcinoma patients. Bloom and Richardson (1957) using a three-stage grading for breast cancer patients found that lymph node involvement increased from 50% in those with the most differentiated tumors to 73% in those with the least differentiated.

Again, an unfavorable tumor–host relationship could result both in a poorly differentiated tumor and in a high likelihood of regional lymph node metastases.

Natural history and anatomic extent of lymph node metastases

It is widely agreed that, when only the lymph nodes adjacent to the tumor contain metastases, survival rates are considerably better than when more distant nodes are involved. Gabriel (1949) observed five-year survival rates for patients with carcinoma of the rectum of 42% when only the nodes adjacent to the rectum were implicated, whereas it fell to 12% when the metastases involved nodes adjacent to the origin of the inferior mesenteric artery. McDivitt *et al.* (1968) observed that patients with breast cancer and Level I axillary node involvement had a 56% five-year survival rate but this fell to 28% for those with Level III metastases. Shields (1980) observed that patients with bronchial carcinoma had worse survival rates when hilar lymph nodes were involved compared to patients with only lobar lymph node involvement. Prognosis was worse still if there were mediastinal lymph node metastases.

More distant regional node metastases are likely to be associated with larger tumors. Berg (1955) reported that breast cancers smaller than 2 cm in size have a 6% incidence of Level III axillary node metastases, whereas if the primary was 6 cm or bigger it was 61%. Berg also reported that Level III metastases were almost always associated with more proximal axillary nodal involvement. This observation was supported by Haagensen (1971).

However, Smith *et al.* (1977) observed that 10% of their radical mastectomy patients had distal lymph node metastases only. Another 10% had middle level node metastases only, and a further 6% had middle and distal nodal involvement without proximal metastases. They concluded that, in a majority of patients, metastases to lymph nodes occur in an orderly manner. Attiyeh *et al.* (1977) also observed a 10% incidence of involvement of more distant axillary lymph nodes without proximal nodal metastases.

Gabriel (1949) reported that patients with carcinoma of the rectum occasionally have distant regional node involvement without proximal metastases but that the majority of patients had proximal metastatic nodes first, and that more distal nodes were rarely involved without the proximal onces being previously invaded. Dukes (1940) observed a single lymph node metastasis in 22% of his rectal cancer specimens, two metastatic nodes in 15%, and three positive nodes in 14.5%. He concluded that spread was from node to node and was slow.

Handley (1964) reported that 31% of breast cancer patients with medial lesions had internal mammary node metastases; 47% of those with central lesions but only 19% of those with lateral lesions. This same ratio persisted in patients with axillary node metastases but was increased respectively to 51% for medial, 59% for central, and 28% for lateral lesions. Handley (1972) reported that only 9% of breast cancer patients with negative axillary lymph nodes had internal mammary lymph node metastases compared to 35% of patients with positive axillary nodes.

More distant regional node involvement is associated with increasing numbers of nodes being involved (Haagensen, 1971; Smith *et al.*, 1977). Berg (1955) observed that while 45% of axillary lymph nodes were situated proximally and 20% distally, 60% of nodes bearing metastases were in the proximal group compared to only 9% of nodal metastases in the more distant level.

Berg and Robbins (1966) have reported that the subsequent 15-year mortality rates for five-year survivors increases with Level III axillary involvement. For patients with no nodes, it was 22%, for patients with Levels I or II involvement, it was 39%, and for Level III involvement, 64%. In the first five years, only 42% of the mortality occurred in patients with no lymph node metastases, 61% in patients with involvement at Level I, 76% at Level II, and 77% at Level III. On the other hand, Langlands *et al.* (1979) reported that after 10 years the original stage of breast cancer appeared to have no effect on survival rates.

Thus, anatomic extent of nodal metastases may be more a manifestation of tumor–host relationship than of tumor duration. If the lymph node metastases are confined to nodes adjacent to the primary tumor, it is because of the tumor–host state, not because time has been insufficient for further spread.

Natural history and degree of regional node involvement

The greater the number of lymph nodes involved, the worse the outcome. Cohen *et al.* (1977) reported that malignant melanoma patients with four or more lymph node metastases had only half the survival rates of those with 1–3 lymph node metastases. Morson and Dawson (1974) observed that colorectal carcinoma patients with one lymph node metastasis had a 60% five-year survival rate which fell to 35% if 2–5 lymph nodes were involved, and 20% if six or more nodes were involved. Fisher *et al.* (1969) have demonstrated how breast cancer patients with four or more lymph node metastases have only half the survival rate of those with 1–3 node involvement. However, patients with one lymph node metastasis have outcomes that are not much worse than those who have no nodes involved.

Morson and Dawson (1974) also noted 60% five-year survival rate for colorectal carcinoma patients with one nodal metastasis compared to 80% for those with no involved nodes. Karakousis *et al.* (1980) reported a five-year survival rate of 41% for malignant melanoma patients with one node metastasis compared to 58% for those with no metastases. Prout *et al.* (1980) reported that a single node metastasis in prostatic carcinoma patients is associated with a not-unfavorable prognosis.

On the other hand, when four or more lymph nodes are involved, the likelihood of control is poor. Attiyeh *et al.* (1977) had no 14-year survival in breast cancer patients with four or more lymph node metastases but most authors show some long-term survivors among such patients (Fisher *et al.*, 1969). Karakousis *et al.* (1980) reported a five-year survival rate for malignant melanoma patients of 18% when three or more lymph nodes were involved with metastases. Morson and Dawson (1974) reported a 20% five-year survival rate for colorectal carcinoma patients when six or more lymph nodes contained metastases. Smith *et al.* (1977) found that the total number of nodes involved was a more important prognosticator for breast cancer patients than was the level of the axillary metastases.

Handley (1972) observed that 10-year survival rates for breast cancer patients were 66% when no regional lymph nodes were involved, 38% when the axilla only was involved, and 35% when internal mammary nodes only were involved. The survival rate fell to 11% when both axillary and internal mammary lymph nodes contained metastases.

Features of the primary tumor that are associated with a poor outcome tend to be associated with a greater number of regional lymph node metastases. Fisher *et al*. (1969) observed that larger primaries are more likely to have four or more lymph node metastases. However, over 40% of the patients with primary tumors smaller than 2 cm who had lymph node metastases had four or more nodes involved. Dukes (1940) commented on the relationship between increasing number of lymph node metastases and the histological grade of rectal cancers.

In the case of breast cancer, the degree of involvement of the axillary regional lymph nodes can be correlated with the likelihood of internal mammary lymph node involvement. Handley and Thackray (1954) and Handley (1964) observed that, in breast cancer patients, when the axillary nodes were not involved, only 9–14% of patients had internal mammary lymph node metastases. If the axilla was lightly involved, 26% had internal mammary node metastases. When axillary involvement was moderate, the internal mammary rate was 37%; and with heavy axillary involvement, 65% of patients had internal mammary metastases.

Thus, patients with unfavorable tumor–host relationships will have regional lymph node metastases in greater number as well as of greater anatomical extent.

Pathological examination of regional lymph nodes is necessary for the identification of metastases because of the inaccuracy of clinical examination. It appears to matter whether the nodal metastases are micrometastases or macrometastases. Attiyeh *et al*. (1977) observed that breast cancer patients with micrometastases (< 2 mm) at Level I had an 85% 10-year survival rate compared to 64% for patients with macrometastases. At all levels, patients with only micrometastases had a 75% 10-year survival rate compared to 40% for patients with macrometastases.

Pickren (1961), by serially sectioning radical mastectomy specimens that had been previously reported as free of nodal metastases, found occult metastases in over 20% of specimens. But he also reported that the survival rate for patients with occult axillary metastases was practically identical to that of patients who had no lymph node involvement. Huvos *et al*. (1971) also could observe no difference in outcome for patients with Level I micrometastases when compared to patients with negative lymph nodes.

While Fisher *et al*. (1969) have repeatedly emphasized the poor outlook of patients with more than four positive axillary nodes, they have also reported (Fisher *et al*., 1981) that the more nodes that are removed, the greater the probability that four or more nodes will be detected. Indeed, Fisher *et al*. (1978) have suggested that the demonstration of occult axillary lymph node metastases in breast cancer has more academic that practical value. From all of these observations it can be concluded that, in breast cancer patients at least, micrometastases in the axillary lymph nodes do not have the same dire significance relative to outcome that macrometastases have (see Chapter 8).

BIOLOGICAL CORRELATIONS

Variable behavior of patients with lymph node metastases

Fisher (1980), based on the results of clinical trials, has suggested that all subgroups of patients, categorized according to aggressiveness and degree of nodal involvement, do not respond to the same extent to a specific therapeutic regimen or to different regimens. He has drawn attention to the NSABP Trials' observation that women under 49 years of age with 1–3 positive lymph nodes have a significant improvement in disease-free probability when treated with an adjuvant course of phenylalanine mustard compared to women over 50 with 1–3 lymph nodes involved or women under 49 with four or more nodes involved. Also, increasing the therapy from one to two or three drugs in patients over 50 increased the disease-free survival late in patients with four or more nodes involved, whereas those with 1–3 nodes involved were unaffected.

Variable behavior of lymph node metastases

Willis (1973) remarks that carcinomas of the tongue, tonsil, and pharynx produce lymph node metastases rather early and in a high proportion of cases. On the other hand, carcinoma of the lip and larynx produce lymph node metastases more tardily and in fewer cases. The sluggish natural history of cervical lymph node metastases of many thyroid cancers is well known.

Sugarbaker (1979) points out that, in malignant melanoma and squamous carcinoma of the tongue, when the incidence of micrometastases in surgical node dissection specimen is compared with the incidence of grossly palpable nodes in observed patients, it is found that microscopic deposits nearly always bloom as macroscopic tumor deposits with time. On the other hand, micrometastatic breast cancer does so in only about 50% of patients while only a small percentage of micrometastatic papillary carcinoma of the thyroid evolves to clinical status.

Devitt (1965) reported the indolent behavior of axillary lymph node metastases in some patients with breast cancer. The nodes may first become apparent 5–10 years after mastectomy. One-third of such recurrences occur concurrently with, or after the appearance of, other distant metastases. Such nodes have apparently remained quiescent for many years in peaceful coexistence with their host. Similar behavior of contralateral axillary lymph node metastases has been observed (Devitt and Mickelchuk, 1969).

Thus, regional lymph node metastases do not have a constant biological significance for carcinomas arising at different sites and in different patients. That this should be so is quite in keeping with the fact that the natural history of the disease is determined by the undoubtedly changeable balance between the tumor's growth potential and the host's restraining capability.

Distant lymph node metastases

In patients succumbing to their cancers, surprising numbers are found to have lymph node metastases at distant sites remote from the primary tumor. Devitt and Mickelchuk (1969) have discussed the significance of contralateral axillary metastases in breast cancer. Viadana *et al.* (1973) and Abrams *et al.* (1950) have observed that 40% of breast cancer patients have abdominal lymph node metastases at autopsy, 55–65% have mediastinal nodes, and 15–36% have cervical nodes. The former authors felt that these represented metastases from organs draining to these areas. Abrams *et al.* (1950) also observed mediastinal metastatic nodes in 30% of autopsy patients dying of carcinoma of the stomach, in 17% of patients dying of carcinoma of the colon or rectum, in 34% of carcinoma of the ovary autopsies, in 40% of renal carcinomas, and in 22% of carcinomas of the pancreas.

Lee (1980) observed that, at autopsy, metastatic melanoma could be found in 56–74% of patients in the abdominal lymph nodes, and in a similar proportion in the thoracic nodes, while other nodes were involved in 42–74% of autopsy studies. Willis (1973) has commented that tumor is transferred from lymph node to lymph node until a whole group or even a large part of the entire lymphatic system of the body is affected. Grinnel (1966) and others have attributed this to lymph blockage and stasis and diversion of lymph flow to other nodes and channels, with the possibility of retrograde flow and sometimes permeation of lymphatic channels.

The alternative possibility exists that in some individuals the lymph nodes, rather than being involved directly by bizarre lymphatic flow, are simply more susceptible to the metastatic process, just as in other patients some specific organs or tissues (liver, lungs or bones) will bear many metastases while others will bear few or none.

Lymph node barrier filter function

In a series of elegant experiments utilizing labeled tumor cells injected into the lymphatics of rabbits, Fisher and Fisher (1967) demonstrated that the majority of labeled tumor cells traversed the lymph nodes to enter either efferent lymph channels or the venous system via nodal lymphaticovenous communications. Many tumor cells initially retained in the nodes following injection, maintained only temporary residence. They concluded that a unification exists between the blood and lymph vascular systems. They also suggested that the characteristics of the tumor cells may be as great as or a greater determinant of their residence in nodes as are the biological and mechanical properties of such nodes (see Chapter 8).

Willis (1973) comments that lymph nodes, far from being the site of annihilation of embolic tumor cells, appear rather to be a hotbed for their successful development. Histologic study fails to reveal any evidence of wholesale destruction of tumor cells in lymph nodes.

Thus, there is little evidence to support the concept of a lymph node barrier. The concept resulted from our limited ability to recognize distant micrometastases and the false assumption that non-recognition meant non-existence.

Immunologic function

Black *et al.* (1955) have reported a correlation between the presence of sinus histiocytosis in axillary lymph nodes of patients with breast cancer and their long-term survival. This has been considered to represent a host immunologic reaction to tumor growth. While many have supported the relationship between the intensity of the nodal reaction and survival rates, others (Berg, 1956) have failed to find any significant correlation.

Since it has been repeatedly shown that regional lymph nodes participate in the initiation of allograft rejection, it has been assumed that these structures have a similar role in tumor immunity mechanisms. There certainly are animal experiments that support such a role. However, in clinical trials the removal of regional lymph nodes in malignant melanoma patients (Veronesi *et al.*, 1980; Sim *et al.*, 1978) in no way prejudiced survival. In breast cancer patients, the irradiation of the regional lymph nodes (Breast Cancer Study Group, 1978) or the surgical removal of the axillary nodes (Fisher, 1980; Fisher *et al.*, 1981) have failed to influence the survival of patients. The results of these trials do not support the assumption that regional lymph nodes make a significant contribution to the host defense, since their removal or irradiation does not compromise survival rates.

THERAPEUTIC IMPLICATIONS

Several clinical trials comparing different techniques of treatment have resulted in observations which are of major significance to the understanding of the biology of the neoplastic process.

Malignant melanoma

Veronesi *et al*. (1980) have reported a prospective randomized clinical trial in which patients with Stage I malignant melanoma of the limbs were assigned to groups receiving either local excision only or local excision plus immediate regional lymph node dissection. For 10 years the survival curves of both groups have been similar. They concluded that immediate lymph node dissection failed to improve the prognosis, in spite of the fact that nearly 20% of the prophylactic dissections contained occult metastases. In the group receiving excision only, 24% of patients developed regional lymph node metastases in the follow-up period.

Sim *et al*. (1978) also have reported a prospective randomized clinical trial of patients with Stage I malignant melanoma who were assigned to groups receiving no lymphadenectomy, immediate lymphadenectomy or delayed lymphadenectomy 2–4 months after the initial primary surgery. There was no difference between the survival rates of the three groups at five years and no difference in the rates of recurrence or metastases. Fourteen percent of those having no initial lymphadenectomy required this operation later. Thus, in these two trials, prophylactic lymphadenectomy did not appear to improve the outcome of patients with malignant melanoma, even though 20% of cases showed occult lymphatic metastases.

Cancer of the breast

The Cancer Research Campaign Working Party (1976, 1980) have compared the outcome of breast cancer patients randomized to receiving simple mastectomy and routine immediate post-operative radiotherapy with that of a group receiving simple mastectomy only, radiotherapy being added only if the disease later recurred. There was no statistically significant difference in survival rates for up to eight years of follow-up. The group receiving radiotherapy had a highly significant decrease in the local recurrence rate but this was not paralleled by a difference in survival, indicating that local 'recurrences' do not act as significant foci for subsequent distant dissemination. Only 110 of the 370 patients that would be predicted to have histologically involved lymph nodes required subsequent treatment for local axillary recurrence.

First reported by Edwards *et al*. (1972) was the observation that clinically positive axillary lymph nodes showed regression and remained dormant in many patients receiving only simple mastectomy. Baum and Coyle (1980) have reported follow-up on 32 patients with clinically positive axillary nodes treated with simple mastectomy alone. Eighteen of these patients showed spontaneous node regression and during the period of follow-up none had developed distant metastases. On the other hand, the nodes remained palpable or had progressed in 14 patients, of whom 10 developed distant metastases and six died.

Of the 62 patients who had clinically negative axillae and were treated by simple mastectomy alone, the axilla in 50 remained negative but four developed distant metastases and died. The axilla in 12 of these 62 patients became clinically positive and six of these developed distant metastases with two deaths. The mean interval between the progression of the axillary nodes and the appearance of metastases was 9.6 months with a median of 8 months. Three developed distant metastases synchronously with the axillary nodes.

Baum and Coyle (1980) have proposed an extended use of axillary node status to predict the outcome in patients with breast cancer. They suggest that those patients who have no enlarged axillary nodes and remain negative, and those who have clinically positive nodes which regress, have tumors which will have a good outcome. On the other hand, those patients whose enlarged axillary nodes either remain or progress, or those with initially negative axillae who later develop positive axillary nodes, have tumors that will likely result in a lethal outcome. Thus, the behavior of the axillary nodes as well as their presence can be used to predict the distant behavior of the tumor.

Veronesi and Valagussa (1981) randomized breast cancer patients to undergo either Halstead mastectomy alone or associated with internal mammary node dissection. In spite of the fact that 20% of the extended mastectomy patients were found to have internal mammary node metastases, there was no difference found after 10 years in either the disease-free or overall survival rates of the two groups. Only 15 Halstead mastectomy patients had a parasternal recurrence compared to an expected number of 75.

Further evidence that failure to treat clinically occult axillary lymph node metastases in women with breast cancer does not affect prognosis has been provided by Fisher (1980). Patients with clinically negative axillae were subjected to radical mastectomy, total mastectomy plus radiotherapy or total mastectomy alone. Survival rates in the groups are not significantly different in spite of the fact that 40% of the radical mastectomy patients were shown to have occult axillary metastases and presumably the same proportion of patients assigned to the other groups would have had a similar likelihood of clinical occult axillary metastases.

Over the years practically every prospective randomized clinical trial has shown that variations in either the technique of surgery or radiotherapy fail to change the survival rates of patients with breast cancer. Gibb (1969) found that routine radiotherapy after radical mastectomy did not improve 10-year survival rates in patients with either negative or positive axillary nodes, although the control patients had a much greater incidence of local recurrence. Kaae and Johannsen (1969) found that 10-year survival rates in patients with either negative or positive nodes were similar in a prospective randomized clinical trial comparing extended radical mastectomy to simple mastectomy and radiation. Brinkley and Haybittle (1971) found survival rates and recurrence-free rates similar at 10 years in a trial comparing radical mastectomy and radiation to modified simple mastectomy and radiation. Bruce (1975) comparing radical mastectomy to simple mastectomy and radiation found five-year survival rates to be not significantly different.

Hayward (1977), comparing wide local excision and radiation to radical mastectomy and radiation, found five to 10-year survival rates similar except for 10-year survival rates in patients with clinical positive axillary lymph nodes. This, in spite of the fact that the patients with wide excision as surgical treatment had a 19% incidence of axillary node recurrence in the clinically Stage I patients and 26% in the clinically Stage II patients. He observed that in almost all cases this local recurrence can be treated successfully by further surgery or radiotherapy and it did not appear to affect survival.

Crile (1966), reporting 12 patients among 40 having a simple mastectomy who developed subseqeunt axillary nodal metastases, observed these to appear after 1 to 72 months with an average of 22 months. At operation, five of these patients were found to have only one node involved and two had three nodes involved. The patient seen after 72 months had only two nodes and only one patient had more than 10 nodes involved. He interpreted this as meaning that metastasis from node to node did not occur frequently. Crile also suggested that the development of these axillary metastases did not influence the ultimate survival. Veronesi and Valagussa (1981) achieved complete long-lasting control in four of 15 parasternal recurrences of breast cancer. Contradicting these observations, Devitt (1965) found recurrence of axillary node metastases to have an ominous prognosis, a view supported by Baum and Coyle (1980).

Burn (1974) reported no difference in local recurrence or survival rates in patients whether treated by radical mastectomy or by simple mastectomy and radiotherapy. Langlands *et al* (1980), comparing radical mastectomy to simple mastectomy and radiotherapy, reported that Stage I patients had better survival rates following radical mastectomy but this did not apply to Stage II or Stage III patients. Lythgoe *et al.* (1978) reported no significant difference in survival between Stage I patients treated either by simple mastectomy alone or by simple mastectomy plus radiotherapy and between Stage II patients treated either by radical or modified mastectomy alone, or simple mastectomy plus radiotherapy. Fisher (1980) found no difference in survival rates when clinical Stage II patients were treated by total mastectomy plus radiotherapy or by radical mastectomy.

On the other hand, Host and Brennhovd (1977) concluded that in Stage I patients, cobalt radiation, roentgen-ray radiation, and no-treatment groups all had similar survival rates, but in Stage II patients, the cobalt radiation groups showed better survival rates than the control and roentgen-ray radiation groups. They attributed this to the higher dose of radiation received by the patients exposed to cobalt radiotherapy. Dwight *et al.* (1972), treating carcinoma of the rectum pre-operatively with radiation, reported that the finding of metastatic cancer in lymph nodes in resected speciments was reduced and that survival was improved.

CONCLUSION

It is probable that lymph node metastases have a different significance in different patients or when associated with primaries at different sites. Nevertheless, the overwhelming majority of prospective randomized clinical trials (mostly in breast cancer but two in malignant melanoma) report no significant improvement in survival time of patients either from surgical excision or irradiation of regional lymph nodes.

These observations have enormous biological significance and confirm earlier suggestions that lymph node metastases are not the cause of the poor prognosis with which they are usually associated. Lymph node metastases are merely indicators of the poor tumor–host relationship. The apparent failure of surgical excision or irradiation of tumor in regional lymph nodes to alter survival rates is explained by the symbolic nature of regional lymph node metastases, indicating how the outcome has already been resolved by the forces of 'biological predetermination'. Is it not likely that these same forces and principles largely account for the favorable outcome of tumors that appear to be confined to the primary site?

REFERENCES

Abrams, H.L., Spiro, R., and Goldstein, N. (1950). Metastases in carcinoma, *Cancer*, **3**, 74.

Adair, F., Berg, J., Joubert, L., and Robins, G.F. (1974). Long-term followup of breast cancer patients: the 30–year report. *Cancer*, **33**, 1145.

Attiyeh, F.F., Jense, M., Huvos, A.G., and Fracchia, A. (1977). Axillary micro-metastases and macrometastases in carcinoma of the breast. *Surg., Gynecol. Obstet.*, **144**, 839.

Bacon, H.E., Dirbas, F., Myers, T.B., and Ponce de Leon, F. (1958). Extensive lymphadenectomy and high ligation of the inferior mesenteric artery for carcinoma of the left colon and rectum. *Dis. Colon Rectum*, **1**, 457.

Berg, C.M., Murad, T.M., Soong, S-J., Ingolls, A.L., *et al.* (1978). A multifactorial analysis of melanoma. *Ann. Surg.*, **188**, 732.

Baum, M., and Coyle, P.J. (1980). The clinical behaviour of untreated axillary nodes following simple mastectomy for early carcinoma of the breast. *Clin. Oncol.*, **6**, 221.

Balch, J.W. (1955). The significance of axillary node levels in the study of breast carcinoma. *Cancer*, **8**, 776.

Berg, J.W. (1956). Sinus histiocytosis: a fallacious measure of host resistance to cancer. *Cancer*, **9**, 935.

Berg, J.W., and Robbins, G.F. (1966). Factors influencing short and long term survival of breast cancer patients. *Surg., Gynecol. Obstet.*, **122**, 1311.

Black, M.M., Kerpe, S., and Speer, F.D. (1955). Survival in breast cancer cases in relation to the structure of the primary tumor and regional lymph nodes. *Surg. Gynecol. Obstet.*, **100**, 543.

Bloom, H.J.G (1965). The influence of delay on the natural history and prognosis of breast cancer. *Br. J. Cancer*, **19**, 22.

Bloom, H.J.G., and Richardson, W.W. (1957). Histological grading and prognosis in breast cancer. *Br. J. Cancer*, **11**, 359.

Breast Cancer Study Group (1978). A report of the primary therapy. *Cancer*, **42**, 2809.

Brinkley, D., and Haybittle, J.L. (1971). Treatment of Stage II carcinoma of the female breast, *Lancet*, **2**, 1086.

Brinkley, D., and Haybittle, J.L. (1977). The curability of breast cancer. *World J. Surg.*, **1**, 287.

Bruce, J. (1975). The treatment of early cancer of the breast. *J. R. Coll. Surg. Edinb.* **20**, 278.

Burn, J.I. (1974). 'Early' breast cancer: the Hammersmith trial. *Br. J. Surg.* **61**, 762.

Cancer Research Campaign Breast Study (1976). Management of early cancer of the breast. *Br. Med. J.*, **1**, 1035.

Cancer Research Campaign Working Party (1980). King's Cambridge trial for early breast cancer, *Lancet*, **2**, 55.

Clarke, E.A., and Spangler, R.F. (1980). Review of Cancer incidence mortality, treatment and survival in Ontario, In *Cancer in Ontario*. The Ontario Cancer Treatment and Research Foundation, Toronto, Ontario, Canada.

Cohen, M.H., Ketcham, A.S., Felix, E.L. *et al.* (1977). Prognostic factors in patients undergoing lymphadenectomy for malignant melanoma. *Ann. Surg.*, **186**, 635.

Copher, G.H., Chenard, J., and Butcher, H.R., Jr. (1962). Factors influencing mortality from mammary cancer. *Arch. Surg.*, **85**, 73.

Crile, G. (1966). Metastases from involved lymph nodes after removal of various primary tumors. *Ann. Surg.*, **163**, 267.

Devitt, J.E. (1962). The influence of conservative and radical surgery on the survival of patients with breast cancer. *Can. Med. Assoc. J.*, **87**, 906.

Devitt, J.E. (1965). The significance of regional lymph node metastases in breast carcinoma. *Can. Med. Assoc. J.*, **93**, 289.

Devitt, J.E. (1967). The clinical stages of breast cancer—what do they mean? *Can. Med. Assoc. J.*, **97**, 1257.

Devitt, J.E. (1971). The enigmatic behaviour of breast cancer. *Cancer*, **27**, 12.

Devitt, J.E., and Mickelchuk, A.W. (1969). Significance of contralateral axillary metastases in carcinoma of the breast. *Can. J. Surg.*, **12**, 178.

Dukes, C.E. (1940). Cancer of the rectum: an analysis of 1000 cases. *J. Pathol. Bacteriol.*, **50**, 527.

Dwight, R.W. Higgins, G.A., Roswit, B., LeVeen, H.H., and Keehn, P.J. (1972). Preoperative radiation and surgery for cancer of the sigmoid colon and rectum. *Am. J. Surg.* **123**, 93.

Edwards, M.H., Baum, M., and Magaray, M.J. (1972). Regression of axillary lymph nodes in cancer of the breast. *Br. J. Surg.*, **59**, 776.

Enker, W.E., Laffer, V.T., and Block, G.E. (1979). Enhanced survival of patients with colon and rectal cancer is based upon wide anatomic resection. *Ann. Surg.*, **190**, 350.

Fisher, B. (1980). Laboratory and clinical research in breast cancer—a personal adventure. *Cancer Res.*, **40**, 3863.

Fisher, B., and Fisher, E.R. (1967). Barrier function of lymph node to tumor cells and erythrocytes. *Cancer*, **20**, 1907.

Fisher, B., Slack, N.H., Bross, I.D.J., *et al.* (1969). Cancer of the breast: size of neoplasm and prognosis. *Cancer*, **24**, 1071.

Fisher, B., Wolmark, N., Bauer, M., Redmond, C., and Gebhardt, M. (1981). The accuracy of clinical nodal staging and of limited axillary dissection as a determinant of histologic nodal status in carcinoma of the breast. *Surg. Gynecol. Obstet.* **152**, 765.

Fisher, E.R., Redmond, C., and Fisher, B. (1977). A perspective concerning the relation of duration of symptoms to treatment failure in patients with breast cancer. *Cancer*, **40**, 3160.

Fisher, E.R., Swamidoss, S., Lee, D.H., *et al.* (1978). Detection and significance of occult axillary node metastases in patients with invasive breast cancer. *Cancer*, **42**, 2025.

Fracchia, A.A., Evans, J.F., and Eisenberg, B.L. (1980). Stage III carcinoma of the breast. *Ann. Surg.* , **192**, 705.

Gabriel, W.B. (1949). Carcinoma of the rectum. In *The principles and practice of rectal surgery*, 4th edn. London: H.K. Lewis. pp. 333–456.

Gibb, R. (1969). Discussion in Breast Cancer Symposium. *Br. J. Surg.* , **56**, 791.

Grinnell, R.S. (1966). Lymphotic block with atypical and retrograde lymphotic metastasis and spread in carcinoma of the colon and rectum. *Ann. Surg.*, **56**, 791.

Haagensen, C.D. (1971). *Diseases of the breast*, 2nd edn. Philadelphia: W.B. Saunders.

Handley, R.S. (1964). The early spread of breast carcinoma and its bearing on operative treatment. *Br. J. Surg.*, **51**, 206.

Handley, R.S. (1972). Observations and thoughts on cancer of the breast. *Proc. R. Soc. Med.* **65**, 437.

Handley, R.S., and Thackray, A.C. (1954). Invasion of internal mammary lymph nodes in carcinoma of the breast. *Br. Med. J.*, **i**, 61.

Hayward, J.L. (1977). The Guy's trial of treatments of 'early' breast cancer. *World J. Surg.*, **1**, 314.

Host, H., and Brennhovd, I. (1977). The effect of post-operative radiotherapy in breast cancer. *Int. J. Radiat. Oncol., Biol. Phys.*, **2**, 1061.

Huvos, A.G., Hutter, R.V.P., and Berg, J.W. (1971). Significance of axillary macrometastases and micrometastases in mammary cancer. *Ann. Surg.*, **173**, 44.

Kaae, S., and Johannsen, H. (1969). Simple versus radical mastectomy in primary breast cancer. In *Prognostic factors in breast cancer* (eds A.P.M. Forrest, and P.B. Kunkler). Edinburgh and London: E & S Livingstone. p. 93.

Karakousis, C.P., Seddiq, M.K., and Moore, R. (1980). Prognostic value of lymph node dissection in malignant melanoma. *Arch. Surg.*, **115**, 719.

Langlands, A.O., Prescott, R.J., and Hamilton, T. (1980). A clinical trial in the management of operable cancer of the breast. *Br. J. Surg.*, **67**, 170.

Langlands, A.O., Pocock, S.J., Kerr, G.R., *et al.* (1979). Long-term survival of patients with breast cancer: a study of the curability of the disease. *Br. Med. J.*, **2**, 1247.

Lee, Y.-T.N. (1980). Malignant melanoma: pattern of metastases. *Cancer*, **30**, 137.

Lythgoe, J.P., Leck, I., and Swindell, R. (1978). Manchester regional breast study. *Lancet*, **i**, 744.

McDermott, F., Hughes, E., Pihl, E., *et al.* (1981). Symptom duration and survival prospects in carcinoma of the rectum. *Surg. Gynecol. Obstet.*, **153**, 321.

McDivitt, R.W., Stewart, F.W., and Berg, J.W. (1968). *Tumors of the breast*. Fascicle 2, Armed Forces Institute of Pathology. p. 112.

Morson, B.C., and Dawson, I.M.P. (1974). Malignant epithelial tumours. In *Gastrointestinal pathology*. Oxford: Blackwell Scientific. p.560.

Pickren, J.W. (1961). Significance of occult metastases. *Cancer*, **14**, 1266.

Prout, G.R., Heaney, J.A., Griffin, P.P., Daly, J.J., and Shipley, W.V. (1980). Nodal involvement as a prognostic indicator in patients with prostatic carcinoma. *J. Urol.*, **124**, 226.

Robbins, G.F., and Bross, I. (1957). The significance of delay in relation to prognosis of patients with primary operable breast cancer. *Cancer*, **10**, 338.

Robbins, S.L., and Cotran, R.S. (1979). Neoplasia. In *Pathologic basis of disease*, 2nd edn. Philadelphia: W.B. Saunders. p.156.

Shields, T.W. (1980). Classification and prognosis of surgically treated patients with bronchial carcinoma: Analysis of VASOG studies. *Int. J. Radiat. Oncol., Biol. Phys.*, **6**, 1021.

Shimkin, M.B., Lucia, E.L., Low-Beer, B.V.A., and Bell, H.G. (1954). Recurrent cancer of the breast. *Cancer*, **7**, 29.

Sim, F.H., Taylor, W.F., Ivins, J.C., Pritchard, D.J., and Soule, E.H. (1978). A prospective randomized study of the efficacy of routine elective lymphadenectomy in management of malignant melanoma. *Cancer*, **41**, 948.

Smith, J.A., Gamez-Aranjo, J.J., Gallagher, H.S., White, E.C., and McBride, C.M. (1977). Carcinoma of the breast. *Cancer*, **39**, 527.

Sugarbaker, E.V. (1979). Cancer metastasis: a product of tumour–host interactions. *Curr. Probl. Cancer*, **3**, no.7.

Veronesi, U., Adamus, J., Bandiera, D.C., Brennhovd, I.O., *et al.* (1980). Stage I melanoma of the limbs. Immediate versus delayed node dissection. *Tumori*, **66**, 373.

Veronesi, U., and Valagussa, P. (1981). Inefficacy of internal mammary nodes dissection in breast cancer surgery. *Cancer*, **47**, 170.

Viadana, E., Bross, I.D.J., and Pickren, J.W. (1973). An autopsy study of some routes of dissemination of cancer of the breast. *Br. J. Cancer*, **27**, 336.

Willis, R.A. (1973). Metastasis via the lymphatics. In *The spread of tumours in the human body*, 3rd edn. London: Butterworths. p.19.

Cancer Treatment: End Point Evaluation
Edited by B.A. Stoll
© 1983 John Wiley & Sons Ltd.

Chapter

10 HAROLD J. WANEBO

Host Immunologic Impairment in Relation to Survival

INTRODUCTION

The immune system is potentially affected by many factors in patients with malignancy. In addition to the immune depressive effects of tumor burden, there are the immune consequences of age, nutrition, carcinogenic factors (or co-factors), and even of the psychologic state. Factors of treatment can also modify the system and surgery, radiation, and chemotherapy all have predictable effects on the host. The final state of immunocompetence is the end result of these numerous interacting factors and it is difficult to assess their relative importance. This complexity may account for the variable results reported in attempts to correlate the level of immune competence with prognosis in the cancer patient.

A factor of possible importance may be tumor type and location because patients with resectable melanoma and sarcoma usually have normal reactivity (Pinsky, 1978), whereas patients with visceral malignancies or head and neck cancer are frequently immunosuppressed (Pinsky, 1978; Pinsky et al., 1974, 1976). Whether the important factor here is tumor type or other associated influence still remains to be established. Although it is presumed that immune suppression is a consequence of malignancy, this may not always be the case, because in certain instances immune depression may *precede* malignancy, as might occur in the malnourished, alcoholic male who ultimately develops squamous cancer of the head and neck (Wanebo et al., 1975).

The role of tumor-specific immunity is controversial and limited to certain tumor types (Old, 1981). Although the importance of tumor-specific immunity to survival is well documented in animal systems, even in these well defined models there is a multiplicity of factors that interfere with an effective antitumor response. The nature and strength of the tumor antigen itself, antigenic modulation or masking by antibody–antigen (or complexes of the two), and other immunoregulating factors all have a role in the complex interaction that is tumor immunity. It is a function only partially understood in animal tumor models, and even less understood in man (Baldwin *et al.*, 1979).

This review will examine the relationship of the immune competent state to prognosis in selected human malignancies which have been adequately staged and have had sufficient follow-up. It will only briefly touch on the topic of tumor-specific immunity and refers the reader to a recent review (Old, 1981). It will include a discussion of the immune system in man, tests of immune function, results of immune testing in cancer patients, and the relation of general immune competence to prognosis.

TESTS OF IMMUNE FUNCTION IN MAN

Most schemes of the immune system divide it into T cell and B cell compartments, with an additional reference to the monocyte macrophage system (Figure 1). The T cell or thymus-derived compartment has a major role in cell-mediated immunity. Lymphocyte maturation occurs under the influence of the thymus gland, either through the lymphocyte circulation or from exposure to thymic hormone. Mature lymphocytes are thought responsible for recognition and destruction of large antigens, alloantigens, and tumor cells. There are also T cells which regulate immune response. Those which augment it are called 'helper cells', and those which depress or turn off the response are termed 'suppressor cells.' These regulating cells are essential for the normal operation of the system.

B cells or bursa-equivalent cells or 'bone marrow-derived cells' make up the other large division. In the chicken there is a well defined 'bursa fabricius' located in the tail gut which is the source of B cells. In the mammal this organ is not identifiable and the actual source of B cells is probably from within the bone marrow. B cells may mature into plasma cells and produce antibody in response to stimuli from certain antigens, viruses, rickettsia, bacteria, etc. Although the role of the B cell has been less emphasized in cancer control, it is obviously essential to tumor immunity and may even play a greater role than commonly recognized.

In addition, there is a third system composed of monocyte macrophage cells which originally were thought to be just scavenger cells, but also have a special role in tumor immunity. Macrophages may exhibit direct cytotoxicity for tumor cells as well as act against opsonized tumor cells. They may release numerous lytic enzymes, as well as producing complement components, reactive oxygen metabolites, prostaglandins, chemotactic factors, and also factors which either promote or inhibit replication of lymphocytes (Nathan *et al.*, 1980).

Also involved as effectors as well as regulators of the immune system are numerous serum components, including not only the immunoglobulins but also probable regulating factors in the alpha I and alpha II globulin region, complement, and in many cases, complexes of complement and antigen. There are other humoral factors, called lymphokines, released by leukocytes or monocytes, which govern lymphocyte function and appear responsible for expansion of certain lymphocytes in response to a stimulus, and which may also inhibit or depress responses.

As can be surmised from the very simplified scheme in Figure 1, this is an interactive and self-regulating system which has many functions to protect the host from invasion by noxious elements of either exogenous or endogenous origin. As can be imagined, the various tests of this system are, at best, limited 'snapshots' of a complex moving picture process.

A variety of *in vivo* and *in vitro* tests have been developed to assess general immune reactivity (Tables 1 and 2). One can evaluate primary delayed hypersensitivity by sensitizing and challenging with *de novo* antigens such as keyhole limpet hemocyanin (KLH) or 2,4–dinitrochlorobenzene (DNCB). Recall delayed hypersensitivity is measured by challenging with common recall antigens such as *Candida albicans*, mumps, streptokinase–

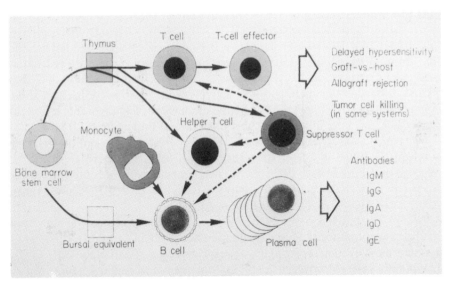

Figure 1 Model of cellular interactions in human lymphocyte differentiation (From Broder and Waldmann, 1978; reprinted by permission of *The New England Journal of Medicine*.)

streptodornase, and tuberculin (Hersh *et al.*, 1976; Pinsky, 1978). The local inflammatory response can be evaluated by cutaneous application of croton oil (Roth *et al.*, 1975) or by the initial response to the concentrated DNCB (2000 μg/ml) used in sensitization (Pinsky, 1978). Humoral immunity can also be evaluated by measuring the primary and secondary antibody responses to various microbial antigens, KLH, or flagellin (Helson, 1976; Lee *et al.*, 1970).

In vitro tests include measurement of monocyte and lymphocyte subpopulations, lymphocyte function (proliferation, cytotoxicity, lymphocyte mediator production), and monocyte–macrophage function (chemotaxis, cytotoxicity, phagocytosis). Serum immunoglobulins (IgG, IgA, IgM) along with primary and secondary antibody responses can also be measured. Serum total complement and component and antigen–antibody complexes can also be predictably assayed.

Lymphocyte–Monocyte Count

The absolute lymphocyte count is of basic importance in cancer patients, and a large body of literature supports a relationship of normal pretreatment lymphocyte counts with improved survival and recurrence rates compared with patients with low values (Fudenberg *et al.*, 1975; McCredie *et al.*, 1973; Papatestas *et al.*, 1976; Riesco, 1970). Lymphocytes are generally segregated into T lymphocytes (cellular immunity) and B cells (basically involved in humoral immunity (Good, 1977). There is much overlap and interaction in this artificially defined system, i.e. B cells also synthesize macrophage-inhibiting factor, a mediator of cellular immunity. T cells are defined as cells that form spontaneous rosettes *in vitro* in the presence of sheep red blood cells (SRBC) usually at 4°C (Fudenberg *et al.*, 1975; Wybran and Fudenberg, 1976). A further distinction is the active rosette that is formed by short contact between lymphocytes and SRBC at elevated, less favorable temperatures (29°C) as initially described by Wybran and Fudenberg (1973).

The active total-rosette-forming cell is considered to represent the immune surveillance function better than just total T-RFC (Kerman *et al.*, 1976; Wybran and Fudenberg, 1973, 1976). The normal levels of total T are 64 ± 6.5% (lower value 51%) and for active T-RFC are 27 ± 6.5% (lower range 15%) according to Wybran and Fudenberg, 1976).

Recent T cell division into helper cell and suppressor cell can be measured by their receptors for the immunoglobulin heavy chain of IgM (termed μ) or IgG (termed γ). These are defined respectively as Tμ (helper cell) or Tγ (suppressor cell) (Moretta *et al.*, 1977). Monocyte–macrophage counts can be measured by enumerating latex-ingesting cells in purified leukocytes (Alexander, 1976; Pitt, 1977). The number of macrophage precursor cells can be counted from long-term cultures of adherent monocytes (Unger *et al.*, 1979).

Table 1   Tests of general immune competence. (From Wanebo, 1979b, reproduced by permission of *Surgical Clinics of North America*)

In vivo tests—delayed hypersensitivity tests

   Primary tests (*de novo* sensitivity)
   DNCB (2,4-dinitrochlorobenzene)
   KLH (keyhole limpet hemocyanin)
   Recall tests
   C. albicans
   Dermatophytin
   Streptokinaese–streptodornase (SK–SD)
   Mumps
   Tuberculin

In vitro tests

(a) Cellular factors
   Total lymphocyte–monocyte levels
      T cells [a] (total-rosette-forming cells; active rosette-forming cells)
      B cells
      Monocytes
   Lymphocyte function
      Blastogenesis
         Mitogens (PHA, PWM, Con A)
         Antigens (*S. aureus*, *C. albicans*, *E. coli*, SK–SD, tuberculin, mumps virus)
         Alloalligens (allogeneic lymphocytes)
      Lymphokine production (MIF)
      Cytotoxicity—direct, antibody-dependent
   Monocyte–macrophage function
      Chemotaxis
      Cytotoxicity (tumor cell, ADCC)
      Phagocytosis
      Enzyme production, i.e. lysozyme
   Granulocyte function
      Nitroblue tetrazolium
      Bacterial phagocytosis—killing
(b) Humoral factors
   Immunoglobulin levels—IgG, IgA, IgM
      Antibody response
         KLH—primary and secondary response
         S. typhi
         Influenza
         Tetanus toxoid
      Complement
         Total
         Components
         Complexes

---

[a] T (helper)—receptor   Ty, Fc–IgM.
T (suppressor)   Tγ, Fc–IgG.
(Also typed by monoclonal antibodies.)

Table 2   Markers for human lymphocyte populations (From Wanebo, 1979b, reproduced by permission of *Surgical Clinics of North America*)

| Thymic origin | | Bone marrow origin | |
T cells	B cells	Null cells (K cells)	Monocyte–macrophage
1 Spontaneous formation of rosettes with SRBC (EA) 2 Respond to phytohemagglutinin and Con A in solution 3 Respond to antigens in solution to which host has been immunized 4 Respond to allogeneic cells 5 Have human T lymphocyte antigen (HTLA) at surface	1 Form spontaneous rosettes with mouse RBC; no rosettes with SRBC 2 Have surface Ig demonstrable with IgG(FAb)$_2$ reagents 3 Have low avidity receptors for Fc of IgG 4 Have receptors for C3b and C3d	1 Non T and non B cell (do not form rosettes with SRBC and do not have detectable surface Ig) 2 Have high avidity receptors for Fc of IgG detected with rosettes with Ripley anti D-coated human red cells 3 Have receptors for C3b and C3d 4 Lack surface marker IgG 5 Do not phagocytose particulates	1 Have receptors for Fc of IgG$_1$ and IgG$_3$ 2 Have receptors for C3 3 Stain with non-specific esterase 4 Have receptors for lymphokines (MIF) 5 Phagocytose particulate matter 6 Migratory response to chemotactic factor

Cell-mediated immunity is measured both by the delayed hypersensitivity tests and in the *in vitro* assays of lymphocyte and monocyte function (Litwin *et al.*, 1977). Humoral immunity is measured by the antibody responses to antigen vaccination, immunoglobulin levels, and complement. T cell function is assessed by certain lymphocyte responses to the mitogens, phyto-hemagglutinin, Con A, and allogeneic lymphocytes, whereas B cell function is, in part, measured by the response to pokeweed mitogen, lipopoly-saccharide (possibly Staphage Lysate), and other antigens (Litwin, 1976; Litwin *et al.*, 1977). Monocyte function can be assayed by various tests including phagocytosis of sensitized cells, cytostasis, or cytotoxicity of tumor cells, and chemotaxis–migration (Alexander, 1976; Evans, 1976; Snyderman and Pike, 1976; Hibbs, 1976; Pitt, 1977; Snyderman *et al.*, 1978).

The status, relevance, and significance of the above tests in cancer patients are, in part, determined by the expertise and interest of those performing the tests and the patient population at their disposal. This review concentrates on selected studies from a rapidly expanding literature and additionally focuses on data previously generated in a single institution (Memorial Sloan Kettering Cancer Center) which can serve as a useful frame of reference.

Delayed hypersensitivity tests in cancer patients

Although patients with early cancer have minimal defects in cell-mediated immunity when skin-tested with DNCB or recall antigens, the proportion of patients who respond is still lower than would be expected in normal individuals (Pinsky, 1978). With progression of disease, the proportion of patients with anergy increases, although, if one examines patients with the same histologic type of malignancy and compares those with localized disease to those with regional metastases, the difference is usually not significant in most series. Only when patients with disseminated disease are included is progressive anergy consistently seen (Catalona and Chretien, 1973; Eilber *et al.*, 1975; Pinsky, 1978).

The relation of delayed hypersensitivity tests to prognosis has been shown with both DNCB and recall antigens (Hughes and Mackay, 1965; Pinsky, 1978; Renaud, 1926; Solowey and Rappaport, 1965; Waldorf *et al.*, 1968) but perhaps has been most clear-cut with DNCB tests (owing to variability in responses to recall antigens) (Levin *et al.*, 1964; Pinsky, 1978; Pinsky *et al.*, 1974; Wanebo *et al.*, 1978a) (Table 3). In one such study, the DNCB response was related to prognosis in a group of 204 patients with a variety of solid tumors who had been followed for a median of two years after complete resection of the malignancy (Pinsky *et al.*, 1976). When the DNCB-positive patients were compared with the DNCB-negative patients, the recurrence rate and survival were poorer in the group who were DNCB-negative (p <0.001). When the patients were further segregated into those with and those

Table 3   Results of skin tests in patients with 'solid' tumours. (From Pinsky, 1978, reproduced by courtesy of Marcel Dekker, Inc.)

Type of cancer	No. of studies	No. of patients	Disease vs. control	Stage of disease	Prognosis
Lung	10	960	8/8	3/4	6/7
Breast	8	781	7/8	2/3	2/3
Head and neck	6	417	6/6	5/6	5/5
Colon	4	319	4/4	2/3	0/2
Melanoma	5	290	4/5	1/1	1/2
Bladder	3	157	3/3	3/3	1/1
Sarcoma	3	92	3/3	1/1	1/2
Prostate	2	83	2/2	0/1	0/1
Stomach	3	75	3/3	1/2	0/1
Neuroblastoma	1	67	1/1	1/1	—
Cervix	2	53	2/2	1/1	1/1
Testis	1	50	1/1	0/1	—

without regional metastases, the recurrence rate and survival were poorer in the DNCB-negative patients with localized disease compared with their DNCB-positive counterparts ($p<0.001$). The presence of regional metastases appears to nullify the beneficial influence of the immune system prognosis, as there was no significant difference in the DNCB-positive versus DNCB-negative patients among those with regional metastases (Pinsky *et al.*, 1976).

Since Renaud's observation that tuberculin sensitivity was depressed or absent in patients with malignant disease (Renaud, 1926), numerous authors have also found depression of delayed hypersensitivity responses to intradermal recall antigens in cancer patients and have generally correlated this depression with worsened prognosis (Eilber *et al.*, 1975; Hersh *et al.*, 1976; Hughes and Mackay, 1965; Israel *et al.*, 1973; Krant *et al.*, 1968; Renaud, 1926; Solowey and Rappaport, 1965; Waldorf *et al.*, 1968). There is considerable variation in the response to recall antigens, e.g. response to tuberculin, in different populations depending on sex, age (Waldorf *et al.*, 1968), and socioeconomic background.

Hersh *et al.* (1976) noted differences in intradermal antigen responses and in their relation to prognosis in patients with melanoma versus those with lung cancer. In general there was significant depression of the responses to *Candida*, streptokinase–streptodornase (Varidase), and mumps in patients with lung cancer compared to the responses in patients with melanoma. Also, significant improvement of median survival in patients with lung cancer correlated with vigorous responses to these antigens (Hersh *et al.*, 1976). Israel has found that tuberculin responses correlated well with prognosis in a large European series of patients with lung cancer (Israel *et al.*, 1973). Pinsky (1978) has recently reviewed the numerous studies of skin tests with either

DNCB or recall antigens in patients with cancer and analyzed the correlations with stage and prognosis in patients with various types of cancer (Table 3).

Basically, most studies have shown normal or near-normal responses in patients with early localized melanoma, sarcoma, and breast cancer, whereas these responses are frequently depressed in cervical, colorectal, head and neck, and lung cancers. There was a general overall correlation of delayed hypersensitivity reactions with stage and prognosis in the studies reviewed. (Anthony *et al.*, 1974; Bolton *et al.*, 1975; Brugarolas *et al.*, 1973; Catalona and Chretien, 1973; Chakravorty *et al.*, 1973; Cunningham *et al.*, 1976; Eilber and Morton, 1970; Eilber *et al.*, 1975; Helson, 1976; Hilal *et al.*, 1977; Holmes and Golub, 1976; Krant *et al.*, 1968; Krown *et al.*, 1978; Liebler *et al.*, 1977; Pinsky *et al.*, 1974; Takita and Brugarolas, 1973; Theofilopoulos *et al.*, 1976; Wanebo *et al.*, 1978a; Wells *et al.*, 1973).

Role of *in vitro* immune tests

The peripheral blood lymphocyte counts have been shown to correlate with stage of disease and prognosis by numerous authors. Cancer patients with low pretreatment counts have higher recurrence rates and lower survival rates than their counterparts with normal pretreatment values (Riesco, 1970). This has been documented in breast cancer (McCredie *et al.*, 1973; Papatestas *et al.*, 1976), colorectal cancer (Evans *et al.*, 1977; Ichiki *et al.*, 1977; Wanebo and Pinsky, 1978), and other solid tumors (Harris *et al.*, 1975).

T and B cell levels have been extensively studied in cancer patients. In general, T cell depression has been observed in most of the patients with carcinoma of visceral origin, whereas T cell levels have been normal in patients with early carcinoma of the breast (Bolton *et al.*, 1976; Stein *et al.*, 1976; Wanebo *et al.*, 1976c), melanoma (Wybran and Fudenberg, 1976), and sarcoma (Pritchard *et al.*, 1976). Although suppressed T cell levels have been noted in patients with early (localized) carcinoma of the head and neck (Deegan and Coulthart, 1977; Wanebo *et al.*, 1975) and lung (Dellon *et al.*, 1975; Gross *et al.*, 1975; Liebler *et al.*, 1977), they are more commonly depressed in patients with more advanced (though still resectable) disease (Anthony *et al.*, 1975; Dellon *et al.*, 1975; Wanebo, *et al.*, 1976a). B cell levels in general have not shown the same correlation with stage of disease, although they may be relevant to prognosis in certain cancer patients receiving treatment with chemotherapy (Hersh *et al.*, 1976). Although some authors have found that the total lymphocyte count provided prognostic information equivalent to T and B cell counts (Harris *et al.*, 1975), recent refinements in testing these subpopulations may provide more relevant information.

The recent development of the active T cell test by Wybran may provide a more sensitive indicator of T cell competence (and indirectly, immunosurveillance) than measuring the total T cell count (Fudenberg *et al.*, 1975; Kerman *et al.*, 1976; Wells *et al.*, 1973; West *et al.*, 1976; Wybran and Fudenberg, 1973, 1976). Wybran, in his analysis of 500 patients with various types of solid tumours, found that 65% of patients with newly diagnosed localized cancer had low active T cells, whereas only 5% had decreased total T cells (Wybran and Fudenberg, 1976). Sixty-nine percent of patients with localized recurrence had depressed active T cells compared with normal total T cells in most patients. In patients with metastatic cancer, about 70% had decreased active T cells and 25% had depressed total T cells. Wybran found that in patients with melanoma and sarcoma, there had been a fall in active T cells without necessarily a decrease in total T cells prior to clinical detection of new lesions (Wybran and Fudenberg, 1976). Similar findings have been shown in patients with carcinoma of the lung and head and neck (Kerman *et al.*, 1976; Stefani *et al.*, 1976; Weese *et al.*, 1977). An unanswered question here is 'Does this represent a qualitative or a quantitative defect in the population of immunocompetent T cells?'

The rosette inhibition tests also gives increased information about T cell competence. Abnormal rosette formation and rosette inhibition by anti-thymic serum globulin have also been observed in patients with head and neck cancer (Deegan and Coulthart, 1977), localized lung cancer (Gross *et al.*, 1975) or colorectal cancer (Ichiki *et al.*, 1977).

K cells are another distinct population of lymphoid cells that can kill target cells by using IgG as a specific sensitizing agent. They are non-phagocytic, lack glass adherence, are not thymic-dependent, and are not involved in antibody production. They appear to be a null cell subset (forming about 20% of those cells) that lacks distinguishing characteristics of T cells (E rosettes) and B cells (surface immunoglobulins). Their role in cancer immunity remains to be defined (Good, 1977; Litwin *et al.*, 1977).

Lymphocyte blastogenesis in response to mitogens and antigens has been extensively studied in cancer patients. Numerous authors have demonstrated depression of the mitogen response, particularly to phytohemagglutinin (Barnes *et al.*, 1975; Ducos *et al.*, 1970; Han and Takita, 1972; Wanebo *et al.*, 1978a), and the added suppressive effect of plasma from cancer patients (Catalona *et al.*, 1973; Glasgow *et al.*, 1974). More recently, authors have added the mixed lymphocyte test using patients' lymphocytes and allogeneic lymphocytes in an effort to find assays more relevant to immune depression in cancer patients. Golub *et al.* (1974) have found that the mixed lymphocyte culture (MLC) assay is more sensitive to immune defects and correlates better with tumor burden and skin tests than did the mitogen responses. Possibly because the MLC assay is an interactive type of test involving participation of several subclasses of T cells, B cells, and adherent cells, it may be a better indicator of recognitive defects than are simple mitogen responses. (Berlinger *et al.*, 1977; Golub *et al*; 1974).

Macrophage function

Macrophages together with polymorphonuclear leukocytes constitute the first line of defense in the body against infections, are also vitally involved in the homograft rejection, and have a major role in tumor immunity in concert with T and B cells (Alexander, 1976; Snyderman and Pike, 1976; Nelson, 1976; Pitt, 1977). Macrophages have been demonstrated in both human and animal tumors (Eccles and Alexander, 1974; Evans, 1976). Their concentration correlated with survival in the animal model, but in man the relation to prognosis remains to be determined. Macrophages have the multi-armed function of chemotaxis, phagocytosis, cytostatis, and cytotoxicity of foreign cells (Hibbs, 1976).

Defective migration of mononuclear cells (chemotaxis) has been demonstrated in cancer patients with malignant tumors in various areas such as breast, lung, kidney, and colorectum (Synderman and Pike, 1976; Kjeldsberg and Pay, 1978). Snyderman *et al.* (1978) have shown that monocyte chemotaxis responses were depressed in patients with active breast cancer but frequently returned to normal after tumor resection. Unger *et al.* (1979) have recently measured multiple facets of monocyte macrophage function in patients with malignancies of the breast, colon, lung, head and neck, and melanoma. Although there was great variability in test results among tumor types, patients with colorectal cancer showed the most consistent abnormalities.

Complement and immune complexes

Hypocomplementemia has been observed in 10% of the sera of patients with various malignancies (Teshima *et al.*, 1977). In general, over 60% of the patients with low levels of total hemolytic complement (serum dilution at which 50% of indicator erythrocytes are hemolyzed) and components C-3 and C1q had high levels of immune complexes using the ^{125}I C1q deviation test. Elevated mean levels of immune complexes (above the upper range in normal individuals) were found in patients with melanoma, cancer of the breast, head and neck, lung, colorectum, and gynecologic malignancy (Teshima *et al.*, 1977). Theofilopoulos *et al.* (1976) had similar findings using the Raji cell radioimmune assay.

Using another assay that measures immune complexes containing IgG by a precipitin test with a monoclonal rheumatoid factor, Samayoa *et al.* (1977) found that 29% of the sera from cancer patients and 35% of the sera from patients with metastatic cancer had elevated immune complex levels compared with 3% of normal controls and 5% of hospitalized patients without malignancy. Baldwin *et al.* (1979) have used the C1q binding test and shown that C1q binding values were higher in breast cancer patients than in controls and that values were highest in patients with 'poorer prognosis' (nodal metastases). Of interest, post-operative values gave clearer prognostic distinctions. Patients with good prognoses had C1q binding values in the normal range, whereas those with poorer prognoses continued to have elevated values (Baldwin *et al.*, 1979; Hoffken *et al.*, 1978). In lung cancer, Rossen *et al.* (1977) found a correlation between increased C1q binding and poor prognosis.

Immunoglobulins

Immunoglobulin levels have not been very useful in patients with solid tumours (Hughes, 1974; Nathanson, 1977). Increased levels of serum IgA have been found in patients with head and neck cancer (Wara *et al.*, 1975) and in patients with bronchopulmonary cancer (Hughes, 1974). Roberts *et al.* (1975) found increased levels of IgA and depressed IgG in patients with breast cancer, although other observers have not (Bolton *et al.*, 1976; Wanebo *et al.*, (1978c). There are no recent extensive kinetic data on humoral antibody formation in patients with solid tumors. Levin *et al.* (1970) have demonstrated delayed induction times in patients with cancer. Impaired capacity to produce IgM and IgG antibodies in response to primary antigenic challenge with *Salmonella adelaide* flagellin has been demonstrated in patients with carcinomas of the pancreas, stomach, and liver (Lee *et al.*, 1970).

MULTIPARAMETER TESTING: RELEVANCE TO STAGE OF DISEASE AND PROGNOSIS

Although individual tests have been useful in measuring certain aspects of immune function in man, they are probably too limited to provide an overall assessment of immunocompetence in patients with cancer. There are numerous studies now which have attempted to measure several aspects of immune function in staged cancer patients and we will cite a few representative ones.

Breast cancer

A detailed review of the literature regarding the immunology and immunotherapy of breast cancer up to 1977 has been published by Nathanson (1977). Major areas discussed included: (1) histologic characterization of a host response in the stroma of primary breast cancer and in the lymph nodes; (2) antigenic studies of breast cancer tissue and circulating tumor antigens; and (3) cellular and humoral immunity studies and effects of radiation, chemotherapy, and immunotherapy. In general, selected measurements of cellular immunity have shown increased recurrence rates in patients with lower pretreatment lymphocyte counts (Papatestas and Kark, 1974) and depressed dermal hypersensitivity to DNCB (Evans *et al.*, 1977; Eilber and Morton, 1970). A general depression of *in vitro* assays of immunity occurs more commonly in patients with advanced disease than in those with localized cancer (Bolton *et al.*, 1976; Stein *et al.*, 1976), but the true relation of recurrence to cell-mediated immunity (CMI) within properly staged patients is not well defined. We will discuss selected studies in this regard.

There are distinctive changes in immune function in breast cancer patients, including the antitumor response by the host to autologous tumor (Black, 1973), the response to a putative cancer-associated antigen (the T antigen), and the general immune response to standardized antigens as assayed by *in vivo* and *in vitro* tests (Bolton *et al.*, 1975, 1976; Hughes and Mackay, 1965; Krown *et al.*, 1978; Stjernsward *et al.*, 1972; Wanebo *et al.*, 1976c, 1978c). Although Black *et al.* (1975) have reported prognostically important changes in skin window and *in vitro* responses by the leukocyte migration inhibition response to cryostat sections of autologous breast cancer, in sequential studies these changes have yet to be duplicated by others. Springer *et al.* (1980) have also shown a high order of responses to the T antigen in breast cancer patients but the relationship to prognosis is not recorded. Although it has been controversial whether there is any impairment of general immuno-competence in early breast cancer (Wanebo *et al.*, 1976c, 1978c), there is general unanimity that immune suppression occurs in patients with more advanced disease. (Adler *et al.*, 1980; Bolton *et al.*, 1976; Hughes and Mackay, 1965; Krown *et al.*, 1978; Nathanson, 1977; Stein *et al.*, 1976; Wanebo *et al.*, 1978c).

A recent report by Adler *et al.* (1980), capitalizing on the combined integrated scores of the *in vivo* response to PPD and DNCB and the *in vitro* response to PPD and PHA, demonstrated an impairment in 51% of patients with early operable tumors versus 11% in controls, 68% in operable patients, and 89% in patients with metastatic disease. Immune depression was not related to age or influenced by mastectomy, nor was it related to tumor size except in patients with large T_4 cancers. Lymph node metastases were associated with greater immune suppression, compared to N_0 patients with smaller tumors (T_1) though not those with larger operable cancers ($T_{2,3}$).

In patients with operable cancer followed for 3–6 years, the predictability of recurrence was highest with *in vitro* stimulation tests (PPD, PHA) compared to cutaneous responses to PPD and DNCB. Conversely, length of disease-free interval and survival correlated best with *in vitro* tests. Probability of recurrence as calculated by actuarial methods at 48 months was 0.26 for optimal responders and 0.61 for suboptimal responders ($p < 0.0001$). Within each stage, patients showing optimal integrated responses to *in vitro* and *in vivo* tests had significantly lower recurrence rates.

The length of disease-free period was significantly greater in patients who were good responders (mean 23.5 months) versus those who were poor responders (mean 12.8 months) ($p<0.01$). Mean survival in patients with metastatic cancer was best in those with pretreatment normal function (29.5 months) versus those with immunosuppression (12.3 months) ($p<0.001$). This study has shown the most clear-cut relation of prognosis to general immune reactivity in breast cancer patients.

In a recent report of breast cancer patients from Memorial Hospital in New York, there was a linear trend to decreasing DNCB with increasing extent of disease ($p<0.01$) (Krown *et al.*, 1980). However, in a limited follow-up of operable breast cancer patients segregated by nodal status, there was a surprising trend to earlier recurrence in the DNCB-positive patients compared to DNCB-negative patients ($p<0.03$). The overall numbers of DNCB-negative patients were only 14, compared to 82 DNCB-positive patients; these small numbers may account for the surprising findings.

Another report with somewhat similar data from the Guthrie and Wainwright Tumor Clinic showed that, in women who had 1–3 positive lymph nodes, 16 of 30 patients who had pre-operative lymphocyte counts greater than 2000/mm^3 recurred by two years, versus two of 44 patients whose lymphocyte count was less than 2000/mm^3. Recurrence in women given radiation was not related to pre-operative count. The change in lymphocyte count from pre-operative value was also related. Patients in whom the lymphocyte count was unchanged or increased by one week after operation had lower recurrence rates (none of 18) than did patients in whom the count decreased (six of 14).($p<0.001$). These findings need to be evaluated in larger series.

The lymphoproliferative response to autologous tumor extracts has been shown to correlate with prognosis in patients with operable breast cancer (Canon *et al.*, 1981). Patients who demonstrated a proliferative response to hypotonic membrane extracts of autologous tumor had a significantly longer disease-free interval than those with a low response to their autologous extract. A low response to the extract was often not accompanied by impaired responses to other antigens. Of interest in this study, patients with low autologous tumor response but normal MLC reaction were at high risk for recurrence, suggesting that the autologous tumor response took priority over non-specific lymphoproliferative responses (Canon *et al.*, 1981). This study essentially complements that of Black *et al.* (1975) who have reported data showing a positive prognostic correlation of immune response to cryostat sections of autologous breast cancer using both the skin window technique and the leukocyte migration inhibition test. Patients who had a particularly favorable prognosis were those showing an active reticuloendothelial response and a positive skin window test or a positive LMI to autologous cryostat sections.

Another test of demonstrated importance in breast cancer patients is the response to the Thomsen–Friedenreich antigen (T) as described by Springer *et al.* (1980). The T antigen is the immediate precursor of the major antigens of the second human blood group system, MN, and is prepared by removal of sialic acid from isolated O, MN antigens. A precursor to the T antigen, termed Tn, is produced by treating with β-galactosidase (Springer *et al.*, 1980). T and Tn antigens are found in reactive form in primary breast adenocarcinoma, but not in healthy or benign breast tissues. Breast carcinoma patients have shown cellular immunity to T antigen *in vivo* and *in vitro*. Delayed-type cutaneous hypersensitivity to the antigen is observed in over 85% of ductal carcinoma patients, but was negative in over 94% of benign breast disease patients and healthy individuals. *In vitro* responses were also significantly different, though of a lower order: 53% of patients with Stages II–IV responded. Thus far, prognostic data have not been reported with this important assay.

Colorectal cancer

Certain immune morphologic features of prognostic significance have been identified in colorectal cancer, such as perivascular lymphocyte cuffing and pericortical hyperplasia, which have been shown to correlate positively with an improved disease-free interval (Pihl *et al.*, 1977). Another, similar study by Nacopoulou *et al.* (1981) has shown a positive correlation of the stage of disease, grade of differentiation of the carcinoma, degree of lympho-plasmocytic infiltration of the tumor, lymphocyte predominance pattern in the lymph nodes, and, to a lesser degree, the germinal center predominance pattern with five-year survival. They failed to show a prognostic relationship with lymph node patterns in colorectal cancer.

Patt *et al.* (1975) also showed a correlation between survival and peri-cortical activity in the lymph nodes. On a more practical basis, measurements of delayed dermal hypersensitivity are perhaps the most reproducible immune reactivity measurement, although selected *in vitro* immune tests may provide complementary information. In a large group of patients with primary and advanced but untreated colorectal cancer, there was a pro-gressive decrease in immune responses to the DNCB skin test, as well as to a panel of recall antigens with increasing stage of disease (Rao *et al.*, 1977).

A detailed additional study of these patients with *in vitro* measurements, including absolute lymphocyte count, mitogen and antigen responses, also showed correlations with tumor burden, but failed to show a prognostic relationship of either the skin test or the *in vitro* tests to time to recurrence in patients with primary operable cancers. (Wanebo *et al.*, 1980). There were positive correlations of survival, however, in patients with advanced disease who were untreated as of time of the primary testing and who did show a correlation of favorable survival with a normal PHA response and lympho-cyte count.

Of interest in this group of patients from the same institution was the correlation between time to recurrence and the pre-operative CEA levels. Patients with an elevated CEA who had Dukes' B or Dukes' C lesions had significantly increased recurrence rates in comparison to their counterparts with normal CEA values (Wanebo *et al.*, 1978b). This test seemed to be more predictable than the non-specific test of cell-mediated immunity. Others have also shown impairment of cell-mediated immune reactions in colorectal cancer patients as measured by dermal antigen testing, lymphocyte stimula-tion, and T rosette measurements (Evans *et al.*, 1977; Goldrosen *et al.*, 1977), but the relation to survival, especially in patients within the same stage, is not defined.

Other tests of cell-mediated immunity have included the immune response as measured by the leukocyte migration inhibition tests to autologous tumor extracts. House and Watt (1979) found that 41 of 107 colorectal cancer patients had a positive LMI response to their autologous tumor and had a survival advantage at the three-year level compared to the non-responders. Patients whose serum contained a factor that inhibited this response had a diminished survival. Although this type of testing provides important biologic information, it is not easily translated to the average clinical practice, as might be some of the more standard tests of general immune function. The most prognostically relevant test is still the carcinoembryonic antigen, as evaluated by numerous workers (Wanebo, 1981).

The numerous CEA studies are beyond the scope of this review, but one study relating the CEA and immune complexes (IC) deserves mention. Staab *et al.* (1980) measured CEA immune complexes and free CEA in 363 patients with carcinoma of the gastrointestinal tract before surgery and in post-operative follow-up. Eighty-nine patients had circulating CEA immune complexes pre-operatively. Patients with pre-operative CEA–IC had poorer prognosis than those without CEA–IC, or those with high levels of free CEA, or those who were CEA-negative. The appearance of CEA–IC in consecutive follow-up tests and a progressive increase during the post-operative follow-up period indicated increased likelihood of disease recurrence. In 32 of 55 recurrence cases, circulating CEA–IC were detected post–operatively; all 32 developed metastatic disease.

Combining CEA measurements with other measurements of immune reactivity may provide additional prognostic information beyond that of standard staging (Wanebo *et al.*, 1980); CEA combined with measurements of other serum glycoproteins such as acute phase reactant proteins (Walker *et al.*, 1981), or other tumor markers as shown by Neville *et al.*, (1978), may also be of importance.

An interesting addition to the T rosette assay for T cells is the rosette inhibition assay using anti-thymocyte globulin (ATG), which has been found to correlate with certain malignant and non-malignant diseases and pregnancy. An increase in the rosette-inhibition titer of anti-thymocyte globulin was correlated with an unfavorable prognosis following surgical resection of colorectal cancer, whereas a decreased ATG titer correlated with a more favorable clinical course. These relationships were not seen with other measurements of T cell function, e.g. PHA and Con A response. This assay may be an indirect measurement of some inhibiting serum factor, possibly even an antibody (Ichiki *et al.*, 1977). Abnormalities in this rosette inhibition test have also been observed in lung cancer patients (Gross *et al.*, 1975).

An extensive study of 400 colorectal cancer patients was carried out by an Australian group who measured pre-operatively the serum antibodies to tumor cell cytoplasm and membrane and the blood lymphocyte cytotoxicity against autochthonous tumor cells and serum blocking activity (Nind *et al.*, 1980). Patients were followed post-operatively for a mean of 35 months. In 345 patients treated by curative resection, a significantly favorable association was found between an autoantibody to the tumor cytoplasm and disease-free interval. In 55 patients treated by palliative resection, there was a positive correlation between the blood lymphocyte cytotoxicity against autochthonous tumor cells and survival. Although this type of testing is difficult and would require the utmost effort by a fine immunologic laboratory, this still represents a monumental study of an effort to measure autologous humoral and cellular immune reactivity in colorectal cancer.

Melanoma

This disease, because of its unique biology, has probably fostered more immunologic studies than any other malignancy. Golub (1977) *et al.* reported a detailed study of lymphocyte function in 94 patients with melanoma and in an equal number of controls. They studied lymphoproliferative responses to mitogens, purified protein derivative (PPD), and allogeneic lymphocytes in addition to DNCB skin tests. There was a general decline of lymphocyte responses according to stage of disease or to tumor burden, but only phytohemagglutinin showed a significant difference between Stages II and III. If comparison was made to controls, the MLC response was significantly different in patients with Stage II or III disease. Overall, only the MLC response was significantly different in the patients with melanoma compared with controls (Golub *et al.*, 1977). None of the *in vitro* tests correlated with DNCB response, nor did any of these tests correlate with clinical outcome (Hibbs, 1976). Pritchard *et al.* (1978), in a similar detailed immunologic study of 262 patients with melanoma, found immune depression in comparison to controls, but no meaningful correlation with clinical status, and questioned the value of such studies in routine monitoring.

It is pertinent here that, in a large study of DNCB reactivity and its relation to prognosis in 419 patients with melanoma reported by Camacho *et al.* (1977), a positive DNCB test was seen in 82% of Stage I patients (localized disease), in 81% of Stage II patients (regional nodes positive), in 70% in Stage III (metastases to a single and visceral organ), and in 68% in Stage IV (metastases in more than one internal organ). This is in contrast to the expected response of about 95% in controls.

In regard to DNCB reactivity related to prognosis in Stage II patients, those who were DNCB-positive had a more favorable course than their DNCB-negative counterparts, i.e. the estimated time to recurrence was 16 months versus 7 months. The survival distribution was also similar. The DNCB-positive patients lived a median of 31 months versus 18 months for the DNCB-negative patients, which was significant ($p<0.05$). In patients with more advanced disease, there was no significant relationship between the DNCB response and survival. The response to common skin test antigens was also examined by Aranah *et al.* (1979) who found that the disease-free interval was longer and the recurrence rates lower in patients demonstrating cutaneous hypersensitivity to common dermal antigens than in those who did not.

Gynecologic malignancy (cervix, ovary, corpus, uterus)

Nalick *et al.* (1974) measured delayed hypersensitivity reactions to 1-nitro-2,4-difluorobenzene (DNFB), and a panel of intradermal antigens in 137 patients with staged gynecologic malignancy, and categorized patients by a combined immunologic index. Patients with *in situ* cancer of the cervix had normal responses, whereas 54% of those with invasive cervical cancer had depressed responses. Immunodepression was found in 33% of the patients with corpus cancer and 65% of those with ovarian cancer.

Patients with squamous cell cancers in the pelvis have also been shown to have depressed cell-mediated *in vitro* responses. Catalona *et al.* (1973) found that 38% of the patients with squamous cell cancer of the cervix had significantly depressed phytohemagglutinin responses and serum inhibitory factors. There were no differences in localized versus metastatic tumors. Similarly, over 40% of these patients were anergic to DNCB (Catalona and Chretien, 1973). In a study by Rao *et al.* (1977) of patients with advanced ovarian cancer who were receiving immunochemotherapy using *C. parvum* and CAF chemotherapy, there was generally a profound depression of DNCB skin testing as well as other immune function tests. Patients who did respond to therapy tended to be DNCB-positive, however, and had improved survival compared to the DNCB-negative patients.

A recent study by Check *et al.* (1980) examined the percentage of lymphocytes found in the Ficoll–Hypaque gradient suspension used for lymphocyte purification, the absolute lymphocyte count, the standard mitogen stimulation, mixed lymphocyte culture, and T and B cell measurements. The percentage of lymphocytes in the gradient-derived cell suspension (termed LG) correlated with survival better than any of the other tests. Low values of the percent LG reflected both a depressed lymphocyte count and altered bouyant density of the leukocytes of many patients with advanced cancer. It was thought that, in part, the depression of the immune function tests may be related to the changes in the percent LG in the lymphocyte count.

DiSaia *et al* . (1978) have noted that, in a follow-up study of 30 patients with Stage III-B cancer of the cervix, there was a significant relation of survival to pretreatment absolute lymphocyte count. Patients were treated primarily by combination external beam and brachytherapy. There were differences in survival according to the lymphocyte count, with significantly improved survival occurring in the group with lymphocyte count greater than 2000 in comparison to the group with measurements between 1000 and 1999, and the worse prognosis occurring in the group with a count less than 1000.

Carcinoembryonic antigen has also been evaluated in patients with gynecologic cancer, specifically cervix and endometrium (Van Nagell *et al.*, 1978). In this study of 300 patients with invasive cervix cancer, 204 had 2–15 follow-up CEA determinations and 30 patients had progressively increasing CEA levels, of whom 29 developed recurrent cervix cancer. The CEA levels were elevated in 48% of the patients overall and varied with stage of disease and with histologic differentiation of the tumor.

A similar study in 60 patients with endometrial cancer showed that the CEA varied with stage and histologic differentiation and that the CEA returned to normal within eight weeks after resection in all but two patients, both of whom later developed recurrent disease. This type of data would need to be expanded to determine its usefulness as a prognostic indicator for early recurrence.

Genitourinary malignancy

Schellhammer *et al.* (1976) measured DNCB and intradermal responses in 192 patients with staged carcinomas of testes, prostate, and bladder. Patients with localized testicular cancer had normal responses, whereas only 50% of those with retroperitoneal nodal metastases and 60% of those with extranodal metastases responded to DNCB. Chemotherapy (in 40% of the latter two groups) was thought to have contributed more to immune depression than did stage of disease. Immune depression existed in the patients with prostatic cancer, whether localized (70% DNCB-positive) or with nodal or extranodal metastases (overall 75% were DNCB-positive).

In patients with bladder disease, those with benign bladder papillomas had normal DNCB tests, whereas only 70% of patients with superficial invasive bladder cancer responded, and only 35% of those with deeply invasive or metastatic bladder cancer responded. Prognostic data were not available. Similar findings in pelvic genitourinary malignancy have been noted by Adolphs and Staffens (1977), Catalona *et al.* (1975), and Olsson *et al.* (1972). The levels of circulating spontaneous T-RFC are significantly depressed in patients with cancer of the bladder and prostate (Catalona, *et al.* 1974a). Phytohemagglutinin responses were normal in early bladder and renal cancer but were depressed in patients with advanced disease. (Catalona *et al.*, 1974b, 1975).

In a review of studies at the National Cancer Institute of patients with genitourinary cancer who were evaluated by delayed hypersensitivity skin tests, lymphocyte blastogenesis, and lymphocyte cell surface markers, there were good correlations between host immune competence and both tumor stage and prognosis in patients with cancers of the bladder, kidney, and in those with advanced prostate cancer not receiving endocrine therapy, but not among patients with prostate cancer receiving endocrine therapy. Although radiation and chemotherapy suppressed T lymphocyte levels, chemotherapy-induced remission resulted in a rebound of T cell counts to above normal, whereas radiation-induced suppression appeared to be more persistent (Catalona *et al.*, 1978).

Of interest in bladder cancer has been the loss of A, B or H blood group antigens on the surface of neoplastic epithelial cells and a correlation of this with aggressive tumor behavior. In a study by Lange *et al* (1978) the absence of these antigens on original or recurrent tumors in patients with low staged transitional cell carcinoma of the bladder correlated with the subsequent development of invasive disease (Stage III or greater), while the presence of the antigens correlated with failure to develop invasive disease. Similar data are presented by Young *et al.* (1979). The carcinoembryonic antigen is also of value in bladder cancer. Generally patients presenting with pre-operative CEA levels above 10 ng/ml are at higher risk recurrence than those with values below 10 ng/ml who had improved survival (Alsabti and Saffo, 1979).

Askari *et al.* (1981), in a controlled blind study of the red cell antigen test in bladder cancer, failed to substantiate the findings of other investigators and did not find evidence that the loss of antigen could be equated with a poor prognosis. They did note that in individuals there was a reduction in the red cell antigen and suggested that further refinement in technique and more data are needed to substantiate the usefulness of this assay (Askari *et al.*, 1981).

Head and neck cancer

Patients with squamous cancer of the head and neck are well known to have marked suppression of cell-mediated immunity and skin reactivity to DNCB is markedly depressed (Hilal *et al.*, 1977; Lundy *et al.*, 1974; Pinsky *et al.*, 1976; Wanebo *et al*, 1975). They also show depression of the *in vitro* cell-mediated tests including T cell levels, T lymphocyte function, and recognitive function of the T lymphocyte, i.e., leukocytes from head and neck cancer patients have a defect in the ability to stimulate or respond to mixed lymphocyte reaction (Berlinger *et al.*, 1976). It is also known that treatment with radiation further inhibits the lymphocyte level (Twomey *et al.*, 1974). Patients with head and neck cancer who have been cured by surgery alone have restoration of lymphocytes to normal or near-normal levels, whereas patients who have been radiated for cure have continued suppression of the T lymphocyte (Twomey *et al.*, 1974). There are also relationships of immune status with immune morphology of the primary tumor or of the lymph nodes, but this topic is beyond the scope of this review (Menzio *et al.*, 1980). The general immunologic test that seems most relevant to prognosis is the DNCB skin test. Several groups have shown prognostic relationships to this test including Hilal *et al.* (1977), Osoba *et al.* (1980), and Maisel and Ogura (1976).

A newer finding, and one which needs to be exploited prognostically in these patients, is monitoring with the use of immune complexes. Veltri *et al* (1978) have documented soluble immune complexes in the circulation of 75% of patients with head and neck cancer using the Raji cell radioimmune assay. Overall there was also depression of the other parameters of cell-mediated immunity in these patients with the elevated complexes. In some patients there was a very close correlation between the elevated levels of soluble IC and depressed lymphocyte reactivity to mitogens during regular monitoring.

Lung cancer

Numerous studies of immune tests in lung cancer patients have shown depression of various parameters including the absolute lymphocyte count (Dellon *et al.*, 1975; Riesco, 1970), cytotoxicity against tumor cells (Vose *et al.*, 1978), skin test responses to tumor cell antigen (Wells *et al.*, 1973), and dermal hypersensitivity to DNCB (Dellon *et al.*, 1975; Liebler *et al.*, 1977; Wanebo *et al.*, 1976a). Several studies have attempted to correlate multiple parameter testing with survival. (Concannon *et al.*, 1977; Liebler *et al.*, 1977; Wanebo *et al.*, 1976a). Concannon *et al.* (1977) assessed an immune profile in 141 lung cancer patients who were referred for radiation therapy and who were studied with a battery of immune tests including DNCB skin testing with microbial antigens, differential blood cell count, enumeration of T and B lymphocytes, and stimulation of lymphocytes with plant mitogens PHA, Con A and PWM. By multivariate analysis using the variables of stage of disease, histologic type of tumor, age, and sex, the stage of disease was shown to be a significant factor in the survival of these patients. The results of this study indicated that significant additional information relative to survival may be obtained from the measurement of the patient's response to DNCB, to skin test antigens, and the proportion of peripheral T lymphocytes.

One study has attempted to correlate IgE and atopy with the clinical course of lung cancer patients (H'allgren *et al.*, 1981). The median total IgE level was significantly increased in the sera of 217 unselected patients with bronchial carcinoma in comparison to the levels in two control populations including 246 normal adults and 143 patients with benign pulmonary disease. The presence of specific IgE antibodies against six common allergens was also increased in the cancer population. In contrast, the incidence of clinical atopy (allergy) was about five times higher in the general population than in the control group. (H'allgren *et al.*, 1981). The actuarial survival rate of patients with squamous cancer, Stages I and II, who had normal IgE levels was significantly better than the rate in patients who had elevated IgE levels. This difference was not evident in patients with adenocarcinoma. It was thought that elevated IgE levels might reflect impaired cellular immunity in the lung cancer patients.

Carcinoembryonic antigen has also been shown to be of prognostic value in primary lung cancer. Vincent *et al.* (1979) found a significantly worse prognosis for patients with preoperative CEA levels greater than 2.5 ng/ml. Ford *et al.*, (1981), using a higher cutoff point, found that a pre-operative serum CEA level greater than 20 ng/ml was associated with poor prognosis in patients undergoing radical surgery for lung cancer ($p=0.043$). This prognostic effect was seen mainly in patients whose tumors showed the greatest immunocytochemical localization of CEA using an anti-CEA antibody and the indirect immunoperoxidase test and in Stage III patients ($p = 0.04$).

Circulating immune complexes and autoantibodies have also been described in lung cancer patients. A recent detailed study using five different assay systems for immune complex measurements in a series of 80 newly diagnosed lung cancer patients found that the Raji cell assay and the *Staphylococcus aureus* binding assay demonstrated a higher prevalence of immune complexes in lung cancer patients and bronchitic patients compared to controls, although there was no difference between the two pulmonary disease populations. Smaller amounts of immune complexes were found when assays were used which depend on complement fixation (C1q assays and conglutinin binding), in which case only 15% of the newly diagnosed lung cancer patients had complexes. No relation to prognosis was shown in this study but it did point out the lack of uniqueness of immune complexes to cancer in patients with either malignant or benign pulmonary diseases (Guy *et al.*, 1981).

A study by Dent *et al.* (1980) evaluated immune complexes by the C1q binding test and carcinoembryonic antigen in 50 patients with lung cancer at the time of or following diagnostic or definitive surgery. The overall incidence of elevated values was 31% for the C1q binding and 34% for the CEA. Elevation of C1q binding activity (C1q-BA) and CEA beyond the immediate post-operative period was predictive of a significantly shorter median survival. The most significant differences in survival were seen between patients with normal values for C1q-BA and CEA and those with elevations of one or both parameters: 6:0 months versus 19.5 months ($p<0.001$). Elevation of either parameter during the immediate pre- and post-operative period was not predictive of a poor survival. It appeared that the CEA estimation had the best predictive value, but the addition of C1q-BA measurement may provide additional prognostic information, particularly in those who do not have elevated CEA values. (Dent *et al.*, 1980).

Inoue *et al.* (1978) of Keio University in Japan studied 137 patients with lung cancer and 50 patients with benign thoracic lesions with DNCB skin testing. Ninety-eight percent of the control patients and 46% of the lung cancer patients were sensitized by 250 μg of DNCB. Whereas 60% of the patients with resectable cancer were DNCB-positive, only 28% of those with unresectable lesions and 29% of those with distant metastases were DNCB-positive, ($p<0.001$). In patients with resectable lung cancer the pre-operative DNCB had no prognostic value. However, an excellent correlation was found between post-operative reactivity and two-year survival. There were 17 patients who were initially DNCB-negative who developed positive reactions on post-operative retesting. Of 12 of these patients followed for two years, only two patients died of disease.

Liebler *et al.* (1977) at the Alleghany General Hospital studied 146 patients, prior to treatment with irradiation, using a battery of tests consisting of dermal responses to DNCB, microbial antigens, peripheral lymphocyte counts and subpopulations (T and B cells), and a response to mitogens. Patients who were DNCB-positive had significantly increased survival in all stages (localized, regional disease, and remote disease). Statistically significant differences in survival were also noted for most of the other immune tests in the same patient groups. Effects of histology, age and sex did not appear to influence survival data as significantly as did the immune status of the patient. Their data indicated that measurements of general immune competence were of significant prognostic value in the management of patients with bronchogenic cancer. Measurement of the DNCB response showed the strongest correlation with survival rate (Liebler *et al.*, 1977)

Cannon *et al.*, (1980) have assessed the prognostic relationship of the lymphocyte proliferative response to alloantigens in the mixed leukocyte response MLC and found a significant relationship between the relative proliferative response and the disease-free interval. In this group the immunologic response predicted subsequent clinical prognosis better than the TNM classification or the histologic type of the tumor, i.e. $T_1N_0M_0$ versus

$T_2N_0M_0$ or $T_1N_1M_0$. The depressed response to the alloantigen was a better discriminator of disease recurrence than the response to PHA (Cannon *et al.*, 1980).

A recent modification of the T rosette test involves sensitizing T lymphocytes to a pooled human lung tumor extract, and is termed the antigen stimulated active rosette-forming T cell. These levels were correlated with the detection of lung cancer, pathologic tumor stage, and post-assay survival of patients with lung cancer. Significant levels of lung tumor antigen-sensitive (LTA) T cells were found in the pre-operative blood of 80% of those with Stage III primary lung cancer. There was a significant correlation of post-operative survival with pre-operative levels of the LTA- sensitive T cells by this assay in Stage I ($p<0.0005$), Stage I + II ($p<0.001$), and Stage III ($p<0.001$) patients who were not treated by chemotherapy (Ramey *et al* ., 1980).

A study by Check *et al.* (1981) evaluated a battery of *in vitro* immune tests including a more recently used test, the percent of lymphocytes (LG) in the gradient-derived cell suspension (using Ficoll–Hypaque separation), and found that this decreased significantly with advancing stage of lung cancer and could predict survival of patients within each stage. The percent LG correlated with survival better than any of the other tests when multivariate analysis of all test combinations were performed. Low values of the percent LG reflected both a depressed lymphocyte count and altered bouyant density of the leukocytes of many patients with advanced cancer. It was concluded that this simple measurement provided valuable information of patients with lung cancer and was probably superior to other assays, including the lymphocyte count, T and B cells, and blastogenesis by planned mitogen stimulation. This assay has also been used in other cancer patient groups (Check *et al.*, 1981).

IMMUNOLOGIC PROFILES IN FOUR COMMON OPERABLE CARCINOMAS

The literature on immune testing in breast, colorectal, lung, and head and neck cancers is extensive and the reader is referred to reviews by Nathanson (1977), Wanebo (1979a), Wanebo and Pinsky (1978), Liebler *et al.* (1977), and Chretien (1977). To simplify this review we will discuss results obtained in a single institution (Memorial Sloan Kettering Cancer Center, New York) with immunologic testing of a large group of patients (839) with primary operable cancers (Wanebo *et al.*, 1978a). This material has been previously reviewed in detail. The group included 190 patients with breast cancer, 312 patients with colorectal cancer, 183 with cancer of the head and neck, and 154 with lung cancer.

Immunologic assessment consisted of skin testing for delayed hypersensitivity with DNCB and a panel of intradermal antigens, total lymphocyte count and enumeration of T and B cells, lymphocyte stimulation with mitogens (phytohemagglutinin, pokeweed mitogen, and Con A) and common antigens (*Candida albicans, Staphylococcus aureus*, streptokinase–streptodornase, PPD, staphage lysate), and determinations of serum immunoglobulin and complement levels.

Basic immune tests and staging

We will initially analyze results of a simplified battery of immune tests including skin testing with DNCB, the absolute lymphocyte count, and lymphocyte blastogenesis with phytohemagglutinin. In order to compare immune function properly in these patients, it is essential to categorize them into homogeneous groups. As the TNM system does not uniformly apply, we have defined a staging system that is based primarily on tumor burden:

> *Stage I*—small (less than 3 cm) primary tumor only.
> *Stage II*—large (greater than 3 cm) primary tumor without nodal metastases.
> *Stage III*—regional lymph node metastases.
> Stage IV—generalized disease.

DNCB response

Different cancers were found to affect the response to DNCB at different stages. In patients with cancer of the head and neck and colon, the response to DNCB was often depressed at an early stage. In patients with cancer of the breast or lung, comparable depression was seen at later stages (Table 4).

Table 4   Percentage of negative responses [a] to DNCB tests in patients with primary cancers of the breast, head and neck, lung, and rectal colon. (From Wanebo, 1979b, reproduced by permission of *Surgical Clinics of North America*)

Stage of disease[b]	Breast cancer	Head and neck cancer	Lung cancer	Rectum or colon cancer
I	11	44[c]	25[c]	24[c]
II	11	25[c]	11	44[c]
III	20	60[c]	24[c]	39[c]
IV	(54)[c,d]	30[c]	33[c]	58[c]
Total patients	190	183	131	237

[a] About 5% of normal individuals are DNCB-negative.
[b] Stage of disease is defined in text.
[c] Significant depression within each cancer group ($p<0.05$).
[d] ( ) Represents an additional 56 patients with Stage IV breast cancer.

Total lymphocyte count and lymphocyte subpopulations

Lymphocyte counts were depressed frequently in patients with early colon cancer, less frequently in patients with early lung and head and neck cancer, and not at all in patients with early breast cancer (Table 5). In Stage III (regional lymph node metastases), only patients with breast cancer showed no depression of lymphocyte counts. All four groups of patients with Stage IV disease (disseminated) showed depressed lymphocyte counts.

Lymphocyte subpopulations were studied in smaller numbers of patients. The T cell count was within normal limits in patients with early breast or lung cancer, but depressed in patients with early head and neck or rectal or colon cancer. When large tumors or lymph node metastases were present, the T cell count was normal in patients with breast cancer but depressed in patients with carcinoma of the lung, head and neck, and rectum or colon (Evans *et al.*, 1977; Wanebo *et al.*, 1975, 1976a; Wanebo and Pinsky, 1978).

Table 5   Lymphocyte levels in patients with primary cancers of the breast, head and neck, lung, and rectal colon. (From Wanebo, 1979b, reproduced by permission of *Surgical Clinics of North America.*)

	Percentage with low lymphocyte counts[a]			
Stage of disease	Breast	Head and neck	Lung	Rectal colon
I (Operable) Small primary <3 cm	<10	21	30	53[b]
II (Operable) Large localized primary <3cm	10	51[b]	—	38[b]
III (Operable) Primary of any size and regional node metastases	20	51[b]	48[b]	30
IV (Inoperable) Very large primary with or without extensive regional or distant metastases	(55)[b,c]	45[b]	<48[b]	45–60[b]
Total number of patients	113	183	70	111

[a] Tenth percentile of controls.
[b] Significant depression within each cancer group ($p < 0.05$).
[c] (a) Represents an additional 42 patients with advanced breast cancer.

Lymphocyte blastogenesis

Discussion will be limited to results obtained by mitogen stimulation, with emphasis on phytohemagglutinin (Table 6). The tenth percentile of the control groups was used as the cutoff point, separating normal from subnormal values. Depression of lymphocyte stimulation with mitogens showed a general correlation with tumor burden, more evident with phytohemagglutinin and Con A than with pokeweed mitogen. The phyto-hemagglutinin response was generally normal in patients with earlier stages of primary operable breast cancer, but did show a general downward trend with increasing extent of disease, and was significantly depressed in Stage IV disease. Patients with cancer of the head and neck or rectum or colon showed a depressed response even in Stage I disease, whereas in lung cancer only patients with Stage III disease had depressed responses. Overall the phytohemagglutinin response was depressed in 60% of patients with advanced disease.

Table 6   Phytohemagglutinin response in patients with primary cancers of the breast, head and neck, lung, and rectal colon. (From Wanebo, 1979b, reproduced by permission of *Surgical Clinics of North America*.)

	Percentage of low response[a]			
Stage of disease	Breast	Head and neck	Lung	Rectal colon
I (Operable) Small primary <3 cm	17	32[b]	25	33[b]
II (Operable) Large primary <3 cm	15	45[b]	—	37[b]
III (Operable) Primary of any size and regional node metastases	28	45[b]	43[b]	25
IV (Inoperable) Very large primary with or without extensive regional metastases or distant metastases	(67)[b,c]	61[b]	55[b]	57[b]
Total number of patients	113	183	70	111

[a] The maximum absolute PHA response of isolated lymphocyte was determined by testing serial dilutions of PHA in triplicate. Low responses were those below the tenth percentile of the control group.

[b] Significant depression within each cancer group ($p < 0.05$).

[c] ( ) represents an additional 42 patients with advanced breast cancer.

Breast cancer

Immunologic studies were performed at the time of surgery in 134 patients with operable breast cancer and in 63 patients with benign breast disease. The DNCB response was normal in patients who had non-infiltrating cancer or infiltrating cancer without regional lymph node metastases (89% were DNCB-positive), and was not significantly depressed in patients with infiltrating cancer who had nodal metastases (80% were DNCB-positive). There were abnormalities, however, in some *in vitro* tests of cellular immune function. While the absolute lymphocyte and T cell counts were normal, there was a small but significant increase in B cells bearing surface immunoglobulins.

Serum immunoglobulin levels (IgA, IgG, and IgM) were normal in patients with benign breast disease as well as in patients with breast cancer. There was no significant difference in the mean lymphocyte response to mitogens and antigens between patients with cancer and those with benign breast disease, but a significantly larger proportion of cancer patients showed lymphocyte responses below the selected cutoff point for the various stimulating agents.

Pathologic studies by Dr Paul Rosen permitted ranking of patients with breast cancer into three groups according to risk of recurrence. The low-risk category included patients with non-infiltrating cancer or infiltrating cancer smaller than 1 cm without lymph node metastases. The intermediate-risk category included patients with infiltrating cancer larger than 1 cm or 1–3 lymph node metastases at Level I only. The high-risk category included patients with four or more lymph node metastases or any macroscopic nodal metastases at Levels II or III. Immunologic function was correlated with risk of recurrence as defined for these categories.

There was no correlation of DNCB reactivity, lymphocyte counts, or proportions of lymphocyte subpopulations with risk of recurrence, but there was a correlation between lymphocyte stimulation response and risk of recurrence. By constructing standardized scores for each of 10 lymphocyte stimulation tests, one could examine them on the same scale and compare trends directly. Only lymphocyte stimulation with phytohemagglutinin showed a continued decrease with progressive disease ($p<0.04$), whereas lymphocyte stimulation with other mitogens and antigens showed a decrease from benign to low-risk patients, and then a 'paradoxical' increase with further progression of disease. A significant linear trend was found for phytohemagglutinin ($p<0.04$), and a significant 'quadratic' trend (V-shaped) was found for the lymphocyte stimulants pokeweed mitogen, *Escherichia coli*, *Staphylococcus aureus*, and MBV ($p<0.05$). Recent extension of these studies showed that, whereas immunologic reactivity decreased with advancing disease and therefore with risk of recurrence of death, patients who were immunodeficient fared as well as those who were immuno-competent within each stage of disease (Krown *et al.*, 1978; Wanebo *et al.*, 1978c).

Bolton *et al.*, (1976) in a similar study found the DNCB response to be more discriminating. These authors, using graded DNCB response, found a significantly depressed DNCB response in patients with early breast cancer compared with controls. Fourteen percent of their patients with Stage I disease versus 4% of controls were DNCB negative. Although DNCB was markedly depressed in patients with advanced disease, patients with locally advanced disease had paradoxically good responses. Stein *et al.* (1976) found depression of delayed hypersensitivity responses and phytohemagglutinin responses in early disease and more profound impairment in metastatic disease. Immune competence was not affected by regional node involvement, nor did the degree of immune impairment correlate with prognosis in equally staged patients.

Head and neck cancer

Immunological studies were performed in 183 patients with mucosal squamous cancer of the head and neck (Hilal *et al.*, 1977). All patients were staged clinically according to the TNM system of the American Joint Committee of Clinical Staging. There was a general depression of immunologic reactivity (except for the lymphocyte response to pokeweed mitogen) even in Stage I. All reactions were significantly depressed in patients with more advanced disease.

Lymphocyte count, phytohemagglutinin response, Con A response, but not DNCB tests nor pokeweed mitogen response, showed progressive depression with increasing extent of disease. There was no correlation with age or sex. Only DNCB reactivity correlated with recurrence, and this was seen only in patients with Stage I and II cancer but not in those with Stage III or IV cancer. None of the *in vitro* tests correlated with prognosis within each stage. Improvements in *in vitro* tests may show better prognostic correlations. Specialized assays for T cells (T cell inhibition test) (Deegan and Coulthart, 1977) and the active T cell test may provide more relevant prognostic information (Golub *et al.*, 1974). Perhaps the relative MLC response, which has shown good correlation with clinical stage and prognosis in patients with head and neck cancer, may be a better prognostic indicator than simple mitogen assays (Berlinger *et al.*, 1977).

Lung cancer

In our investigation of lung cancer, 154 patients with lung cancer, 20 patients with benign pulmonary lesions, and 109 healthy persons were examined. Patients were staged clinically and pathologically according to the staging system established by the American Joint Committee for Lung Cancer. The DNCB test was positive in only 73% of patients with lung cancer but was positive in all 20 patients with benign thoracic disease ($p<0.05$). The incidence of positive tests was 78% for Stages I and II (37 patients), 73% for resectable Stage III (37 patients), and 66% for unresectable or inoperable Stage III (57 patients). DNCB reactivity showed a relationship to the histologic type. The incidence of positive tests was 80% in patients with epidermoid carcinoma, 57% in patients with oat cell carcinoma, and 80% in those with terminal bronchiolar carcinoma. Results of *in vitro* tests correlated best with stage of disease. They included the lymphocyte count, T cell count, and lymphocyte stimulation with phytohemagglutinin, pokeweed mitogen, and Con A (Table 7). Results of these tests were in the normal range in patients with Stage I cancer, but were significantly depressed in patients with Stage III cancer.

Survival of patients with Stage I and II disease was not shortened when DNCB reactivity, lymphocyte counts, or phytohemagglutinin response were depressed (combined disease). This may change as the number of patients increases, follow-up time becomes longer, and the number of patients with recurrent disease is greater. In patients with Stage III disease (resectable as well as operable but non-resectable), only the phytohemagglutinin response correlated with survival. The lymphocyte count correlated with prognosis only in patients with non-resectable Stage III disease. The difference in survival between DNCB-positive and DNCB-negative patients (Stage III, resectable) shows a trend but is not yet significant.

Similar multiparameter data in primary operable patients have been generated by Holmes and Golub (1976) and Liebler *et al* (1977). In general, these studies showed good immune function in patients with local or Stage I disease and impairment of immune parameters in patients with unresectable or advanced disease. Holmes found that, generally, resectability correlated with DNCB response in 33 patients tested pre-operatively. Sixteen of 17 DNCB-positive patients had resectable disease, whereas 14 of 16 DNCB-negative patients had unresectable disease. Liebler studied patients with lung cancer referred for radiation therapy and found that, although there was general impairment of *in vivo* and *in vitro* parameters with progression of disease, the DNCB response correlated best with survival rate (Liebler *et al.*, 1977).

Rectal or colon cancer

Multiparameter immune tests were performed in 312 patients with rectal or colon cancer, including 181 patients with primary resectable cancer, 53 patients with advanced primary operable cancer, and 96 patients with recurrence (Rao *et al.*, 1977; Wanebo and Pinsky, 1978; Wanebo *et al.*, 1976b). Immune reactivity was measured by the DNCB skin test (219 patients) and by *in vitro* tests (111 patients), including lymphocyte count, T and B cell count, lymphocyte stimulation tests with mitogens and antigens, serum immunoglobulin levels, and complement levels. Levels of carcino-embryonic antigen in the blood were also determined before surgery.

There was a linear depression of immune reactivity as measured by DNCB tests, phytohemagglutinin response, and lymphocyte count, with increasing stage of disease. Immune functions were depressed even in patients with Dukes' A cancer (24% were DNCB-negative, 33% had low phytohemag-glutinin responses), more so in patients with Dukes' B and C lesions (40% were DNCB negative, 30% had low phytohemagglutinin responses), and were profoundly depressed in patients with advanced primary cancer or recurrence (60% showed depressed DNCB responses, phytohemagglutinin responses, and lymphocyte counts).

Follow-up of 54 Dukes' C patients over 24 months showed no significant difference in recurrence rate between DNCB-positive (16 of 32) and DNCB-negative (14 of 22) patients. Only patients with advanced disease showed a correlation of depressed immune response (phytohemagglutinin and lymphocyte count, but not DNCB) with shorter survival ($p>0.05$) (Table 7). In contrast, a significant correlation of early recurrence with increased

Table 7 Correlation of normal pretreatment immune respone to prolongation of disease-free survival or overall survival

	Patients	Pos. DNCB	Normal lymphocyte count	Normal PHA response
Breast cancer				
Resectable	96	↓ survival in DNCB$^+$	N.A.	N.A.
Advanced	106	↓ survival in DNCB$^+$	N.A.	N.A.
Colorectal cancer				
Resectable				
(Dukes A, B, C)	181	none	none	none
Advanced disease	126	none	$p<0.05$	$p<0.05$
Head and neck cancer				
Resectable				
(for cure Stage IV)	160	Stage I and II:$p<0.05$ Stage III: N.S.	none	none
Advanced (Stage IV)	23	none	none	none
Lung cancer				
Stage I and II	37	N.A.	N.A.	N.A.
Stage III (resectable)	29	$p<0.10$	none	$p<0.05$
Unresectable	22	N.S.	$p<0.05$	$p<0.05$

N.A. = not available
N.S. = not significant

levels of carcinoembryonic antigen (<5 ng/ml) was found in patients with Dukes' C lesions ($p<0.001$), but no correlation with survival was seen in patients with advanced disease (Wanebo *et al.*, 1978b).

In a study from Roswell Park comparing lymphocyte blastogenesis in colon cancer patients and age-matched controls, there was an age-related and tumor-related decline in immune function (Goldrosen *et al.*, 1977). In another study from the same institution, there were suggestive data that recurrence rates are lower in patients with colorectal cancer with B_2 and C_2 lesions who have positive delayed hypersensitivity reaction to *Monilia* and DNCB, a lower B cell level (EAC rosette), and a normal level of carcinoembryonic antigen (Evans *et al.*, 1977). The T cell rosette inhibition test has also been shown to be a good indicator of T cell function in these patients (Ichiki *et al.*, 1977).

CONCLUSION

Immunologic testing as a guide to cancer management is still under development and selected immune tests show good correlation with prognosis in certain diseases but not in others. A critical problem is in obtaining adequate studies of carefully staged, homogeneous groups of cancer patients who have been followed over adequate periods of time. The more recent studies are attempting to do this. Another problem is the standardization of the tests, and reproducibility in the *in vitro* assays with sequential testing. There is also the added problem of age, which is often not well controlled in many of these studies.

Immune testing has provided important information regarding the biology of various cancers. As seen in this review, especially in the examination of patients from a single institution, there are differences in the degree of immune impairment seen in the different cancers. In general, patients with resectable breast cancer have a relatively intact immune system which does show progressive depression with advancing disease. In contrast, patients with even early stages of head and neck cancer are already immunologically depressed (as measured by several different parameters both *in vivo* and *in vitro*) and there is further progression with advancing disease. As was pointed out, there are environmental factors that may have an impact here. These patients are frequently malnourished, alcoholic, heavy smokers, and elderly, all of which add to the immunologic impairment. Patients with colorectal cancer are also immunologically depressed if measured prior to surgical resection. If the patients are tested following adequate resection and restoration of normal function, they then appear to be relatively normal as a group (Wanebo *et al.*, 1980).

Patients with Stage I and II lung cancer have relatively intact immunity but show progressive immune depression with Stage III cancer, which is even more marked if they have unresectable disease. As a rule, patients with unresectable disease are significantly more immunologically depressed than their resectable counterparts (Inoue *et al.*, 1978). Patients whose DNCB test returns to normal after tumor resection appear to have an improved survival rate compared to the group whose DNCB remains negative (Inoue *et al.*, 1978). Thus, with certain diseases, immunologic testing may provide an additional stratifying point separating patients of similar stages into high- and low-risk groups.

It is imperative in this respect that the test involved be sufficiently precise and reproducible to be applicable. The carcinoembryonic antigen test is such an example of a well developed immunologically derived test which has good precision, appears to correlate with tumor burden or stage of disease, and in several diseases appears to have prognostic predictive value (Vincent *et al.*, 1979; Wanebo *et al.*, 1978b). The addition of immune complex testing may add value to the CEA test, as shown by Dent *et al.*, (1980). It is possible that combining the CEA test with selected general immune function tests may also sharpen the biologic relevance of these tests. One might speculate that the CEA would register the extent of tumor burden, whereas the other immune profile tests would register the host response, and the results of the two tests should give an indication of the patient's ultimate prognosis with treatment.

As a reasonable immune profile for patients with solid tumor, the writer would suggest the use of DNCB, total lymphocyte and monocyte count, a lymphocyte subpopulation measurement (T cell rosette count, both active and standard), B cell measurement, lymphocyte proliferation tests using well defined stimulants (e.g. plant mitogens, selected antigens, and pooled allogeneic lymphocytes), and an assessment of the effect of the patient's serum versus standard AB sera. Immune complex measurements should include the Raji cell, C1q binding assay or one of the newer assays, C1q deviation test.

Tests of monocyte–macrophage function are probably also important, although the results are variable in some hands (Unger *et al.*, 1979). Tests of migration (Snyderman *et al.*, 1978) appear to show correlation with prognosis and could be of value. Other tests under current consideration include the typing of lymphocytes by monoclonal antibodies and inserting them into the pre-thymocyte suppressor and helper cell moieties. Testing with human tumor extracts is more strictly a research tool and not readily available to the conventional immunobiology laboratory.

An additional use for immune testing is as an indicator of the effects of cancer management. These tests have been found useful in assessing the consequences of treatment of surgery (Dellon *et al.*, 1975; Holmes and Golub, 1976; Israel *et al.*, 1973; Liebler *et al.*, 1977; Wanebo *et al.*, 1978a), radiation (Stefani *et al.*, 1976; Stjernsward *et al.*, 1972), chemotherapy (Hersh *et al.*, 1976; Roth *et al.*, 1978), and, of course, immunotherapy (Helson, 1976;

Hersh *et al.*, 1976; West *et al.*, 1976). Such tests provide information on the host's ability to deal with tumor during treatment, and may suggest areas for immune reinforcement in addition to conventional therapy.

REFERENCES

Adler, A., Stein, J.A., and Ben-Efraim, S. (1980). Immunocompetence, immuno-suppression, and human breast cancer. *Cancer*, **45**, 2061–2073.

Adolphs, S.D., and Staffens, L (1977). Evaluation of the immunocompetence of patients with transitional cell carcinoma of the bladder. *Urol. Res.*, **5**, 29–33.

Alexander, P. (1976). The functions of the macrophage in malignant disease. In *The macrophage in malignant disease* (ed. S. Alexander). New York: Raven Press. pp. 207–223.

Alsabti, E.A., and Saffo, M.H. (1979). Plasma levels of CEA as a prognostic marker in carcinoma of urinary bladder. *Urol. Int.*, **34**, 387–392.

Anthony, H.M., Kirk, J.A., Madsen, K.E., *et al.* (1975). E and EAC rosetting lymphocytes in patients with carcinoma of bronchus. *Clin. Exp. Immunol.*, **20**, 29.

Anthony, H.M., Templeman, G.H., Madsen, K.E., *et al.* (1974). The prognostic significance of DHS skin tests in patients with carcinoma of bronchus. *Cancer*, **34**, 1901–1906.

Aranah, G.V., McKhann, C.F., Simmons, F.L., and Grage, T.B. (1979). Recall skin-test antigens and the prognosis of stage I melanoma. *J. Surg. Oncol.*, **11**, 13–16.

Askari, A., Colmenares, E., Saberi, A., and Jarman, W. (1981). Red cell surface antigen and its relationship to survival of patients with transitional cell carcinoma of the bladder. *J. Urol.*, **125**, 182–184.

Baldwin, R.W., Hoffken, K., and Robins, R.A. (1979). *Recent results in cancer research*. Heidelberg: Springer Verlag.

Barnes, E.W., Farmer, A., Penhale, W.J., *et al.* (1975). Phytohemagglutinin-induced lymphocyte transformation in newly presenting patients with primary carcinoma of the lung. *Cancer*, **36**, 187.

Berlinger, N.T., Hilal, E.Y., Oettgen, H.F., *et al.* (1977). Deficient cell mediated immunity in head and neck cancer patients secondary to autologous suppressive immune cells. *Laryngoscope*, **88**, 470.

Berlinger, N.T., Lopez, C., and Good, R.A. (1976). Facilitation or attenuation of mixed leukocyte culture responsiveness by adherent cells. *Nature*, **260**, 145–146.

Black, M.D., Barclay, T.H.C., and Hankey, B.F. (1975). Prognosis in breast cancer utilizing histologic characteristics of primary tumor. *Cancer*, **36**, 2048–2054.

Black, M.M. (1973). A model for cancer surgery. *Isr. J. Med. Sci.*, **9**, 284–299.

Bolton, P.M., Mander, A.M., Davidson, H.M., *et al.* (1975). Cellular immunity in cancer: Comparison of delayed hypersensitivity skin tests in three common cancers. *Br. Med. J.*, **3**, 18–20.

Bolton, P.M., Teasdale, C., Mander, A.M., *et al.* (1976). Immune competence in breast cancer—relationship of pretreatment immunologic tests to diagnosis and tumor stage. *Cancer Immunol. Immunother.*, **1**, 251–268.

Broder, S., and Waldman, T.A. (1978). The suppressor-cell network in cancer (Part 1). *New Engl. J. Med.*, **299**, 1281–1284.

Brugarolas, A., Han, T., Takita, H., *et al.* (1973). Immunologic assays in lung cancer. *N.Y. State J. Med.*, **73**, 747.

Camacho, E.S., Pinsky, C.M., Wanebo, H.J., *et al.* (1977). DNCB reactivity and prognosis in 358 patients with malignant melanoma (Abstract). *Proc. AACR and ASCO.* p.115.

Cannon, G.B., Dean, J.H., Herberman, R.B., *et al.* (1980). Association of depressed postoperative lymphoproliferative responses to alloantigens with poor prognosis in patients with stage I lung cancer. *Int. J. Surg.,* **25,** 9–17.

Cannon, G.B., Dean, J.H., Herberman, R.B., Keels, M., and Alford, C. (1981). Lymphoproliferative responses to autologous tumor extracts as prognostic indicators in patients with resected breast cancer. *Int. J. Cancer,* **27,** 131–138.

Catalona, W.J., and Chretien, P.B. (1973). Abnormalities of quantitative dinitrochlorobenzene sensitization in cancer patients: correlation with tumor stage and histology. *Cancer,* **31,** 353–356.

Catalona, W.J., Potvin, C., and Chretien, P.B. (1974a). T lymphocytes in bladder and prostatic cancer patients. *J. Urol.,* **112,** 378.

Catalona, W.J., Sample, W.F., and Chretien, P.B. (1973). Lymphocyte reactivity in cancer patients: correlation with tumor histology and clinical stage. *Cancer,* **31,** 65–71.

Catalona, W.J., Smolev, J.K., and Harty, H.I. (1975). Prognostic value of host immunocompetence in urologic cancer patients. *J. Urol.,* **114,** 922–926.

Catalona, W.J., Tarpley, J.L., Chretien, P.B., *et al.* (1974b). Lymphocyte stimulation in urologic cancer patients. *J. Urol.,* **112,** 373.

Catalona, W.J., Tarpley, J.L., Potvin, C., and Chretien, P.B. (1978). Host immunocompetence in genitourinary cancer: relation to tumor stage and prognosis. *Natl Cancer Inst. Monogr.,* **49,** 105–110.

Chakravorty, R.C., Curutchet, H.P., Coppolla, F.S., *et al.* (1973). The delayed hypersensitivity reaction in the cancer patient; observations on sensitization by DNCB. *Surgery,* **73,** 730–735.

Check, I.J., Hunger, R.L., Karrison, T., *et al.* (1981). Prognostic significance of immunological tests in lung cancer. *Clin. Exp. Immunol.,* **43,** 362–369.

Check, I.J., Hunger, R.L., Rosenberg, K.D., and Herbst, A.L. (1980). Prediction of survival in gynecological cancer based on immunological tests. *Cancer Res.,* **40,** 4612–4616.

Chretien, P.B. (1977). Immunology of head and neck cancers. *Semin. Oncol.,* **4,** 172.

Concannon, J.P., Dalbow, M.H., Eng, C.P., and Conway, J. (1977). Immunoprofile studies for patients with bronchogenic carcinoma. I. Correlation of pretherapy studies with stage of disease. *Int. J. Radiat. Biol. Phys.,* **2,** 447.

Cunningham, T.J., Daut, D., Wolfgang, P.E., *et al.* (1976). A correlation of DNCB-induced delayed cutaneous hypersensitivity reactions and the course of disease in patients with recurrent breast cancer. *Cancer,* **37,** 1696–1700.

Deegan, M.J., and Coulthart, S.W. (1977). Spontaneous rosette formation and rosette inhibition assay in patients with squamous cell carcinoma of head and neck. *Cancer,* **39,** 2137–2141.

Dellon, A., Potvin, C., and Chretien, P.B. (1975). Thymus dependent lymphocyte levels in bronchogenic carcinoma: correlations with histology, clinical stage and clinical course after surgical biopsy. *Cancer,* **35,** 687.

Dent, P.B., Louis, J.A., McCulloch, P.B., Dunnett, C.W., and Gerottini, J. (1980). Correlation of elevated C1q binding activity and carcinoembryonic antigen levels with clinical features of prognosis in bronchogenic carcinoma. *Cancer,* **45,** 130–136.

DiSaia, P.J., Morrow, C.P., Hill, A., and Mittelstaedt, L. (1978). Immune competence and survival in patients with advanced cervical cancer: peripheral lymphocyte counts. *Int. J. Radiat. Oncol., Biol. Phys.,* **4,** 449–451.

Ducos, J., Migueres, J., Colombies, P., *et al.* (1970). Lymphocyte response to PHA in patients with lung cancer. *Lancet*, **i**, 1111.

Eccles, S.A., and Alexander, P. (1974). Macrophage content of tumours in relation to metastatic spread and host immune reaction. *Nature*, **250**, 667–669.

Eilber, F.R., and Morton, D.L. (1970). Impaired immunologic reactivity and recurrence following cancer surgery. *Cancer*, **25**, 362–367.

Eilber, F.R., Nizze, J.A., and Morton, D.L. (1975). Sequential evaluation of general immune competence in cancer patients: correlation with clinical course. *Cancer*, **35**, 660–665.

Evans, J.T., Goldrosen, M.H., Tin, H., *et al.* (1977). Cell-mediated immune status of colon cancer patients. Evaluation by dermal antigen testing, measurement of lymphocyte stimulation and counts of peripheral blood rosette-forming cells. *Cancer*, **40**, 2716–2725.

Evans, R. (1976). Tumor macrophages in host immunity to malignancies. In *The macrophage in neoplasia* (ed. M.A. Fink). New York: Academic Press.

Ford, C.H., Stokes, J.H., and Newman, C.E. (1981). Carcinoembryonic antigen and prognosis after radical surgery for lung cancer: immunocytochemical localization and serum levels. *Br. J. Cancer*, **44**, 145–153.

Fudenberg, H.H., Wybran, J., and Robbins, D. (1975). T-rosette-forming cells, cellular immunity and cancer. *New Engl. J. Med.*, **292**, 475.

Glasgow, A.H., Nimberg, R.B., Menzoian, J.O., *et al.* (1974). Association of anergy with an immunosuppressive peptide fraction in the serum of patients with cancer. *New Engl. J. Med.*, **291**, 1263–1267.

Goldrosen, H.H., Han, T., Jung, O., Smolur, J., and Holyoke, E.D. (1977). Impaired lymphocyte blastogenic response in patients with colon adeno-carcinoma: effects of disease and age. *J. Surg. Oncol.*, **9**, 229–234.

Golub, S.H., O'Connell, T.X., and Morton, D.L. (1974). Correlation of *in vivo* and *in vitro* assays of immunocompetence in cancer patients. *Cancer Res.*, **34**, 183–187.

Golub, S.H., Rangel, D.M., and Morton, D.L. (1977). *In vitro* assessment of immunocompetence in patients with malignant melanoma. *Int. J. Cancer*, **20**, 873–880.

Good, R.A. (1977). Biology of the cell-mediated immune response: a review. In *Malnutrition and the immune response* (ed R.M. Suskind). New York: Raven Press.

Gross, R.L., Latty, A., Williams, E.A., *et al.* (1975). Abnormal spontaneous rosette formation and rosette inhibition in lung carcinoma. *New Engl. J. Med.*, **292**, 439.

Guy, K., Mario, U.D., Irvine, W.J., Hunter, A.M., Hadley, A., and Horne, N.W. (1981). Circulating immune complexes and autoantibodies in lung cancer. *Br. J. Cancer*, **43**, 276–283.

H'allgren, R., Arrendal, H., Hiesche, K., Lundquist, G., N'ou, E., and Zetterstr'om, O. (1981). Elevated serum immunoglobulin E in bronchial carcinoma: its relation to the histology and prognosis of cancer. *J. Allergy Clin. Immunol.*, **67**, 398–406

Han, T., and Takita, H. (1972). Immunological impairment in bronchogenic carcinoma: a study of lymphocyte response to phytohemagglutinin. *Cancer*, **30**, 616.

Harris, J., Stewart, T., Sengar, D.P.S., *et al.* (1975). Quantitation of T- and B-lymphocytes in peripheral blood of patients with solid tumours. I. Relation to other parameters of *in vivo* and *in vitro* immune competence. *Can. Med. Assoc. J.*, **112**, 948–952.

Helson, L. (1976). Reactions to dinitrochlorobenzene in patients with neuroblastoma and survival. *J. Natl Cancer Inst.* **57**, 723–724.

Hersh, E.M., Gutterman, J.U., and Mavligit, G.M. (1976). Immunocompetence, immunodeficiency and prognosis in cancer. Proc. Int. Conf. on Immunobiology of Cancer. *Ann. N. Y. Acad. Sci.,* **276**, 386–406.

Hibbs, J.B., Jr (1976). The macrophage as a tumoricidal effector cell: a review of *in vivo* and *in vitro* studies on the mechanism of the activated macrophage nonspecific cytotoxic reaction. In *The macrophage in neoplasia* (ed. M.A. Fink). New York: Academic Press.

Hilal, E.Y., Wanebo, H.J., and Pinsky C.M. (1977). Immunologic evaluation and prognosis in patients with head and neck cancer. *Am. J. Surg.,* **134**, 469–473.

Hoffken, K., Meredith, I.D., Robins, R.A., Baldwin, R.W., Davies, C.J., and Blamey, R.W. (1978). Immune complexes and prognosis of human breast cancer. *Lancet,* **i**, 672.

Holmes, E.C., and Golub, S.H. (1976). Immunologic defects in lung cancer patients. *J. Thorac. Cardiovasc. Surg.,* **71**, 161–168.

House, A.K., and Watt, A.G. (1979). Survival and the immune response in patients with carcinoma of the colorectum. *Gut,* **20**, 868–874.

Hughes, L.E., and Mackay, W.D. (1965). Suppression of the tuberculin response in malignant disease. *Br. Med. J.,* **2**, 1346–1348.

Hughes, N.R. (1974). Serum concentrations of γG, γM immunoglobulins in patients with carcinoma, melanoma and sarcoma. *J. Natl. Cancer Inst.,* **46**, 1015.

Ichiki, A.T., Collmann, R., Sonoda, T., *et al.* (1977). Inhibition of rosette formation by antithymocyte globulin: an indicator for T-cell competence in colorectal cancer patients. *Cancer Immunol. Immunother.,* **3**, 119–124.

Inoue, H., Ishikara, T., Kobayashi, K, *et al.* (1978). Sequential evaluation of DNCB reactivity in patients with primary lung cancer: correlation with prognosis. *J. Thorac. Cardiovasc. Surg.,* **76**, 479–482.

Israel, L., Mugica, J., and Chahinian, P.H. (1973). Prognosis of early bronchogenic carcinoma. Survival curves of 451 patients after resection of lung cancer in relation to the results of preoperative tuberculin skin tests. *Biomedicine,* **19**, 68.

Kerman, R.H., Smith, R., Stafani, S.S., *et al.* (1976). Active T-rosette forming cells in the peripheral blood of cancer patients. *Cancer Res.,* **36**, 3274.

Kjeldsberg, C.R., and Pay, G.D. (1978). A qualitative and quantitative study of monocytes in patients with malignant solid tumors. *Cancer,* **41**, 2236–2241.

Krant, M.J., Manskopf, G., Brandrup, C.S., *et al.* (1968). Immunologic alterations in bronchogenic cancer. Sequential study. *Cancer,* **21**, 623–631.

Krown, S.E., Pinsky, C.M., Wanebo, H.J., *et al.* (1980). Immunologic reactivity and prognosis in breast cancer. *Cancer* **46**, 1746–1752.

Krown, S.E., Pinsky, C.M., Wong, P.P., *et al.* (1978). Immune reactivity and prognosis in patients with breast cancer (Abstract). *Proc. Am. Soc. Clin. Oncol.,* **19**, 351.

Lange, P.H., Limas, C., and Fraley, E.E. (1978). Tissue blood-group antigens and prognosis in low stage transitional cell carcinoma of the bladder. *J. Urol.,* **119**, 52–55.

Lee, A.K.Y., Rowley, M., and Mackay, I.R. (1970). Antibody-producing capacity in human cancer. *Br. J. Cancer,* **24**, 454.

Levin, A.G., Cunningham, M.P., Steers, A.K., *et al.* (1970). Production of 19S and 7S antibodies by cancer patients. *Clin. Exp. Immunol.,* **7**, 839.

Levin, A.G., McDonough, E.F., Jr, Miller, D.G., *et al.* (1964). Delayed hypersensitivity response to DNCB in sick and healthy persons. *Ann. N. Y. Acad. Sci.*, **120**, 400–409.

Liebler, G.A., Concannon, J.P., Magovern, G.J., *et al.* (1977). Immunoprofile studies for patients with bronchogenic carcinoma. I. Correlation of pretherapy studies with survival. *J. Thorac. Cardiovasc. Surg.*, **74**, 506–518.

Litwin, S.D. (1976). *In vitro* evaluation of pokeweed mitogen activated human B lymphocytes. In *Clinical evaluation of immune function in man.* New York: Grune and Stratton. pp. 133–149.

Litwin, S.D., Christian, C.L., and Siskind, G.W. (1977). *Clinical evaluation of immune function in man.* New York: Grune and Stratton.

Lundy, J., Wanebo, H.J., Pinsky, C.M., *et al.* (1974). Delayed hypersensitivity reactions in patients with squamous cell cancer of the head and neck. *Am. J. Surg.*, **128**, 530.

McCredie, J.A., Inch, W.R., and Sutherland, R.M. (1973). Peripheral blood lymphocytes and breast cancer. *Arch. Surg.*, **107**, 162–165.

Maisel, R.H., and Ogura, J.H. (1976). Dinitrochlorobenzene skin sensitization and peripheral lymphocyte count: predictors of survival in head and neck cancer. *Ann. Otol., Rhinol. Laryngol.*, **85**, 517–623.

Menzio, P., Cortesina, G., Sartoris, A., Morra, B., Bussi, M., and Tabaro, G. (1980). Relationships between cervical node histological patterns and rosette test scores: possible prognostic value in laryngeal cancer. *Laryngoscope*, **90**, 1032–1038.

Moretta, L., Webb, S.R., Grassi, G.E., Lidyard, P.M., *et al.* (1977). The functional analysis of two human T-cell subpopulations: help and suppression of B-cell responses by cells bearing receptors for IgM or IgG. *J. Exp. Med.*, **146**, 184–200.

Nacopoulou, L., Azaris, M., Papacharalampous, N., and Davaris, P. (1981). Prognostic significance of histologic host response in cancer of the large bowel. *Cancer*, **47**, 930–936.

Nalick, N.H., *et al.* (1974). Immunocompetence and prognosis in patients with gynecological cancer. *Gynecol. Oncol.*, **2**, 81–92.

Nathan, C., Murray, H.W., and Cohn, Z.A. (1980). The macrophage as an effector cell. *New Engl. J. Med.*, **303**, 622–626.

Nathanson, L. (1977). Immunology and immunotherapy of human breast cancer: a review. *Cancer Immunol. Immunother.*, **2**, 209–224.

Nelson, D.S. (1976). *Immunobiology of the macrophage.* New York: Academic Press.

Neville, A.M., Patel, S., Capp, M., Laurence, D.J., Cooper, E.H., Tuberville, C., and Coombes, R.C. (1978). The monitoring role of plasma CEA alone and in association with other tumor markers in colorectal and mammary carcinoma. *Cancer*, **42**,1448–1151.

Nind, A.P.P., Nairn, R.C., Pihl, E., Hughes, E.S.R., Cuthbertson, A.M. and Rollo, A.J. (1980). Autochthonous humoral and cellular immunoreactivity to colorectal carcinoma: prognostic significance in 400 patients. *Cancer Immunol. Immunother.*, **7**, 257–261.

Old, L.J. (1981). Cancer immunology: the search for specificity. *Cancer Res.*, **41**, 361–375.

Olsson, C.A., Rao, C.N., Menzoian, J.O., *et al.* (1972). Immunologic unreactivity in bladder cancer patients. *J. Urol.*, **107**, 607–609.

Osoba, D., Kersey, P.A., Clark, R.M., and Rosen, I.B. (1980). Prognostic value of skin testing with dinitrochlorobenzene in patients with head and neck cancer. *Can. J. Surg.*, **23**, 43–44.

Papatestas, A.E., and Kark, A.E. (1974). Peripheral lymphocyte counts in breast carcinoma. An index of immune competence. *Cancer*, **34**, 2014–2017.

Papatestas, A.E., Lesmick, G.J., Jenkins, G., *et al.* (1976). The prognostic significance of peripheral lymphocyte counts in patients with breast cancer. *Cancer*, **37**, 164–168.

Patt, D.J., Brynes, R.K., Vardiman, J.W., and Coppleson, L.W. (1975). Mesocolic lymph node histology as an important prognostic indicator for patients with carcinoma of the sigmoid colon: an immunomorphologic study. *Cancer*, **35**, 1388–1397.

Pihl, E., Malahy, M.A., Khankhanian, N., Hersh, E.M., and Mavligit, G.M. (1977). Immunomorphological features of prognostic significance in Dukes' class B colorectal carcinoma. *Cancer Res.*, **37**, 4145–4149.

Pinsky, C.M. (1978). Skin tests. In *Immunodiagnosis of cancer* (eds R.B. Heberman, and K.R. McIntire). New York: Marcel Dekker.

Pinsky, C.M., El Domiere, A., Caron, A.S. *et al.* (1974). Delayed hypersensitivity reactions in patients with cancer. In *Recent results in cancer research* (eds G. Mathe, and R. Weiner). New York: Springer Verlag.

Pinsky, C.M., Wanebo, H.J. Mike, V., *et al.* (1976). Delayed cutaneous hypersensitivity reactions and prognosis in patients with cancer. *Ann. N. Y. Acad. Sci.*, **276**, 407–410.

Pitt, J. (1977). Biology of the monocyte and macrophage: a review. In *Malnutrition and the immune response* (ed. R.M. Suskind). New York: Raven Press.

Pritchard, D.J., Ivins, J.C., and Ritts, R.E., Jr (1976). Immunologic aspects of human sarcoma. *Recent Results Cancer Res.*, **54**, 185–196.

Pritchard, D.J., Ritts, R.E., Jr, Taylor, W.F., *et al.* (1978). Prospective study of immune responsiveness in human melanoma. I. Assessment of initial pretreatment status with stage of disease. *Cancer*, **41**, 2165–2173.

Ramey, W.G., Fitzpatrick, H.F., Hashim, G.A., *et al.* (1980). Diagnosis, stage, and prognosis of lung carcinoma by preoperative assay of lung tumor antigen-sensitive T lymphocytes. *J. Thorac. Cardiovasc. Surg.*, **80**, 656–660.

Rao, B., Wanebo, H.J., Pinsky, C.M., Stearns, M., and Oettgen, H.F. (1977). Delayed hypersensitivity reactions in colorectal cancer. *Surg. Gynecol. Obstet.*, **144**, 677–681.

Renaud, M. (1926). La cuti réaction à la tuberculine chez les chandereux. *Bull. Soc. Med.* (Paris), **50**, 1441–1442.

Riesco, A. (1970). Five year cure: relation to total amount of peripheral lymphocyte and neutrophils. *Cancer*, **25**, 135.

Roberts, M.M., Bathgate, E.M., and Stevenson, A. (1975). Serum immunoglobulin levels in breast cancer. *Cancer*, **36**, 211.

Rossen, R.D., Reisberg, M.A., Hersh, E.M., and Gutterman, J.V. (1977). The C1q binding test for soluble immune complexes: clinical correlations obtained in patients with cancer. *J. Natl Cancer Inst.*, **58**, 1205–1215.

Roth, J.A., Eilber, F.R., and Morton, D.L. (1978). Effect of adriamycin and high-dose methotrexate chemotherapy on *in vivo* and *in vitro* cell-mediated immunity in cancer patients. *Cancer*, **41**, 814–819.

Roth, J.A., Eilber, E.R., Nizze, J.A., *et al.* (1975). Lack of correlation between skin reactivity to dinitrochlorobenzene and croton oil in patients with cancer. *New Engl. J. Med.*, **293**, 388–389.

Samayoa, E.A., McDuffie, F.C., Nelson, A.M., *et al.* (1977). Immunoglobulin complexes in sera of patients with malignancy. *Int. J. Cancer*, **19**, 12–17.

Schellhammer, P.F., Bracken, R.B., Bean, M.A., *et al.* (1976). Immune evaluation of patients with genitourinary cancer with skin testing. *Cancer*, **38**, 149–156.

Snyderman, R., and Pike, M.C. (1976). Defective macrophage function produced by neoplasms: identification of an inhibitor of macrophage chemotaxis. In *The macrophage in neoplasia* (ed. M.A. Fink). New York: Academic Press.

Snyderman, R., Meadows, L., and Holder, W. (1978). Abnormal monocyte chemotaxis in patients with breast cancer: evidence for a tumor-mediated effect. *J. Natl. Cancer Inst.*, **60**, 737–740.

Solowey, A.C., and Rappaport, F.T. (1965). Immunologic responses in cancer patients. *Surg. Gynecol. Obstet.*, **121**, 756–760.

Springer, G., Murthy, S., DeSai, P., and Scanlon, E. (1980). Breast cancer patient's cell mediated immune response to Thomsen-Friedenreich (T) antigen. *Cancer*, **45**, 2949–2954.

Staab, H.J., Anderer, F.A., Stumpf, E., and Fischer, R. (1980). Are circulating CEA immune complexes a prognostic marker in patients with carcinoma of the gastrointestinal tract? *Br. J. Cancer*, **42**, 26–33.

Stefani, S., Kerman, R., and Abbate, J. (1976). Immune evaluation of lung cancer patients undergoing radiation therapy. *Cancer*, **37**, 2792.

Stein, J.A., Adler, A., Efraim, S.B., *et al.* (1976). Immunocompetence, immuno-suppression and human breast cancer. I. An analysis of their relationship by known parameters of cell-mediated immunity in well-defined clinical stages of disease. *Cancer*, **38**, 1171–1187.

Stjernsward, J., *et al.* (1972). Lymphopenia and change in distribution of human B and T lymphocytes in peripheral blood induced by irradiation for mammary carcinoma. *Lancet*, **i**, 1352–1356.

Takita, H., and Brugarolas, A. (1973). Skin test in bronchogenic carcinoma. I. Correlation of the immunological status and the extent of the disease. *J. Surg. Oncol.*, **5**, 315.

Teshima, H., Wanebo, H., Pinsky, C., *et al.* (1977). Circulating immune complexes detected by [125] I-C1q deviation test in sera of cancer patients. *J. Clin. Invest.*, **59**, 1134–1142.

Theofilopoulos, A.N., Wilson, C.B., and Dixon, F.J. (1976). The Raji cell radio-immune assay for detecting immune complexes in human sera. *J. Clin. Invest.*, **57**, 169–182.

Twomey, P.L., Catalona, W.J., and Chretien, P.B. (1974). Cellular immunity in cured cancer patients. *Cancer*, **33**, 435–440.

Unger, S.W. Bernhard, M.I., Pace, R.C., and Wanebo, H.J. (1979). Alterations of monocyte function in neoplastic diseases. *Surg. Forum*, **30**, 142–144.

van Nagell, J.R., Jr, Donaldson, E.S., Gay, E.C., Rayburn, P., Powell, D.F., and Goldenberg, D.M. (1978). Carcinoembryonic antigen in carcinoma of the uterine cervix. I. The prognostic value of serial plasma determinations. *Cancer*, **42**, 2428–2434.

van Nagell, J.R., Jr, Donaldson, E.S., Wood, E.G., Sharkey, R.M., and Goldenberg, D.M. (1977). The prognostic significance of carcinoembryonic antigen in the plasma and tumors of patients with endometrial adenocarcinoma. *Am. J. Obstet. Gynecol.*, **128**, 308–313.

Veltri, R.W., Sprinkle, P.M., Maxim, P.E., Theofilopoulos, A.N., Rodman, S.M., and Kinney, C.L. (1978). Immune monitoring protocol for patients with carcinoma of the head and neck. *Ann. Otol.*, **87**, 692–700.

Vincent, R.G., Chu, T.M., and Lane, W.W. (1979). The value of carcinoembryonic antigen in patients with carcinoma of the lung. *Cancer*, **44**, 685.

Vose, B.M., Vanky, F., Fopp, M., and Klein, E. (1978). Restricted autologous lymphocytotoxicity in lung neoplasia. *Br. J. Cancer*, **38**, 375.

Waldorf, D.S., Willkens, R.F., and Decker, J.L. (1968). Impaired delayed hyper-sensitivity in an aging population. *J. Am. Med. Assoc.*, **203**, 111–114.

Walker, C., Gray, B.N., and Barnard, R. (1981). Serum glycoproteins in diagnosis and monitoring of patients with large-bowel cancer. *Dis. Colon Rectum*, **24**, 171–175.

Wanebo, H.J. (1979a). Immunobiology of head and neck cancer; basic concepts. *Head Neck Surg.* Sept/Oct, 42–55.

Wanebo, H.J. (1979b). Immunologic testing as a guide to cancer management. *Surg. Clin. N. Am.*, **59**, 323–347.

Wanebo, H.J. (1981). Are carcinoembryonic antigen levels of value in the curative managment of colorectal cancer? *Surgery*, **89**, 290–295.

Wanebo, H.J., Jun, M.Y., Strong, E., *et al.* (1975). T-cell deficiency in patients with squamous cell cancer of the head and neck. *Am. J. Surg.*, **130**, 445.

Wanebo, H.J., and Pinsky, C. (1978). A review of immunologic reactivity in patients with colorectal cancer. In *Carcinoma of the colon and rectum* (ed. W. E. Enker). Chicago: Year Book Medical Publishers.

Wanebo, H.J., Pinsky, C.M., Beattie, E.J., *et al.* (1978a). Immunocompetence testing in patients with one of the four common operable cancers. A review. *Clin. Bull.*, **8**, 15–22.

Wanebo, H.J., Rao, B., Attiyeh, F., Pinsky, C., Middleman, P., and Stearns, M. (1980). Immune reactivity in patients with colorectal cancer: assessment of biologic risk by immunoparameters. *Cancer*, **45**, 1254–1263.

Wanebo, H.J., Rao, B., Bhaskar, R., *et al.* (1978b). Carcinoembyronic antigen: prognostic and therapeutic guidelines in the management of colorectal cancer. *New Engl. J. Med.*, **299**, 448–451.

Wanebo, H.J., Rao, B., Miyazawa, N., *et al.* (1976a). Immune reactivity in primary carcinoma of the lung and its relation to prognosis. *J. Thorac. Cardiovasc. Surg.*, **72**, 339–347.

Wanebo, H.J., Rao, B., Pinsky, B., *et al.* (1976b). Delayed hypersensitivity reactions in patients with colorectal cancer. In *Neoplasm immunity, mechanisms* (ed. R. G. Crispen). Chicago: Institute for Tuberculosis Research. pp. 157–166.

Wanebo, H.J., Rosen, P.P., Thaler, T., *et al.* (1976c). Immunobiology of operable breast cancer: an assessment of biologic risk by immunoparameters. *Ann. Surg.*, **184**, 258.

Wanebo, H.J., Thaler, H.T., Hansen, J.A., *et al.* (1978c). Immunologic reactivity in patients with primary operable breast cancer. *Cancer*, **41**, 84–94.

Wara, W.M., Wara, D.W., Phillips, T.L., *et al.* (1975). Elevated IgA in carcinoma of the nasopharynx. *Cancer*, **35**, 1313.

Weese, J., West, W., Herberman, R., *et al.* (1977). Depression of 'high affinity' T-cell rosettes indicative of recurrent carcinoma. *Surg. Forum*, **28**, 155–157.

Wells, S.A., Jr, Burdick, J.F., Joseph, W.L., *et al.* (1973). Delayed cutaneous hypersensitivity reactions to tumor cell antigens and to nonspecific antigens. Prognostic significance in patients with lung cancer. *J. Thorac. Cardiovasc. Surg.*, **66**, 557–562.

West, W.H., Sienknecht, C.W., Townes, A.S., *et al.* (1976). Modification of the rosette assay between lymphocytes and sheep erythrocytes to study patients with cancer, systemic lupus erythematosus and other diseases. *J. Clin. Immunol. Immunopathol.*, **5**, 60–66.

Wybran, J., and Fudenberg, H.H. (1973). Thymus derived rosette forming cells in various disease states: cancer, lymphoma, bacterial and viral infections and other diseases. *J. Clin. Invest.*, **52**, 1026.

Wybran, J., and Fudenberg, H.H. (1976). T-cell rosettes in human cancer. In *Clinical tumor immunology* (ed. J. Wybran, and M. Staquet). New York: Pergamon Press.

Young, A.K., Hammond, E., and Middleton, A.W., Jr (1979). The prognostic value of cell surface antigens in low grade, non-invasive, transitional cell carcinoma of the bladder. *J. Urol.*, **122**, 462–464.

Chapter

11 BERTIL BJÖRKLUND

Tumor Products Reflecting Growth Activity

INTRODUCTION

The search continues for a general marker for cancer which will identify individuals with cancer at an early stage. This goal has not been attained so far and emphasis has shifted toward tests which can identify and measure growth products which reflect tumor growth activity. During recent years an increasing number of such tests have been described (Björklund, 1973; Schönfeld, 1978; Lehmann, 1979; Herberman and McIntire, 1979; von Kleist and Breuer, 1981). Only a few have been carefully evaluated and become generally available, but more tests are being studied for potential usefulness or for expansion of their applicability (Table 1). Panels of two or more different tests have also been devised which seem to offer discriminatory advantages over a single test (Schlegel et al., 1981; Lüthgens and Schlegel, 1981).

Tumor growth products are defined here as chemicals which are produced and released at supranormal concentrations by cells involved in the formation of tumors. Under normal conditions, such products are produced scarcely or not at all by adult, differentiated human cells. They may be produced by fetal tissue cells (Gold and Freedman, 1965), by trophoblasts of the placenta (Björklund et al., 1981) or by the endoderm of the yolk sac (Nørgaard-Pedersen and Gaede, 1975).

Since proliferation is an essential element of malignant progression, methods of measuring proliferation products should be of considerable value

Table 1. Categories of tumor growth products, applications, and references.

Tumor growth product	Application	References
Tumor-associated antigens		
Carcinoembryonic antigen (CEA)	General (colorectal, breast, lung)	Gold and Freedman (1965), Hansen *et al.* (1974), Zamcheck (1981), Martin *et al.* (1977), Lokish *et al.* (1978), Vincent and Chu (1973)
Tissue polypeptide antigen (TPA)	General (colorectal, breast, urinary bladder)	Björklund and Björklund (1957), Björklund (1981), Schlegel *et al.* (1981), Lüthgens and Schlegel (1981)
Alpha-fetoprotein (AFP)	Endodermal sinus tumor of the testis and ovary, liver cancer	Abelev (1968), Nørgaard-Pedersen *et al.* (1975), Talerman (1981)
Pancreatic oncofetal antigen (POA)	Pancreas cancer	Gelder *et al.* (1978)
Tennessee antigen (TAG)	General	Potter *et al.* (1980)
Human casein	Breast cancer	Zangerle *et al.* (1978)
Gastric fetal sulfoglycoprotein antigen (FSA)	Gastric cancer	Häkkinen (1966, 1978)
Ferritin	Hodgkin's disease, AML, myeloproliferative diseases, hepatoma, germ cell tumors, breast and lung cancer	Lamerz (1981)
Lung tumor-associated antigen (LTAA)	Lung cancer	Braatz *et al.* (1979), McIntire *et al.* (1979)
Serum β_2-microglobulin (β_2-m)	Leukemia, lymphoma, myelomatosis	Cooper and Plesner (1980)
Pregnancy-specific β_1-glycoprotein (SP$_1$) (also TBG, PAPP-C, PSβG)	Choriocarcinoma	Horne *et al.* (1976)
Non-specific cross-reacting antigen (NCA)	CML and AML	von Kleist *et al.* (1972)
Hormones		
Human chorionic gonadotropin (HCG; β-HCG)	Trophoblastic neoplasms, embryonal cell carcinoma of the testis	Vaitukaitis *et al.* (1972), Vaitukaitis (1979)
Calcitonin	Medullary thyroid cancer (C cells)	Silva *et al.* (1974), Calmettes *et al.* (1978)

Tumor growth product	Application	References
Ectopic ACTH	Bronchial cancer (oat cell, carcinoid), ectopic syndrome	Gewirtz and Yalow (1974), Podmore *et al.* (1979)
Insulin	Insulinoma	
Enzymes		
Acid phosphatase	Prostatic cancer, metastases	Schwartz (1975)
Serum prostatic acid phosphatase (PAP)	Prostatic cancer	Foti *et al.* (1977), Chu *et al.* (1975), Chu (1978)
Placental alkaline phosphatase (Regan isoenzyme)	Adenocarcinoma of the ovaries, testis tumors, pancreatic cancer	Fishman *et al.* (1968a, b, 1976), Stolbach *et al.* (1972)
Lactic dehydrogenase (LDH)	Hemoblastic disease, lymphomas	Prochazka *et al.* (1968), Pfleiderer and Wachsmuth (1961)
γ-Glutamyltranspeptidase (GGTP)	Pancreatic cancer	
Galactosyl-, sialyl-, glycosyl- and fucosyltransferases	Various malignancies	
Immune complexes		
Circulating immune complexes (CIC)	Various malignancies	Gauci *et al.* (1981), Day *et al.* (1981)
Neurogenic amines and serotonin metabolitis		
Catecholamines Vanilmandelic acid Metanephrine	Neuroblastoma	Schwartz (1975)
Cystathionine Dopamine Dopamine β-hydroxylase Homovanillic acid Metanephrine	Pheochromocytoma	
5-Hydroxyindole acetic acid	Carcinoid	

to the oncologist. For convenience, tumor growth products are divided into five categories:

Tumor-associated antigens.
Hormones.
Enzymes.
Immune complexes.
Neurogenic amines.

TUMOR-ASSOCIATED ANTIGENS

Conceputal basis

The conceptual basis for interpreting the presence of tumor-associated antigens in clinical specimens has long been discussed (Vygodchikov, 1959; Day, 1965; Takeda, 1969; Fishman and Sell, 1976, Manes, 1979). How specific are tumor antigens and how specific can they be? The answers to these questions depend on the validity of the dogmas of 'variable gene expression' and 'constancy of the genome'. If the dogma is true, it would be expected that proliferation of cells either into tumors *or* into normal structures should lead to synthesis of identical proteins.

The total concentration of antigen would be the sum of the normal and tumor growth products. An increase above the normal level should indicate increased proliferation, which (if no other explanation is to hand) should point to cancer growth activity. Clinical studies of carcinoembryonic antigen (CEA) (Reynoso and Keane, 1979) and tissue polypeptide antigen (TPA) (Björklund, 1981) support this line of reasoning. There is a highly significant correlation between elevated concentrations of CEA and/or TPA and proliferative activity.

If 'oncogenes' exist (i.e. genetic information encoded in the normal genome and expressed by all malignant cells of whatever phenotype), they should not be silent during development. Such genes are not proven, but the existence of oncodevelopmental gene products has been firmly established.

Studies of molecular hybridization and nuclear transplantation have given support to the dogma that all differentiated cells of an organism contain equivalent genetic information (Kohne and Byers, 1973), but it should be borne in mind that differences below the level of 5% cannot be detected (Manes, 1979). If the total mammalian genome contains $3–5 \times 10^9$ base pairs, it is evident that even 1–2% of this DNA could carry with it special genetic information. Therefore, the dogma may not represent the whole truth.

Manes (1979) considers that, on the basis of molecular hybridization experiments, the absolute constancy of the genome throughout development must still remain an open issue. As for nuclear transplantation studies, the lower success rate with nuclei obtained later during development suggests that DNA is being modified with advancing development. Therefore, even if the total genetic information is constant, it should not be called 'equivalent'.

There is also evidence from work with prokaryotes and plants that regulatory DNA sequences, termed 'insertion elements', are excised from the chromosomal DNA and reintegrated at other sites, thereby altering gene expression (Manes, 1979). It is also known that extreme selective pressure against dividing mammalian cells can amplify certain genetic sequences of survival value (Alt *et al.*, 1978).

Should there exist genes which promote tumor growth and which are never expressed during normal development, they could give rise to gene products like antigenic proteins. Such products would then be truly cancer-specific and not found in any other condition, but nonetheless still arise from the host genome. So far, no antigenic product has been found which would fit into this category.

From the above it seems that if the key to malignancy does not lie in phenotype alterations, we have to look at malignant functions of the *regulatory systems* and at *proliferation* as such. An example of the role of proliferation for antigenic expression on leukemic cells was described by Newman (1981), who found that four antigens pseudospecific for leukemia were representative of normal differentiation of proliferation-linked antigens. Their presence on normal lymphoprogenitors supported the hypothesis that leukemic cells continue to express normal gene products that have a transient expression on normal cells.

From the field of bacteriology it is well known that few characteristics of microorganisms are so markedly affected by the microenvironment as is chemical composition, including antigens. Lacey (1961) listed 137 published instances of 'non-generic variation' of surface antigens with environment. A theoretical attempt to align these findings with those from tumor antigenicity studies has been made by Björklund (1963). It is possible that the antigenic variation of proliferating cells is the result of an interplay between the cell and a changing surrounding fluid. The cell is dependent on the composition of the fluid and reacts accordingly.

Carcinoembryonic antigen (CEA)

This cancer-associated antigen described by Gold and Freedman (1965) was first thought to be specific for colon cancer and fetal gut, but is now known to represent a wide variety of cancers (Menendez-Botet *et al.*, 1978; Reynoso and Keane, 1979). It may be considered a general marker but has special reference to tumors of the colon–rectum, breast, pancreas, and lung.

CEA is a 7–8 S glycoprotein of around 180 000 daltons which is stable to heating. It is soluble in perchloric acid (PCA) and is hence left in the supernatant when plasma proteins are precipitated by PCA. The carbohydrate part of CEA is of the order of 40–60%. Blood group A antigen binds anti-CEA antibodies. Lectins like Concanavalin A (Con A), wheat germ agglutinin (WGA), and phytohemagglutinin (PHA) bind CEA.

For some years it was thought that the immunologic specificity resided in the polysaccharide moiety, but it has been shown (Hammarström *et al.*, 1975; Coligan *et al.*, 1975; Coligan and Todd, 1975) that most of the carbohydrate can be removed from CEA yet retain its activity. Therefore, it seems that the antigenicity is carried by determinant groups of the protein part of CEA. The amino acid sequence of the 30 N-terminal amino acids reported by Shively *et al.* (1979) is in agreement with the one reported by Terry *et al.* (1974) for positions 1 through 24. Sequencing more than 24 amino acids has encountered technical problems, probably due to the high degree of glycosylation.

CEA preparations from different tumors contain similar if not identical sequences, and the tumor-associated site(s) may comprise a relatively small portion of the CEA molecule (Krantz *et al.*, 1979). Other portions seem to be responsible for cross-reactions with 12 different antigens which were found by the use of antisera to CEA. Of special interest is the non-specific cross-reacting antigen (NCA) (von Kleist *et al.*, 1972; Mach and Puztaszeri, 1972), because NCA also bears a specific determinant not present in CEA which has found use in studies of the differentiation of myeloid cells in myeloid leukemia (see later).

Because of the numerous cross-reacting antigens with one or more determinants in common with CEA, the full usefulness of CEA may be obscured. The heterogeneity which characterizes CEA and the different assay procedures have also contributed to variation of results. Improved diagnostic assays may be obtained by the introduction of monospecificity, either by exhaustive absorption with normal tissue antigens, or by finding the pertinent antigenic site of CEA and producing corresponding monoclonal antibodies, or by using synthetic antigen based on the pertinent amino acid sequence as immunogen.

Nevertheless, with standardized procedures and reagents, the CEA assay can be used to follow patients with certain types of cancer. In general, the higher the level of CEA the poorer the prognosis, and assay of the level may predict the effect of chemotherapy. A rising CEA level seems to be incompatible with disease regression; it may pre-date clinical signs of tumor progression or resistance to treatment and thus at an early stage may indicate the need for other therapy.

In colorectal cancer, serial CEA assays are important in assessing the status of patients during therapy and initial values may give a guide to the prognosis. If the level of CEA in serum continues to be high following surgery, it indicates failure of therapy, and if a low level of CEA is followed by increasing levels, recurrent disease should be suspected (Zamcheck, 1981). Martin *et al.* (1977) have used the CEA level to detect recurrent gastrointestinal tumor and as an indication for second-look procedures. Staab *et al.* (1978) and Wanebo *et al.* (1978) also advocate CEA as a guide to this procedure, but supporting evidence other than elevated CEA needs to be available (Minton *et al.*, 1978).

In breast cancer, decreasing serial CEA levels seem to correlate with response to treatment while rising values indicate lack of response and relapse (Lokish *et al.*, 1978; Tormey and Waalkes, 1978). In lung cancer, the CEA assay is capable of indicating the result of thoracotomy and also the response to radiotherapy and chemotherapy (Vincent and Chu, 1973). There is probably a pre-operative level of CEA above which operations is likely to be ineffectual.

Normal, healthy blood donors show low levels of CEA in more than 90% of cases, and patients with a variety of benign diseases exhibit moderately elevated values in 20–30% of cases. Such elevations, which are often temporary, are seen in inflammatory conditions such as gastritis, hepatitis, pancreatitis, colitis, obstructive liver disorders, and cirrhosis.

In animal experiments the liver was shown to be responsible for the removal of CEA from the plasma (Shuster *et al.*, 1973). The highest CEA levels clinically encountered occur in patients with metastatic disease of the liver and may be due to failure of the liver to metabolize or excrete CEA. Therefore, careful monitoring of liver function is important for a correct interpretation of observed CEA values.

The methodology of determining the concentration of CEA in clinical specimens is based on immunological techniques. Most used are radioimmunoassays with separation of free and bound radioligand by second antibody or zirconyl gel. More recently, a radiometric method has been introduced employing solid phase anti-CEA and ^{125}I-labelled anti-CEA antibodies. There is also an enzyme-linked immunoassay.

Normal values for CEA in plasma or serum may vary from one laboratory to another and so does reproducibility. Strict control and serial testing are advocated, and so is the saving of frozen (-70°C) aliquots of serum from previous bleedings which can be used to determine if observed changes reflect altered proliferative activity or are due to methodological variation.

CEA is expressed as ng/ml or mg/l and, depending upon technique and laboratory standards, the cut-off point is usually set at 2.5 ng/ml (Roche original method with perchloric acid extraction) or 3–5 mg/l (Abbott solid-phase technique). Regular assay of control sera from the local population ensures clinical usefulness of the test. Most laboratories describe their results in terms of specificity (% true negatives) and sensitivity (% true positives). By using the sensitivity of a test at a predetermined specificty, results are obtained which can be compared with results from other areas which have the same criteria for specificity.

The cut-off point recommended is the one which results in 95% specificity (i.e. 95% of healthy or non-cancerous subjects are set to be negative by the test). Oehr *et al.* (1981b,c) has drawn attention to a practical way of plotting and reading sensitivity at any chosen percentage of specificity. In this way valid comparisons of data by various investigators can be made.

Tissue polypeptide antigen (TPA)

TPA, being the oldest human tumor antigen, represents an isolated protein member of the common human tumor antigenic principle (Björklund and Björklund, 1957, 1981; Björklund *et al.*, 1958, 1961; Lang, 1963). TPA is a non-species-specific proliferation antigen which has been found in various species down to fishes, indicating its existence for approximately 400 million years (Björklund *et al.*, 1976).

TPA is an unbranched, elongated single chain protein with a molecular weight of 43 000 daltons (subunit $TPA:B_1$) (Lüning *et al.*, 1980). It contains no measurable sugar, lipid or other prosthetic group. The major part of the amino acid sequence is known and the antigenic, repeated determinant group is known by its unique amino acid sequence; it has been synthesized and found to exhibit specific activity of TPA *in vitro* (Lüning *et al.*, 1979; Redelius *et al.*, 1980). No other antigenic determinants have been demonstrated in TPA. The sedimentation constant is 4.5 S and the IP is 4.5.

The amino acid sequence of TPA derived from a pool of many carcinomatous tumors was found to be indistinguishable from that of TPA derived from one single bronchial cancer and also from that of TPA from a pool of human placentae (Redelius *et al.*, 1980). In the latter, TPA occurs exclusively in the trophoblast layer and in the syncytiotrophoblats.

Anti-TPA antibodies can be made in rabbits and horses against pure TPA or TPA-containing cancer cells from tumors or cancer cell lines cultivated *in vitro*. These antibodies can be absorbed by pure, solid-phase TPA and isolated by elution.

Absorption by pure TPA but not by other antigens removes anti-TPA antibodies as tested by hemagglutination inhibition, radioimmunoassay, immunohistochemistry, gel diffusion, and immunoelectrophoresis. All these activities are restored with affinity purified anti-TPA antibody which comprises less than 0.1% of the protein in antiserum to TPA. The antibodies, which are of IgG nature, show complete cross-reactivity between species and give reactions of identity with TPA of various origins. Thus, the specificity of TPA is established by amino acid sequence and immunochemical analysis of antigenic activity (Björklund and Björklund, 1981).

Clinical studies have been performed by the hemagglutination inhibition technique using TPA-labelled tannic acid-treated sheep red blood cells (Björklund, 1978). Later, a double antibody radioimmunoassay was developed which is now the method of choice for determining TPA in serum and other body fluids (Björklund *et al.*, 1980).

In the first clinical study of TPA (Björklund *et al.*, 1973), 1483 individuals with cancer and other conditions were analysed by blind and double-blind techniques. A significant correlation was found between elevated TPA levels in the serum and the presence of cancer, with higher values in metastatic disease than in primary cancer. Similar results were obtained by others in cancers at various sites (Menedez-Botet *et al.*, 1978; Hagbard and Sorbe, 1978; Nemoto *et al.*, 1979; Holyoke and Chu, 1979).

Skryten *et al.* (1981) studied 2028 serum specimens from 1060 patients with various types of malignancy. They found significant differences in TPA levels between patients with progressive disease as compared to those with stable disease or no evidence of disease. Nine major cancer sites were involved— breast, corpus uteri, cervix uteri, ovary, kidney, testis, prostate, urinary bladder, and head and neck (see Figure 1).

A raised TPA level in the urine may be associated with the presence of urothelial cancer (Isacson and Andrén-Sandberg, 1978; Kumar *et al.*, 1981).

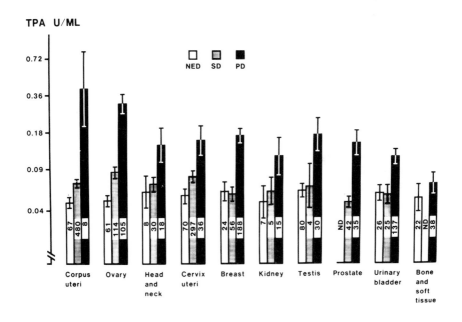

Figure 1 Geometrical mean values and standard errors for TPA in 2028 serum specimens from 1060 patients with cancerous disease. NED = no evidence of disease; SD = stable disease; PD = progressive disease; ND = not done. (Skryten *et al.*, 1981.)

In the study by Kumar *et al.*, 18 of 19 patients with bladder cancer showed a mean TPA of 524 ± 392 U/l and 15 cases with tumor absent showed a mean TPA of 34 ± 27 U/l. The assay, to be of practical value, has to be carried out on 24 h urine samples.

Elevations of TPA have been recorded in patients hospitalized for a variety of infectious or inflammatory conditions. In influenza, urinary infections, and upper respiratory infections, Lundström *et al.* (1973) found elevated levels in about 20% of 613 hospitalized patients. In hepatitis, frequent TPA elevations were seen by Sylvan (1977). In certain autoimmune diseases with a proliferative element (LED, chronic acute hepatitis, rheumatoid arthritis), moderate TPA elevations have also been observed (Ruibal *et al.*, 1982). In 422 patients of whom 253 had operations for malignant disease and the remainder for benign disease, it was found that the TPA level was not influenced by surgical trauma (Andrén-Sandberg and Isacson, 1975).

The level of TPA in serum in patients with an established diagnosis of cancer seems to have a prognostic significance. Eklund (1977) studied a total of 352 cancer cases for a mean follow-up period of 27 months (among them, 190 died from their disease). All patients were grouped from A to D according to increasing level of TPA values. Each group included patients with various types, stages, and sites of cancer and different types of therapy. It was found that 70% of group D died within 5 months and that, while high values of TPA in cancer predicted a high rate of mortality, low values of TPA predicted a low mortality rate. The correlation between mortality and TPA was statistically highly significant ($p = 0.001$).

For comparison, Eklund studied 470 non-cancerous subjects (mainly with infectious disease). In class A with negative TPA values, the mortality rate was 5% within 12 months while for classes B, C, and D with positive TPA values, mortality was about 25% in 12 months. This study demonstrated that TPA values represented an indicator of mortality in malignant disease and in some non-malignant diseases as well.

Cytochemical interpretation of biopsies should benefit from immunocytochemical staining for TPA (Björklund and Björklund, 1979).

Correlation between CEA and TPA

In comparative studies of TPA and CEA assays, the correlation coefficient (r) between the two tests has been of the order of 0.6–0.7. This indicates that additional discriminatory information should be possible by the combined use of TPA and CEA. Simultaneous testing of TPA and CEA has been carried out (Menendez-Botet *et al.*, 1978; Nemoto *et al.*, 1979; Holyoke and Chu, 1979; Lüthgens and von Jürgensonn, 1979; Lüthgens and Schlegel, 1980; Oehr *et al.*, 1980, 1981a, c; Lüthgens *et al.*, 1981).

Schlegel *et al.* (1981) published a study of 274 cases, mainly of breast cancer, ranging from those with no evidence of recurrence (NED) to progressive disease (PD). The discriminatory value of TPA and CEA was compared to 18 common laboratory tests comparing NED and PD. These tests were: blood levels of IgE, creatinine, LDH, CHE (cholinesterase), AP (alkaline phosphatase), γ-GT, Cu, Fe, total protein and albumin, α_2-globulin, γ-globulin, hematocrit, Hb, levels of erythrocytes, leukocytes, thrombocytes, and sedimentation rate (SR). Regression analysis showed that individuals with a product of TPA × CEA below a certain value (450) had a probability of 5.6% of belonging to the group PD and a probability of 94% of belonging to the group NED. For product values above 1200, the probability of belonging to the group PD was 96%. The total number of variables from the 18 common laboratory tests contributed less than the product of TPA and CEA, and even TPA or CEA alone was better than the sum of all other variables.

These results with CEA and TPA were obtained by introducing a 'grey zone' between the two populations NED and PD, corresponding to an overlap of about 12%. In this area no predictions can be made. This is a more reasonable technique than using a single cut-off line. Figure 2 shows the actual values for the 176 cases of mammary cancer. The authors concluded that neither TPA nor CEA separately provided sufficient discrimination, but that a 95% discrimination was obtained by combining TPA and CEA.

In a report on CEA and TPA assays in 307 cases of breast cancer (Lüthgens and Schlegel, 1981), the previous results were borne out. Negative TPA and CEA findings were seen in 1.2% of 83 PD group cases, and positive TPA and/or CEA in 98.8%. In 159 NED cases, TPA was negative in 91.2% and CEA in 91.8%. Both TPA and CEA were negative in 86.2% of the NED cases.

It is often difficult to compare results from different studies. Some of the difficulties can be overcome by using inverse distribution function values (Oehr *et al.*, 1981c) or by specificity–sensitivity diagrams (Oehr *et al.*, 1981b). The advantage of such techniques is that sensitivities can be compared at the same level of specificity.

In order to elucidate the role of TPA and CEA in tissue cells, immunohistochemical methods have been worked out using both indirect techniques with peroxidase, and peroxidase–antiperoxidase (PAP) complexes. In recent work (Björklund *et al.*, 1982), staining for TPA and CEA in breast cancer showed an overall concordance of 58% and differences *within* as well as *between* tumors. It is therefore possible that TPA and CEA are synthesized during different phases of the proliferative cycle.

TPA seems to be the most general of the tumor markers. CEA adds significantly to sensitivity and specificity in a wide range of applications but there are variations from one type of malignancy to another (see Table 2). Figures estimated from diagrams by Oehr *et al.* (1981b) indicate that TPA +

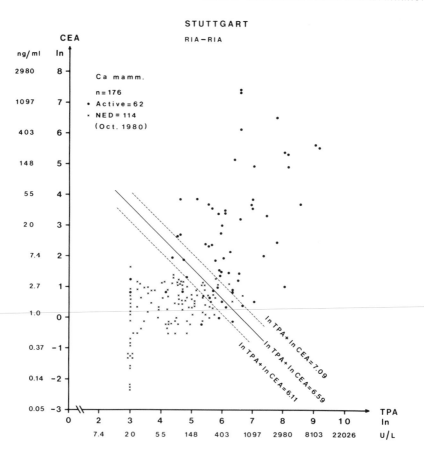

Figure 2 Simultaneous CEA and TPA assay in serum from 176 patients with breast cancer. Between ln TPA + ln CEA=6.11 and 7.09 there is a 'grey zone'. Above and below this zone, the discrimination for active cancer and NED is 95% (Schlegel *et al.*, 1981).

CEA is more useful in cancer of the lung and in colorectal cancer, but in non-seminomatous malignancy of the testis β-HCG and AFP are the methods of choice. In carcinoma of the bladder, assay of TPA in serum gives a satisfactory result with a sensitivity of 93% at 95% specificity.

Alpha-fetoprotein (AFP)

This antigen, discovered by Abelev *et al.* (1963), is an adequate marker in patients with germ cell tumours of the gonads or in extragonadal sites

Table 2. Comparison of sensitivity of tests at a false positive rate of 5% (specificity 95%) in various malignant conditions. Data derived from specificity–sensitivity diagrams by Oehr *et al.* (1981b)

Malignant condition	Sensitivity (%) at 95% specificity of					
	TPA	CEA	AFP	β-HCG	TPA	SP$_1$
Bladder carcinoma, $n=75$ ($P_{1S}=9$; $P_1=29$; $P_2=15$; $P_3=17$; $P_4=7$; TX=5)	93	27				
Lung cancer, $n=120$ ($S_I=9$; $S_{II}=9$; $S_{III}=64$; $S_{unknown}=38$)	47	62.5				
Non-seminomatous tumors of the testis, $n=59$ ($T_{1-4} N_0 M_0 = 4$; T_{1-4} N only bulky disease $M_0 = 19$; $T_{1-4} N_{1-4} M_1 = 26$; unknown=6)	47	9	70	75	42	1
Colorectal carcinoma, $n=54$ (Dukes' A=9; B=19; C=15; D=11)	57	49				

(Nørgaard-Pedersen *et al.*, 1975; Nørgard-Pedersen, 1981). It has reasonable specificity, the level is to a certain degree proportional to the viable tumor mass, and the assay is specific, sensitive, and simple. Simultaneously and independently Abelev (1968) and Masopust (1968) found raised levels of serum AFP in patients with teratocarcinoma of the ovary and testis.

It had previously been found by Abelev *et al.* (1963) that AFP was produced by hepatocellular hepatomas and this fetal protein has since been demonstrated in the serum of patients with primary liver cancer. The increased sensitivity of new assay techniques has increased the percentage of false positives in control populations and has led to a significant decrease of the specificity of the AFP assay in primary cancer of the liver.

AFP is relatively well characterized. It resembles albumin (about 50% homology) but differs in being a glycoprotein with 4–5% carbohydrate. AFP is composed of a single polypeptide chain with a molecular weight of about 70 000 daltons. The half-life is 5 days. The amino acid composition of AFP is similar in various species and resembles that of albumin (Ruoslahti, 1979). Structural data on AFP are fragmentary. Fragments of human AFP obtained by cleavage with cyanogen bromide have been subjected to amino acid sequence analysis. Different N-terminal sequences have indicated heterogeneity of the fragments, the significance of which is difficult to understand.

The assay of AFP in serum is carried out by immunodiffusion, hemagglutination, immunoradioautography (Nørgaard-Pedersen and Gaede, 1975), and radioimmunoassay (sensitivity about 5 µg/l). Immunohistochemical techniques are also available for examination of cell and tissue specimens.

Assay of AFP in serum is recommended in hepatoma and in embryonal malignant teratoblastoma of the testis and ovary, i.e. germ cell tumors with endodermal sinus and yolk sac elements. Studies of AFP in pregnancies with neural tube defects have been reported (Seppälä and Ruoslahti, 1972) and examination of natural serum AFP early in pregnancy is claimed to detect 80–90% of cases of open fetal neural tube defect at the 95th percentile of the normal range (Brock *et al.*, 1978).

Other antigenic tumor growth products

Pancreatic oncofetal antigen (POA)

POA, a glycoprotein of 800 000–900 000 daltons, has been found at elevated concentrations in the serum of about 50% of patients with pancreatic cancer (Gelder *et al.*, 1978). POA was also elevated in 13–36% of patients with some other types of cancer (biliary tract, lung, stomach, breast, and colon) and in fetal serum. Twelve percent of cases in pancreatitis and 30% in gastric ulcer had increased POA. Further studies are being carried out to evaluate POA by rocket immunoelectrophoresis.

Tennessee antigen (TAG)

TAG was found by Jordon and developed with Potter *et al.* (1980). It is described as a glycoprotein distinct from CEA and with properties of a general tumor marker. A special assay which included precipitation with perchloric acid and dialysis followed by titration and hemagglutination was introduced, but considered too difficult for the average laboratory. The assay needs more characterization of the antigen, additional clinical studies, and a more generally acceptable method.

Human casein

Human casein derived from breast milk can be determined in serum by radioimmunoassay. Significant elevations are seen in the first clinical stages of breast cancer and also later when metastases occur (Zangerle *et al.*, 1978). Further follow-up casein determinations are necessary before the value of the test can be assessed in breast cancer.

Gastric fetal sulfoglycoprotein Antigen (FSA)

FSA has been assayed in gastric juice from more than 40 000 persons with the aim of diagnosing early gastric cancer (Häkkinen, 1966). The test is by immunodiffusion in gel following a number of chemical separation steps in each case. Progress has since been made toward a radioimmunoassay. In a study of 28 642 individuals, 2246 were positive by FSA assay. Among these, over 1% had gastric cancer, 7–8% had advanced atrophic gastritis, and more than 20% presented a picture of gastritis.

Polyposis and peptic ulcer were also found among the FSA-positive cases (Häkkinen, 1978), and the method thus seems to be capable of picking up not only early gastric cancer but also a variety of other gastric conditions. It would however mean that about 8% of an FSA-screened population, 40–70 years of age, would be subjected to gastroscopy and other measures.

Ferritin

Ferritin is an iron storage protein which is present especially in the liver, spleen, and bone marrow. Ferritin is well characterized as a spherical shell with inorganic iron within the core of the molecule. The monomer has a molecular weight of about 500 000 daltons. Tissue ferritins from certain tumors have been separable into multiple isoferritins, and of interest is ferritin purified from HeLa cells and human hepatoma. There is some evidence for a change in ferritin with malignancy, and antibodies to acidic HeLa cell ferritin recognize acidic isoferritins.

Ferritin is present in small amounts in all human sera (10–200 ng/ml) but its level may be elevated in a variety of diseases including some malignant conditions. The latter are represented by Hodgkin's disease, acute myeloid leukemia, myeloproliferative diseases, pancreatic cancer, hepatoma, terato-blastoma, malignant germ cell tumors, breast and lung cancer (Lamerz, 1981).

Lung tumor-associated antigen (LTAA)

LTAA has been studied by Braatz *et al.*(1979) and a radioimmunoassay described by McIntire *et al.* (1979). LTAA is reported to consist of three subunits, each with a molecular weight of 25 000 daltons. LTAA has been found in serum from patients with lung cancer and further evaluation is in progress.

Pregnancy-specific β_1-glycoprotein (SP$_1$)

SP$_1$ (or TBG, PAPP-C, PSβG) has been identified in normal and malignant trophoblastic cells (Horne *et al.*, 1976), and in choriocarcinoma serum SP$_1$

levels are found to be elevated. Proteins from the placenta (Bohn and Winckler, 1977) are also being investigated for their potential clinical usefulness.

Serum β_2-microglobulin (β_2-m)

β_2-m is a low molecular weight protein of 11 400 daltons. It forms the light chain of HLA on the surface of all nucleated cells. Elevated levels of β_2-m may occur irregularly in a variety of advanced adenocarcinomas but they do not appear to be related to cancer as such. The assay is undergoing investigation as an aid in the management of chronic lymphocytic leukemia, lymphomas, and multiple myelomatosis (Cooper and Plesner, 1980).

Non-specific cross-reacting antigen (NCA)

NCA is an antigen whose presence is helpful in the differentiation between acute and chronic myeloid leukemia (von Kleist *et al.*, 1972; von Kleist, 1979). The characterization of NCA may serve as a model for further work on carcinoembryonic antigens.

HORMONES

Human chorionic gonadotropin (HCG)

This glycoprotein of about 45 000 daltons is normally produced by syncytiotrophoblastic cells of the placenta. It possesses two subunits, α and β, which are shared with luteinizing hormone (LH), synthesized by the human pituitary. The subunits are essentially similar but the β subunit exhibits different immunologic specificities (Vaitukaitis *et al.*, 1972; Vaitukaitis, 1979) which have made it possible to assay β-HCG without interference from other hormones.

Although HCG is normally found in serum and urine during pregnancy, HCG-like substances have been found in urinary extracts in non-pregnant subjects. The assay for β-HCG is essential in monitoring therapy in trophoblastic tumors but elevations of the level are also seen in other cancers. Serum or urine from women with chemotherapy-responsive gestational trophoblastic disease has only HCG and no free subunits, while women with unresponsive gestational disease usually exhibit altered forms of HCG with subunits similar to those from patients with ectopic secretion of HCG (Vaitukaitis and Ebersole, 1976).

In men with non-seminomatous germ cell tumors, 60–90% have an increased AFP level in the serum. If both HCG and AFP are assayed, more than 90% of the patients exhibit raised levels of at least one marker (Scardino *et al.*, 1975).

The radioimmunoassay for β-HCG, which has a molecular weight of 23 000 and a half-life of 45 min, can detect levels down to 1 μg/1. This assay is, so far, the one that comes closest to being tumor-specific for choriocarcinoma and ovarian and testicular germ cell tumors (Braunstein, 1979).

Calcitonin

This hormone is synthesized by C cells in the thyroid. Its serum level is often elevated in medullary thyroid carcinoma, which arises from the calcitonin-secreting C cells. The tumors comprise about 10% of all thyroid neoplasms and usually develop through a phase of C cell hyperplasia. During this early stage, calcitonin levels may be elevated in the serum but elevations of CEA are not seen. Later, when the tumor becomes malignant, both calcitonin and CEA levels increase (Rule *et al.*, 1979). The correlation coefficient (r) for the two tests in medullary cancer is of the order of 0.46.

Ectopic production of calcitonin has been observed in 35–75% of patients with lung cancer (Silva *et al.*, 1974). Little is known about the significance of this finding.

Ectopic ACTH

The presence of this peptide hormone has been reported in oat cell carcinoma, carcinoid tumors and in 70–80% of breast cancers (Podmore *et al.*, 1979). Tumors associated with the ectopic ACTH syndrome almost always make lipotrophin, often produce growth hormone, and sometimes also prolactin. Tumors with amine precursor uptake and decarboxylation charac-teristics are regularly devoid of ACTH, while oat cell and carcinoid tumors usually contain ACTH (70–76%). However, benign breast lesions may also contain ACTH and it is not impossible that some breast tissues may contain receptors for peptide hormones such as ACTH.

Insulin

This hormone may be produced by tumors derived from the islets of Langerhans in the pancreas. About 80–90% of these tumors have no endocrine function, but in those cases where hyperinsulinemia occurs the patient suffers hypoglycemia and hypoglycemic shock. Low blood sugar and increase of immunologically detectable insulin in serum are important for the diagnosis.

Hormones of various types may be produced by tumors derived from hormone-producing cells but may also have an ectopic origin. Cushing's syndrome can result from tumors located in the ovaries, pancreas, thyroid, breast, lung, prostate, and thymus. Hypercalcemia has been described in cancers of the kidney, uterus, urinary bladder, ovaries, lung, and in lymphosarcoma. Hypoglycemia has been observed not only in tumors of the islets of Langerhans but also in association with retroperitoneal fibromas and sarcomas, in tumors of the adrenal cortex, neuroblastoma, mesothelioma, and in pseudomyxoma derived from peritoneum.

ENZYMES

Acid phosphatase

Elevation of the acid phosphatase level in the serum is seen in not more than 30% of patients without bone metastases and in 60–90% of patients with such metastases. When it became possible to raise antibodies to acid phosphatase from prostatic fluid, there developed sensitive detection methods such as counter-immunoelectrophoresis and a solid-phase radioimmunoassay (Foti *et al.*, 1977; Chu *et al.*, 1975; Chu, 1978). With the latter assay, positive reactions (≥80 ng/ml) are seen in about one-third of patients with Stage I prostatic cancer, 80% of Stage II, 70% of Stage III, and 90% of Stage IV.

Placental alkaline phosphatase (Regan isoenzyme)

This enzyme has been evaluated in patients with different types of malignancy but mainly in advanced cases (Fishman *et al.*, 1976). The assay measures the ability to hydrolyze phenyl phosphate at pH 10.7, expressed as KA (King–Armstrong) units, following incubation at 65°C for 5 min in order to eliminate non-placental isoenzymes. Elevations of Regan isoenzyme in serum is found in 30–40% of patients with adenocarcinoma of the ovary, testicular tumors, and carcinoma of the pancreas.

Determination of the Regan isoenzyme may help to distinguish a raised alkaline phosphatase level due to bone metastases. If the elevated alkaline phosphatase level can be shown to be due to Regan isoenzyme, surgery or radiotherapy can be contemplated (Stolbach *et al.*, 1972).

Lactic dehydrogenase (LDH)

Isoenzyme patterns seem to vary with the morphological composition of human tissues, and special types of isoenzyme patterns have been observed during ontogeny (Pfleiderer and Wachsmuth, 1961). It is possible that the different patterns of isoenzymes characterize phases of development and differentiation. Changes to a more immature pattern could reflect redifferentiation of adult tissues. Serial assays of LDH levels have been carried out for many years and elevations are most often seen in hemoblastic diseases and in malignant lymphomas.

A number of other enzymes have been investigated in the management of malignant diseases, including γ-*glutamyl transpeptidase (GGTP), galactosyl-, sialyl-, glycosyl-* and *fucosyltransferases.* At present, it is difficult to evaluate their role in tumor development.

IMMUNE COMPLEXES

Information on tumor antigens comes also from studies of circulating immune complexes (CIC) in serum from cancer patients. They contain hitherto mostly unknown antigens, representing a host of tumor growth products which can be dissociated from their corresponding antibodies and studied. There is now abundant evidence that malignancy in both humans and experimental animals can elicit the formation of antibodies toward tumor antigens resulting in the formation of CIC. In some cases, part of the antigenic content has been identified (Kapsopoulou-Dominos and Anderer, 1979; Papsidero *et al.*, 1978; Strobel *et al.*, 1979).

The interaction between the malignant cells and the immune system is an immunologically hyperreactive situation where large amounts of antibody are synthesized. The measurement of CIC serves as an indicator of the antibody response to tumor growth products. Sequential measurements of CIC prior to treatment may serve as a prognostic indicator, while a rising titer later may predict a relapse.

Many investigators have shown elevated CIC in patients with a variety of cancers (Gauci *et al.*, 1981; Day *et al.*, 1981). Antitumor antibodies have been demonstrated in human tumors which carry receptors for the Fc region of immunoglobulins and CICs are bound to the receptors. This has been thought to increase the likelihood of tumor cell survival, and reduction of CIC in serum might therefore promote tumor cell destruction.

Limited studies have shown that plasmapheresis was followed by temporary objective evidence of tumor regression in 30% of 45 patients with widely disseminated malignant disease of various origins including breast, lung, cecum, colon, rectum, stomach, kidney, thyroid, head and neck, melanoma, and fibrosarcoma (Israel *et al.*, 1981). Since plasmapheresis results in removal of many products, the explanation of the improvement is far from clear.

The method for detection of CIC may vary from one laboratory to another. Two methods are preferred: either radiolabelled C1q binding assay (Zubler *et al.*, 1976) or Raji cell radioimmunoassay (Theophilopoulos *et al.*, 1976). It has been proposed that measurement of CIC in cancer patients may be useful to evaluate the activity and extent of the malignancy. Clearly, it would be of significant additional value if the composition of the CICs could be elucidated.

NEUROGENIC AMINES AND SEROTONIN METABOLITES

In certain rare tumors, well defined biochemical products are clinically useful for diagnosis and management. They include (Schwartz, 1975, 1981) neurogenic amines and their metabolites in neuroblastoma (including catecholamines, vanilmandelic acid, metanephrine, cystathionine, dopamine, dopamine β-hydroxylase, and homovanillic acid). Also useful are metanephrine in pheochromocytoma, and catecholamines, vanilmandelic acid, and serotonin metabolites (5-hydroxyindole acetic acid) in carcinoid.

CONCLUSION

Some assays of tumor products which express tumor growth activity seem to be of special value:

CEA was originally claimed to be specific for colorectal cancer, but time has shown that CEA is useful in an increasing variety of tumors.

TPA is the most general and the oldest of the markers.

AFP has a place in primary liver cancer and in endodermal sinus tumors of the testes and ovaries.

β-*HCG* is employed in trophoblastic neoplasms (choriocarcinoma) and in ovarian and testicular germ cell tumors.

In certain rare malignancies, critical information can be obtained by specific markers: by assay of *neurogenic amines* and their metabolites in pheochromocytoma and neuroblastoma, and of *serotonin metabolites* in carcinoid tumors.

In prostatic cancer, assay of *serum prostatic acid phosphatase* may have useful applications.

The writer recommends for general use the combined assay of CEA and TPA (using the product value), and for selected sites AFP, β-HCG, neurogenic amines, serotonin, and perhaps serum prostatic acid phospatase assay.

Other tumor growth products are subject to investigation but there is a long road between the first reports of a promising laboratory test and its general application. Necessary steps include chemical isolation and characterization, extensive clinical evaluation, satisfaction of the requirements of national authorities, controlled production, and making test materials available to hospitals, laboratories, and practitioners. This is a long and expensive road which takes a good deal of conviction, work, collaboration, and investment.

REFERENCES

Abelev, G.I. (1968). Production of embryonal serum α-globulin by hepatomas: review of experimental and clinical data. *Cancer Res.*, **28**, 1344–1350.

Abelev, G.I., Perova, S.D., Khramkova, N.I., Postnikova, Z.A., and Irlin, I.S. (1963). Production of embryonal α-globulin by transplantable mouse hepatomas. *Transplant. Bull.*, **1**, 174–180.

Alt, F.W., Kellems, R.E., Bertino, J.R., and Schimke, R.T. (1978). Selective multiplication of dihydrofolate reductase genes in methotrexate-resistant variants of cultured murine cells. *J. Biol. Chem.*, **253**, 1357–1370.

Andrén-Sandberg, Å., and Isacson, S. (1975). Tissue polypeptide antigen (TPA) i serum vid kirurgiskt trauma [Tissue polypeptide antigen (TPA) in serum in connection with surgical trauma] (Abstract). *Acta Soc. Med. Suecanae*, **84**, 254, häfte 4.

Björklund, B. (1963). Antigenicity of human carcinoma cells in the light of an alternative conceptual approach to neoplasia. In *Conceptual advances in immunology and oncology*. New York:. Hoeber Medical. pp. 503–520.

Björklund, B. (ed.) (1973). *Immunological techniques for detection of cancer.* Stockholm: Bonniers.

Björklund, B. (1978). Tissue polypeptide antigen (TPA): biology, biochemistry, improved assay methodology, clinical significance in cancer and other conditions, and future outlook. In *Laboratory testing for cancer* (ed. H. Schönfeld). Basel: Karger. *Antibiotics Chemother.*, **22**, 16–31.

Björklund, B. (1981). Tissue polypeptide antigen. Review and recent progress. In *Critical evaluation of tumor markers* (eds S. von Kleist, and H. Breuer). Basel: Karger. *Contr. Oncol.*, **7**, 73–87.

Björklund, B., and Björklund, V. (1957). Antigenicity of pooled human malignant and normal tissues by cyto-immunological technique: presence of an insoluble, heat-labile tumor antigen. *Int. Arch. Allergy*, **10**, 153–184.

Björklund, V., and Björklund, B. (1979). Localization of synthesis of TPA in normal and malignant human tissues by immunohistological techniques. In *Protides of the biological fluids* (ed. H. Peeters). Oxford: Pergamon Press. pp. 229–232.

Björklund, B., and Björklund, V. (1981). Specificity of tissue polypeptide antigen (TPA) and its relation to proliferative activity. In *Proc. 2nd Int. Congr. Inst. Clin. Pathol.*, Madrid. London and Madrid: Editorial Garsi. pp. 57–61.

Björklund, B., Björklund, V., and Hedlöf, I. (1961). Antigenicity of pooled human malignant and normal tissues by cytoimmunological technique. III. Distribution of tumor antigen. *J. Natl. Cancer Inst.*, **26**, 533–545.

Björklund, B., Björklund, V., Lundström, R., and Eklund, G. (1976). Tissue polypeptide antigen (TPA) in human cancer defense responses. In *The reticuloendothelial system in health and disease: immunologic and pathologic aspects* (eds H. Friedman, and M.R. Escobar). New York:. Plenum. pp.357–370.

Björklund, B., Björklund, V., Wiklund, R., Lundström, R., Ekdahl, P.H., Hagbard, L., Kaijser, K., Eklund, G., and Lüning, B. (1973). A human tissue polypeptide related to cancer and placenta: I. Preparation and properties; II. Assay technique; and III. Clinical studies of 1483 individuals with cancer and other conditions. In *Immunological techniques for detection of cancer* (ed. B. Björklund). Stockholm:. Bonniers. pp. 133–187.

Björklund, V., Björklund, B., Wittekind, Ch., and von Kleist, S. (1982). Immunohistochemical localization of tissue polypeptide antigen (TPA) and carcinoembryonic antigen (CEA) in breast chancer. *Acta Path. Scand.*, A6, 471–476.

Björklund, B., Lundblad, G., and Björklund, V. (1958). Antigenicity of pooled human malignant and normal tissues by cyto-immunological technique. II. Nature of tumor antigen. *Int. Arch. Allergy,* **12,** 241–261.

Björklund, B., Wiklund, B., Lüning, B., Andersson, K., Kallin, E., and Björklund, V. (1980). Radioimmunoassay of TPA. A laboratory test in cancer. *TumorDiagnostik,* **2,** 78–84.

Bohn, H., and Winckler, H. (1977). Isolierung und Characterisierung des Placenta-Proteins PP5. *Arch. Gynaekol.,* **223,** 179–186.

Braatz, J.A., Gaffar, S.A., Princler, G.L., Kortright, K.H., and McIntire, K.R. (1979). Isolation and characterization of a human lung tumor associated antigen. In *Carcino-embryonic proteins,* vol. II, (ed. F.-G. Lehmann). Amsterdam: Elsevier/North-Holland Biomedical Press. pp. 523–532.

Braunstein, G.D. (1979). Use of human chorionic gonadotropin as a tumor marker in cancer. In *Immunodiagnosis of cancer.* vol. I (eds R.B. Herberman, and K.R. McIntire). New York: Marcel Dekker. pp. 383–409.

Brock, D.J.H. Scrimgeour, J.B., Steven, D.J. Barron, L., and Watt, J. (1978). Maternal plasma α-fetoprotein screening for fetal neural tube defects. *Br. J. Obstet. Gynecol.,* **85,** 575–581.

Calmettes, C., Maukhtar, M.S., and Milhaud, G. (1978). Plasma carcinoembryonic antigen versus plasma calcitonin in the diagnosis of medullary carcinoma of the thyroid. *Cancer Immunol. Immunother.,* **4,** 251–256.

Chu, T.M. (1978). Serum acid phosphohydrolase (phosphatase) and ribonuclease in diagnosis of prostatic cancer. In *Laboratory testing for cancer* (ed. H. Schönfeld). Basel: Karger. *Antibiotics Chemother.,* **22,** 98–104.

Chu, T.M., Bhargava, A.K., Barnard, E.A., Ostrowski, W., Varkarakis, M.J., Merrin, C., and Murphy, G.P. (1975). Tumor antigen and acid phosphatase isoenzymes in prostate cancer. *Cancer Chemother. Rep.,* **59,** 97.

Coligan, J.E., Egan, M.L., Guyer, R.L., and Terry, W.D. (1975). Structural studies on the carcinoembryonic antigen. *Ann. N. Y. Acad. Sci.,* **259,** 355.

Coligan, J.E., and Todd, C.W. (1975). Structural studies of carcinoembryonic antigen. Periodate oxidation. *Biochemistry,* **14,** 805–810.

Cooper, E.H., and Plesner, T. (1980). Beta 2 microglobulin review: its relevance in clinical oncology. *Med. Pediatr. Oncol.,* **8,** 323.

Day, E.D. (1965). *The immunochemistry of cancer.* Springfield: Charles T. Thomas. pp. 5–149.

Day, N.K., Good, R.A., and Witkin, S.S. (1981). Circulating immune complexes and complement in human malignancy. In *Immune complexes and plasma exchanges in cancer patients* (eds B. Serrou, and C. Rosenfeld). Amsterdam: Elsevier/North-Holland Biomedical Press. pp. 99–110.

Eklund, G. (1977). TPA-värden som mått på överlevnad [TPA-values as a measure of survival; English translation available]. In *Laboratorietester vid cancer [Laboratory testing in cancer]* (eds H. Hautkamp, and A. Högman). Stockholm: Folksam. pp. 17–19.

Fishman, W.H., Inglis, N.R., Green, S., Antiss, C.L., Ghosh, N.K., Reif, A.E., Rustigian, R., Krant, M.J., and Stolbach, L. (1968). Immunological and biochemistry of the Regan isoenzyme of alkaline phosphatase in human cancer. *Nature,* **219,** 697–699.

Fishman, W.H., Ingris, N.I., Stolbach, L.L., and Krant, M.J. (1968). A serum alkaline phosphatase isoenzyme of human neoplastic cell origin. *Cancer Res.,* **28,** 150–154.

Fishman, W.H., Nishiyama, T., Rule, A., Green, S., Inglis, N.R., and Fishman, L.

(1976). Onco-developmental alkaline phosphatase isozymes. In *Onco-developmental gene expression* (eds W.H. Fishman, and S. Sell). New York: Academic Press. pp. 165–176.

Fishman, W.H., and Sell, S. (eds) (1976). *Onco-developmental gene expression.* New York: Academic Press.

Foti, A.G., Cooper, J.F., Herschman, H., and Malvaez, R.R. (1977). Detection of prostatic cancer by solid-phase radioimmunoassay of serum prostatic acid phosphatase. *New Engl. J. Med.,* **297**, 1357–1361.

Gauci, L., Caraux, J., and Serrou, B. (1981). Immune complexes in the context of the immune response in cancer patients. In *Immune complexes and plasma exchanges in cancer patients* (eds B. Serrou, and C. Rosenfeld). Amsterdam: Elsevier/North-Holland Biomedical Press. 37–98.

Gelder, F.B., Resse, C.J., Moossa, A.R., Hall, T., and Hunter, R. (1978). Purification, partial characterization and clinical evaluation of a pancreatic oncofetal antigen (POA). *Cancer Res.,* **38**, 313–324.

Gewirtz, G., and Yalow, R.S. (1974). Ectopic ACTH production in carcinoma of the lung. *J. Clin. Invest.,* **53**, 1022–1032.

Gold, P., and Freedman, S.O. (1965). Demonstration of tumor-specific antigens in human colon carcinomata by immunological tolerance and absorption techniques. *J. Exp. Med.,* **122**, 467–481.

Hagbard, L., and Sorbe, B. (1978). Preliminary experiences of TPA (tissue polypeptide antigen) in cancer of the ovary [in Swedish with summary in English]. *Läkartidningen,* **75**, 3433–3435.

Häkkinen, I. (1966). An immunochemical method for detecting carcinomatous secretion from human gastric juice. *Scand. J. Gastroenterol.,* **1**, 28.

Häkkinen, I. (1978). Gastric fetal sulfoglycoprotein antigen. In *Laboratory testing for cancer* (ed. H. Schönfeld). Basel: Karger. *Antibiotics Chemother.,* **22**, 132–140.

Hammarström, S., Engvall, E., and Johansson, B.G. (1975). Nature of the tumor-associated determinants of carcinoembryonic antigen. *Proc. Natl Acad. Sci.,* **72** (4), 1528–1532.

Hansen, H.J., Snyder, J.J., Miller, E., Vandervoorde, J.P., Miller, O.N., Hines, L.R., and Burns, J.J. (1974). Carcino-embryonic antigen (CEA) assay. A laboratory adjunct in the diagnosis and management of cancer. *Human Pathol.,* **5**, 139–147.

Herberman, R.B., and McIntire, K.R. (eds) (1979). *Immunodiagnosis of cancer,* Vols I and II. New York and Basel: Marcel Dekker.

Holyoke, E.D., and Chu, T.M. (1979). Tissue polypeptide antigen. In *Immunodiagnosis of cancer* (eds R.B. Herberman, and K.R. McIntire). New York and Basel: Marcel Dekker. pp. 513–521.

Horne, C.H.W., Towler, C.M., Pugh-Humphreys, R.G.P., Thomson, A.W., and Bohn, H. (1976). Pregnancy-specific β_1-glycoprotein. A product of the syncytio-trophoblast. *Experientia,* **32**, 1177–1199.

Isacson, S., and Andrén-Sandberg, Å. (1978). Tissue polypeptide antigen (TPA) and cytology in cancer of the urinary bladder. In *Clinical application of carcino-embryonic antigen assay* (eds B.P. Krebs, C.M. Lalanne, and M. Schneider). Amsterdam and Oxford: Excerpta Medica. pp. 374–377.

Israel, L., Edelstein, R., Samak, R., Baudelot, J., McDonald, J., Breau, J.L., Manonni, P., and Radot, E. (1981). Clinical results of multiple plasmaphoresis in patients with advanced cancer. In *Immune complexes and plasma exchanges in cancer patients* (eds. B. Serrou, and C. Rosenfeld). Amsterdam: Elsevier/North-Holland Biomedical Press. pp. 309–327.

Kapsopoulou-Dominos, K., and Anderer, F.A. (1979). Circulating carcinoembryonic antigen immune complexes in sera of patients with carcinomata of the gastrointestinal tract. *Clin. Exp. Immunol., 35*, 190.

Kohne, D.E., and Byers, M.J. (1973). Amplification and evolution of deoxyribonucleic acid sequences expressed as ribonucleic acid. *Biochemistry, 12*, 2373–2378.

Krantz, M., Ariel, N., and Gold, Ph. (1979). CEA biology and chemistry: characterization of partial proteolysis fragments. In *Carcino-embryonic proteins*, vol.I (ed. F.-G. Lehmann). Amsterdam: Elsevier/North-Holland Biomedical Press. pp. 17–24.

Kumar, S., Costello, C.B., Glashan, R.W., and Björklund, B. (1981). The clinical significance of tissue polypeptide antigen (TPA) in the urine of bladder cancer patients. *Br. J. Urol., 53*, 578–581.

Lacey, B.W. (1961). Non-generic variations of surface antigens in *Bordetella* and other micro-organisms. In *Microbial reaction to environment* (eds G.G. Neynell, and H. Gooder). London: Cambridge University Press. pp. 343–390.

Lamerz, R. (1981). Ferriton and cancer. In *Proc. 2nd Int. Congr. Inst. Clin. Pathol.*, Madrid. London and Madrid: Editorial Garsi. pp. 63–67.

Lang, N. (1963). Immunologie des Karzinoms als Grundlage therapeutischer Überlegungen. *Med. Welt*, 2538–2545.

Lehmann, F.-G. (ed.) (1979). *Carcino-embroyonic proteins*, vols I and II. Amsterdam: Elsevier/North-Holland Biomedical Press.

Lokish, J.J., Zamcheck, N., and Loewenstein, M. (1978). Sequential carcinoembryonic antigen levels in the therapy of metastatic breast cancer. *Ann. Intern. Med.,*

Lundström, R., Björklund, B., and Eklund, G. (1973). A tissue-derived polypeptide antigen: its relation to cancer and its temporary occurrence in certain infectious diseases. In *Immunological techniques for detection of cancer* (ed. B. Björklund). Stockholm: Bonniers. pp. 243–247.

Lüning, B., Redelius, P., and Björklund, B. (1979). Amino acid sequence identity of TPA fragments from different sources. In *Protides of the biological fluids* (ed. H. Peeters). Oxford: Pergamon Press. pp. 67–69.

Lüning, B., Wiklund, B., Redelius, P., and Björklund, B. (1980). Biochemical properties of tissue polypeptide antigen (TPA). *Biochim. Biophys. Acta, 624*, 90–101.

Lüthgens, M., and Schlegel, G. (1980). CEA + TPA in clinical tumor diagnosis with special reference to breast cancer. [in German and English]. *TumorDiagnostik, 2*, 63–77.

Lüthgens, M., and Schlegel, G. (1981). Verlaufskontrolle mit Tissue Polypeptide Antigen and Carcinoembryonalem Antigen in der radioonkologischen Nachsorge und Therapie [Follow-up by tissue polypeptide antigen and carcinoembryonic antigen in radioncologic surveillance and therapy; with summary in English]. *TumorDiagnostik, 2*, 179–188.

Lüthgens, M., Schlegel, G., Schoen, H.-D., and Kruse-Jarres, J.D. (1981). Simultaneous follow-up of breast cancer patients by carcinoembryonic antigen and tissue polypeptide antigen (Abstract). *UICC Conf. on Clinical Oncology*, Lausanne, Switzerland, 28–31 October.

Lüthgens, M., and von Jürgensonn, H. (1979). TPA-RIA in clinical cancer diagnostics. In *Protides of the biological fluids* (ed. H. Peeters). Oxford: Pergamon Press. pp. 263–266.

Mach, J.-P., and Puztaszeri, G. (1972). Carcinoembryonic antigen (CEA): demonstration of a partial identity between CEA and a normal glycoprotein. *Immunochem., 9*, 1031–1034.

McIntire, K.R., Braatz, J.A., Gaffar, S.A., Princler, G.L., and Kortright, K.H. (1979). Development of a radioimmunoassay for a lung tumor associated antigen. In *Carcino-embryonic proteins,* vol. II (ed. F.-G. Lehmann). Amsterdam: Elsevier/North-Holland Biomedical Press. pp. 533–540.

Manes, C. (1979). Current concepts in onco-developmental gene expression. In *Carcino-embryonic proteins,* Vol. I (ed. F.-G. Lehmann). Amsterdam: Elsevier/North-Holland Biomedical Press. pp. 1–6.

Martin, E.W., Jr, James, K.K., Hurtubise, P.E., Catalano, P., and Minton, J.P. (1977). The use of CEA as an early indicator for gastrointestinal tumor recurrence and second-look procedures. *Cancer,* **39,** 440–446.

Masopust, J. (1968). Occurrence of fetoprotein in patients with neoplasms and non-neoplastic diseases. *Int. J. Cancer,* **3,** 364–373.

Menendez-Botet, C.J., Oettgen, H.F., Pinsky, C.M., and Schwartz, M.K. (1978). A preliminary evaluation of tissue polypeptide antigen in serum or urine (or both) of patients with cancer or benign neoplasms. *Clin. Chem.,* **24,** 868–872.

Minton, J.P., James, K.K., Hurtubise, P.E., Rinker, L., Joyce, S., and Martin, E.W., Jr (1978). The use of serum CEA determinations to predict recurrence of carcinoma of the colon and time for a second-look operation. *Surg., Gynecol., Obstet.,* **147,** 208–210.

Nemoto, T., Constantine, R., and Chu, T.M. (1979). Human tissue polypeptide antigen in breast cancer. *J. Natl Cancer Inst.,* **63,** 1347–1350.

Newman, R.A. (1981). Leukaemia-associated antigens. In *CEA und andere Tumor-marker* (eds G. Uhlenbruck, and G. Wintzer). Leonberg: TumorDiagnostik Verlag. pp. 315–319.

Nørgaard-Pedersen, B., and Gaede, P. (1975). Immunoelectrophoretic quantitation of maternal serum human placental lactogen hormone and alpha-fetoprotein in the same electrophoretic run. *Scand. J. Immunol.,* **4,** Suppl. 2, 19–24.

Nørgaard-Pedersen, B. (1981). Alpha-fetoprotein in the diagnosis, therapy and monitoring of infantile and adult germ cell tumors (teratocarcinomas) of gonadal and extragonadal origin. In *Critical evaluation of tumor markers* (eds S. von Kleist, and H. Breuer). Basel: Karger. *Contr. Oncol.,* **7,** 39–49.

Nørgaard-Pedersen, B., Albrechtsen, R., and Theilum, G. (1975). Serum alpha-fetoprotein as a marker for endodermal sinus tumor (yolk-sac tumor) or a vitelline component of a teratocarcinoma. *Acta Pathol. Microbiol. Scand.,* **83,** 573–589.

Oehr, P., Adolphs, H-D., Wustrow, A., Klar, R., Schlösser, T., and Winkler, C. (1981a). Simultanbestimmung von CEA, TAG und TPA im Serum von Harn-blasencarcinom-Patienten: Analyse von Markerfrequenz und Markerunabhängig-keit unter Berücksichtigung von Tumorstadium, Malignitätsgrad und Krankheits-verlauf [Serum concentrations of CEA, TAG and TPA with regard to stage, grade and course of disease in bladder carcinoma patients; with summary in English]. *TumorDiagnostik,* **2,** 27–33.

Oehr, P., Derigs, G., and Altmann, R. (1981b). Evaluation and characterization of tumor-associated antigens by conversion of inverse distribution function values into specificity–sensitivity diagrams. *TumorDiagnostik,* **2,** 283–290.

Oehr, P., Hamann, D., Klar, R., Schlösser, T., and Winkler, C. (1980). Serumkon-zentrationen von Tissue Polypeptide Antigen und Tennessee-Antigen im Ver-gleich zu CEA, AFP und beta-HCG bei Patienten mit Harnblasen- und Hodencar-cinomen [Serum concentrations of tissue polypeptide antigen (TPA) and Tennes-see-antigen in comparison with CEA, AFP and beta-HCG in patients with cancer of the urinary bladder and testis]. *Nucl. Compact.,* **11,** 223–227.

Oehr, P., Wustrow, A., Derigs, G., and Bormann, R. (1981c). Evaluation and characterization of tumor-associated antigens by the inverse distribution function. *TumorDiagnostik*, **2**, 195–198.

Papsidero, L.D., Harvey, S.R., Synderman, M.C., Nemoto, T., Valenzuela, L., and Chu, T.M. (1978). Characterization of immune complexes from the pleural effusion of breast cancer patient. *Int. J. Cancer*, **21**, 675.

Pfleiderer, G., and Wachsmuth, E.D. (1961). Alters- und funktionsabhängige Differenzierung der Lactatedehydrogenase menschlicher Organe. *Biochem. Z.*, **334**, 185–198.

Podmore, J., Wilson, B., Cowden, E.A., Beastall, G.H., and Ratcliffe, J.G. (1979). Multiple hormones in human tumours. In *Carcino-embryonic proteins*, vol. I (ed. F.-G. Lehmann). Amsterdam: Elsevier/North-Holland Biomedical Press. pp. 457–463.

Potter, Th. P., Jr. Jordan, T., Jordan, I.D., and Lasater, H. (1980). TennaGen, a new tumor associated antigen. In *Prevention and detection of cancer*, vol. II (ed. H.E. Nieburgs). New York: Marcel Dekker. p. 467.

Prochazka, B., Jirasek, V., Barta, V., Kohout, J., Korbova, L., Schlupek, A., and Slezak, Z. (1968). Differences in lactate dehydrogenase isoenzyme patterns in fundus and pylorus of rat stomach. *Gastronenterology*, **54**, 60–64.

Redelius, P., Lüning, B., and Björklund, B. (1980). Chemical studies of tissue polypeptide antigen (TPA). II. Partial amino acid sequences of cyanogen bromide fragments of TPA subunit B_1. *Acta Chem. Scand. B*, **34**, 265–273.

Reynoso, G., and Keane, M. (1979). Carcinoembryonic antigen in prognosis and monitoring of patients with cancer. In *Immunodiagnosis of cancer* (eds R. Herberman, and K.R. McIntire). New York: Marcel Dekker. pp. 239–254.

Ruibal, A., Clotet, B., Pigrau, C., Durán Bellido, P., Fraile, M., and Roca, I. (1982). Tissue polypeptide antigen in autoimmune diseases. *TumorDiagnostik*, **3**, 40–45.

Rule, A.H., De Lellis, R.A., Tashjan, A.H., Spiler, I., Feldman, Z., Reichlin, S., Nathanson, L., and Wolfe, H.J. (1979). Calcitonin and carcinoembryonic antigen: tumor markers in medullary thyroid carcinoma. In *Carcino-embryonic proteins*, vol. II (ed. F.-G. Lehmann). Amsterdam: Elsevier/North-Holland Biomedical Press. pp. 781–785.

Ruoslahti, E. (1979). Structure-function relationships in alpha-fetoprotein. In *Carcino-embryonic proteins*, vol. I (ed. F.-G. Lehmann). Amsterdam: Elsevier/North-Holland Biomedical Press. pp. 153–163.

Scardino, P.T., Cox, D., and Waldemann, T.A. (1975). The value of serum tumor markers in the staging and prognosis of germ cell tumors of the testis. *Urology*, **6**, 382.

Schlegel, G., Lüthgens, M., Eklund, G., and Björklund, B. (1981). Correlation between activity in breast cancer and CEA, TPA, and eighteen common laboratory procedures and the improvement by the combined use of CEA and TPA. *TumorDiagnostik*, **2**, 6–11.

Schönfeld, H. (ed.) (1978). *Laboratory testing for cancer*. Basel: Karger. *Antibiotics Chemother.*, **22**, 1–184.

Schwartz, M.K. (1975). Biochemical procedures as aids in diagnosis of different forms of cancer. *Ann. Clin. Lab. Sci.*, **4**, 95–403.

Schwartz, M.K. (1981). Biochemical markers in cancer. In *Critical evaluation of tumor markers* (eds. S. von Kleist, and H. Breuer). Basel: Karger. *Contr. Oncol.*, **7**, 3–11.

Seppälä, M., and Ruoslahti, E. (1972). Alpha-fetoprotein in normal and pregnancy sera. *Lancet*, **i**, 375–376.

Shively, J.E., Glassman, J.N.S., Engvall, E., and Todd, C.W. (1979). Amino acid sequence of CEA and CEA related antigens. In *Carcino-embryonic proteins*, vol.

I (ed. F.-G. Lehman). Amsterdam: Elsevier/North-Holland Biomedical Press. pp. 9–15.

Shuster, J., Silverman, M., and Gold, Ph. (1973). Metabolism of human carcinoembryonic antigen in xenogenic animals. *Cancer Res.*, **33**, 65–68.

Silva, O.L., Becker, K.L., and Primack, A. (1974). Ectopic production of calcitonin by oat-cell carcinoma. *New Engl. J. Med.*, **290**, 1222–1224.

Skryten, A., Unsgaard, B., Björklund, B., and Eklund, G. (1981). Serum TPA related to activity in a wide spectrum of cancer conditions. *TumorDiagnostik*, **3**, 117–120.

Staab, H.J., Anderer, F.A., Stumpf, E., and Fischer, R. (1978). Carcinoembryonic antigen follow-up and selection of patients for second-look operation in management of gastrointestinal carcinoma. *Oncology*, **10**, 273–282.

Stolbach, L.L., Skillman, J., and Goodman, R. (1972). Increase in serum alkaline phosphatase due to Regan isoenzyme in a patient with localized jejunal lymphoma. *Arch. Surg.*, **105**, 491–493.

Strobel, P., Daugherty, H., Rule, A., Fitzgerald, K., Smith, F., Inglis, N., and Stolbach, L. (1979). Presence of immune complexes in ascites fluids: relationship to CEA. In *Carcino-embryonic proteins*, vol.II (ed. F.-G. Lehmann). Amsterdam: Elsevier/North-Holland Biomedical Press. pp. 69–73.

Sylvan, S. (1977). TPA vid akut hepatit [TPA in acute hepatitis]. In *Laboratoriestester vid cancer [Laboratory Testing in Cancer]*. (eds H. Hautkamp, and A. Högman). Stockholm: Folksam. pp. 35–36.

Takeda, K. (ed.) (1969). *Immunology of cancer with special reference to tumor immunity in the primary autochthonous host*. Hokkaido University School of Medicine.

Talerman, A. (1981). Alpha-fetoprotein and germ cell tumors. In *Critical Evaluation of Tumor Markers* (eds. S. von Kleist and H. Breuer), *Contr. Oncol.*, vol. 7, pp. 50–60, Basel: Karger.

Terry, W.E., Henkart, P.A., Coligan, J.E., and Todd, C.W. (1972). Structural studies of the major glycoprotein in a preparation with carcinoembryonic antigen activity. *J. Exp. Med.*, **136**, 200–204.

Theophilopoulos, A.N., Wilson, C.B., and Dixon, F.J. (1976). The Raji cell radioimmunoassay for detecting immune complexes in human sera. *J. Clin. Invest.*, **57**, 169.

Tormey, D.C., and Waalkes, T.O. (1978). Clinical correlation between CEA and breast cancer. *Cancer*, **42**, Suppl. 1507–1511.

Vaitukaitis, J.L. (1979). Secretion of human chorionic gonadotropin by tumors. In *Carcino-embryonic proteins*, vol. I (ed. F.-G. Lehman). Amsterdam: Elsevier/North-Holland Biomedical Press. pp. 447–456.

Vaitukaitis, J.L., Braunstein, G.D., and Ross, G.T. (1972). Radioimmunosassay which specifically measures human chorionic gonadotropin in the presence of human luteinizing hormone. *Am. J. Obstet. Gynecol.*, **113**, 751–758.

Vaitukaitis, J.L., and Ebersole, E.R. (1976). Evidence for altered synthesis of human chorionic gonadotropin in gestational trophoblastic tumors. *J. Clin. Endocrinol. Metab.*, **42**, 1048–1055.

Vincent, R.G., and Chu, T.M. (1973). Carcinoembryonic antigen in patients with carcinoma of the lung. *J. Thorac. Cardiovasc. Surg.*, **66**, 320–328.

von Kleist, S. (1979). Antigens crossreacting with CEA. Evaluation of their interrelationship and clinical role. In *Carcino-embryonic proteins*, vol. I (ed. F.-G. Lehmann). Amsterdam: Elsevier/North-Holland Biomedical Press. pp. 35–39.

von Kleist, S., and Breuer, H. (eds) (1981). *Critical evaluation of tumor markers*. Basel: Karger. *Contr. Oncol.*, **7**, 1–120.

von Kleist, S., Chavanel, G., and Burtin, P. (1972). Identification of an antigen from normal human tissue that crossreacts with the carcinoembryonic antigen. *Proc. Natl Acad. Sci.*, **69**, 2492–2494.

Vygodchikov, G.V. (ed) (1959). *Pathogenesis and immunology of tumors.* Oxford: Pergamon Press. pp. 1–254.

Wanebo, H.J. Sterns, M., and Schwartz, M.K. (1978). Use of CEA as an indicator of early recurrence and as a guide to a selected second-look procedure in patients with colorectal cancer. *Ann. Surg.*, **188**, 481.

Zamcheck, N. (1981). Clinical use of carcinoembryonic antigen. In *Critical evaluation of tumor markers* (eds S. von Kleist, and H. Breuer). Basel: Karger. *Contr. Oncol.*, **7**, 25–38.

Zangerle, P.F., Thirion, A., Hendrick, J.-C., and Franchimont, P. (1978). Casein and other tumor markers in relation to cancer of the breast. In *Laboratory testing for cancer.* (ed. H. Schönfeld). Basel: Karger. *Antibiotics Chemother.*, **22**, 141–148.

Zubler, R.H., Lange, G., Lambert, P.H., and Miescher, P.A. (1976). Detection of immune complexes in unheated sera by a modified ^{125}I-Clq binding test. *J. Immunol.*, **116**, 232.463

Chapter

12 ALEXANDER W. PEARLMAN

Doubling Time and Survival Time

The clinical significance of survival statistics should be critically assessed on the basis of measurements which reflect the biologic behavior of tumors. One such unit is the growth rate of the tumor as expressed numerically by the doubling time (T_d). The measurement of survival in multiples of tumor doublings takes account of differences in growth rate between tumors and the effect of growth rate on survival.

This chapter investigates the clinical growth rates of various human malignant tumors and their implication for the evaluation of treatment and prognosis. It postulates that the effect of treatment on the disease-free interval and duration of survival in a patient should be considered in terms of the individual tumor doublings.

It was shown by Breur (1966) that resumption of exponential growth after the irradiation of a tumor was at the same rate as prior to treatment. The radiation did not alter the growth rate of the tumor, but merely retarded its progress by the amount of time required for the tumor to attain its original size. For slowly growing tumors, this can represent a considerable increase in longevity. This observation may also have considerable clinical implications for systemic cancericidal treatment.

CONCEPTS OF DOUBLING TIME

An estimate of a malignant tumor's potential for growth can be deduced from its duration, size, and degree of histological differentiation. Even when taken together, these variables yield an imprecise clinical index of tumor aggressiveness. Collins *et al.* (1956) published the first of a series of papers on the biomathematics of tumor growth rate. They and others (Berkson, 1962; Nathan *et al.*, 1962; Krutova and Korman, 1976) advanced the concept that tumor growth in humans is essentially exponential and that the evolution of a tumor during its preclinical phase, as well as its rate of metastatic spread, could be reflected in its clinical doubling time (that period of time during which there is a twofold increase in volume).

Rapidly growing tumors, if untreated or unsuccessfully treated, would tend to metastasize or reach a size incompatible with host survival sooner than a slowly growing tumor (Breur, 1966). Prolonged survival after therapy does not therefore necessarily imply therapeutic benefit. Survival statistics are traditionally recorded in units of time, usually at intervals of five years or multiples thereof. For some patients this may be the only practicable yardstick, but it can be misleading because the concept of survival time does not incorporate the growth rate of the tumor.

Experimental evidence that a tumor may exhibit a constant growth rate during both its visible and invisible phases has been presented by Mottram (1935, 1936). He induced cutaneous epitheliomas in mice by the application of tar. Serial measurements of the diameters of the tumors were plotted on a semi-logarithmic graph and the growth rate was found to be constant. Backward extrapolation of the growth curve through the period of microscopic growth indicated that the *induction of the tumor coincided with the earliest application of the irritant*. These experiments suggested that the tumor could have arisen from a single cell or clone and that the growth rate during the entire period of the experiment was exponential. Brues *et al.* (1939) demonstrated that, in chemically induced tumors in animals, there was a high degree of correlation between the tumor growth rate and the duration of the latent period preceding the appearance of a palpable tumor.

A model of exponential growth is illustrated in Figure 1, based mainly upon the contributions of Collins *et al.* (1956) and Schwartz (1961). The clinical diagnosis of cancer is merely an event in the course of the disease. It has been preceded by a silent preclinical phase and will be followed by a variable, though shorter, interval if growth is unrestrained. Should growth continue at the same rate after diagnosis, it would require few additional doublings for the tumor to become huge, so that by the 47th doubling, tumor size would be incompatible with survival by the host. The preclinical phase in the untreated patient may occupy as much as three-quarters of the entire lifespan of the tumor. It requires approximately 30 tumor doublings for a single cell $10\mu m$ in diameter to reach a diameter of 1 cm, generally accepted as the smallest diagnosable tumor.

The influence of diagnostic delay on treatment and prognosis has been the subject of considerable controversy. The diagnostic gap consists of two parts. The true diagnostic gap is that between the earliest diagnosable tumor and the onset of symptoms, and this will be shortened by the development of more refined methods of diagnosis. The apparent diagnostic gap, or patient delay before presentation, may yield some information about the growth rate of the

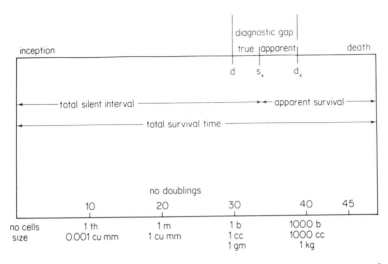

Figure 1 Model of growth in a hypothetical tumor illustrating the sequence of events when growth is exponential. (Reproduced by permission of American Cancer Society.)

tumor. Taken together, the true and apparent diagnostic gaps usually occupy a relatively small portion of the entire life-cycle of the tumor. Considering the long preclinical growth period, clinical diagnosis can hardly be considered an early event even under the most optimal conditions.

Since diagnosis is not an early event, metastasis may occur before the clinical onset and yet not become evident until some time after treatment has been completed. Survival statistics survey only that limited portion of the life-cycle that can be observed after diagnosis.

The measurement of survival time in a patient cannot be meaningfully evaluated without considering the biologic nature of the tumor as reflected in its growth rate. When the change in the volume of a tumor during a measured interval is known, the average growth rate can be calculated and expressed in terms of its doubling time, i.e. the number of days required for a twofold increase in volume. Estimates of volume doubling times for human tumors indicate a range varying from a few days to years (Table 1). In calculating the doubling times in the authors' series, we have used the Gerstenberg formula (Philippe and Le Gal, 1968):

$$T_d = \frac{0.1(t - t_o)}{\log d_t - \log d_o}$$

Table 1. Tumor doubling times in days

Author(s)	Testis No.	Testis Mean	Testis Range	Breast No.	Breast Mean	Breast Range	Colorectal No.	Colorectal Mean	Colorectal Range	Sarcoma No.	Sarcoma Mean	Sarcoma Range	Type[c]
Collins et al. (1956)	9	36	11–153	2	56	28–84	4	84	93–103				
Spratt and Spratt (1964)	10	48	13–58	29	82	11–100	10	109	11–150	23	42		
Joseph et al. (1971)	7			9			15			64		5–34	O
Chahinian (1972), Chahinian and Israel (1976)	2	24	22–26	1	100		4	63	42–90	1	40		
Breur (1966)	9	40	4–205	6	196	23–745	2	94	63–135	16	104	20–212	F
										13	50	17–253	O
Brenner et al. (1967)				4	170	31–355	1	59					
Plesnicar et al. (1976)										18	40	3–200	O
Band and Kocandrle (1975)										8	44	11–79	O
										2	17	11–23	F
										2	31	25–37	E
										3	58	14–120	Me
Tubiana and Malaise (1976)	16	19								12	30		H
										41	35		Me
Gershon-Cohen et al. (1962)				18[a]	102	23–209							
Philippe and Le Gal (1968)				78[b]	44	5–210							
							72[b]	44	3–235				
Pearlman (1973, 1976, 1979)	22	35	4–43							11	33	15–65	O
										9	195	30–270	F
										16	23	4–59	E
										17	48	11–122	Mi

[a] Growth rate based on mammography.
[b] Growth rate based on mastectomy scar recurrences.
[c] O=osteogenic sarcoma; F=fibrosarcoma; E=Ewing's sarcoma; Mi=miscellaneous sarcomas; H=hematosarcoma; Me=mesenchymal sarcomas.

where t is the time of the first measurement and t_o the final measurement, the difference being recorded in days; and d_t is the diameter of the tumor at time t and d_o the diameter at time t_o.

A growth curve that plots as a straight line on a semi-log graph represents a constant rate of change in volume or an exponential growth pattern. The duration of the tumor and its probable time of inception can be estimated by backward extrapolation of the growth curve (Collins *et al.*, 1956; Schwartz, 1961). Though there are no uniform criteria for classifying tumor doubling times, the authors have chosen to follow the recommendations of Collins *et al.* (1956). Growth is rapid if the T_d is 25 days or less, intermediate between 26 and 75 days, and slow when it exceeds 75 days (Table 2).

Table 2. Growth rate of 483 malignant tumors

	T_d(days)	Number	Percent
Rapid	<25	237	49
Intermediate	26–75	184	38
Slow	> 76	62	13

Until recent years, published studies of the rate of growth of many human tumors suggested that a constant growth rate during the period of observation is characteristic of tumor growth dynamics (Breur, 1966; Pearlman, 1973; 1979; Spratt and Ackerman, 1961). Recently however, the biomathematical concept that the evolution of malignant tumors follows a pattern of exponential growth for their entire life-cycle has been challenged, mainly on the basis of experimental studies on cell cultures and in animals. It is now generally agreed that exponential growth occurs for at least a period, but that eventually there is deceleration of growth (Bagshawe, 1968; Laird, 1965; Mayneord, 1932; Patt and Blackford, 1954).

As pulmonary metastases from osteogenic carcinomas increase in size, a slowing of growth has been recorded when the diameter exceeds 20 mm (Plesnicar *et al.*, 1976). A plot of the diameters of a solid tumor over a relatively short time span may closely approximate a straight line on a log scale, but this may reflect small inaccuracies in mensuration (Laird, 1965). In practice it may be impossible to distinguish an exponential growth curve from a Gompertzian curve over a short period of observation, but in experimental tumors a small portion of the growth curve always appears exponential (Tubiana and Malaise, 1976).

Tumors are composed of proliferating and non-proliferating fractions, the relative sizes of which may vary from time to time. Smithers (1968) has pointed out the paucity of available experimental data on the growth rate of tumors of microscopic size, and implies that assigning exponential growth to the silent interval is no more than an assumption. Human tumors display a wide range of changing behavior patterns, and the effect on growth rate of such phenomena as hormonal dependence, maturation, spontaneous regression, necrosis, degeneration, and metaplasia needs to be evaluated. It is probable that no single mathematical model can explain all of the variations observed in tumor growth (Weiss, 1973).

Although exponential growth may not necessarily be present during the entire life of the tumor, it can be assumed that, for moderate-sized tumors (up to approximately 2 cm diameter), constant growth rates prevail over a significant portion of the life-cycle of the tumor (Garland *et al.*, 1963; Garland, 1966).

RELATION TO CYTOKINETIC ACTIVITY

Investigations of cell kinetics have demonstrated a discrepancy between the volume doubling time and the potential doubling time of a tumor. The latter is calculated on the assumption that each mitosis produces two viable daughter cells capable of further division and therefore is always less than the clinical tumor doubling time. The potential doubling time of a tumor reflects only the growth fraction while the volume growth of a tumor is a balance of three factors: the proportion of cells actively engaged in cell division, the length of the cell cycle and (of most significance) the rate of cell loss (Hewitt and Wilson, 1959; Iverson, 1967; Mendelsohn *et al.*, 1960 Steel, 1967, 1968).

The difference between clinical and potential doubling times represents cell loss due to cell death, the migration of cells out of the tumor, and the inability of some cells to reproduce (the resting fraction) (Bagshawe, 1968; Frindel *et al.*, 1968). Other factors possibly involved are long periods of quiescence or the effect of hormonal imbalance upon the growth rate of hormone-dependent tumors. Cell production rates vary greatly among the considerable range of tumor doubling times (Lamberton, 1972).

Cytokinetic profiles of malignant tumors may be able to provide a rational basis for devising treatment strategies. The mitotic index (MI) counts the ratio of cells undergoing mitosis in the entire population and represents the rate of cell production (Rosenoer and Curby, 1975). The MI is constant in an exponentially growing population. An advantage of determining the MI is that it does not require the injection of radioactive material, but multiple large biopsies are required, limiting its use to large tumors.

Though the MI has been measured for many tumors, its practicability and clinical usefulness are limited (Tubiana and Malaise, 1976). Breur (1966) was unable to show any significant correlation between the growth rate and the number of mitoses in primary tumors, though he did observe a trend toward fewer mitoses in more slowly growing tumors.

The labeling index (LI) is determined by cell labeling with radioactive thymidine. Actively dividing cells in the phase of DNA synthesis will incorporate the label (Fabrikant, 1971; Tubiana *et al.*, 1975). Incorporation of DNA precursors makes possible the recognition of S phase cells by auto-radiography as the non-cycling quiescent cells are unable to incorporate DNA precursors. The DNA content of a cell may be determined by either cytophotometry or autoradiography.

The LI is used to evaluate the growth fraction and thus the potential doubling time of the tumor. There is a significant correlation between the T_d and the LI (Bresciani *et al.*, 1974; Friedman *et al.*, 1973), suggesting that variations in T_d among different histological types is due mainly to differences in the growth fraction (Lamerton, 1972). The clinical value of measuring doubling times is clear, yet it remains only a crude measure of cell kinetics, since it reveals little about the rates of proliferation or death of subpopula-tions of cells, or the response to treatment of these subpopulations (Straus, 1974).

Relating cell kinetics, especially the growth fraction, to clinical events presents difficulties, though some correlations have been suggested (Shack-ney, 1976). It has been noted, for instance, that the only tumors capable of control by chemotherapy, namely malignant lymphoma and certain embryon-al tumors, have a high rate of cell loss (Tubiana and Malaise, 1976). A correlation between doubling times and the growth fraction has been observed and the LI is highest in rapidly growing tumors (Tubiana *et al.*, 1975).

However, Silvestrini *et al.* (1974) and Tubiana and coworkers (Tubiana, 1971; Tubiana and Malaise, 1976; Tubiana *et al.*, 1975) were unable to find a correlation between the growth fraction of primary breast cancer and its histological type or the presence of lymph node metastases in the axilla. Campeljohn *et al.* (1956) could find no correlation between the Dukes' stage of a rectal cancer and either the rate of cellular proliferation or the proportion of cells in mitosis.

In their study of head and neck tumors, Friedman *et al.* (1973) were able to accumulate considerable information about the doubling time of tumors by daily measurement of cell kinetics in serial biopsies. This is limited to large accessible tumors.

PERIOD OF RISK

Collins *et al.* (1956) and Collins (1958) defined the 'period of risk' as the interval after which the patient, free of disease, may be assumed to have been cured of certain tumors. It is based on the postulate that the growth rate of a given malignant tumor is essentially constant from the time of inception and that any metastases or recurrences would grow at approximately the same rate as the original tumor. The maximum total duration of a malignant tumor in a child cannot exceed the chronological age at the time of treatment plus the nine months of intrauterine life. Recurrence at the primary site, or microscopic metastases present at the time the primary tumor was treated, will therefore grow to a diagnosable size during this length of time—the maximum period of risk.

Collins' (1958) original series of 340 patients with Wilms' tumor had only two instances of recurrence or metastasis after the risk period. Pollack *et al.* (1960) found no exceptions to the rule amongst 68 patients with Wilms' tumor. Knox and Pillars (1958) had no recurrences in 206 patients with Wilms' tumor, neuroblastoma, and rhabdomyosarcoma after completion of the risk period. Similar results have been reported by others (Bodian, 1959; Kieswetter and Mason, 1960; Sutow, 1958).

The 'period of risk' has special applicability to childhood cancer because the total time span involved is relatively short. The potentially long risk period in adults would make the application of this concept cumbersome, unless the growth rate of the individual tumor was known. However, reasonable estimates of the risk period can be made, and have been established by experience.

If the doubling time of a tumor is known, the period of risk would approximate 30 tumor volume doublings, the time required to establish a diagnosable tumor size. It has been observed that local recurrence in oral cavity cancer is unusual after a disease-free interval of two years. Few recurrences are seen in patients with osteogenic sarcoma who remain disease-free for two years after definitive treatment. Five-and 10-year survivals tend to be equal in corpus carcinoma, allowing for age-adjusted mortality.

THE LETHAL LIMIT

Spratt and Spratt (1964) introduced the concept of the lethal limit which is defined as the maximum limit of survival of untreated patients from the time of discovery of pulmonary metastases. It is recorded in multiples of doubling time for pulmonary nodules, the most rapidly growing metastasis being chosen as the yardstick for measuring survival. The lethal limit is the number of tumor volume doublings required to reach the largest size that a pulmonary tumor may attain before it is no longer compatible with life.

When an intrathoracic neoplasm has reached a diameter of 200 mm (equivalent to 40.8 doublings of a single cell), the next doubling of volume would be incompatible with survival in the host (Spratt *et al.*, 1963b). Survival time is the product of the doubling time in days and the number of doublings survived. The larger the pulmonary metastasis is at its first observation, the fewer the number of doublings required to reach the lethal limit.

Growth rates, which reflect the relative malignancy of a tumor, have been shown to have a log-normal distribution. Survival in multiples of tumor volume doublings have a similar log-normal distribution. The probability that an untreated patient will survive beyond the lethal limit, based on the log-normal distribution of growth rates and survival, is only 0.05 (one in 20). There is a 95% probability that the patient will die within the lethal limit (Spratt and Spratt, 1964).

The major contribution of the lethal limit concept is that the results of palliative treatment in individual patients can be evaluated against the maximum probability of survival of untreated patients.

The lethal limit as originally proposed applies only to patients with pulmonary metastases.

CLINICAL APPLICATION OF TUMOR DOUBLING TIMES

Most investigations on tumor doubling times are based on measurement of acccessible soft tissue lesions or of pulmonary metastases. One inherent

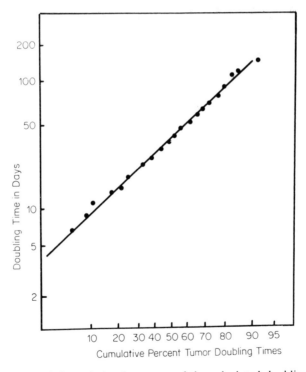

Figure 2 The cumulative relative frequency of the calculated doubling times of 211 tumors in the author's series plotted successively on a log-probit graph. The cumulative percentage of each doubling time is indicated by the dots. (Reproduced by permission of American Cancer Society.)

disadvantage of such selected material is the preponderance of biologically aggressive and advanced tumors. The interval of clinical observation represents only the terminal part of the tumor's life-cycle. A second point is that there is no certainty that the growth rate of a metastasis is similar to that of the primary tumor. These observations do not, however, negate the overall clinical usefulness of such growth rate investigations.

Figure 2 shows doubling times for 211 such cases in the author's series. The calculated growth rates form a continuous spectrum of tumor doubling times. A log-normal frequency distribution of randomly observed tumor diameters in primary and metastatic cancers supports the concept that tumor growth is by geometric progression.

Growth rates are not discontinuous as might be implied by an arbitrary classification into slow, intermediate, and rapid. The variability of growth

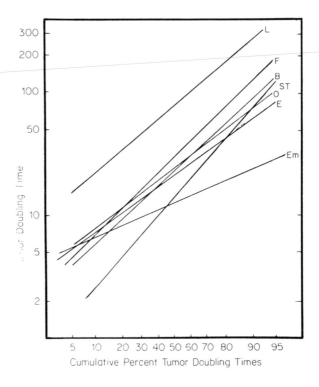

Figure 3 The cumulative relative frequency of the calculated doubling times of seven histopathological groups plotted on a log-probit graph. (F=fibrosarcoma, 29; B= breast cancer, mastectomy scar recurrence, 72; ST = soft tissue sarcoma, 70; O=osteogenic sarcoma, 158; E=Ewing's sarcoma, 21; E=embryonal cancer, testis, 35. The numbers indicate the number of observations.)

rates most likely represents a predetermined biological property of the tumor, modified to some degree by the tumor bed and the availability of nutrients. A specific growth rate is characteristic of an individual tumor (Charbit *et al.*, 1971; Pollack *et al.*, 1960; Spratt and Spratt, 1964; Spratt *et al.*, 1963a, b).

Survival time is the product of doubling time and the number of doublings. Survival time, therefore, is not a suitable yardstick by which to compare the results of treatment in different series of patients, without stratification by tumor growth characteristics of the samples under consideration.

The distribtion of tumor doubling times for seven histopathological types of cancer have been assembled in a log-probit graph (Figure 3). The distribution is log-normal for each type, though the slopes of the curves and their relative position vary. Charbit *et al.* (1971) recorded the doubling times of a number

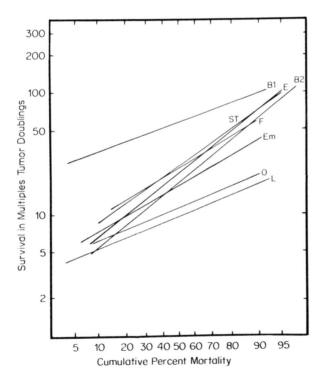

Figure 4 The cumulative mortality (survival) of the same histolpathological groups whose growth rates were plotted in Figure 3. These are assembled in a log-probit graph. Survival is recorded in multiples of tumor volume doublings for each tumor. (B1=breast cancer, survival from mastectomy; B2=breast cancer, survival from mastectomy scar recurrence; E=Ewing's sarcoma; ST= soft tissue sarcoma; F=fibrosarcoma; Em=embryonal carcinoma, testis; O=osteogenic sarcoma; L=lung cancer.)

of tumors in a similar manner. The distribution was log-normal and the plot of his curves fell into a series of parallel lines, suggesting that the growth pattern for each type was similar, varying only in the relative position of the curve (faster or slower growth rates). We were unable to confirm this relationship. Though the tumor growth curves are log-normal in distribution, each entity has a different slope, indicating a different spectrum of growth rates for each tumor type.

If relative malignancy depends upon the growth rate, then survival which is influenced by the rate of progression of the tumor should also be log-normal in distribution. The survival curves of the same group of patients, whose growth rate curves are illustrated in Figure 3 have been assembled in Figure 4. Survival has been recorded in multiples of tumor doublings. Survival follows a log-normal distribution when measured in this manner. Comparison of series of patients by their survival in terms of multiples of tumor doublings may be a better way to evaluate treatment.

The application of this principle to the analysis of a clinical problem is illustrated by the author's investigation of a group of 82 patients whose first evidence of spread following mastectomy for cancer of the breast was a scar recurrence. These patients fulfilled the following criteria. The recurrence was within the mastectomy scar or the graft; the area of recurrence was not within a previously irradiated field; and none of the patients received therapy other than routine post-operative irradiation. The interval between mastectomy and the scar recurrence was known. The tumor volume doubling time was calculated on the assumption that the first implant of a cell or clone occurred at the time of mastectomy. This would represent the shortest possible doubling time for the recurrent tumor.

Studies of the growth rate of breast cancer have been assembled in Table 3. Growth rates in two studies are based on mastectomy scar recurrence (Pearlman, 1976; Philippe and Le Gal, 1968) and in another two on the

Table 3 Breast cancer: tumor growth rates [a]. (Reproduced by permission of the Editors of *Cancer*)

Author(s)	Method of study	Growth rate		
		Rapid	Intermed.	Slow
Pearlman (1976	Scar recurr.	44(53%)	27(33%)	11(14%)
Philippe and Le Gal (1968)	Scar recurr.	33(42%)	34(42%)	11(16%)
Rigby-Jones (1962)	History	139(47%)	104(35%)	55(18%)
Charlson and Feinstein (1974)	History	121(55%)	66(30%)	33(15%)
Kusama *et al.* (1972)	Metastases	37(19%)	61(31%)	101(51%)

[a] For definition of growth rate see text.

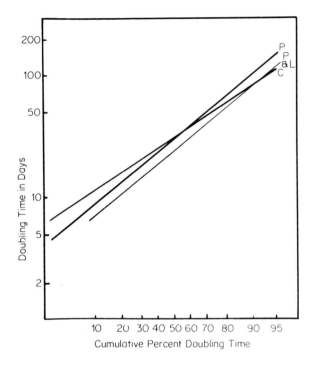

Figure 5 The cumulative relative frequency of the calculated doubling times of three series of breast cancer patients are assembled in a log-probability graph. (Pearlman (1976) (P) and Phillipe and Le Gal (1968) (P&L) are based on mastectomy scar recurrences but Charbit *et al.* (1971) (C) is based on primary breast cancer.)

analysis of the history (Charlson and Feinstein, 1974; Rigby-Jones, 1962). The latter groups are unselected, in contrast to the highly selected groups with scar recurrence. The series of Kusama *et al* (1972) had a preponderance of slowly growing tumors and differs from the others in that the patients had far advanced disease at first observation. The table shows that the other four studies have a similar distribution of the three categories of growth rate.

Calculated doubling times in three series of breast cancer are assembled in Figure 5. Two studies are based on mastectomy scar recurrences (P and P&L), and one on primary breast cancer (C). The distribution of the growth rates and the slopes of the curves are essentially similar.

The importance of recording survival in units of tumor doublings is further illustrated in Figure 6. The survival curves of groups of patients have been assembled, all with advanced disease and a uniformly poor prognosis. One group had mastectomy scar recurrence, and the other had sarcoma of soft tissue or bone. All were therapeutic failures. There was practically no

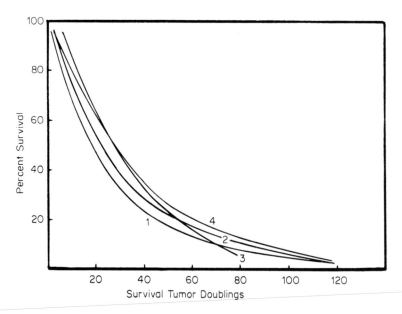

Figure 6 Survival as measured in tumor doublings are assembled in an arithmetical graph for two groups of patients. Curve 1, survival of breast cancer group after mastectomy scar recurrence; curve 2, sarcoma group—soft tissue and osseous, followed to death; curve 3, breast cancer subgroup, less than five-year survival from mastectomy; curve 4, breast cancer subgroup, over five–year survival after mastectomy.

difference in survival in terms of multiples of tumor doublings, despite differences in the growth rates of individual tumors and a wide range of survival times. The analysis of survival statistics in units of tumor doublings is therefore useful when comparing groups of patients with different histopathological types of tumor.

If doubling time truly influences survival, there should be a demonstrable difference in the distribution of growth rates between patient groups whose survival time differs. Tumor doubling times for the entire group of 211 patients in the author's series have been assembled in a log-probit curve (Figure 7, curve 3). The group was subdivided on the basis of survival time, i.e. five years or longer, 3–5 years, and less than three years and the distribution of the T_ds for each subgroup is shown (curves 1, 2 and 4). The relationship between growth rate and survival time is evident from the position of the curves. The breast cancer group alone was treated statistically in the same manner and the relationship is similar (curves 5, 6, and 7). There is a direct relationship between survival time and growth rate.

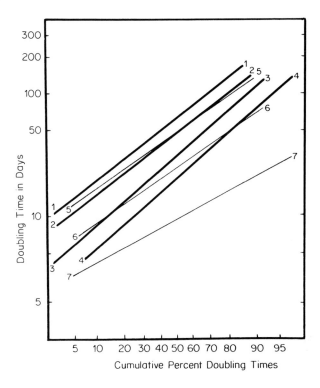

Figure 7 Cumulative mortality (survival) curves to demonstrate the influence of growth rate on survival. Curve 3 represents the distribution of the doubling times for the entire group of 211 patients (as Figure 2) and represents an average baseline. The group of patients has been divided into three subgroups based on survival times: curve 1, survival five years or longer; curve 2, survival 3–5 years; and curve 4, less than three years. Curves 5, 6, and 7 represent a similar analysis for breast cancer cases alone: curve 5, survival five years or longer; curve 6, survival 3–5 years; and curve 7, less than three years.

Charlson and Feinstein (1974), in their analysis of growth rates of breast cancer based on anamnesis, concluded that TNM staging does not provide a homogenous group of patients but contains proportions of each of the three growth rate categories in both Stages I and II. Five-year survivals in Stage I could range from 96% for slowly growing tumors to 75% for intermediate, and 50% for rapidly growing tumors (Figure 8). They showed that the influence of growth rate on prognosis is reflected in the five-year survival rates and is independent of treatment, whether simple or radical mastectomy.

Bloom (1965), in analyzing the influence of delay in seeking treatment upon prognosis, found that delays of less than three months and up to one

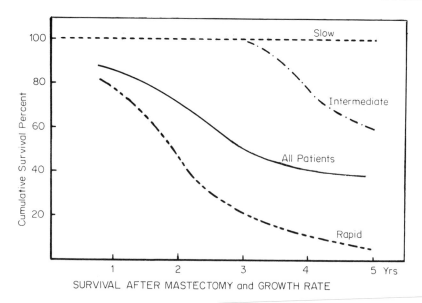

Figure 8 The cumulative percent of survivors for each yearly interval up to five years is correlated with the growth rate: slow, intermediate or rapid. (Reproduced by permission of American Cancer Society.)

year did not significantly influence survival rates at 5, 10, 15 or 20 years. There was little difference in the proportion of Stage I and II patients. The group with shortest delay presumably have more rapidly growing tumors which bring them to the physician earlier. Rigby-Jones (1962) correlated the influence of delay and tumor size with prognosis. There was no significant difference in survival with delays of less than three months as compared to 3–8 months, until the tumor size reached a diameter of 6 cm or larger. The latter obviously represent the more rapidly growing tumors.

The relationship between growth rates and five-year survival is illustrated in Table 4. Whether patients are selected or unselected, slowly growing tumors are associated with a five-year survival of 80–100%. Approximately two-thirds of the patients with intermediate growth also survive five years, while patients with rapidly growing tumors fare poorly (Figure 8). It is obvious that five years is insufficient follow-up for statistical purposes.

There were 67 patients in the author's series (Pearlman, 1976) whose course could be followed to death. The tumor growth rate was based on the known time interval between mastectomy and the first diagnosis of a scar recurrence of measurable size. Survival curves for those who survived more than five years are compared with those of patients who survived less than

Table 4 Breast cancer: Five-year survival and growth rate [a]. (Reproduced by permission of the Editors of *Cancer*)

Author(s)	Growth rate		
	Rapid	Intermed.	Slow
Pearlman (1976)	5%	62%	100%
Rigby-Jones (1962)	18%	63%	84%
Charlson and Feinstein (1974)	37%	64%	82%

[a] Includes all stages.

five years (Figure 9). Survival in multiples of tumor doublings was similar for both groups despite the variation and range of survival time.

Survival as measured in units of tumor doublings appears to be influenced to a minor degree by the growth rate of the tumor. Patients with rapidly growing tumors survive a greater number of doublings despite the shorter survival time (Figure 10). This was noted at all levels of survival. The same observation was made by Malaise *et al.* (1973, 1974) in a more heterogeneous group of patients.

The reason for this phenomenon is not clear, but a number of possible explanations have been advanced: (1) Calculation of the growth rate for rapidly growing tumors is probably less accurate than for slowly growing tumors, where slight inaccuracies in calculating time or mensuration errors are less critical. (2) Rapidly growing tumors are apt to be diagnosed earlier, when still small, and it requires a longer growth period for small tumors to reach the critical cell number. (3) The more rapid is the growth, the sooner will the tumor outgrow its blood supply. This would probably result in a slowing of the growth rate in the later stages, thus increasing the number of doublings the patient can survive.

CONCLUSION

(1) A constant growth rate (or doubling time) is characteristic of many malignant human tumors over a large part of their clinical history. But the period of clinical observation represents only a fraction of the entire life span of a tumor. An essential question is whether the total natural history of a tumor corresponds to an estimate based upon constant growth during the clinical phase.

(2) In a study of patients whose first evidence of recurrence after mastectomy was in the scar, it was found that recording survival as the number of tumor doublings brought the wide range of survival times into line.

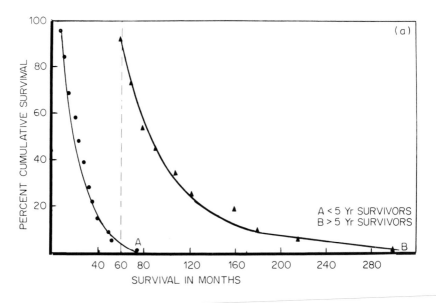

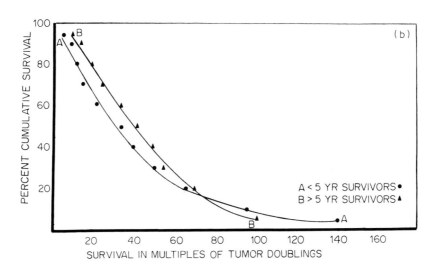

Figure 9 (a) Survival of two groups of patients with breast cancer, mastectomy scar recurrence. Survival has been recorded in months. Those surviving less than five years (curve A) are compared with those surviving more than five years (curve B). (b) The same group of patients whose survival has been recorded in Figure 9 (a). Survival is now measured in units of tumor doublings.

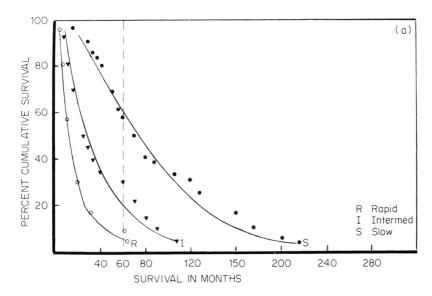

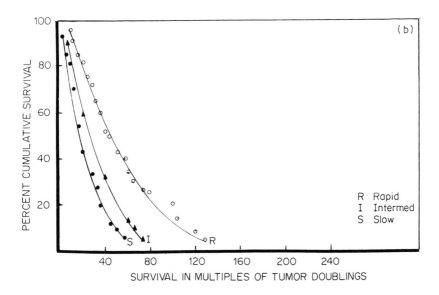

Figure 10 (a) Survival of the same group of patients as in Figure 9 (a). Survival is recorded in months. The patients have been subdivided into three groups based on the rate of tumor growth, i.e. rapid, intermediate, and slow. (b) Survival of the same groups as in Figure 10(a) now measured in units of tumor doublings.

The difference in survival of three groups (rapid, intermediate, and slow growth) was found to reflect their tumor doubling times. Whether patients survived more or less than five years, survival, as measured in terms of tumor doublings, was the same. It was independent of therapy.

The distribution of doubling times (T_d) within one histopathological type of cancer, and the survival of the same group recorded in multiples of tumor volume doublings, is log-normal. The individual's survival time is the product of the T_d and the number of T_ds the patient lives. Patients surviving the same number of tumor doublings may have a large range of survival times depending on the magnitude of the T_d.

(3) The concept of 'early' diagnosis needs to be qualified because of the existence of a long preclinical silent period preceding diagnosis. 'Early' diagnosis is not synonymous with a small tumor, and during the preclinical phase events may occur which will affect the patient's survival despite treatment, and biologically aggressive tumors tend to metastasize. Survival statistics which are based solely on clinical observations encompass only a limited portion of the life-cycle of the tumor.

(4) It has repeatedly been observed that survival rates do not necessarily decline with increasing delay in presentation. On the contrary, when patients with aggressive tumors have been eliminated, there remains a group whose longevity is greater than average. This phenomenon has been shown for many tumors, but especially those of lung, stomach, and breast. Large tumors may be present for many years, yet remain localized to the organ of origin. The clinical behavior of these tumors and the long survival of the patients reflects an indolent behavior, little influenced by treatment.

Acknowledgements

The author is grateful to Dr Milton Friedman, who reviewed and corrected the manuscript. His critical comments were incorporated into the text. Many of the patients included in this study were treated under the guidance of Dr Friedman.

REFERENCES

Bagshaw, K.D. (1968). Tumor growth and anti-mitotic action. *Br. J. Cancer*, **22**, 698.

Band, P.R., and Kocandrle, C. (1975). Growth rate of pulmonary metastases in human sarcoma. *Cancer*, **36**, 471.

Berkson, J. (1962). Prognosis of malignant tumors of the breast. *Acta Union Int. Contra Cancer*, **18**, 1003.

Bloom, H.J.G. (1965). The influence of delay on the natural history and prognosis of breast cancer. *Br. J. Cancer*, **19**, 228.

Bodian, M. (1959). Neuroblastoma. *Pediatr. Clin. N. Am.*, **6**, 449.

Brenner, M.W., Holsti, L.R., and Perttala, Y. (1967). The study by graphical analysis of the growth of human tumors and metastases of the lungs. *Br. J. Cancer*, , **22**, 1.

Bresciani, F., Pavluzi, R., Benassi, M., *et al.* (1974). Cell kinetics and growth of squamous cell carcinoma in man. *Cancer Res.*, **34**, 2405.

Breur, K. (1966). Growth rate and radiosensitivity of human tumors. *Eur. J. Cancer*, **2**, 157, 173.

Brues, A.M., Wenger, A.E., and Andervont, H.B. (1939). Relation between latent period and growth rate in chemically induced tumors. *Proc. Soc. Exp. Biol. Med.*, **43**, 374.

Campeljohn, R.S., Bone, G., and Aherne, W. (1956). Cell proliferation in rectal carcinoma and rectal mucosa. *Eur. J. Cancer*, **9**, 577.

Chahinian, A.P. (1972). Relationship between tumor doubling time and anatomo-clinical features in 50 measurable pulmonary cancers. *Chest*, **61**, 340.

Chahinian, A.P., and Israel, L. (1976). Rates and patterns of growth in lung cancer. *Curr. Artic. Neoplasia*, **97**, 10, 95.

Charbit, A., Malaise, E.P., and Tubiana, M. (1971). Relation between the pathologic-al nature and the growth rate of human tumors. *Eur. J. Cancer*, **7**, 307.

Charlson, M.E., and Feinstein, A.R. (1974). The auxometric dimension. *J. Am. Med. Assoc.*, **228**, 180.

Collins, V.P. (1958). The treatment of Wilms' tumor. *Cancer*, **11**, 89.

Collins, V.P., Loeffler, R.K., and Tivey, H. (1956) Observations on growth rates of human tumors. *Am. J. Roentgenol.*, **Radium Ther. Nucl. Med.**, **11**, 988.

Fabrikant, J.I. (1971). The kinetics of cellular proliferation in normal or malignant tissues. *Radiology*, **111**, 700.

Friedman, M.F., Nervi, C., Casale, C., *et al.* (1973). Significance of growth rates, cell kinetics and histology in the irradiation and chemotherapy of squamous cell carcinoma of the mouth. *Cancer*, **31**, 10.

Frindel, E., Malaise, E., and Tubiana, M. (1968). Cell proliferation kinetics in five solid human tumors. *Cancer*, **22**, 611.

Garland, H.L. (1966). The rate of growth and natural duration of primary bronchial cancer. *Am. J. Roentgenol.*, *Radium Ther. Nucl. Med.*, **96**, 604.

Garland, L.H., Coulson, W., and Wolin, E. (1963). The rate of growth and apparent duration of untreated primary bronchial carcinoma. *Cancer*, **16**, 694.

Gershon-Cohen, J., Berger, S.M., and Klickstein, H.S. (1962). Reontgenography of breast cancer moderating concept of biologic predeterminism. *Cancer*, **16**, 961.

Hewitt, H.B., and Wilson, C.W. (1959). A survival curve for mammalian leukemia cells irradiated *in vivo*. *Br. J. Cancer*, **13**, 69.

Iverson, O.H. (1967). Kinetics of cellular proliferation and cell loss in human carcinomas. *Eur. J. Cancer*, **3**, 389.

Joseph, W.L., Morton, D.L., and Adkins, P.C. (1971). Prognostic significance of tumor doubling time in evaluating operability in pulmonary metastatic disease. *J. Thorac. Cardiovasc. Surg.*, **61**, 23.

Kieswetter, W.B., and Mason, E.J. (1960). Malignant tumors in childhood. *J. Am. Med. Assoc.*, **172**, 1117.

Knox, W.E., and Pillars, E. (1958). Time of recurrence and cure of tumors of childhood. *Lancet*, **i**, 188.

Krutova, T.V., and Korman, D.B. (1976). Correlation between doubling time of volume of human lung tumors. *Bull. Exp. Biol. Med.*, **81**, 73

Kusama, S., Spratt, J.S., Donegan, W.L., *et al.* (1972). The gross rates of growth of human mammary cancer. *Cancer*, **25**, 594.

Laird, A.K. (1965). Dynamics of tumor growth. Comparison of growth rates and extrapolation of growth curve to one cell. *Br. J. Cancer*, **19**, 278.

Lamerton, L.F. (1972). Cell proliferation and the differential response of normal and malignant tissues. *Br. J. Radiol.*, **45**, 161.

Malaise, E.P., Chavaudra, N., Charbit, A., and Tubiana, M. (1974). Relationship between growth rate of human metastases survival and pathological type. *Eur. J. Cancer,* **10**, 451.

Malaise, E.P., Chavaudra, N., and Tubiana, M. (1973). The relationship between growth rate, labeling index, and histological type of human solid tumor. *Eur. J. Cancer,* **9**, 305.

Mayneord, W.V. (1932). On law of growth of Jensen's rat sarcoma. *Am. J. Cancer,* **16**, 841.

Mendelsohn, M.L., Dohan, F.C., and Moore, H.A. (1960). Autoradiographic analysis of cell proliferation in spontaneous breast cancer of C3H mouse. *J. Natl. Cancer Inst.,* **25**, 477, 485.

Mottram, J.C. (1935). On origin of tar tumors in mice. *J. Pathol. Bacteriol.,* **40**, 407.

Mottram, J.C. (1936). Further considerations of growth rates in tar warts in mice and their antigrafts. *Am. J. Cancer,* **28**, 115.

Nathan, M.H., Collins, V.P., and Adams, R.A. (1962). Differentiation of benign and malignant pulmonary nodules by growth rate. *Radiology,* **79**, 221.

Patt, H.M., and Blackford, M.E. (1954). Quantitative studies of growth response of Krebs ascites tumor. *Cancer Res.,* **14**, 391.

Pearlman, A.W. (1973). Growth rate investigations and tumor lethal dose in Ewing's sarcoma. *Acta Radiol.,* **12**, 57.

Pearlman, A.W. (1976). Breast cancer: influence of growth rate on prognosis and treatment evaluation. *Cancer,* **38**, 1826.

Pearlman, A.W. (1979). Fibrosarcoma—the biomathematical approach to late metastases. *Mt Sinai J. Med,* **46**, 255.

Philippe, E., and Le Gal, Y. (1968). Growth of 78 recurrent mammary carcinomas. *Cancer,* **21**, 461.

Plesnicar, S., Klanjscek, G., et al. (1976). Signficance of doubling time vaslues in patients with pulmonary metastases of osteogenic sarcoma. *Cancer Lett.,* **1**, 351.

Pollack, W.F., Hastings, N., and Snyder, W.H. (1960). The Collin's period of risk formula for malignant tumors in children. *Surgery,* **48**, 606.

Rigby-Jones, P. (1962). Prognosis of malignant tumors of the breast in relation to rate of growth and axillary lymph nodes observed clinically. *Acta Union Int. Contra Cancer,* **18**, 815.

Rosenoer, V.M., and Curby, W.A. (1975). Growth kinetics of solid tumours. *Med. Clin. N. Am.,* **59**, 339.

Schwartz, M. (1961), A biomathematical approach to clinical tumor growth. *Cancer,* **14**, 1272.

Shackney, S.E. (1976). Role of radioautographic studies in clinical investigative oncology and chemotherapy *Cancer Treat. Rep.,* **60**, 1873.

Silvestrini, R., Sanfillipo, L., et al. (1974). Kinetics of human mammary carcinomas and their correlation with the cancer and the host characteristics. *Cancer,* **34**, 1252.

Smithers, D.W. (1968). Clinical assessment of growth rate in human tumors. *Clin. Radiol.,* **19**, 113.

Spratt, J.S., and Ackerman, L.V. (1961). The growth of a colonic adenocarcinoma. *Am. J. Surg.,* **27**, 23.

Spratt, J.S., Spjut, H.J., and Roper, Ch. L. (1963a). The frequency distribution of the growth rates and the estimated duration of primary pulmonary carcinomas. *Acta Union Int. Contra Cancer,* **19**, 6.

Spratt, J.S., and Spratt, Th. L. (1964). Rates of growth of pulmonary metastases and host survival. *Am. J. Surg.,* **159**, 161.

Spratt, J.S., Ter-Pergossian, M., and Long, R.T.L. (1963b). The detection and growth of intrathoracic neoplasms. *Arch. Surg.*, **86**, 283.

Steel, G.G. (1967). Cell loss as a factor in the growth rate of human tumors. *Eur. J. Cancer*, **3**, 381.

Steel, G. G. (1968). Cell loss from experimental tumors *Cell Tissue Kinet.*, **3**, 193.

Straus, M.J. (1974). Growth characteristics of lung cancer and its application to treatment design. *Semin. Oncol.*, **3**, 167.

Sutow, W.W. (1958). Prognosis in neuroblastoma of childhood. *Am. Med. Assoc. J. Dis. Childh.*, **96**, 299.

Tubiana, M. (1971). Kinetics of tumor cell proliferation and radiotherapy. *Br. J. Radiol.*, **44**, 325.

Tubiana, M. and Malaise, E.P. (1976). Growth rate and cell kinetics in human tumors. *Scientific foundations of oncology* (eds E. Symington, and R.L. Carter). London: Heinemann Medical. p. 126.

Tubiana, M., Richard, J.M., and Malaise, E.P. (1975). Kinetics of tumor growth and of cell proliferation. *Laryngoscope,* **85**, 1039.

Weiss, W. (1973), The growth rate of bronchogenic carcinoma. Is it constant? *Cancer,* **32**, 167.

Cancer Treatment: End Point Evaluation
Edited by B.A. Stoll
© 1983 John Wiley & Sons Ltd.

Chapter

13 K.-R. TROTT

In Vivo Measurements on the Tumour Predicting Response

INTRODUCTION

This chapter will review attempts to recognize early tissue changes in human cancer, in the hope of identifying those responses to therapy which can predict local cure. It is important to gain information during therapy on the individual sensitivity of each tumour, so that we can give the dose the tumour needs, instead of the dose that most normal tissues tolerate.

In order to allow alternative treatment to be initiated in time, information on the individual tumour sensitivity has to be available early. This is either in the first few weeks of therapy if the alternative is to change to another treatment, at completion of the prescribed treatment dose if the intention is to increase the dose further, or within the first few weeks after completion of therapy if the alternative is elective surgery of the residual tumour or other therapy. (In the case of radiotherapy, response of a tumour would need to be analysed about two weeks after the start of treatment, or at the completion of therapy, or at 1–3 months later).

The methods of assesment which may be applied during the first few weeks of therapy are:

The rate of tumour shrinkage.
Histological changes in biopsies.
Proliferative and other changes in the tumour, studied in biopsies by special methods.

At completion of therapy or a few weeks after therapy, the prognosis might be predicted from studying:

Residual macroscopic tumour.
Residual microscopic tumour.

THE HETEROGENEITY OF RESPONSE

The sensitivity of different tumours to chemotherapy varies widely, but this is less so in the case of radiotherapy. Local control doses for tumours of similar size but different histological groups show little variation in clinical radiotherapy, and squamous cell carcinomas and adenocarcinomas have about the same radiosensitivity (Trott, 1982), On the other hand, variability in chemosensitivity between different histological groups and subgroups is generally much greater, even between different individuals with apparently identical tumours.

Much more than for chemotherapy, the site seems to be of particular importance for the radiosensitivity of some tumours. Especially for squamous cell carcinomas of the head and neck, small changes in anatomical extension may influence radiosensitivity considerably (Suit and Walker, 1980). More often, however, the radiosensitivity of the neighbouring normal tissues influences the dose which can be safely given in any tumour site and thus leads to the marked influence of tumour localization on radiocurability. In chemotherapy, these factors are of relatively minor importance.

Tumour size may be the most important prognostic factor assessable before initiating radiotherapy and chemotherapy. Local cure results from the inactivation of all clonogenic tumour cells: if more tumour cells have to be inactivated, a higher dose of radiation or drug is needed. Experiments by Steel and Adams (1975) demonstrated that the probability of control of induced lung metastases by a tolerated dose of cyclophosphamide decreased rapidly as the tumour load increased. Similarly in radiotherapy, Suit (1973) showed that the radiation dose necessary to cure murine adenocarcinomas increases by about 2.5 Gy for each doubling of the tumour volume.

Data on human tumours are scarce. Hjelm-Hansen *et al.* (1979) showed that the local control rate of squamous cell carcinomas treated with the same dose decreased as their diameter increased. In order to compensate for the increased tumour volume, each increase in diameter of 1 cm requires an additional dose of 3–5 Gy to be given (Figure 1).

Tumours are often graded by the pathologist according to their degree of anaplasia and proliferative activity. In some tumours the influence of tumour anaplasia on prognosis is very pronounced but, often, it is the mode of tumour growth and tumour spread which is influenced by the degree of anaplasia, rather than its radiosensitivity (Trott, 1982).

Even if allowance is made for these various factors before radiotherapy, one cannot define one 'curative' dose for any type of cancer. In a homogeneous group of tumours such as cancer of the larynx stage $T_{3-4}N_0M_0$,

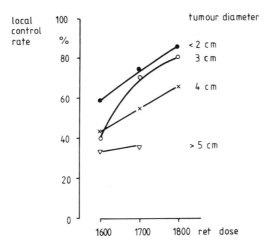

Figure 1 The dependence of local control rates in carcinomas of the larynx of different size, on NSD-dose of irradiation. (Data from Hjelm-Hansen *et al.*, 1979.)

treated in 40–50 days with 27–29 fractions, the chances of local tumour control depends on radiation dose, and increases with increasing dose according to an S-shaped dose–response curve (Figure 2). In practice, this means that 20% of all patients could be treated successfully with a dose of 55 Gy whereas another 20% would need more than 59 Gy. In other tumours, the spread of individual radiosensitivity is even bigger, the dose differences between the most sensitive 20% and the most resistant 20% being more than 20 Gy (Thames *et al.*, 1980).

THE RELATION OF TUMOUR REGRESSION TO TUMOUR CURE

Radiosensitivity of a malignant tumour is thought to be associated with prompt regression *during* radiotherapy. Tumours which do not shrink or even progress in size during radiotherapy are regarded as being radioresistant. In the pioneering days of radiotherapy, individual tumour radiosensitivity was assessed by giving a large single dose, and deciding further treatment according to the volume response of the tumour after the test dose (Kienböck, 1907), and much the same principle is often used in chemotherapy today.

In some radiotherapy departments, head and neck tumours are still treated according to such a schedule, i.e. by normal fractionation to a dose of 40 or 50 Gy, and the regression pattern recorded. Those tumours which respond well get further radiotherapy to the full 'curative' dose, whereas those which do not shrink sufficiently are sent for elective surgery or receive palliative

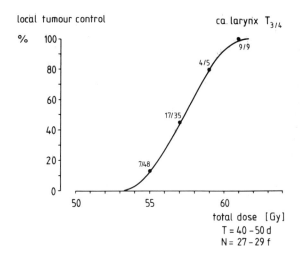

Figure 2 The dependence on total dose of local control rate in T_{3-4} carcinomas of the larynx treated by radiotherapy in 27–29 fractions in 40–50 days. (Data from Maciejewski *et al.*, 1983.)

treatment because they are regarded as basically radioresistant (Lederman, 1972; Bohndorf, 1981; Walther *et al.*, 1982). Even now, regression during therapy is the most common criterion for defining tumour radiosensitivity, for assessing prognosis, and for selecting treatment policy for the individual patient. However, there is little experimental and clinical basis for thus assessing individual radiosensitivity by recording the macroscopic tumour response.

Even radioresponsive tumours usually regress slowly during radiotherapy compared to the rate at which the number of surviving clonogenic tumour cells decreases (Figure 3). Therefore, after the first few radiation doses in a course of fractionated irradiation, any assessment of macroscopic or microscopic tumour deals predominantly with doomed cells. If there is any correlation with the processes leading to tumour control, it has to be indirect, rather than a causative relation.

In Chapter 3, animal experiments on tumour regression after fractionated radiotherapy have indicated that the regression pattern is an inherent biological characteristic of every tumour and is only loosely related to the radiosensitivity of the tumour. From these animal experiments it may be concluded that tumour regression during the course of fractionated radiotherapy is not likely to be a reliable predictor of the risk of local tumour recurrence after attempts of curative radiotherapy. Although for some tumours and some fractionation schedules there is a significantly faster or

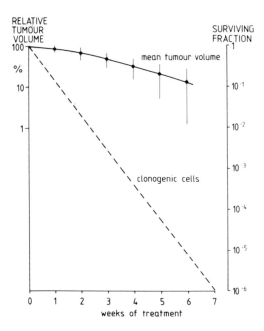

Figure 3 Comparison of volume regression in a series of 12 oropharyngeal carcinomas during radiotherapy (data from Fletcher *et al.*, 1963), with the decrease in the fraction of tumour cells with unlimited proliferative capacity. Tumour cure is assumed to occur at a surviving fraction of less than 10^{-6}.

more extensive regression in those tumours which are eventually cured, it is far from being clinically useful and could not be generalized from one tumour to another or from one schedule to another.

In chemotherapy, regression of the tumour is a basic criterion for assessing response. The same type of mouse tumour treated with different effective cytotoxic drugs responds consistently with the same regression pattern, proving that tumour regression reflects processes involved in cell removal rather than in cell killing. In breast cancer patients too, it has been shown that the regression rate is the same for cytotoxic and radiation treatment in the same individual, although there are 30-fold differences between individuals (Thomlinson, 1982). This means that the curative effectiveness of cytotoxic agents in different patients cannot be meaningfully compared, using the local rate of tumour regression as a criterion.

Individual correlation between human tumour regression and local control by radiotherapy has so far been studied at three tumour sites, all involving squamous cell carcinomas — in the oropharynx (and other head and neck sites), uterine cervix, and bronchus. The selection of these sites was probably

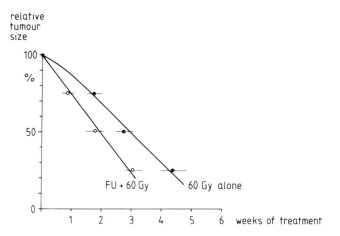

Figure 4 Regression of carcinomas of the oropharynx treated either by radiotherapy alone or radiotherapy plus fluorouracil. (Data from Fletcher *et al.*, 1963.) The points are the geometric means of the times to shrink to the stated volume ± their standard error.

due to the accessibility of these tumours to inspection or palpation. The experience gained in these tumours cannot, however, be extrapolated to other histology or to other sites where the tumour can now be measured with improved imaging techniques (Husband, 1980; Quivey *et al.*, 1980).

Head and neck cancers

In the first analysis of tumours of the oropharynx, Suit *et al.* (1965) concluded that regression rate was independent of the outcome of treatment. Moreover, increasing the speed of regression by adding fluorouracil did not increase local control rate (Fletcher *et al.*, 1963) (Figure 4). However, the data on which the original analysis of Suit was based were reviewed later by Barkley and Fletcher (1977). They contended that in the original study a bias was working against any prognostic correlation, since at that time total dose was based on tumour regression: slowly regressing tumours were generally given higher doses since they were regarded as more radioresistant.

As a result of the first analysis, subsequent patients received the same dose irrespective of the individual regression rate. In the new series of 125 patients, Barkley and Fletcher (1977) reported a statistically significant correlation between local control and absence of palpable or detectable tumour at completion of treatment. Of 22 patients (T_{2-3}) showing residual disease, 12 had a recurrence, while of 68 patients showing no apparent residual tumour at completion of therapy, only 15 had a local recurrence.

Despite statistical significance, the prognostic accuracy in this study is not very good, as less than 50% of the recurrences were detected in this way, and its application depends very much on the conclusions that are drawn from this information. The most important lesson from this study may be that, if the radiation dose for the individual patient is based on the assumption that rapidly shrinking tumours are more radiosensitive and therefore need a lower radiation dose, fatal underdosage will occur in those patients who display rapid tumour regression.

Fazekas *et al.* (1972) grouped a series of 49 patients with squamous cell carcinoma of the oral cavity and oropharynx according to whether the clinical impression of tumour clearance or of residual disease at termination of radiotherapy was correct or not. They concluded that there was no correlation between long-term tumour control and the presence or absence of residual local induration.

Sobel *et al.* (1976) reported a study on the relation of initial tumour response to long-term control after radiotherapy in 124 patients with cancer of the oral cavity and oropharynx. Tumour clearance was assessed at four different intervals: 30 days after the start of treatment, at completion of treatment, about two months and about six months after completion of treatment. The following questions were studied:

> Does the rate of regression predict local control or recurrence?
> Does the complete clearance of a tumour predict local control?
> Does persistence of induration predict local failure or recurrence?

In 60 patients with tumours of the oral cavity, the regression rate during radiotherapy was identical for cures and failures, but complete clearance at completion of radiotherapy carried a significantly better prognosis than persistent disease. However, the prognostic accuracy of tumour persistence is poor, and 38% of patients with residual disease at the end of the treatment course eventually attained local control. It was not until the end of a three-month follow-up interval that persistence of induration could reliably (in about 90% of cases) predict later recurrence. Results in 64 patients with carcinomas of the oropharynx were similar, with tumour persistence at three months again carrying a very poor prognosis (100% local recurrence rate).

Sobel *et al.* (1976) concluded that the clinical parameters for the assessment of tumour response at completion of treatment are *not* accurate enough to predict the final outcome. The decision whether to proceed with irradiation after test doses (of 50–60% of the initially prescribed dose) or to perform surgery should not be based on the degree of tumour regression. Moreover, salvage surgery in patients with tumour persistence after irradiation did not improve prognosis.

Mäntylä *et al.* (1979) measured tumour regression at mid-treatment and at the end of treatment in 110 patients with head and neck cancer (mostly carcinomas of the larynx). Local control rates in tumours showing complete regression either at mid-treatment or after treatment were significantly better than in those who showed only partial remission. Yet the *practical* prognostic value of either early shrinkage or persistent tumour at the end of treatment was poor. In small tumours (T_{1-2}, N_0), 50% of the tumours persistent at the end of the radiotherapy course were controlled locally, and more than 50% of the advanced tumours (either T_{3-4} or N_{1-3}) with complete remission at the end of treatment developed a local recurrence within two years. The histological differentiation did not correlate with tumour regression either at mid-treatment or end of radiotherapy.

Another study on over 500 cases of various head and neck tumours was published by Dawes (1980), who confirmed that patients with incomplete tumour response one month after completion of treatment had a much poorer prognosis than patients showing complete response. However, the 'false positive rate' was over 20%, which was regarded by Suit and Walker (1980) as the limit of clinical usefulness. Only three months after treatment was the predictive accuracy of persistent tumour better, as the 'false positive rate' had decreased to less than 15%.

Cancer of the uterine cervix

Three studies have been published on the relation of initial tumour response to long-term control in carcinoma of the uterine cervix. Marcial and Bosch (1970) concluded from a retrospective analysis of 469 patients with various stages of cervical cancer treated by external radiotherapy followed by intracavitary radium that patients with tumours regressing completely by the end of external radiotherapy showed excellent survival. However, less than 15% of all patients had complete tumour clearance after external radiotherapy, and 90% of them were Stage I and IIa. Therefore, rapid tumour clearance was merely an indicator of a small tumour mass with the associated good prognosis of small tumours!

Except for this favourable response of small tumours, no prognostic value could be assigned to tumour clearance rates during treatment or even one month after radiotherapy. Late complete tumour regression was not associated with a worse prognosis than early regression.

Similar conclusions have to be drawn from data published by Grossman *et al.* (1973) on 526 patients with various stages of cancer of the uterine cervix. Tumour size was assessed in a semiquantitative way at bi-weekly intervals during radiotherapy and three, six, and 12 months after radiotherapy. The mean tumour size decreased during radiotherapy and reached a plateau about three months after completion (Figure 5).

The degree of tumour regression during and soon after the completion of radiotherapy was closely related to five-year survival: cancer-free survival was

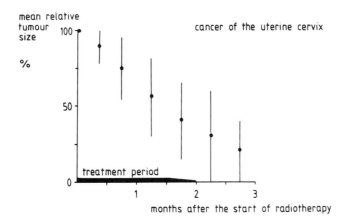

Figure 5 Regression of carcinomas of the uterine cervix during radiotherapy (6–8 weeks) and after radiotherapy. (Data from Grossman *et al.*, 1973.)

69% in patients with excellent early response but only 29% in patients with poor early response. However, as in the study of Marcial and Bosch (1970), this effect was mostly due to the better initial response of small tumours. Except for Stage II there was *no* statistically significant influence of tumour response on prognosis stage by stage. Even in Stage II, despite its statistical significance, quantitation of response at completion of treatment (6–8 weeks after the start of radiotherapy) was practically useless for determining prognosis (Suit and Walker, 1980), despite the optimistic conclusions drawn by Grossman *et al.* (1973) from their data.

The third study on 116 patients with advanced carcinoma of the uterine cervix was published by Dische and Saunders (1980) and Dische *et al.* (1980). They were the only ones to find a highly significant association between local tumour control and reduction in bulk of tumour at the cervix, measured 1–2 weeks after external radiotherapy (given either in air or high-pressure oxygen). In contrast to the studies of Marcial and Bosch (1970) and Grossman *et al.* (1973), no gross influence of tumour size or tumour stage on regression was found.

The interpretation of this study is complicated by the fact that it was part of a randomized clinical trial on the use of radiotherapy with high-pressure oxygen (HPO). Dische (1974) had shown previously that HPO radiotherapy was associated with better initial response, as well as better long-term control and survival. In the HPO group 80% of the patients had more than 50% tumour regression, while about 55% of the air group had a similar response. The difference in initial response between both treatment modalities was more significant than in local tumour control.

Dische *et al.* (1980) claimed that HPO was the reason for the improvement of local control in the randomized trial, which showed up already two weeks after external radiotherapy by increased tumour regression rate. Stratification of the tumours according to regression rates abolishes the positive effect of HPO on local control and survival. The correlation of HPO to regression rate *and* local control warns us against using these data in the final conclusions on the predictive value of tumour regression. No data on tumour regression rates in HPO trials in head and neck cancer are available. However, increasing the regression rate of head and neck tumours by adding fluorouracil (Figure 4) did not significantly increase the local tumour control rate (Fletcher *et al.*, 1963).

Apart from carcinoma of the uterine cervix and some head and neck sites, no association between initial volume response and prognosis has been reported. Dische and Saunders (1980) did not observe any correlation in 35 patients with carcinoma of the bronchus.

Summarizing the clinical evidence in squamous cell carcinomas at two sites treated by radiotherapy, it is evident that regression rate *during* treatment usually gave no prognostic information, but some sort of correlation between tumour regression and long-term prognosis was demonstrated in most studies soon *after* treatment. Reliable prediction of local failure, however, was not possible earlier than 1–3 months after completion of therapy. This is too late to consider alternative primary treatment modalities. Moreover, it appears that, in any case, elective surgery for residual disease does not have any significant influence on prognosis. Modulation of regression rate by combined treatment modalities (e.g. chemotherapy or HPO) may or may not influence long-term prognosis.

HISTOLOGICAL CHANGES IN BIOPSIES

Various attempts have been made to assess the treatment response of human tumours by biopsies taken during or after radiotherapy, but very few animal experiments have been performed to validate the applied criteria. Quantitative histological analysis was the most frequently used technique in biopsies taken either after about one-third of the total dose had been given, or at completion of radiotherapy.

The criteria for analysis and the prognostic value in carcinoma of the uterine cervix were recently analysed by Trott (1980). As with macroscopic tumour response, the predictive value of the histological assessment depended very much on the timing of the assay: yet, whereas for macroscopic assessment it was better at the end of or after treatment, the histological assessment was best predictive early in the course of radiotherapy.

Histology during treatment

Dubrauszky (1966), Glücksmann (1941), and Gusberg and Herman (1962) proposed radiosensitivity tests based on a biopsy taken 1–2 weeks after a radiation dose of 10–20 Gy. The most widely discussed assay, developed by Glücksmann and Spear (1945), compared a biopsy taken before radiotherapy with another one taken one week after radium treatment. In an area of growing tumour near normal tissues tumour cells were differentially counted according to four cell types.

The presence of viable, resting, and interphase cells and of normal mitoses indicated a poor prognosis. Only if their frequency decreased to less than 30% of the total cell count one week after the first radium treatment was the response called favourable. On the other hand, both degenerating and differentiating cells were regarded as signs of a favourable response, and for this their number had to show an increase by the first week of radiotherapy.

Glücksmann (1974) summarized his experience on more than 1100 patients with carcinoma of the uterine cervix. The prognosis in those patients who showed an unfavourable histological response was generally very poor, with five-year survival rates in Stages II and III of 11% and 12% respectively, whereas for those patients responding favourably, survival rates were 68% and 74% respectively. Elective surgery after radiotherapy of Stage II carcinoma of the uterine cervix was more beneficial to those patients who had an unfavourable radiation response than to those who had a favourable radiation response in the biopsy. Whereas McGarrity and Garvan (1961) confirmed the prognostic value of Glücksmann's assay, Limburg *et al.*, (1972) did not find a statistically significant correlation of histological response with survival.

Similar assays developed independently by Gusberg and Herman (1962) and by Dubrauszky (1966) for quantitating the response of carcinoma of the cervix to radiotherapy have been compared to that of Glücksmann and Trott (1980). All methods involve differential counting of either degenerate cells (Dubrauszky) or of cells with prominent nucleoli (Gusberg) or of differentiating, keratinizing cells (Glücksmann), and comparing this count with the number of small, viable, undifferentiated cells (which was the common denominator in all three assays). The prognostic value of the methods employed by Glücksmann and Dubrauszky in Stage III cannot be compared directly since the overall treatment results were very different (Trott, 1980), yet favourable histological response was associated in both studies with long-term control in 74% and 80% respectively whereas unfavourable response predicted failure in the majority of cases (89% and 60% respectively).

Histology after treatment

Dische and Saunders (1980) observed that the histological evaluation of biopsies from carcinomas of the uterine cervix taken *after* radiotherapy did not yield useful prognostic information. It was less than that from assessing the degree of clinical regression.

In histological tests performed after radiotherapy, the criterion of response is the presence or absence of viable-looking tumour cells. This examination is made routinely by pathologists on specimens after pre-operative radiotherapy but its prognostic and therapeutic implications have only rarely been investigated (Tohorst, 1981). Eichhorn and Hüttner (1982) studied the effectiveness of different pre-operative radiotherapy schedules in carcinoma of the bronchus by comparing the frequency of histologically negative specimens, and observed that multiple small doses gave superior results to few large doses. Total doses were equivalent to more than 1800 ret, which might be sufficient to sterilize small carcinomas of the bronchus, yet local clearance rates at operation were below 20% from doses per fraction of 4–5 Gy. However, the long-term predictive value of histological tumour clearance soon after radiotherapy for bronchial carcinoma has not been investigated.

Autopsy findings have been analysed at variable intervals after radiotherapy for carcinoma of the bronchus, in those patients who died from distant metastasis. Eichhorn (1981) tested different fractionation schemes with this end-point, and found better clearance with small doses than with large doses per fraction. Eichhorn and Lessel (1977) recorded better response of carcinoma of the bronchus to neutrons than to photons. Holsti *et al.*, (1980) compared the 'curative' doses for small cell and squamous cell tumours of the bronchus.

In animal experiments, Suit and Gallager (1964) demonstrated residual foci of viable-looking tumour cells in locally controlled adenocarcinomas of the mouse. Trott (1983) described similar viable foci in mouse tumours of different histology, weeks and months after radiation doses which prevented local recurrence with above 90% probability.

In human adenocarcinomas, similar observations after radiotherapy were reported. Biopsies performed after radical radiotherapy of the prostate were positive for many months without indicating local failure of treatment. The positive biopsy rate correlated only with the interval after irradiation but not with prognosis (Cox and Stoffel, 1977; Kagan *et al.*, 1977; Perez *et al.*, 1980). Similar observations after pre-operative radiotherapy for adenocarcinomas of the uterus (Wilson *et al.*, 1980) and of the rectum (Rider, 1977) suggest a common biological behaviour of irradiated adenocarcinomas which limits the predictive information of post-irradiation histology.

On the other hand, after pre-operative radiotherapy of bladder cancers, the histological response observed in the surgical specimen may give valuable prognostic information (van der Werff-Messing, 1979). In those tumours (T_3)

treated with 40 Gy/4 weeks with no tumour cells left in the histological specimen, the long-term survival rate was over 50% compared to 20% in those who showed no change compared to the pre-irradiation biopsy. A similar correlation of tumour control with histological tumour clearance after pre-operative radiotherapy in bilharzial bladder cancer was reported by Awwad *et al.*, (1979). No correlation was shown with the histopathological classification of radiation damage of tumour cells.

These differences between tumours in the predictive value of tumour histology after radiotherapy reflect the fact that effective radiotherapy schedules leave only very few clonogenic cells in the uncontrolled tumours, and they cannot be identified under the microscope within the rapidly or slowly disintegrating bulk of doomed tumour cells.

OTHER BIOLOGICAL INVESTIGATIONS

In order to improve the prognostic accuracy of information gained from looking at a biopsy during or after radiotherapy, various additional tests have been performed on the biopsy material to quantitate its viability. The methods range from primary culture to clonogenic survival *in vitro* and xenograft growth in immunosuppressed mice (Tohorst, 1981). These methods are discussed in other chapters.

Some authors have looked at cell proliferation after *in vitro* incubation with ^{3}H-TdR and observed some prognostic correlation with the decrease in labelling index during radiotherapy in carcinoma of the cervix (Fettig *et al.*, 1973; Tatra and Breitenecker, 1975). Courdi *et al.*, (1980) found a progressive decrease of the labelling index in adenocarcinomas of the rectum with increasing radiation dose but obtained no prognostic information. Moreover, the low labelling index after pre-operative radiotherapy rose rapidly back to normal values if surgery was delayed after pre-operative radiotherapy, even for only a few days (Metzger and Kummermehr, 1981).

Autoradiography of biopsies during radiotherapy does not appear to improve the prognostic information which can be derived from routine histological examination. Yet data from serial labelling experiments during chemotherapy may be more promising, since some suggest a positive correlation with tumour remission (Murphy *et al.*, 1975).

More attention should be given to flow cytofluorometry (FCF) techniques which are presently developing very rapidly. Several studies have demonstrated changes in the DNA distribution pattern during radiotherapy but their clinical and prognostic implications are still unknown (Linden *et al.*, 1980). In chemotherapy, the response of leukaemic stem lines in the bone marrow can be quantitated during therapy and might have prognostic implications (Hiddemann *et al.*, 1982). However, so far, sound data on the relation of FCF data to long-term control of tumours are lacking.

CONCLUSION

It would be very useful to be able to identify, in a group of cancer patients, those needing high radiation or chemotherapy doses, and those who could be spared high doses with their accompanying risk of complications. As long as the possibility of selecting patients according to their individual tumour sensitivity does not exist, treatment doses are prescribed to the maximum which normal tissues tolerate without excessive damage. This implies that a large number of patients are given higher doses than those necessary for cure, while other patients are underdosed.

Tumour regression reflects processes involved in cell removal rather than in cell killing. There may be, in some tumours, an indirect association between inherent sensitivity to treatment and the speed and mode of tumour cell clearance, and this may allow predictions to be made. But so far, we are unable to determine in which tumours this end-point may be relevant or not, as we do not know the mechanisms underlying such an apparent association.

To establish a predictive test, it is not sufficient to demonstrate macroscopic or microscopic changes occurring during radio- or chemotherapy or to show differences between different tumour types. We are aiming at the early identification of those individuals who will fail to be cured among a group of patients stratified according to our best knowledge of risk factors. Some clinical or pathological methods are already of some help in some tumours, but no new method has been shown to give any better results. Yet, the individualization of treatment is critically dependent on the validity of prognostic tests.

REFERENCES

Awwad, H., El-Baki, H.A., El-Bolkainy, N., Burgers, M., El-Badawy, S., Mansour, M., Soliman, O., Omar, S., and Khafagy, M. (1979). Preoperative irradiation of T_3-carcinoma in bilharzial bladder. A comparison between hyperfractionation and conventional fractionation. *Int. J. Radiat. Oncol., Biol. Phys.*, **5**, 787.

Barkley, H.T., and Fletcher, G.H. (1977). The significance of residual disease after external irradiation of squamous cell carcinoma of the oropharynx. *Radiology*, **124**, 493.

Bohndorf, W. (1981). Zur Vorbestrahlung bei Hals-Nasen-Ohren-tumoren. In *Kombinierte chirurgische und radiologische Therapie maligner Tumoren*. (ed. M. Wannenmacher). München, Wien, Baltimore: Urban and Schwarzenberg.

Courdi, A., Tubiana, M., Chavaudra, N., LeFur, R., and Malaise, E.P. (1980). Changes in labeling indices of human tumors after irradiation. *Int. J. Radiat. Oncol., Biol. Phys.*, **6**, 1639.

Cox, J.D., and Stoffel, T.J. (1977). The significance of needle biopsy after irradiation for stage C adenocarcinoma of the prostate. *Cancer*, **40**, 156.

Dawes, P.J.D.K. (1980). The early response of oral, oropharyngeal, hypopharyngeal and laryngeal cancer related to local control and survival. *Br. J. Cancer*, **41**, Suppl. IV, 14.

Dische, S. (1974). The hyperbaric oxygen chamber in the radiotherapy of carcinoma of the uterine cervix. *Br. J. Radiol.*, **47**, 99.

Dische, S., Bennett, M.H., Saunders, M.I., and Anderson, P. (1980). Tumour regression as a guide to prognosis: a clinical study. *Br. J. Radiol.*, **53**, 454.

Dische, S., and Saunders, M.I. (1980). Tumour regression and prognosis: a clinical study. *Br. J. Cancer*, **41**, *Suppl.* IV, 11.

Dubrauszky, V. (1966). Assessment of radiosensitivity of carcinoma of the cervix. *J. Obstet. Gynaecol. Br. Commonw.*, **73**, 41.

Eichhorn, H.J. (1981). Different fractionation schemes tested by histological examination of autopsy specimens from lung cancer patients. *Br. J. Radiol.*, **54**, 132.

Eichhorn, H.J., and Hüttner, J. (1982). Der Einfluss unterschiedlicher Einzeldosen und Fraktionszahlen auf die Strahlenwirkung. *Strahlentherapie*, **158**, 151.

Eichhorn, J.J., and Lessel, A. (1977). Four years experiences with combined neutron–telecobalt therapy. Investigations on tumour reaction of lung cancer. *Int. J. Radiat. Oncol., Biol. Phys.*, **3**, 277.

Fazekas, J.T., Green J.P., Vaeth, J.M., and Schroeder, A. (1972). Post-irradiation induration as a prognosticator. *Radiology*, **102**, 409.

Fettig, O., Kaltenbach, F.B., and Kloke, W.D. (1973). Der '3H-Thymidin-Test' zur Beurteilung der Strahlensensibilität des Collum Carcinoms. *Arch. Gynäkol.*, **213**, 283.

Fletcher, G.H., Suit, H.D., Howe, C.D., Samuels, M., Jesse, R.H., and Villareal, R.U. (1963). Clinical method of testing radiation-sensitizing agents in squamous cell carcinoma. *Cancer*, **16**, 355.

Glücksmann, A. (1941). Preliminary observation on the quantitative examination of human biopsy material taken from irradiated carcinomata. *Br. J. Radiol.*, **14**, 187.

Glücksmann, A. (1974). Histological features in the local radiocurability of carcinomas. In *The biological and clinical basis of radiosensitivity* (ed. M. Friedman). Springfield: C.C. Thomas.

Glücksmann, A., and Spear, F.G. (1945). The qualitative and quantitative histological examination of biopsy material from patients treated by radiation for carcinoma of the cervix uteri. *Br. J. Radiol.*, **18**, 313.

Grossman, I., Kurohara, S.S., Webster, J.H., and George, F.W. (1973). The prognostic significance of tumor response during radiotherapy in cervical carcinoma. *Radiology*, **107**, 411.

Gusberg, S.B., and Herman, G.G. (1962). Radiosensitivity testing of cervix cancer by the test dose technique. *Am. J. Roentgenol.*, **87**, 60.

Hiddemann, W., Clarkson, B.D., Büchner, T., Melamed, M.R., and Andreeff, M. (1982). Bone marrow cell count per cubic millimeter bone marrow: a new parameter for quantitating therapy-induced cytoreduction in acute leukemia. *Blood*, **59**, 216.

Hjelm-Hansen, M., Jorgenson, K., Anderson, A.P., and Lund, C. (1979). Laryngeal carcinoma – II. Analysis of treatment results using the Ellis model. *Acta Radiol. Ther., Biol. Phys.*, **5**, 385.

Holsti, L.R., Rissanen, P.M., Torsti, R., and Kairento, A.L. (1980). Autopsy analysis of the effective radiation dose sterilizing bronchial carcinoma. *Br. J. Cancer*, **41**, Suppl. IV, 48.

Husband, J. (1980). Diagnostic techniques: their strengths and weaknesses. *Br. J. Cancer*, **41**, Suppl. IV, 21.

Kagan, A.R., Gordon, J., Cooper, J.R., Gilbert, H., Nussbaum, H., and Chan, P. (1977). A clinical appraisal of post-irradiation biopsy in prostatic cancer. *Cancer*, **39**, 637.

Kienböck, R. (1907). *Radiotherapie. Ihre biologischen Grundlagen, Anwendungsmethoden und Indikationen.* Stuttgart : Enke.

Lederman, M. (1972). Radiation therapy in cancer of the larynx. *J. Am. Med. Assoc.,* **221**, 1253.

Limburg, H., Napp, J.H., and Wilbrand, V. (1972). Die prognostische Beurteilung des Kollumkarzinoms nach Strahlenbehandlung durch Probeentnahme und Scheidenabstrich. *Geburtshilfe Frauenheilkunde*, **12**, 723.

Linden, W.A., Köllermann, M., and König, K. (1980). Flow cytometric and autoradiographic studies of human kidney carcinomas surgically removed after preirradiation. *Br. J. Cancer*, **41**, Suppl. IV, 177.

McGarrity, K.A., and Garvan, J.M. (1961). Results of assessment of irradiation response in the treatment of carcinoma of the uterine cervix by evaluation of serial biopsies. In *Radiobiology. Proceedings of the Third Australasian Conference.* London: Butterworths.

Maciejewski, B., Preuss-Bayer, G., and Trott, K.-R. (1983). The influence of the number of fractions and of overall treatment time on local control and complication rate in squamous cell carcinoma of the larynx. *Int. J. Radiat. Oncol., Biol. Phys.,* (in press).

Mäntylä, M., Kortekangas, A.E., Valavaara, R.A., and Nordman, E.M. (1979). Tumour regression during radiation treatment as a guide to prognosis. *Br. J. Radiol.,* **52**, 972.

Marcial, V.A., and Bosch, A. (1970). Radiation-induced tumor regression in carcinoma of the uterine cervix: prognostic significance. *Am. J. Roentgenol.,* **108**, 113.

Metzger, H., and Kummermehr, J. (1981). Vergleich der Proliferationsmuster nach Kurzzeit- und Langzeitvorbestrahlung beim colorectalen Karzinom. In *Kombinierte chirurgische und radiologische Therapie maligner Tumoren* (ed. M. Wannenmacher). Urban and Schwarzenberg. München, Wien, Baltimore:

Murphy, W.K., Livingston, R.B., Ruis, V.G., Gercovich, F.G., George, S.L., Hart, J.S., and Freireich, E.J. (1975). Serial labeling index determination as a predictor of response in human solid tumors. *Cancer Res.,* **35**, 1438.

Perez, C.A., Walz, B.J., Zivnuska, F.R., Pilepich, M., Prasad, K., and Bauer, W. (1980). Irradiation of carcinoma of the prostate localized to the pelvis: analysis of tumor response and prognosis. *Int. J. Radiat. Oncol., Biol. Phys.,* **6**, 555.

Quivey, J.M., Castro, J.R., Chen, G.T.Y., Moss, A., and Marks, W.M. (1980). Computerized tomography in the quantitative assessment of tumour response. *Br. J. Cancer*, **41**, Suppl. IV, 30.

Rider, W.D. (1977). Radiation for rectal cancer. *J. Can. Med. Assoc.,* 117, 1119.

Sobel, S., Rubin, P., Keller, B., and Poulter, C. (1976). Tumor persistence as a predictor of outcome after radiation therapy of head and neck cancers. *Int. J. Radiat. Oncol., Biol. Phys.,* **1**, 873.

Steel, G.G., and Adams, K. (1975). Stem cell survival and tumor control in the Lewis lung carcinoma. *Cancer Res.,* **35**, 1530.

Suit, H.D. (1973). Radiation biology: a basis for radiotherapy. In *Textbook of radiotherapy,* 2nd edn. (ed. G.H. Fletcher). Philadelphia: Lea and Febiger.

Suit, H.D., and Gallager, H.S. (1964). Intact tumor cells in irradiated tissue. *Arch. Pathol.,* **78**, 648.

Suit, H.D., Lindberg, R., and Fletcher, G.H. (1965). Prognostic significance of extent of tumor regression at completion of radiation therapy. *Radiology,* **84**, 1110.

Suit, H.D., and Walker, A.M. (1980). Assessment of the response of tumours to radiation: clinical and experimental studies. *Br. J. Cancer,* **41**, Suppl. IV, 1.

Tatra, C., and Breitenecker, G. (1975). Der klinische Wert histoautoradiographischer Untersuchungen während der Strahlentherapie des Zervixkarzinoms. *Strahlentherapie*, **150**, 487.

Thames, H.D., Peters, L.J., Spanos, W., and Fletcher, G.H. (1980). Dose response of squamous cell carcinomas of the upper respiratory and digestive tracts. *Br. J. Cancer*, **41**, Suppl. IV, 35.

Thomlinson, R.H. (1982). Measurement and management of carcinoma of the breast. *Clin. Radiol.*, **33**, 481.

Tohorst, J. (1981). Aussagemöglichkeiten der Pathologie nach Bestrahlungsbehandlung maligner Tumoren. In *Kombinierte chirurgische und radiologische Therapie maligner Tumoren* (ed. M. Wannenmacher). München, Wien, Baltimore: Urban and Schwarzenberg.

Trott, K.R. (1980). Can tumour response be assessed from a biopsy? *Br. J. Cancer*, **41**, Suppl. IV, 163.

Trott, K.R. (1983). Prognostic value of tumour pathology. In *Biological bases and clinical implications of tumor radioresistance* (eds. C. Nervi, G. Archangeli, and G.H. Fletcher). Springfield: C.C. Thomas.

van der Werff-Messing, B. (1979). Preoperative irradiation followed by cystectomy to treat carcinoma of the urinary bladder category T3, Nx 0–4, M0. *Int. J. Radiat. Oncol., Biol. Phys.*, **5**, 394.

Walther, E., Hünig, R., Wey, W., Krauer, W., and Roth, J. (1982). Die präoperative Radiotherapie von Pflasterzellkarzinomen im Oropharynx und Cavum oris. In *Verhandlungsberichte der Deutschen Krebsgesellschaft*. München: G. Schwabe Verlag.

Wilson, J.F., Cox, J.D., Chabazian, C.M., and del Regato, J.A. (1980). Time dose relationship in endometrial adenocarcinoma: importance of the interval from external pelvic irradiation to surgery. *Int. J. Radiat. Oncol., Biol. Phys.*, **6**, 597.

Cancer Treatment: End Point Evaluation
Edited by B.A. Stoll
© 1983 John Wiley & Sons Ltd.

Chapter

14 H.B. KAL and G.W. BARENDSEN

In Vitro Methods for Predicting Response

INTRODUCTION

Tumours of different types show differing degrees of response to radiation or chemical agents, and this applies to a lesser extent also to tumours of similar type. It would be useful to have reproducible quantitative assays of tumour responsiveness to specific treatments, which could then be used as a guide to such therapy.

Experimental developments in this field depend to a large extent on the availability of experimental tumours in inbred strains of animals, which can be transplanted and studied by a variety of methods. The manifestations of response which are of most clinical interest are tumour volume reduction, growth delay, and local control, and these depend on changes in cell proliferation and reproductive death. However, tumour growth rate and its modification depend not only on cell division and the cell cycle time of proliferating cells but also on the fraction of these cells, the life span of non-proliferating cells, and cell loss. Consequently, volume changes in tumours after treatment do not directly reflect the fraction of cells inactivated (see Chapter 3).

By contrast, the eradication of a tumour is clearly dependent on cell death, since it requires permanent abolition of the reproductive capacity of all malignant cells. Therefore, the dose of an agent required to achieve tumour control is determined by the sensitivity of the individual cells or subpopulations of cells. Quantitative information on this point can be obtained by excision of the tumour and the inoculation or transplantation of cells into a new host or by assay with techniques involving *in vitro* cultures.

The technique of disaggregation of solid tumours and the preparation of monodispersed cell suspensions was developed by Reinhold (1965a). Assay techniques which can be applied to study the reproductive capacity of these cells include the end-point dilution assay (Hewitt and Wilson, 1959), the growth latency assay (Clifton and Draper, 1963), the lung colony assay (Hill and Bush, 1969), and the *in vitro* colony assay (Barendsen and Broerse, 1969).

In all studies in which tumours are excised and cells are studied by various techniques, three main criteria must be satisfied. First, it is necessary to ascertain that the cell suspension obtained provides a representative sample of the cells initially present in the tumour. Secondly, the assay of the properties of cells should be performed in such a way that the conditions are optimal for the expression of these properties. Thirdly, it is necessary to investigate whether the characteristics analysed are relevant for cells in undisrupted tumours.

If the conditions for a relevant assay are met, excision and *in vitro* assay techniques can provide information on the mechanisms which determine malignant growth of solid tumours and on their reaction to various treatments. Furthermore, for experimental tumours, *in vitro* methods are more rapid and far more economical than *in vivo* assay procedures.

In the application of *in vitro* assay methods to the prediction of response by human tumours, especially to chemotherapeutic drugs, progress has generally been slow. Low plating efficiency and the long culture periods required are responsible for ambiguity in predicting response to treatment in the patient. Further improvements (e.g. using agar culture conditions) are required to improve the correlation with clinical tumour sensitivity.

In the following sections, various aspects of *in vitro* techniques for assessment of tumour response will be evaluated under the headings of:

> Experimental tumour models developed for *in vitro* assays.
> Relevance of information from *in vitro* assays.
> *In vitro* assays of response by human tumours.

EXPERIMENTAL TUMOUR MODELS DEVELOPED FOR *IN VITRO* ASSAYS

Selection of tumours and hosts

Commonly used experimental tumours are generally rapidly growing and have growth rates and cell proliferation patterns different from those of the primary tumour or human tumours. These biological differences must be considered critically when experimental tumours are used as models for human cancer. Therefore, radiobiological data on response in animal tumours cannot be as readily extrapolated to clinical situations as those on radiation response in normal tissues. Nevertheless, studies of response in experimental tumours can provide important insights into biological processes in tumours at the cellular level, and these insights may result in improved treatment of cancer in man.

Experimental tumours induced by chemicals (e.g. benzopyrene) or by viruses are frequently immunogenic. Results obtained from studies in which immunogenic tumours are employed are generally difficult to interpret. This is especially true when different end-points, such as tumour growth delay or local control, and *in vitro* survival are compared. Therefore, experimental tumours must be carefully selected to assure that they are not immunogenic (Rasey *et al.*, 1977; Reinhold, 1965b).

In addition, to minimize the individual variations in reactions to experimental conditions and treatment, highly inbred animals must be used to provide syngeneic hosts for tumour transplantion.

Selection of *in vivo* – *in vitro* tumours

The first experimental solid tumour which allowed quantitative plating of cells *in vitro* with a high plating efficiency was derived from a rat rhabdomyosacroma by the application of a controlled selection procedure (Barendsen and Broerse, 1969). First, a cell suspension of the BA 1112 tumour (Reinhold, 1965a) was cultured in MEM medium. A fraction of the cells adhered to the culture dish and a few clones developed with growth as monolayers. A single clone was isolated and inoculated into the flank of a rat of the WAG/Rij inbred strain in which the BA 1112 tumour had originally developed. Cells from the tumour resulting from this inoculum were again cultured and a single clone was selected for inoculation into a WAG/Rij rat. This procedure was repeated several times and resulted in the *in vivo* – *in vitro* system designated as R-1 in 1966.

The *in vivo* – *in vitro* system has subsequently been developed for other types of transplantable tumours and they are being used for a variety of quantitative studies (Rockwell, 1977). The cloning efficiencies of these *in vivo* – *in vitro* tumours range from a few per cent to 30 or 40%; the cloning efficiencies of the original donor tumours, in general, are only a few per cent or less.

It is important to note that the tumours selected for *in vitro* quantitative analysis may have features which are significantly different from those of the donor tumours (Kal *et al.*, 1983). Thus, although they are useful for experimental studies, the results should not be considered applicable to the original primary tumour. In addition, during continued culturing, changes can occur in culture or in transplanted tumours which make the properties of the subsequent generations significantly different from the preceding tumour transplants (Jung *et al.*, 1980; Beck *et al.*, 1981).

Sample requirement

A basic requirement of *in vivo* – *in vitro* assays for solid tumours is that the cell suspensions prepared from the tumours should provide a representative sample of the cells present in the donor tumour, and that cells of subpopulations are not selectively lost due to the disaggregation procedure. The cell yield is generally significantly less than 50% and may be as low as 1%.

Several subpopulations of cells can be distinguished in a tumour according to their various characteristics. Tumours contain both malignant cells and cells of normal origin which form blood vessels and other structural elements. For some tumours, the malignant cells have a different DNA content from that of normal ones and this can be analysed (e.g. by flow cytofluorimetry techniques). However, an increased DNA content is by no means a general characteristic difference between tumour and normal cells (Kal, 1973a; Beck *et al.*, 1981).

Another problem is that cells in tumours may be present in a resting state (G_0 phase). This may be due to conditions in the microenvironment (e.g. inadequate supply of oxygen and nutrients), but other tumour characteristics (e.g. differentiation properties) might also increase the fraction of non-cycling cells. Cells in different proliferative states may be differentially susceptible to damage by the enzyme procedure employed to obtain a single cell suspension and this may result in selection of cells. In addition, it is known that tumours may contain fractions of hypoxic cells. If lack of oxygen or nutrients causes cells to be in a non-proliferating phase, a correlation between hypoxic fractions and the proportion of cells in G_0 should be expected. Finally, among the population of cells in progress through the proliferative cycle, cells in G_1, S, G_2, and M can be distinguished (Kal, 1973b).

It is evident, therefore, that it is not possible to establish in all experiments with cells from excised tumours whether certain subpopulations of cells are selectively lost due to the disaggregation procedure. Furthermore, grossly haemorrhagic and necrotic tissue from tumours are generally discarded before preparing the tumour cell suspension, yet these regions contain viable cells (Jirtle and Clifton, 1978). Thus, an unrepresentative sample of the tumour will be obtained if these necrotic regions are not included.

Nevertheless, for each type of tumour to be studied for its response to radiation or drugs, at least some experiments on this sampling problem should be carried out. For example, labelling of cells with ^{3}H-TdR to distinguish G_0, S, and G_2 cells or employing flow cytofluorimetry techniques.

With the R-1 tumour, repeated injections of ^{3}H-TdR at 4 h intervals have been used to label all proliferating cells and to distinguish these from non-proliferating cells (Barendsen *et al.*, 1973; Hermens and Barendsen, 1979). After the last injection, tumours were excised, cell suspensions prepared, and cells were cultured for different time intervals up to 120 h. The labelling index of cells in 12 h cultures was 0.48, which was not significantly different from the value of 0.51 for cells in the tumour. This indicates that the cell dispersion technique employed to prepare cell suspensions from these R-1 tumours did not exclusively select proliferating or non-proliferating cells (Barendsen *et al.*, 1973). Comparable data have been obtained for the mouse EMT6 tumour system (Kallman *et al.*, 1980).

A similar conclusion could be drawn concerning the distribution of cells over the cell cycle phases. DNA histograms obtained with flow cyto-fluorimetry of the cells in suspension can provide an indication of whether the distribution of cells over the cell cycle phases is normal. However, this can be deduced only from DNA histograms for which the DNA content of tumour cells differs from that of the normal cells present in the tumour.For the R-1 rat rhabdomyosarcoma, the DNA contents of tumour cells and normal cells differ by a factor of 1.4. It was shown that a radiation dose of 20 Gy administered to R-1 cells *in vitro* and to R-1 tumours *in situ* induced similar changes in the distributions of cells over the cell cycle phases as a function of time after treatment (Kal, 1973a). This also indicates that no preferential selection of cells occurred in the suspension.

RELEVANCE OF INFORMATION FROM *IN VITRO* ASSAYS

To assess the relevance of information obtained from *in vitro* assays on cells from experimental solid tumours, it is important to study different types of responses to treatment. For irradiation of some tumours, good agreement has been observed between the degree of cell kill and cure rate, but in comparing these end-points with growth delay, the discrepancies observed could only be resolved by detailed studies of cell proliferation (Barendsen, 1980). For some chemical agents (particularly in combination with radiation) discrepancies between results obtained for different end-points are as yet unresolved (Kal and Barendsen, 1980). A few examples of results and problems will be presented below.

Quantitative *in vitro* culturing of isolated tumour cells

The technical procedure for the quantitative culturing of tumour cells *in vitro* involves the following steps:

> The preparation of a cell suspension according to the cell dispersion technique described by Reinhold (1966).
> Determination of the concentration of cells in the cell suspension by use of a Bürke chamber or electronic cell counter.
> Plating of a known number of cells into culture dishes.
> Culturing of cells in a 37°C incubator for a period of 8–10 days.
> Fixing and counting of colonies.

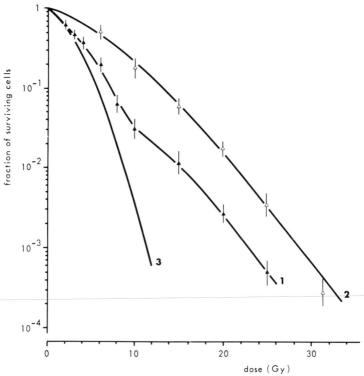

Figure 1 Survival curves obtained by irradiation of R–1 rhabdomyosarcomas growing in the flanks of WAG/Rij rats followed by excision of the tumour and plating of cells *in vitro*. Curves 1 and 2: tumours irradiated with 300 kV x-rays in anaesthetized and dead (to obtain anoxia) animals (closed and open diamonds, respectively). Curves 2 and 3: R–1 cells irradiated *in vitro* in equilibrium with nitrogen and oxygen, respectively (included for comparison).

Using this technique for cells derived directly from a tumour, the fractions of clonogenic cells can be determined for tumours which have been treated with various single or fractionated doses of radiation or drugs. With this assay method, survival curves for tumour cell populations irradiated *in vivo* can be derived (Figure 1). The assay is not complicated by host factors operating against the tumour cells. A disadvantage of the technique is that accurate and reproducible results are obtained only for doses where the surviving fractions of cells range between 1 and 10^{-4}. However, for the interpretation of results obtained after treatment, this range is useful.

The disaggregation procedure using trypsin developed by Reinhold (1965a) has been used for many tumour systems. In addition, an enzyme 'cocktail' containing collagenase, pronase, and DNAse has been applied (Brown *et al.*,

1979). It has been shown that different enzyme treatments used for the disaggregation of the tumours result in different cell yields. For the mouse EMT6/UW tumours, the cell yield was increased from $(2-3) \times 10^6$ cells/g to 4×10^7 cells/g, i.e. about 20% of the total tumour cell population was obtained with the enzyme cocktail as compared with a few per cent by the trypsin method (Rasey and Nelson, 1980).

The trypsin and enzyme cocktail procedures yielded equally representative samples of the total tumour cell populations as demonstrated by the survival data obtained after radiation treatment. However, tumours treated with cyclophosphamide showed a lesser cell survival when cells were isolated with the enzyme cocktail than with trypsin, whereas the opposite result was obtained for bleomycin-treated tumours. This indicates that different tumour disaggregation methods can influence survival of tumour cells after cytotoxic treatment, presumably due to interaction of drug-caused damage and enzyme injury (Rasey and Nelson, 1980).

Several corrections are necessary to relate the cloning efficiency observed to the fraction of surviving cells following treatment. In general, after a single dose of radiation, the fraction of surviving cells can be calculated from the ratio of the cloning efficiencies of the treated and control tumour cells. However, when fractionated irradiation is used, the cell yield and the tumour volume are generally different from those of control tumours at the time of the start of treatment.

Figure 2 illustrates changes occurring in cell yield and volume after treatment of a rat rhabdomyosarcoma with a dose of 10 Gy of x-rays or methotrexate at 3×10 mg/kg at 4 h intervals. To correct for these differences, the fraction of surviving cells as a result of the treatment can be calculated (Barendsen and Broerse, 1970; Kal and Barendsen, 1972).

With the *in vitro* assay, direct determination of tumour cell survival can be made but these data are generally not sufficient to describe the course of events in the undisturbed tumour. By contrast, *in situ* assays preserve the tumour environment but give only indirect estimates of tumour cell survival. The relations between results of *in vitro* assays and *in situ* responses may differ among various experimental tumours. For the rat rhabdomyosarcoma R-1, however, the fraction of surviving cells could be directly correlated with tumour cure rates (Barendsen and Broerse, 1970).

A major cause of discrepancies between different methods of assay in several experimental tumour systems is recovery from potentially lethal damage (PLD). Little *et al.* (1973) and Hahn *et al.* (1974) showed that, for the EMT6 and NCTC tumours, there was an increase in cell survival with time of excision, the increase reaching a peak within 6–24 h after a dose of radiation. Shipley *et al.* (1975) and McNally and Sheldon (1977) later demonstrated a similar phenomenon in the Lewis lung carcinoma and the carcinoma MT, respectively.

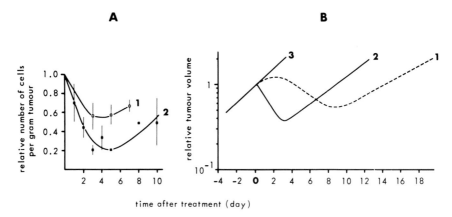

Figure 2 (A) Relative number of R–1 rhabdomyosarcoma cells per gram tumour obtained with the disaggregation method as a function of time after treatment with a dose of 10 Gy of 300 kV x-rays (curve 1) or methotrexate administered i.p. three times at 10 mg/kg, 4 h interval (curve 2). (B) Tumour volume changes in R–1 rhabdomyosarcomas as a function of time after treatment with a dose of 10 Gy of 300 kV x-rays (curve 1) or methotrexate administered i.p. three times at 10 mg/kg, 4 h interval (curve 2); the control tumour is also indicated (curve 3).

Comparison of *in situ* assays and *in vitro* clonogenic assays

The simplest technique for assessment of response to radiation or drugs is the determination of tumour volume at a specified time interval after treatment in comparison with that at the start of treatment (Bogden *et al.*, 1978). In general, this method is useful for screening purposes, i.e. to investigate after a short time interval whether there is a significant response to a treatment.

Transplants into animals may be used in this way for screening the sensitivity of surgically obtained human tumour material (Figure 3). The relevance of the data obtained for the prediction of growth delay and control is difficult to assess and may relate to: uncertainties about the contribution of inactivated cells which are not immediately eliminated but may produce a limited number of progeny; non-cycling cells and their life span; blood vessels and other stromal elements. For experimental tumours, it is therefore not sufficient to limit observations to one or a few measurements at specific time intervals after treatment, but volume changes should be determined until the tumour has regrown to at least the volume at the start of the treatment.

The second method used for analysis of tumour response *in situ* is volume measurement during the entire period of regression and recurrence, and this provides adequate data for the calculation of growth delay. This method has been employed for a very large number of animal tumours treated by

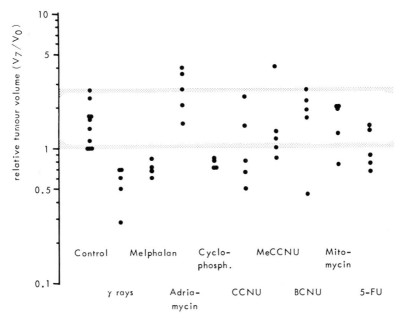

Figure 3 Relative tumour volumes of human colon tumour transplants following different treatments. Drugs were administered 24 h after transplantation of the tumour fragment under the kidney capsule of mice. Irradiations were performed on days 1 and 5 after transplantation. Tumour volumes were measured on day 0 (V_0) and on day 7 (V_7) (T. Smink, personal communication).

radiation, drugs, hyperthermia, and combinations of these modalities. Using this tumour growth delay end-point, it is of great importance to determine whether immunological differences exist between the tumour and its host, as these may influence the outcome of the treatment. In addition, factors not directly related to cell reproductive death can result in delayed recurrence. Damage to the tumour 'bed' including the vasculature may result in slower regrowth, while slow removal of dead cells can also influence changes in the volume depending on the time at which growth delay is assessed (Begg, 1980).

In Figure 4 examples are presented of data on volume responses of an experimental rat rhabdomyosarcoma, R-1, treated with different doses of x-rays. The curves show that after single doses in excess of 30 Gy the tumours disappear but recur after intervals which increase with the dose. At doses in excess of 60 Gy, a fraction of the tumours does not recur. The rate at which the tumours regress is independent of the dose, for doses in excess of 30 Gy. The numerical quantity commonly derived from these curves is the number of

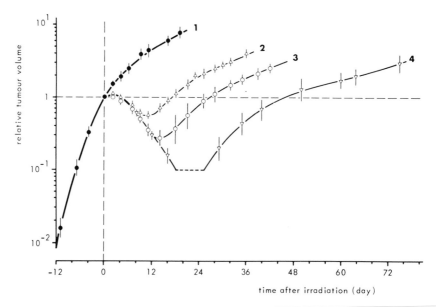

Figure 4 Tumour volume changes in R–1 rhabdomyosarcomas as a function of time after irradiation. Curve 1: the growth of unirradiated tumours. Curves 2 to 4: obtained after irradiation with doses of 20, 30, and 40 Gy of 300 kV x-rays, respectively.

days required by the tumour to regrow to the same volume that it had at the start of the treatment.

The third end-point used for experimental studies of tumour responses *in situ* is the local control probability. This probability increases only for doses in excess of a threshold value. As illustrated in Figure 4, the R-1 tumours all recur after doses of up to 40 Gy. The probability of local control increases with dose for the rat rhabdomyosarcoma. The TCD_{50}, i.e. the dose to obtain 50% cure, is 61.5 ± 2 Gy (Barendsen and Broerse, 1969). In Figure 5, tumour growth delay is presented as a function of the accumulated dose of 300 kV x-rays. This figure also indicates the single dose required for obtaining 90% local control (TCD_{90}), calculated by extrapolation of the survival curve obtained for the R-1 tumour with the *in vitro* assay (arrow a) and the observed TCD_{90} for 300 kV x-rays (arrow b).

Data on local control of tumours can be considered an extension of those on growth delay and, in general, conclusions from experiments on growth delay agree with those from experiments on local control. Local control of experimental tumours is equivalent to the end-point of major interest to clinicians, but because of the many differences in growth characteristics between experimental tumours in animals and primary cancer in man,

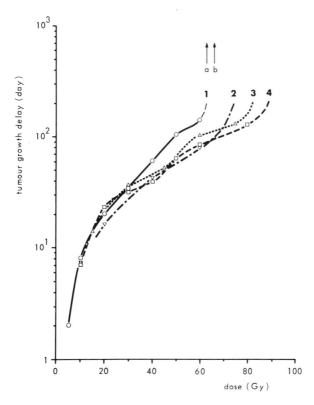

Figure 5 Tumour growth delay of R–1 rhabdomyosarcomas as a function of accumulated dose of 300 kV x-rays. Curve 1: single doses. Curves 2 to 4: daily doses of 4, 3, and 2 Gy, respectively, applied five times a week for different numbers of weeks. Arrow 'a' indicates the single dose of 300 kV x-rays calculated on the basis of a survival curve required for attaining a cure rate of 90%; arrow 'b' indicates the observed TCD_{90}.

conclusions from experimental data on local control should not be considered as more relevant to the clinical situation than data on growth delay.

IN VITRO ASSAYS OF RESPONSE BY HUMAN TUMOURS

In vitro methods of assessing the clonogenic capacity of cells from experimental tumours treated *in vivo* have been applied to assess the responsiveness of human tumour cells to treatment. These methods aim to determine the sensitivity (specifically to chemotherapeutic drugs) of tumour cells derived from fresh human tumour material, in the hope that the responsiveness *in vitro* has a predictive value with respect to clinical response.

Long-term cultures; Clonogenic cell assay

Interest in the use of clonogenic cell assays to study the chemosensitivity of solid human tumours was stimulated by the work of Hamburger and Salmon (1977). They showed that it is possible to obtain useful information from cultured human tumour cells, although plating efficiencies in the order of 0.1–0.01% were observed. As a result of their observations, the technique is now being widely studied, both to develop methodology and to attempt to validate the original premises (Pavelic *et al.*, 1980).

Salmon *et al.*, (1978) collected bone marrow cells from patients with myeloma, malignant ovarian effusions, and tumour nodules obtained by laparotomy. Single cell suspensions of these cell populations were made. Cell suspensions were transferred to tubes and adjusted to a final concentration of 1×10^6 cells per millilitre. These cells were then exposed to a variety of chemotherapeutic drugs. To obtain a dose–effect relationship, each drug was tested at a minimum of three dose levels for 1 h at 37°C in Hanks' balanced salt solution. The cells were then centrifuged, washed, and suspended in agar medium supplemented with horse serum and the addition of 2-mercaptoethanol. One millilitre of the mixture was added to a petri dish containing conditioned medium in a 1 ml agar feeder layer. Cultures were incubated at 37°C. Colonies appeared in 10–21 days. Plates were examined for drug effects after about 14 days.

This clonogenic assay used accessible tumours that could readily be converted into single cell suspensions containing a sufficient number of viable tumour cells. However, the cloning efficiency of human tumours is low (about 0.01% to a few per cent), comparable to that observed for normal human bone marrow granulocytic and erythroid progenitors *in vitro* (Pike and Robinson, 1970: Tepperman *et al.*, 1974).

Alberts *et al.* (1980) reported on the application of this clonogenic cell assay to tumour material from 40 patients with overian cancer, and 13 of 21 patients responded clinically to drugs predicted to be effective *in vitro*. Prediction of *in vitro* resistance was 99% accurate. They concluded that this assay can be effectively used to plan a suitable chemotherapy regimen for ovarian cancer patients. Since drug sensitivity testing with this method usually requires two or three weeks, the test is of optimal use in adjuvant chemotherapy for cancers with a high probability of occult metastases.

The results with the *in vitro* clonogenic cell assay can be summarized as follows:

(a) Cells from most sponteneous human carinomas and sarcomas can form colonies in soft agar, although at low plating efficiencies. Lymphomas are an exception, with plating efficiencies of at least 0.01% achieved in only a small percentage of cases.

(b) These clonogenic cells are representative of tumour stem cells which are responsible for sustained malignant growth *in vivo*. The ultimate test of whether they are representative with regard to drug sensitivity will be the finding of a correlation between *in vitro* effects and *in vivo* treatment results.

This human tumour clonogenic assay may have clinical applications for both established drugs and agents undergoing development, and also provides a tool for studying cellular pharmacology, mechanisms of drug resistance, and drug interactions. The diversity of methodological approaches and applications is illustrated in the proceedings of the International Symposium on this assay (*Cancer Chemother. Pharmacol.*, **6**, 1981).

Short-term cultures

Assays for assessing the responsiveness of human tumour cells to anticancer drugs in a shorter period of time than that needed for the clonogenic assay may be divided into three categories. Drug effects have been assessed either by morphologic assessment of cellular damage in monolayer or organ culture, tests of inhibition of cellular respiration, or measurement of inhibition of radioactive precursor incorporation.

Morphologic assessment of cellular damage

Wright *et al.* (1957) reported on this approach in which fresh human tumour fragments were set up as explant cultures in chick embryo plasma extract clots on cover slips. They were supplied with media supplemented with autologous or pooled human sera. After growth was established, the effects of anticancer drugs were evaluated by light microscope assessment of damage, scored on a scale graded from 1 to 4. The initial report was encouraging but later reports were less so (Plummer Cobb *et al.*, 1961; Wright *et al.*, 1962).

These authors warned that 'cautious clinical extrapolation for tissue culture data is in order pending additional clinical correlation results' and both short-term explant cultures and organ cultures were tried by many others in the early 1960s. More recently, Limburg (1976), Waverius (1976), Lickiss *et al.* (1974), and Holmes and Little (1974) have used the *in vitro* culture technique and reported positive clinical correlations.

The development of this assay has been pursued by Dendy (1976) and by Wheeler *et al.*, (1974). They minced biopsy specimens to provide monolayer cultures. Cell death was initially assessed morphologically. More quantitative methods were subsequently used, i.e. ^{3}H-thymidine or ^{125}I-5-iodo-2'-deoxyuridine incorporation, autoradiography, and cell counting. It was found that 31 patients treated in accordance with predictions of the *in vitro* test

survived for significantly longer times than did 32 others treated by standard
protocols.

Although encouraging results have been obtained, the applicability of the
in vitro assay is hampered by two problems: the first is the inability to
standardize the cultures or quantitate the results (Lickiss *et al.*, 1974). The
second problem is that both malignant and non-malignant cells grow in
explant cultures; growth of fibroblasts can invalidate many monolayer tests in
a relatively short time (Hamburger, 1981).

Attempts have been made to render morphologic assessment of cell kill less
subjective by determining the proportion of cells in culture that can exclude
vital dyes such as trypan blue, eosin or nigrosin. Most authors have observed,
however, that vital dyes are not reliable indicators of drug-induced cytotoxicity (Durkin et al., 1979; Roper and Drewinko, 1976; Rupniak and Hill, 1980).

Inhibition of cellular respiration

The test using the inhibition of cellular respiration was described by Arai and
Suzuki (1956), Buskirk *et al.* (1973), Di Paolo and Dowd (1961), and Kondo
(1971). Arai and Suzuki (1956) reported on a simplified agar dilution method
in which serial dilutions of potential antitumour agents were incubated in
direct contact with freshly isolated Ehrlich ascites tumour cells. The effect of
the agent was determined by the decrease in dehydrogenase activity as a
direct reflection of decreased respiration, with methylene blue as the indicator. The test could be performed in less than 3 h.

Buskirk *et al.*, (1973) described a modified test based on this respiration-
related cytotoxicity and stated that the *in vitro* test correlated well with *in vivo*
results. In addition, tests that monitor changes in oxygen consumption have
been used (Laszlo, *et al.*, 1958; Dickson and Suzanger, 1976). The technical
difficulties of determining this parameter have prevented its widespread use.

Problems with these tests on the inhibition of cellular respiration or
changes in oxygen consumption are the qualitative nature of the results and
the fact that the metabolism of both malignant and non-malignant cells is
measured.

Inhibition of radioactive precursor incorporation

The work of Bickis *et al.*, (1966) provides a model of this type of assay. Slices
of fresh human tumours were incubated in the presence of radioactive tracers
and cytostatic agents. Drug effects were estimated from the changed rate of
incorporation of radioactive precursors into DNA, RNA, and protein.

Yarnell *et al.*, (1964) measured incorporation of ^{32}P into trichloroacetic
acid-precipitable materials after growth of cells in organ culture. Volm *et al.*,

(1979) described a short-term test that involved inhibition of incorporation of tritiated thymidine or uridine. The incorporation of precursors into trichloro-acetic acid-precipitable material was measured after 1 h of incubation. Good correlation was observed in a prospective trial. Other authors using similar systems noted similar correlations (Bech-Hansen *et al.*, 1977; Raich, 1978; Shrivastan and Paulson, 1980).

An accurate measure of cell survival, however, may not be obtained with the precursor incorporation test. One problem is the lack of incorporation of DNA precursors by cells with a long cycle time. Precursor incorporation into cells may be temporarily halted due to damage to cells in the isolation process. Also, most drugs have profound effects on nucleotide synthesis.

Decreased DNA synthesis may be due to drug-induced depression of labelled nucleoside transport or changes in nucleotide pools. Increased DNA synthesis may be due to increased use of salvage pathways in the presence of drugs such as methotrexate or 5-fluorouracil that affect the *de novo* pathway (Wolberg, 1972). Finally, the problem of incorporation of DNA precursors by a heterogeneous mixture of cells is encountered. Some of these problems might be circumvented by the use of the labelling index technique (Living-stone *et al.*, 1980). In order to improve the usefulness of the *in vitro* assay for clinical application, it will be necessary to compare its results with the effects of treating the same tumours *in vivo*.

For a detailed review of the use of *in vitro* tests as predictors of clinical response, see von Hoff and Weisenthal (1982), Dendy (1976), Hamburger (1981), and the proceedings of the International Symposium on the stem cell assay (*Cancer Chemother. Pharmocol.*, **6**, 1981).

CONCLUSION

As a general conclusion, it can be stated that the application of *in vitro* assays to cells from human tumours is still hampered by problems of selection of subpopulations of cells, the presence of both malignant and non-malignant cells, relevance of the response, and quantification of dose–response rela-tions.

Studies of response of experimental solid tumours by use of *in vitro* assays have provided important information on cellular factors which determine volume reduction, growth delay, and local control. A number of problems concerning resting and proliferating cells, repair of damage, and the influence of the microenvironment remain to be solved.

With respect to the predictive value of *in vitro* assays for responses of human cancer, further studies are required to make improvements in plating efficiency and to determine correlations between *in vitro* sensitivity and *in vivo* results of treatments.

REFERENCES

Alberts, D.S., Salmon, S.E., Chen, H.S.G., Surwit, E.A., Soehnlen, B., Young, L., and Moon, T.E. (1980). *In-vitro* clonogenic assay for predicting response of ovarian cancer to chemotherapy. *Lancet*, **ii**, 340.

Arai, T., and Suzuki, M. (1956). A rapid agar dilution technique for the estimation of antitumor cell activity. *J. Antibiot. A* (Tokyo), **9**, 169.

Barendsen, G.W. (1980). Analysis of tumour responses by excision and *in vitro* assay of cellular clonogenic capacity. *Br. J. Cancer*, **41**, Suppl. IV, 209.

Barendsen, G.W., and Broerse, J.J. (1969). Experimental radiotherapy of a rat rhabdomyosarcoma with 15 MeV neutrons and 300 kV x-rays. I. Effects of single exposures. *Euro. J. Cancer*, **5**, 373.

Barendsen, G.W., and Broerse, J.J. (1970). Experimental radiotherapy of a rat rhabdomyosarcoma with 15 MeV neutrons and 300 kV x-rays. II Effects of fractionated treatments, applied five times a week for several weeks. *Eur. J. Cancer*, **6**, 89.

Barendsen, G.W., Roelse, H., Hermens, A.F., Madhuizen, H.T., van Peperzeel, H.A., and Rutgers, D.H. (1973). Clonogenic capacity of proliferating and nonproliferating cells of a transplantable rat rhabdomyosarcoma in relation to its radiosensitivity. *J. Natl. Cancer Inst.*, **51**, 1521.

Bech-Hansen, N.T., Sarangi F., Sutherland, D.J., and Ling, V. (1977). Rapid assays for evaluating the drug sensitivity of tumor cells. *J. Natl. Cancer Inst.*, **59**, 21.

Beck, H.-P., Brammer, I., Zywietz, F., and Jung, H. (1981). The application of flow cytometry for the quantification of the response of experimental tumors to irradiation. *Cytometry*, **2**, 44.

Begg, A.C. (1980). Analysis of growth delay data: potential pitfalls. *Br. J. Cancer*, **41**, Suppl. IV, 93.

Bickis, I.J., Henderson, M.D., and Quastel, J.J. (1966). Biochemical studies of human tumors. II. *In vitro* estimation of individual tumor sensitivity to anticancer agents. *Cancer*, **19**, 103.

Bogden, A.E., Kelton, D.E., Cobb, W.R., and Esber, H.J. (1978). A rapid screening method for testing chemotherapeutic agents against human xenografts. In *Use of athymic (nude) mice in cancer research* (eds. D.P. Houchens, and A.A. Ovejera). New York: Gustav Fischer. p.231.

Brown, J.M., Yu, N.Y., and Workman, P. (1979). Pharmacokinetic considerations in testing hypoxic cell radiosensitizers in mouse tumours. *Br. J. Cancer*, **39**, 310.

Buskirk, H.H., Crim, J.A., van Giessen, G.J., and Petering, H.G. (1973). Rapid *in vitro* method for determining cytotoxicity of antitumor agents. *J. Natl. Cancer Inst.*, **51**, 135.

Clifton, K.H., and Draper, N.R. (1963). Survival-curves of solid transplantable tumour cells irradiated *in vivo*: a method of determination and statistical evaluation; comparison of cell survival and ^{32}P-uptake into DNA. *Int. J. Radiat. Biol.*, **7**, 515.

Dendy, P.P. (ed.) (1976). *Human tumors in short-term culture*. New York: Academic Press.

Dickson, J.A., and Suzanger, M. (1976). *In vitro* sensitivity testing of human tumor slices to chemotherapeutic agents. In *Human tumors in short-term culture* (ed. P.P. Dendy). New York: Academic Press. p.107.

Di Paolo, J.A., and Dowd, J.E. (1961). Evaluation of inhibition of human tumor tissue by cancer chemotherapeutic drugs with an *in vitro* test. *J. Natl. Cancer Inst.*, **27**, 807.

Durkin, W.J., Ghanta, V.K., Balch, C.M., Dorris, D.W., and Humamoto, R.N. (1979). A methodological approach to the prediction of anticancer drug effects in humans. *Cancer Res.*, **39**, 402.

Hahn, G., Rockwell, S., Kallman, R.F., Gordon, L.F., and Frindel, E. (1974). Repair of potentially lethal damage *in vivo* in solid tumour cells after x-irradiation. *Cancer Res.*, **34**, 351.

Hamburger, A.W. (1981). Use of *in vitro* tests in predictive cancer chemotherapy. *J. Natl. Cancer Inst.*, **66**, 981.

Hamburger, A.W., and Salmon, S.E. (1977). Primary bioassay of human tumour stem cells. *Science*, **197**, 461.

Hermens, A.F., and Barendsen, G.W. (1979). The proliferative status and clonogenic capacity of tumour cells in a transplantable rhabdomyosarcoma of the rat before and after irradiation with 800 rad of x-rays. *Cell Tissue Kinet.*, **11**, 83.

Hewitt, H.B., and Wilson, C.W. (1959). A survival curve for mammalian cells irradiated *in vivo*. *Nature*, **183**, 1060.

Hill, R.P., and Bush, R.S. (1969). A lung-colony assay to determine the radiosensitivity of the cells of a solid tumour. *Int. J. Radiat. Biol.*, **15**, 435.

Holmes, J.L., and Little, J.M. (1974). Tissue culture microtest for predicting response of human cancer to chemotherapy. *Lancet*, **ii**, 985.

Jirtle, R., and Clifton, K.H. (1978). The effect of tumor size and host anemia on tumour cell survival after irradiation. *Int. J. Radiat. Oncol. Biol. Phys.*, **4**, 395.

Jung, H., Beck, H.-P., Brammer, I., and Zywietz, F. (1980). Factors contributing to tumour growth after irradiation. *Br. J. Cancer*, **41**, Suppl. IV, 226.

Kal, H.B. (1973a). Proliferation behaviour of P and Q cells in a rat rhabdomyosarcoma after irradiation as determined by DNA measurements. *Eur. J. Cancer*, **9**, 753.

Kal, H.B. (1973b). Distributions of cell volume and DNA content of rhabdomyosarcoma cells growing *in vitro* and *in vivo* after irradiation. *Eur. J. Cancer*, **9**,77.

Kal, H.B., and Barendsen, G.W. (1972). Effects of continuous irradiation at low dose rates on a rat rhabdomyosarcoma. *Br. J. Radiol.*, **45**, 279.

Kal, H.B., and Barendsen, G.W. (1980). Cell survival and growth delay in rat R-1 tumours after radiation and vinblastine treatment. *Br. J. Cancer,* **41**, Suppl. IV, 275.

Kal, H.B., Barendsen, G.W., Reinhold, H.S., and Hermens, A.F. (1983). The rat rhabdomyosarcoma: cell kinetics *in vivo* and *in vitro* and its responses to treatments. In *Methods in tumor biology, tissue culture and animal tumor models* (ed. R. Sridhar). New York: Marcel Dekker. (in press).

Kallman, R.F., Combs, C.A., Franko, A.J., Furlong, B.M., Kelley, S.D., Kemper, H.L., Miller, R.G., Rapacchietta, D., Schoenfeld, D., and Takahashi, M. (1980). Evidence for the recruitment of noncycling clonogenic tumor cells. In *Radiation biology in cancer research* (eds. R.E. Meyn, and H.R. Withers). New York: Raven Press. p.397.

Kondo, T. (1971). Prediction of response of tumor and host to cancer chemotherapy. *Natl. Cancer Inst. Monogr.,* **34**, 251.

Laszlo, J., Stengle, J., Wight, K., and Burk, D. (1958). Effects of chemotherapeutic agents on metabolism of human acute leukemia cells *in vitro*. *Proc. Soc. Exp. Biol. Med.,* **97**, 127.

Lickiss, J.N., Cane, K.A., and Barkie, A.G. (1974). *In vitro* selection in antineoplastic chemotherapy. *Eur. J. Cancer*, **10**, 809.

Limburg H. (1976). Individualised chemotherapy of ovarian cancer by means of the tissue culture method. In *Human tumors in short-term culture* (ed. P.P. Denby). New York: Academic Press. p. 293.

Little, J.B., Hahn, G.M., Frindel, E., and Tubiana, M. (1973). Repair of potentially lethal damage *in vitro* and *in vivo*. *Radiology*, **106**,689.

Livingstone, R.B., Titus, G.A., and Heilbrum, I.K. (1980). *In vitro* effects of DNA synthesis as a predictor of biological effect from chemotherapy. *Cancer*, **40**, 2209.

McNally, N.J., and Sheldon, P.W. (1977). The effect of radiation on tumour growth delay, cell survival and cure of the animal using a single tumour system. *Br. J. Radiol.*, **50**, 321.

Pavelic, Z.P., Slocum, H.K., Rustum, Y.M., Creaven, P.J., Karakousis, C., and Takita, H. (1980). Colony growth in soft agar of human melanoma, sarcoma, and lung carcinoma cells disaggregated by mechanical and enzymatic methods. *Cancer Res.*, **40**, 2160.

Pike, B.L., and Robinson, W.A. (1970). Human bone marrow colony growth in agar gel. *J. Cell Physiol.*, **76**, 77.

Plummer-Cobb, J., Walker, D.G., and Wright, J.C. (1961). Comparative chemotherapy studies on primary short-term cultures of human normal benign and malignant tumor tissues — a five-year study. *Cancer Res.*, **21**, 583.

Raich, P.C. (1978). Prediction of therapeutic response in acute leukemia. *Lancet*, **i**, 74.

Rasey, J.S., Carpentier, R.E., and Nelson, N.J. (1977). Response of EMT-6 tumors to single fractions of x-rays and cyclotron neutrons. *Radiat. Res.*, **71**, 430.

Rasey, J.S., and Nelson, N.J. (1980). Response of an *in vivo–in vitro* tumour to x-rays and cytotoxic drugs: effect of tumour disaggregation method on cell survival. *Br. J. Cancer*, **41**, Suppl. **IV**, 217.

Reinhold, H.S. (1965a). A cell dispersion technique for use in quantitative transplantation studies with solid tumours. *Eur. J. Cancer*, **1**, 67.

Reinhold, H.S. (1965b). *Stralingsgevoeligheid van tumoren. Een experimenteel onderzoek bij de rat*. Radiobiological Institute, TNO, Rijswijk, the Netherlands.

Reinhold, H.S. (1966). Quantitative evaluation of the radiosensitivity of cells of a transplantable rhabdomyosarcoma in the rat. *Eur. J. Cancer*, **2**, 33.

Rockwell, S. (1977). *In vivo–in vitro* tumor systems: new models for studying the response of tumors to therapy. *Lab. Animal Sci.*, **27**, 831.

Roper, P., and Drewinko, B. (1976). Comparison of *in vitro* methods to determine drug-induced cell lethality. *Cancer Res.*, **36**, 2181.

Rupniak, H.T., and Hill, B.T. (1980). Studies with a clonogenic assay for tumour cells from human biopsy material and its comparison with other survival assays. *Br. J. Cancer*, 41, Suppl. **IV**, 255.

Salmon, S.E., Hamburger, A.W., Soehnlen, B., Durie, B.G.M., Alberts, D.S., and Moon, T.E. (1978). Quantitation of differential sensitivity of human tumor stem cells to anti-cancer drugs. *New Engl. J. Med.*, **298**, 1321.

Shipley, W.U., Stanley, J.A., Courtenay, V.D., and Field, S.B. (1975). Repair of radiation damage in Lewis lung carcinoma cells following *in situ* treatment with fast neutrons and x-rays. *Cancer Res.*, **35**, 932.

Shrivastan, S., and Paulson, D. (1980). *In vitro* chemotherapy testing of transitional cell carcinoma. *Invest. Urol.*, **40**, 395.

Tepperman, A.D., Curtis, J.E., and McCulloch, E.A. (1974). Erythropoietic colonies in cultures of human marrow. *Blood*, **44**, 659.

Volm, M., Wayss, K., Kaufman, M., and Mattern, J. (1979). Pretherapeutic detection of tumour resistance and the results of chemotherapy. *Eur. J. Cancer*, **15**, 983.

Von Hoff, D., and Weisenthal, L. (1982). *In vitro* methods to predict for patient responses to chemotherapy. In *Advances in pharmacology and chemotherapy*. New York: Academic Press. (in press)

Waverius, H.M. (1976). Detection of acquired resistance to cytotoxic drugs *in vivo* by short-term cultures of human tumors. In *Human tumors in short-term culture* (ed. P.P. Dendy. New York: Academic Press. p.311.

Wheeler, T., Dendy, P., and Dawson, A. (1974). Assessment of an *in vitro* screening test of cytotoxic agents in the treatment of adrenal malignant disease. *Oncology*, **30**, 362.

Wolberg, W.H. (1972). Response of DNA thymine synthesis in human tumor and normal tissue to 5-fluorouracil. *Cancer Res.*, **32**, 130.

Wright, J.C., Plummer-Cobb, J., Gumport, S., Golomb, F.M., and Safadi, D. (1957). Investigation of the relation between clinical and tissue culture response to chemotherapeutic agents on human cancer. *New Engl. J. Med.*, **257**, 1207.

Wright, J.C., Plummer-Cobb, J., Gumport, S.L., Safadi, D., Walker, D.G., and Golomb, F.M. (1962). Further investigations of the relation between the clinical and tissue culture response to chemotherapeutic agents on human cancer. *Cancer*, **15**, 284.

Yarnell, M., Ambrose, E.J., Shepley, K., and Tchao, R. (1964). Drug assays on organ culture of biopsies from human tumours. *Br. Med. J.*, **2**, 490.

Part 3

Predictive Factors and Selective Treatment

Cancer Treatment: End Point Evaluation
Edited by B.A. Stoll
© 1983 John Wiley & Sons Ltd.

Chapter

15 OLEG S. SELAWRY

Selective Treatment in Lung Cancer

INTRODUCTION

Selective treatment aims at adapting the best therapy to the clinical condition, personal needs, tumor response, and specific tolerance of each individual patient. This chapter will discuss selective therapy, against the background of the natural history of lung cancer, according to cell type and stage of the cancer, respiratory function, and other host factors. These lead to the development of a comprehensive treatment plan such as that described in recent reviews (Minna *et al.*, 1982; Selawry and Hansen, 1982; Matthews, 1982). The discussion will follow the usual course of clinical decision-making, and is colored by the author's experience as a practising pulmonary oncologist.

Individual tumor characteristics can be defined according to cell type, volume doubling time and stage of disease, and by its interactions with the host.

TUMOR CELL TYPE

The cell type classification adopted by the World Health Organization (1982) is congruent with the clinical characteristics of the tumor, its expected response to treatment, and end-results. However, the tumor can be composed of more than one cell type and the extent of differentiation can vary at different sites. It is important, therefore, to provide the pathologist with an adequate tumor sample and it is helpful to discuss with the pathologist the microscopic sections of each tumor, before accepting the responsibility for treatment planning.

Squamous cell carcinoma

This morphologic type of tumor starts usually in a segmental or lobar bronchus and has a median volume doubling time of 3–4 months. It eventually spreads to the locoregional hilar, mediastinal and possibly cervical lymph nodes but, even at autopsy, only about 50% of the patients show distant metastases. The diagnosis is frequently established by sputum cytology or transbronchial biopsy. This tumor predominates in surgical series, because surgery offers the best end-results when compared to the other common cell types (Table 1).

Table 1. Characteristics of the four major cell types of lung cancer

Cell type	Cell type			
	Squamous	Small	Adeno-	Large
Predominant location	Central	Central	Peripheral	Any
Distant metastases(%)	20–50	99+	20–90	20–90
Volume doubling (median, months)	3–4	0.7	5–6	3–4
Median survival (months)				
Resected patients	23	6–8	18–19	15(AJC)[a]
Regional disease	3–4	3	1–6	4(VALG)[b]
Extensive disease	3	2	4	3(VALG)

[a] AJC = American Joint Committee
[b] VALG = Veteran's Association Lung Group.

   Poor vascularization (and hence poor oxygenation) of the central core of larger tumors can lead to necrosis and occasional cavitation. Poorly differentiated squamous cell carcinoma has a substantially higher propensity for distant metastases. It may require electron microscopy and/or cytogenetic studies (Whang Peng *et al.*, 1982) to distinguish squamous cell cancer from small cell carcinoma in some cases.

Small cell carcinoma

This type of tumor spreads rapidly to hilar and mediastinal nodes and beyond, so that virtually every patient has widespread metastatic disease at the time of diagnosis. The volume doubling time is by the far the fastest of any lung cancer, with a median of 21 days, because of a high growth fraction. The microscopic diagnosis is most commonly established by transbronchial or mediastinal biopsy, lymph node or bone biopsy or aspirate.

The need for adequate tumor samples is emphasized by the finding of other cell types in 6% of small cell cancers at the time of diagnosis, increasing to 35% at autopsy (Matthews, 1982). Electron microscopy and, where available, cytogenetic studies for establishment of 3p(14–23) chromosomal deletion (Whang Peng *et al.*, 1982), are helpful, especially for patients with the intermediate cell subgroup of small cell carcinoma.

This highly malignant tumor requires prompt therapy because of the propensity for life-threatening complications such as obstruction of the superior vena cava or brain metastases. Chemotherapy, using a combination of two or more drugs, is the treatment of choice and 80–90% of the patients achieve at least 50% shrinkage of the primary tumor with 30–60% complete tumor regression within 6–8 weeks. Duration of response shows a median of 9–12 months, and 5–10% of the patients survive 2–7 years (or more) free of symptomatic cancer.

Radiotherapy is equally as effective for local treatment, but does not prolong median survival. Nevertheless, five-year survival has been observed occasionally after such treatment (Hansen, 1982). Surgery might be used for the uncommon T_1 or T_2 N_0 M_0 Stage I peripheral lesion. As with radiotherapy, there are occasional long-term survivors, without prolongation of median survival time. Hence, surgery is not at present the standard treatment for small cell carcinoma of the lung.

Adenocarcinoma

This tumor type is more commonly peripherally located, frequently with extension toward the pleura or actual pleural invasion and effusion. Sputum cytology and bronchoscopy are not as commonly diagnostic as in the other cell types, especially in the early stages of the disease. Transthoracic (Rotex-) needle biopsy will be of help for the diagnosis of peripheral lesions.

The volume doubling time and the natural history are the slowest of all the tumor types, with a median of 5–6 months. The propensity for distant metastases in patients beyond Stages I and II is the highest next to small cell carcinoma, especially in the case of poorly differentiated tumors. Bronchioloalveolar carcinoma is an important subtype and is the only type of lung cancer with no apparent increase in relation to cigarette-smoking, and the only one with claim of intraluminal dissemination.

As for all other 'non-small cell lung cancers' (NSCLC), an increasingly fashionable term, surgery is the treatment of choice for resectable disease in this group. Details are discussed later.

Large cell carcinoma

This morphologic type of tumor has the same volume doubling time as squamous cell carcinoma but a higher propensity for distant metastases. It encompasses a variety of distinct tumor types, including the highly malignant giant cell carcinoma and the well differentiated clear cell carcinoma, in addition to a major component of undifferentiated carcinomas. Resectability in this group is slightly better than that found in adenocarcinoma while response to chemotherapeutic agents shows some differences from that of other cell types. The giant cell tumors generally run a short clinical course similarly to untreated small cell carcinomas, and are generally resistant to chemotherapy.

STAGE OF DISEASE

Five-year survival of patients with Stage I disease exceeds 50% (80–90% in some series) for certain $T_1 N_0 M_0$ tumors. Surgery is, therefore, the treatment of choice except for small cell carcinoma. For Stage II disease, five-year survival drops to 30%, for Stage III disease to about 15%. Thorough presurgical staging will improve the end-results by exclusion of patients with unsuspected metastases.

For Stage I, all non-small cell carcinomas have similarly favorable end-results after resection. For Stages II and III, older series showed the best results for squamous cell carcinoma, and worse results for the adenocarcinoma group. The difference is decreasing in recent surgical series, probably because of improved presurgical staging.

VOLUME DOUBLING TIME (VDT)

It would be reasonable to assume that rapid VDT of a tumor correlates to short survival and slow growth to a better prognosis. Further, one might assume that the fastest growing tumors, with many actively growing cells, would be the most vulnerable to chemo- and radiotherapy. In practice, these assumptions are of limited value and do not, at present, help toward selection of treatment. The VDT is usually variable for one and the same untreated lesion and for different metastatic lesions in the same patient. The extent and duration of response to treatment and longevity showed no significant relation to VDT in a series of patients with small cell carcinoma (Bakhtar and Selawry, unpublished data).

A therapy regimen which includes cyclophosphamide, lomustine, and methotrexate is effective in small cell carcinoma (the fastest growing) and adenocarcinoma (the slowest growing) cell types of lung cancer, but relatively ineffective in squamous and large cell carcinoma. This treatment regimen with the addition of vincristine was used in 11 patients with small cell carcinoma, with 14 metastases permitting flow-cytometric DNA analysis before and during chemotherapy (Vindeloer *et al.*, 1982). Kinetic parameters were found to be insufficient to predict the extent and duration of response and survival, confirming the results of a broader review (Tannock, 1978). These data imply that the cytogenetic and pharmacokinetic heterogeneity of tumor cell populations will frequently override the initial cytokinetic status, presumably due to selection and eventual overgrowth by resistant clones of cells.

However, combining VDT with staging may help in the selection of treatment. For example, the appearance of a single metastatic lesion more than one year after surgery (with or without subsequent single lesions at spaced intervals) occasionally permits useful palliation or even long-term control by resection of intensive radiotherapy, without elective chemotherapy.

INTERACTIONS BETWEEN TUMOR AND HOST

The neutral term 'interactions' is used in this context because it can be difficult to assign certain influences exclusively to the tumor or to the tumor-bearing host.

Performance status

This factor is an important determinant of prognosis. Asymptomatic patients have a much better prognosis than semi-ambulatory or bedridden patients and are better candidates for treatment. Thus, the median survival in a group of 5022 inoperable male patients was 34, 14–21, and 3–5 weeks for asymptomatic, semi-ambulatory, and bedridden patients, respectively (Stanley, 1980).

The asymptomatic patient with distant metastases and non-small cell lung carcinoma might choose to delay chemotherapy until he becomes symptomatic. The bedridden patient might prefer symptomatic treatment at home to intensive chemotherapy and the risk of pronounced toxicity.

Body weight

In a major study, patients with more than 4.5 kg (=10 lb) weight loss had a median life expectancy of 11 weeks, as compared to 22 weeks for those with a lesser or nil weight loss (Stanley, 1980). Such weight loss might occur without apparent reason or might be influenced by fever, pain, dysphagia or extensive hepatic metastases. As with performance status, development of anorexia and weight loss militate against heroic treatment.

Sex and age

Major studies show a consistent, 50–90% better five-year survival for women compared to men with resectable and locoregional disease. To a lesser extent, this applies also to patients with distant metastases. The reason for this difference is unknown and treatment by estrogens or progestational agents has failed to prolong survival in randomized trials of male patients with lung cancer. Age (above or below 70) seems not to affect post-surgical survival and end-results (Stanley, 1980), nor response to chemotherapy. Biologic rather than chronologic age should be used to decide treatment planning.

Elderly patients may be more sensitive to chemotherapy, requiring lower starting doses of chemotherapy. Decreased creatinine clearance is associated with slower clearance of methotrexate, hence longer serum half-life time and greater toxicity. The bone marrow reserve (stem cells) may be decreased, leading to slower recovery from hematologic toxicity. Patients with marginal cardiac function might not be able to tolerate the increased myocardial fibrosis induced by anthracyclines such as doxorubicin.

Some of the younger patients (< 50) with non-resectable tumors are thought to have more aggressive disease. This is not predictable however and does not influence selection of treatment.

Hemogram

A normal hemogram is prognostically and therapeutically favorable. Anemia requires investigation and treatment, with the possible exception of the terminal case. Leukocytosis may be an expression of post-obstructive pneumonitis and indicates a possible need for treatment. A leukemoid reaction spells an ominous prognosis.

Leukopenia in itself might be a prognostically favorable sign (Selawry and Hansen, 1982), but might also reflect extensive osseous metastases or prior myelosuppressive treatment. Leukopenia will then interfere with myelosuppressive chemo- and/or radiotherapy. Lumphocytopenia below 1000/mm^3 is associated with short survival (Stanley, 1980). Thrombocytopenia secondary to extensive osseous metastases or myelosuppressive treatment might suggest preferential use either of platelet-stimulating (vinblastine, vincristine) or platelet-sparing drugs (cyclophosphamide, semi-weekly methotrexate), especcially in patients with hemoptysis.

Respiratory function

Impaired respiratory function can strongly influence the selection of treatment, as potentially curative resection or intensive radiotherapy might not be possible. On the other hand, acute respiratory distress (due to obstruction of a major airway by tumor, extensive pleural or pericardial effusion) or hemoptysis might require immediate therapeutic action.

Marginal respiratory function might make it difficult to use drugs with known pulmonary toxicity (bleomycin, alkylating agents, methotrexate, mitomycin, nitrosoureas). The debilitated immuno- and myelosuppressed patient is prone to opportunistic lung infections, requiring vigorous treatment.

Other factors which might influence the choice of treatment include the presence of unrelated diseases and the presence of certain marker substances in the blood. Their detailed discussion exceeds the scope of this chapter.

COMPREHENSIVE TREATMENT PLANNING

The comprehensive treatment plan offers the greatest possible and likely benefit at the least risk, and provides contingency plans in case of treatment failure. On the basis of the baseline clinical data, the feasibility of surgery, radiotherapy, and chemotherapy is considered, alone or in combination. (Experimental treatments, e.g. immunostimulation or hyperthermia are not discussed in this chapter). Supportive and symptomatic treatment will be mentioned later.

Cure is the most desirable end-result, and failing that, the longest possible prolongation of life in comfort. Symptomatic treatment is stressed when the former two aims are not achievable. First, second and third choices of treatment by stage of disease and by cell type are listed in Table 2.

Resectable disease

Stages I, II, and III (T_{1-2}, N_{1-2}, M_0) are best resected. Current five-year survival figures for Stage I disease of NSCLC exceed 50%. The end-results of the American Joint Committee for patients with Stage II disease are 35% for squamous and 18% for adeno- plus large cell carcinoma, but decreasing to 13, 11, and 2% respectively for Stage III squamous cell, large cell, and adenocarcinoma with positive mediastinal nodes (T_{1-2}, N_2, M_0) (Mountain, 1980).

Another group has observed 44% and 56% *three*-year survival in 25 squamous and 44 adenocarcinomas respectively, after resection in T_{1-2}, N_2, M_0 disease (Martini *et al.*, 1978). Most of these patients had 1–2 ipsilateral mediastinal nodes, mostly below the upper paratracheal and above the paraesophageal level. Furthermore, most of these patients received intensive, post-surgical radiotherapy.

Bronchioloalveolar carcinoma had a favorable 51% five-year survival rate in 76 patients in five recent surgical series (Minna *et al.*, 1982). For small cell carcinoma, surgery must remain experimental despite a reported 36% five-year survival in 11 patients who presented with asymptomatic solitary pulmonary nodules. These patients were among 887 males who underwent thoracotomy for diagnosis, and among 309 patients with T_{1-2}, N_0, M_0, Stage I disease who were resected for cure (Higgins, *et al.*, 1975).

Table 2 Treatment of first, second, and third choice by stage and cell types.

Stage	Squamous cell	Large cell	Adenocarcinoma	Small cell
Local I II III $T_2\,N_1\,M_0$	1. Surgery 2. Radiotherapy 3. Chemotherapy (upon relapse after no.2)	1. Surgery 2. Radiotherapy 3. Chemotherapy (upon relapse after no. 2)	1. Surgery 2. Radiotherapy 3. Chemotherapy (upon relapse after no.2)	1. Chemotherapy (drug combinations) ± radiotherapy (?) ± surgery (?)
$T_2\,N_2\,M_0$	1. Surgery followed by radiotherapy 2. Radiotherapy 3. Chemotherapy	1. Surgery followed by radiotherapy 2. Radiotherapy 3. Chemotherapy	1. Surgery followed by radiotherapy 2. Chemotherapy, then radiotherapy (?)	
Regional III $T_3\,N_0\,M_0$	Superior sulcus tumor: 1. Radiotherapy 2. Chemotherapy with single drugs	Superior sulcus tumor: 1. Surgery or Radiotherapy followed by surgery 2. Radiotherapy 3. Chemotherapy		1. Chemotherapy with drug combination such as (a) cyclophosph. + lomustine + methotrexate (b) cyclophosph. + doxorubicin + vincristine or cisplatin + etoposide ± radiotherapy(?)
$T_3\,N_{1-2}\,M_0$ M_1 supraclav. nodes	1. Radiotherapy 2. Chemotherapy with single drugs	1. Radiotherapy 2. Chemotherapy with drug combination	1. Radiotherapy or chemotherapy followed by radiotherapy 2. Chemotherapy	
Extensive M_1 distant metastases	1. Chemotherapy with single drugs such as (a) vinblastine (b) methotrexate (c) cisplatin (d) cyclophosph.	1. Chemotherapy with drug combinations such as cisplatin + cyclophosph. + doxorubicin	1. Chemotherapy with drug combinations such as cyclophosph. + lomustine + methotrexate 2. VLB or VCR 3. Mitomycin	1. Chemotherapy as above 2. Non-cross-resistant drug combinations 3. Single drugs not yet used in combinations.

Pre-operative and post-operative radiotherapy have failed to improve surgical end-results in major randomized clinical trials. Utilization of presurgical radiotherapy for superior sulcus tumors (Paulson, 1979) and of post-surgical radiotherapy after mediastinal node disection (Martini *et al.*, 1978) was elective, not randomized. Except for these two situations, elective adjuvant radiotherapy is not indicated.

Adjuvant chemotherapy was clearly unsuccessful in randomized clinical trials, with the possible exception of cyclophosphamide or cyclophosphamide plus methotrexate after resection of small cell carcinoma. Hence, the routine use of adjuvant chemotherapy is not recommended.

Radiotherapy with intent to cure resulted in 5-6% five-year survival in three major series, including 1050 patients with inoperable or unresectable lung cancer (Minna *et al.*, 1982). Again, addition of chemotherapy to radiotherapy in randomized trials failed to improve survival in extensive randomized trials, except for small cell carcinoma (*vide infra*). Chemotherapy alone is rarely associated with five-year survival and is not used electively for this purpose, with the possible exception of patients with small cell carcinoma (*vide infra*).

Non-resectable locoregional cancer

Locoregional tumors are defined as those confined to one hemithorax, the ipsilateral pleura and chest wall, the mediastinum and ipsi- or bilateral supraclavicular, scalene and cervical nodes.

Small non-resectable tumors in ambulatory patients can be treated with intent to cure, even though the five-year survival salvage is at best 5–6%. Expertly planned radiotherapy to maximal safely tolerated dosage is the treatment of choice. The simultaneous administration of chemotherapy has failed to improve median or long-term survival in prospective, randomized trials. Trials of chemotherapy to maximal tumor shrinkage followed by radiotherapy remain experimental but worth exploring, especially in patients with adenocarcinoma.

Fifty percent tumor shrinkage or better was noted following radiotherapy in 77% of 71 patients with small cell carcinoma, and in 23% of 292 patients with squamous and 85 patients with large cell carcinoma. Only 13% of 68 patients with adenocarcinoma responded, despite the usually peripheral location, which permits delivery of higher radiation doses (Selawry and Hansen, 1982). Median survival is not significantly changed in responding cases, but a subgroup of patients will experience gratifying palliation for many months.

The above considerations apply to NSCLC but for small cell carcinoma it is preferable not to initiate treatment with radiotherapy as chemotherapy is the mainstay of treatment. Initial radiotherapy makes it difficult to evaluate the antineoplastic effect of chemotherapy, and reduces drug tolerance as it suppresses hematopoiesis in the radiation field (Selawry, 1982; Hansen, 1982). Treatment details are discussed later.

Radiotherapy which shrinks the tumor will relieve symptoms and signs of local tumor pressure but symptomatic relief occurs even with lesser tumor shrinkage and is therefore more common. Cough, dyspnea, hemoptysis, pain, and superior vena caval obstruction are temporarily relieved in 60-80% of the patients. Atelectasis clears in only 20–25%, and hoarseness from recurrent nerve paralysis clears in less than 10% of the patients (Minna *et al.*, 1982).

Cerebral metastases usually respond to radiotherapy. The entire brain should be irradiated to the highest safely tolerated dose, with extra dosage to major tumor lesions. This may palliate symptoms for the balance of the patient's life. Resection of a solitary cerebral metastasis is a possible alternative, using radiotherapy as a second line of defense. This approach may be advised when the solitary cerebral lesion occurs several years after surgery to the primary tumor, in an otherwise 'cured' patient.

On the other hand, bedridden or semi-ambulatory patients with widely disseminated disease and an expected survival of less than three months are usually well palliated by corticosteroid therapy. They may not require radiotherapy, as has been shown in a randomized trial (Selawry and Hansen, 1982).

Combination of intensive radiotherapy with palliative resection (to 'debulk' the primary tumor) has been shown to be no more effective than radiotherapy alone. Nor does simultaneous administration of chemotherapy improve the results of optimal radiotherapy alone. However, patients who fail on radiotherapy might experience transient, worthwhile improvement on subsequent chemotherapy (*vide infra*).

Extensive disease

Median survival is notoriously short at this stage (Table 1). Chemotherapy offers possible prolongation of life at the risk of toxicity, and the chance of benefit and choice of drugs depends on the cell type (Table 2). Each drug or drug combination is started at a safely tolerated dose and is increased to cause moderate, safely reversible toxicity for the best therapeutic results.

Squamous cell carcinoma

This is the only cell type where drug combinations have not proved to be superior to single drugs, despite repeated claims to the contrary. Vinblastine and methotrexate are the drugs of choice, each with response rates between

20% and 40%, well manageable toxicity and prolongation of survival to 8–12 months in responders.

Methotrexate is best given at twice weekly increments of 10–15 mg/m^2 body surface area or about 15–20 mg total in one single oral increment. This regimen is platelet-sparing and rarely causes diarrhea, in contrast to daily medication. Mucositis and leukopenia are the most common dose-limiting factors. Impaired renal function, edema, and effusions delay drug excretion and lead to inordinate toxicity, unless the starting dose is drastically reduced.

In such cases it might be preferable to initiate treatment with i.v. vinblastine 5 mg/m^2 or 7–10 mg total every two weeks. Leukopenia is the most common dose-limiting toxicity but constipation or ileus can occur in delibated patients. The drug is predominantly excreted by the liver and an elevated serum bilirubin level calls for reduced dosage.

The individual tolerance for methotrexate and for vinblastine varies considerably. Thus, some patients might develop dose-limiting toxicity at the starting dose while others might tolerate 2–3 times that much. At a later stage, non-cross-resistant drugs such as cyclophosphamide, cisplatin, lomustine, and mitomycin (in order of decreasing activity) may still offer the chance of a short respite.

Small cell carcinoma

This type is the most chemosensitive tumor, as noted earlier. The smaller the tumor and the less overt the metastatic spread, the better is the disease-free survival with intensive treatment. Thus 15% of 540 expertly treated patients with 'locoregional' tumors had a 2½-year disease-free survival, compared to only 2.3% of 95 patients with extensive disease (Minna *et al.*, 1982).

Two-drug combinations such as cisplatin and etoposide, or doxorubicin and lomustine are reported to give as good a response as the more widely used three-drug combinations, such as cyclophosphamide, lomustine, and methotrexate; cisplatin, doxorubicin, and vincristine; or cyclophosphamide, doxorubicin, and vincristine (Selawry, 1982). It is critically important for comprehensive treatment planning to group the available drugs into non-cross-resistant drug combinations.

It is equally desirable to use each component of a drug combination to its own maximal safely tolerated dose. The combination of cyclophosphamide, lomustine, methotrexate, and vincristine will be used to illustrate this point:

> Leukopenia calls for reduction or cessation of all drugs except for vincristine, which is less myelosuppressive.
> Thrombocytopenia necessitates reduction or omission of lomustine as the most likely culprit, with corresponding increase in dose of the other drugs.

Nausea and vomiting after cyclophosphamide or lomustine are rarely dose-limiting. Cyclophosphamide can be given in subdivided daily doses, and lomustine in subdivided fortnightly (not daily) doses, when antiemetics are insufficient for control of emesis.

Mucositis suggests the reduction or interruption of methotrexate as the offending agent, with augmentation of the dose of the other agents.

Debilitating paresthesias of the distal extremities may occur within weeks after initiation of vincristine, and this agent should then be discontinued.

Constipation or ileus and hemorrhagic cystitis are uncommon sequelae of vincristine and cyclophosphamide, respectively, and require interruption or cessation of treatment.

Intensive study is still continuing as to (1) the best initial drug combinations; (2) optimal time for change to a non-cross-resistant regimen (either electively, at the time of maximal response or upon relapse); (3) best use of radiotherapy (? to be given to the tumor bed after complete, or close to complete, regression in patients who presented without overt distant metastases; (4) timing and dosage of radiotherapy to the brain; (5) possible use of surgery in complete responders who presented with resectable disease, because more than 50% of these eventually relapse at the primary tumor site after radiotherapy.

Patients whose response to drug combinations is exhausted may still respond to single drugs which are non-cross-resistant or have been given inadequate trial. Response rates at this stage are low and short-lived. Etoposide, vincristine, cyclophosphamide, and cisplatin are worth a trial, their overall response rates being 46, 42, 38, and 19%, respectively (Selawry, 1982). Procarbazine has been found ineffective in this situation (Hansen, 1982; Selawry, 1982), as is also lomustine. The bone marrow reserve is usually insufficient in the advanced, extensively pretreated patient for the use of strongly myelosuppressive drugs such as doxorubicin and mitomycin. Unfortunately, drugs with a low order of myelotoxicity (such as bleomycin and streptozotocin) are ineffective against small cell carcinoma (Selawry, 1982).

Adenocarcinoma

Response rates of 40–50% are seen with drug combinations such as cyclophosphamide 5–600 mg/m^2 i.v. and lomustine 40–50 mg/m^2 p.o. at three-week intervals plus methotrexate 10–15 mg/m^2 twice weekly (single dose per day p.o.) with flexible dose adjustment as described above. In a series of 45 patients, two manifested complete tumor regression and the median survival of responders was 11.5 months as compared to 5 months for the non-responders (Kocha *et al.*, 1982). Cisplatin, cyclophosphamide, and doxorubicin is an alternative and effective drug combination.

Patients who fail to respond or who relapse have a further chance of short-term response to mitomycin, vinblastine, or cisplatin, with overall response rates of 26, 23, and 21%, respectively. Doxorubicin, fluorouracil, and procarbazine are usually ineffective in this situation.

Large cell carcinoma

Doxorubicin-based drug combinations (e.g. doxorubicin, cisplatin, and cyclophosphamide) afford transient and partial tumor regression in some 40% of these patients. Treatment might therefore be reserved for the symptomatic patient. The combination of cyclophosphamide, lomustine, and methotrexate is no better than the single-component drugs, in contrast to the findings in the case of small cell and adenocarcinoma. The effect of single drugs after combination chemotherapy is unimpressive, although cisplatin and cyclophosphamide might be worth trying. Bleomycin, fluorouracil, and vincristine are useless in this situation.

Supportive and symptomatic treatments

These are the very basis for more specific and selective therapy. The available measures are similar for all organ sites and will therefore not be discussed in detail.

The patient's role in the selection of the treatment

The comprehensive treatment plan is an integration of the best available knowledge as applied to the patient's physical problems. The patient may accept the plan without asking for detailed information, and then the treatment plan is advanced without modification.

In the author's practice, the vast majority of patients wish to know their diagnosis in terms which are meaningful to them. They wish to know the nature of the problem ('a growth', 'cancer', or the specific type of cancer). They ask about their chances of cure or palliation, about the risks and discomforts of treatment, about alternatives, and, if everything else fails, whether they 'will have to suffer'. Their own priorities are stated. A thorough discussion, often in the presence of a close relative or friend, leads in one or more sessions to the patient's informed consent, against the background of a realistic appraisal of his options, an assurance of his comfort by symptomatic treatment, and advice concerning work, exercise, diet, and the like.

The patient might express the feeling that he is a fighter and is willing to endure considerable discomfort and risk in order to have an outside chance of cure or long-term palliation. Alternatively another patient might wish to finish an important project and avoid immediate risk to his life (e.g. complete his will or hand his business over). He might feel that he has lived a full and happy life and wishes to continue to do so for as long as possible, but not at the expense of major risk or discomfort, and he rejects surgery of moderate or high risk.

Some patients initially (or permanently) reject a good chance of cure or palliation, because of depression or because of escape to some 'miracle therapy'. Another patient (or his referring physician) might be so deeply convinced that the cancer will relentlessly progress, that he closes his mind to treatment of established value. He might have seen or heard of frightful toxicity in patients on chemotherapy, and might regard the treatment as more threatening than the disease.

Finally, there comes a time in the evolution of advanced cancer when chances of a clinically meaningful improvement are minimal. A consensus develops between the patient, those closest to him, and the medical team, to concentrate on comfort. At this point, selective measures are those which apply to terminal disease in general.

Follow-up of the 'cured' patient

Little selectivity occurs in this area. Follow-up of patients after resection for cure, or after radiotherapy with intent to cure, or after complete tumor regression from chemotherapy, is at increasing time intervals. Symptoms, signs, appropriate laboratory tests, and chest films are used to monitor the patient for the possibility of recurrent or metastatic disease, or the development of a second primary tumor. Scans and repeat bronchoscopy with biopsy or brushing are done at less frequent intervals (annually in patients with small cell carcinoma or as clinically indicated for the other cell types).

A general rehabilitation program is worked out, as full recovery might take many months. Where necessary, pulmonary function is improved with supportive measures, and smokers are encouraged to 'kick' their habit. Passive smoke inhalation also is reduced to a minimum. Among the author's last 500 patients, there are less than 5% who were unable to discontinue smoking on a permanent basis.

Last but not least, apparently cured patients are invaluable counsellors to the concerned and often frightened, newly diagnosed patient. Their graciously offered advice carries the weight of personal experience.

Acknowledgements

This work was supported in part by the Henrietta Appelbaum and the Harold Lamotte Fund.

REFERENCES

Hansen, H.H. (1982). Management of small-cell anaplastic carcinoma, 1980–1982. In *Lung cancer* (eds S. Ishikawa, Y. Hayata, and K. Suemasu), Int. Congr. Ser. 569. Amsterdam: Excerpta Medica. pp. 31–54.

Higgins, G.A., Shields, T.W., and Keehn, R.J. (1975). The solitary pulmonary nodule. Ten-year follow-up of the Veterans' Administration–Armed Forces cooperative study. *Arch. Surg.*, **110**, 570–575.

Kocha, W., Selawry, O., and Broder, L. (1982). 1-(2-Chloroethyl)–3–cyclohexyl–1–nitrosourea, cyclophosphamide and methotrexate combination chemotherapy for adenocarcinoma of the lung (Abstract). *Proc. 3rd World Conf. on Lung Cancer*, Tokyo, p.194.

Martini, N., Flehinger, B.J., Zaman, M.B., and Beattie, E.J. (1978). Prospective study of 445 lung carcinomas with mediastinal lymph node-metastases. *J. Thorac. Cardiovasc. Surg.*, **80**, 390–399.

Matthews, M.J. (1982). In *Lung cancer* (ed. R.B. Livingston). Boston: Martinus Nijhoff. pp.283–306.

Minna, J.D., Higgins, G.A., and Goldstein, E.J. (1982). Cancer of the lung. In *Principles and practice of oncology* (eds V.T. DeVita, S. Hellman, and S.A. Rosenberg). Philadelphia: Lippincott. pp. 396–473.

Mountain, C. (1980). In *Surgery of lung cancer* (eds H.H. Hansen, and M. Roerth). Amsterdam: Excerpta Medica. p. 1.

Paulson, D.L. (1979). Carcinoma in the superior pulmonary sulcus. *Ann. Thorac. Surg.*, **28**, 44–47.

Selawry, O.S. (1982). Small cell carinoma of the lung. *Semin. Respir. Med.*, **4**, 56–63.

Selawry, O.S., and Hansen, H.H. (1982) Lung cancer. In *Cancer medicine* (eds. J.F. Holland, and E.T. Frei). Philadelphia: Lea and Febiger.

Stanley, K.E. (1980). Prognostic factors for survival in patients with inoperable lung cancer. *J. Natl Cancer Inst.*, **65**, 25–32.

Tannock, I. (1978). Cell kinetics and chemotherapy. A critical review. *Cancer Treat. Rep.*, **62**, 1117–1133.

Vindeloer, L.L., Hansen, H.H., Gersel, A., Hirsch, F.R., and Nissen, N.I. (1982). Treatment of small cell carcinoma of the lung monitored by sequential flow cytometric DNA analysis. *Cancer Res.*, **42**, 2499–2505.

Whang Peng, J., Kao-Shan, C.S., Lee, E.C., Bunn, P.A, P.A, Corney, D.N., Gazdar, A.F., and Minna, J.D. (1982). Specific chromosome defect associated with human small-cell lung cancer: deletion 3p(14–23). *Science*, **215**, 181–182.

World Health Organization (1982). Histological typing of lung tumors—second edition. *Am. J. Clin. Pathol.*, **77**, 123–136.

Cancer Treatment: End Point Evaluation
Edited by B.A. Stoll
© 1983 John Wiley & Sons Ltd.

Chapter

16 M. ADAMS AND I.J. KERBY

Selective Treatment in Uterine Cancer

INTRODUCTION

The results of treatment of uterine cancer depend largely on the extent of the disease and the biology of the tumour. Results are also influenced by factors affecting the ability of the patient to tolerate treatment. In each patient, treatment needs to be individualized according to these prognostic variables. The aim is to ensure adequate treatment but avoid unnecessary morbidity for good prognosis patients, and to recognize those poor prognosis groups possibly requiring more aggressive treatment.

In both cervical and endometrial cancer, the factors affecting treatment selection will be considered under the following headings:

Extent of disease
Biology of the tumour.
Effectiveness and morbidity of treatment.
Patient factors affecting treatment choice.
Individual selection of treatment.

CERVICAL CANCER

EXTENT OF DISEASE

Staging

Cervical cancer spreads locally towards the pelvic wall and can be assessed by vaginal and rectal examination. This forms the basis of the FIGO staging

Table 1 Correlation of stage of cervical carcinoma and survival rate.

Stage		Definition (FIGO system)	Five-year actuarial survival [a](no. of patients)	
I		*Invasive cancer confined to cervix*		
	a	Micro-invasive cancer (carcinoma *in situ* with early stromal invasion)	93%	(15)
	b	Invasive cancer beyond early stromal invasion including:		
		occult Stage Ib,		
		clinically demonstrable cancer	80%	(121)
II		*Lesion beyond cervix but has not reached pelvic side walls, bladder or rectal mucosa*		
	a	Proximal two-thirds of vagina only	72%	(82)
	b	Clinically detectable in parametrium	47%	(82)
III		*Disease has extended to pelvic side wall or lower third of vagina*		
	a	Lower one-third of vagina only		
	b	Extension to pelvic side wall/hydronephrosis or non-functioning kidney due to ureteral stenosis	30%	(127)
IV		*Carcinoma has extended beyond true pelvis or has involved bladder or rectum*		
	a	Spread to adjacent organs	0%	(3)
	b	Distant metastasis	0%	(10)
All stages		*Overall actuarial five-year survival*	55%	(242/440)

[a] From an analysis of 440 patients treated with radiotherapy at Velindre Hospital, Cardiff (1974–1978)

system which correlates well with survival (Table 1). However, clinical staging is inaccurate in approximately one-third of patients. Averette *et al.* (1972) pioneered surgical staging and found discrepancy between clinical and surgical staging in 38% of 317 patients. Clinical staging tended to underestimate the extent of the disease in all clinical stages.

It is not certain how far this would affect treatment results from radiotherapy, since, in most of those understaged, disease would in any case be ecompassed in pelvic radiotherapy ports and treatment would not be altered significantly. Moreover, van Nagell *et al.* (1971) found that clinical findings of parametrial invasion of tumour was considerably increased when examination was performed under anaesthesia, and this may increase the accuracy of staging without the inevitable morbidity of surgical staging.

Metastastic spread to lymph nodes tends to be orderly, involving first the para-uterine, obturator, internal and external iliac, and common iliac nodes before finally involving the para-aortic nodes. There is considerable variation in the incidence of pelvic node metastases reported but there is a consistent increase in incidence with stage. Morton *et al.* (1961) averaged the incidence from a number of surgical studies comprising nearly 5000 patients, and found 16.5% of Stage I, 31.9% of Stage II, and 46.7% of Stage III patients had pelvic nodal metastases. More recently Boronow (1977) found that as many as 20.7% of patients with occult Stage Ib carcinoma and 29.5% of clinically detectable Stage Ib tumours had pelvic lymph node metastases at lymphadenectomy. Therefore, pelvic nodal metastases can be assumed to be present in a significant proportion of patients even in the early stages.

The incidence of para-aortic nodal metastases similarly increases with stage but incidence data are scanty and very variable. Averaging reported series, the incidence is 2.5–5% in Stage I rising to 10–18.2% in Stage IIa, 5–44% in Stage IIb, and 25–38% in Stage III (Averette *et al.*, 1975; Bucksbaum, 1972; Nelson *et al.*, 1977; Piver *et al.*, 1977b; Delgado *et al.*, 1977). The incidence variation probably results from random sampling in small numbers of patients, and microscopic foci of tumour may often have been missed. *Post-mortem* studies on patients dying from cervical cancer indicate that 70% have para-aortic disease when distant metastases are present (Sotto *et al.*, 1960). However, we do not know how often distant metastases are the result of lymphatic or of haematogenous spread.

The presence of pelvic node metastases, irrespective of stage, reduces survival rate considerably. Mitani *et al.* (1962) found that five-year survival in a group of surgically treated Stages I and II patients was 70% if nodes were negative, 50% if one nodal metastasis was found, and 37% if two or more nodes were present. Averette and Jobson (1979) reported a 51% five-year survival after irradiation in patients found to have occult pelvic metastases at surgical staging. Therefore, pelvic treatment salvages approximately one-half of patients with Stages I or II disease with pelvic node metastases. However, it is not clear how many patients with proven para-aortic node metastases are salvageable with current treatment (discussed below).

Tumour size

The relationship between tumour size, prognosis, and risk of metastases is well recognized in breast or head and neck cancers, but its importance is ignored in all recognized staging systems for carcinoma of the cervix. Nevertheless, when tumour size exceeds 4 cm in Stages Ib or IIa, the risk of pelvic node metastases increases (Table 2) and prognosis deteriorates in surgically treated patients (Piver and Chung, 1975) (Table 3). We have noted a similar relationship of tumour size to prognosis in radiotherapeutically

Table 2 Relationship of size of cervical carcinoma to pelvic node metastasis. (Modified from Piver and Chung, 1975)

Tumour	Proportion with pelvic nodal metastases	
	Stage Ib	Stage IIa
Up to 3 cm	20/94 (21.2%)	8/38 (21%)
4 to 6+ cm	19/51 (35.2%)	24/57 (42%)
All sizes	39/145 (26.8%)	32/95 (33.6%)

Table 3 Relationship of tumour size to prognosis in cervical carcinoma treated by surgery or radiotherapy

Tumour size	Prognosis (five-year survival)			
	Stage Ib		Stage IIa	
	Radiotherapy[a]	Surgery[b]	Radiotherapy[a]	Surgery[b]
Up to 3 cm	85/100 (85%)	85/102 (83%)	39/46 (87%)	27/40 (68%)
4 cm – 6 cm	11/21 (52%)	34/55 (62%)	20/36 (61%)	22/59 (37%)

[a] Velindre Hospital Cardiff
[b] Piver and Chung (1975).

treated patients at Velindre Hospital, Cardiff (Table 3). Therefore, patients presenting with bulky Stages Ib and 2a tumours have a high risk of local recurrence and nodal metastases, and this should be considered in treatment planning.

TUMOUR BIOLOGY

A number of histological factors have been shown to reflect the likelihood of tumour metastasis and risk of recurrence, and host reaction factors may also be important in this respect.

Grade and histological type of tumour

Classifying squamous cell cancers on the basis of differentiation has little bearing on prognosis (Kistner and Hertig, 1951; Linnell and Maansson, 1952; Ng and Atkin, 1973). Division into large cell and keratinizing squamous cell cancer and small cell cancer is a more useful classification (Reagan *et al.*,

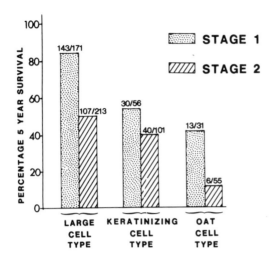

Figure 1 Relationship of cell type to prognosis in cervical carcinoma. (Modified from Reagan and Fu, 1979.)

1957). Reagan and Fu (1979) grouped together five reported series of patients treated with radiation, and showed there was a consistent relationship between cell type and survival, irrespective of stage (Figure 1).

Although van Nagell *et al.* (1979) suggested that keratinizing cancers were more resistant to radiotherapy, there is as yet insufficient evidence to prove that survival in such cases is significantly increased if treated surgically. Oat cell carcinoma occurs in only 4% of patients with carcinoma of the cervix, but is important because it is an aggressive tumour.

In a series of 41 patients, van Nagell *et al.* (1977) found that 70% were Stages I or II but only 46% remained alive at an average follow-up of over five years. There was no increased incidence of bulky tumours, and pelvic node metastasis was found in eight of 13 (62%) treated with lymphadenectomy. Pelvic recurrence was seen in four of 13 surgically treated patients compared to one of 28 treated with radiotherapy. However, 37% of patients developed distant metastases within one year, and it is therefore not clear to what extent pelvic control increases survival.

Adenocarcinoma constitutes 5% of carcinoma of the cervix. Kottmeier (1979) reported that five-year survival (48.4%) is slightly lower than for squamous cell carcinoma (57%) irrespective of treatment. Adenocarcinoma is no longer believed to be radioresistant, and Bush (1979) reported that survival of Stage Ib squamous and adenocarcinoma treated with radiation therapy was identical, while Weiner and Wizenberg (1975) reported that the results of radiation were not improved if combined with surgery.

Nevertheless, van Nagell et al. (1979) reported a higher recurrence rate in Stage Ib adenocarcinoma than in those with squamous cell tumours, and a third of the cases developed distant metastases. In our experience, seven of 12 patients with Stages I or IIa adenocarcinoma had lesions of 4 cm or more, suggesting that these tumours tend to be more bulky, possibly because they arise in the endocervix and form a barrel-shaped bulky lesion before they present clinically.

Vascular invasion

Vascular invasion by tumour cells has been reported to be an adverse prognostic factor by several observers (Barber et al., 1978; van Nagell et al., 1979). It is associated with an increased incidence of pelvic nodal metastases and local recurrence. It is seen in only 29% of surgically treated Stage Ib patients but in 63% of those who recur (van Nagell et al., 1979). Interestingly, it was noted in 93% of the aggressive oat cell carcinoma cases (van Nagell et al., 1977). Vascular invasion therefore is a feature to be considered in planning treatment, since it implies high risk of pelvic and distant metastases in apparently early disease.

Lymphocytic infiltration

Lymphocytic infiltration of tumour has been noted to be a good prognostic factor in gastric cancer (Black *et al.*, 1971), breast cancer (Bloom and Field, 1971), and Hodgkin's disease (Lukes *et al.*, 1966). Van Nagell *et al.* (1979) have also reported it to be associated with a low incidence of pelvic node metastases (9%), low recurrence rate after surgery (7%), and a five-year survival of 90% in Stage Ib cancer of the cervix.

Micro-invasive carcinoma

The natural history of micro-invasive cancer has, until recently, been ill defined and this has led to widely differing views on its management. An extensive study by Lohe *et al.* (1978) has helped to clarify the position. Two main prognostic groups were defined:

Early stromal invasion

This is characterized by *in situ* carcinoma with isolated tumour projections in continuity with the epithelium. In this group there were no cancer deaths in 285 patients, despite 72% having conservative treatment with cone biopsy or simple hysterectomy. A review of a further 895 cases in the literature revealed only four who died from cancer (0.04%).

Micro-carcinoma

This is characterized by confluent masses of tumour no longer connected to the surface epithelium. Being at most 10 mm wide and 5 mm in depth, it is a lesion requiring very careful histological diagnosis. In this group, Lohe *et al.* (1978) found that three out of 134 (2%) died of cancer, and a similar number of cancer deaths (3%) was noted in a review of 435 patients in the literature. Interestingly, all cancer deaths in Lohe's study had histological evidence of vascular invasion by tumour cells, and tumour recurrence was on the pelvic wall and not in the parametrium.

Averette *et al.* (1976) observed that between 3 to 5 mm deep to the surface the histological picture of micro-invasive cancer changes. Tumour fingers become confluent and often separated from the epithelium, and when this occurs there is a risk of pelvic nodal metastases. Boronow (1977) reported no nodal metastases at lymphadenectomy when invasion was 3 mm or less, and there was no evidence of vascular invasion.

There is therefore no evidence to justify treating the pelvic lymph node region when the histological picture is consistent with early stromal invasion of no greater than 3 mm. However, the picture is not so clear in micro-carcinoma because, when the depth of penetration is 5 mm, the incidence of nodal metastases may be as high as 3.5%. Tumour vascular invasion or oat cell type suggests an increased risk of pelvic wall nodal metastases.

EFFECTIVENESS AND MORBIDITY OF TREATMENT

Curative treatment must eradicate the primary tumour and nodal metastases with a minimum of complications. Fletcher (1973) has shown that tumour curability with irradiation is determined by tumour size and the dose that can be safely given. Nodal metastases, size for size, will respond in the same way as the primary. Microscopic disease will be controlled in 90% of cases by 5000 rad, but 2–4 cm tumours will need 7000 rad to attain the same degree of control. However, a large treatment volume will not tolerate such high doses without prohibitive complications.

The effectiveness of radical surgery is similarly limited by tumour size since it is difficult to remove large tumours with an adequate margin without damaging vital structures. There is consequently the dilemma as to what is adequate treatment and what is an unacceptable level of complications. Treatment options are as follows:

Intracavitary treatment alone

Intracavitary treatment enables a very high dose to be given to a pear-shaped volume around the cervix. There is a rapid fall-off of dose with increasing distance from the sources and, consequently, complications are confined to midline structures, mainly the rectum and bladder. A remote, high-dose-rate, after-loading system (cathetron) achieves comparable levels of tumour control to low-dose radium insertions (Joslin *et al.*, 1972; O'Connell *et al.*, 1967; Berry, 1980). Cathetron therapy has also been found to have fewer normal tissue complications (Berry, 1980), but the reasons for this are not clear.

Hamberger *et al.* (1978) found that, with intracavitary radium alone, 96% of 93 patients with Stage Ib carcinomas (1 cm or less) were controlled locally and only 2% of cases developed severe complications resulting from excessive radiation dosage.

Intracavitary and external radiation

Intracavitary radiation alone will not deliver a cancericidal dose to the pelvic wall. Therefore, if there is a significant risk of nodal metastases at the pelvic wall or when the primary is large, external radiation is needed to increase the pelvic wall radiation dose or to shrink the tumour prior to intracavitary treatment. This means an inevitable risk of small bowel damage.

In the case of small tumours, intracavitary radiation with concurrent external radiation to the whole pelvis (Joslin *et al.*, 1972) enables the pelvic wall dose to be raised to 5000 rad or more, whilst avoiding overdosage of the intracavitary high-dose volume which contains the primary tumour. If the tumour is large (4 cm or more), a greater emphasis has to be placed on external radiation to shrink the tumour sufficiently to carry out intracavitary treatment with good distribution.

Our experience shows that in the case of small tumours (3 cm or less), local control is achieved in 90%, while 6% developed severe complications (4% small bowel damage and 2% large bowel damage). Results are similar for Stages I and IIa if tumour size is 3 cm or less. As tumour size increases (Stages Ib and IIa), local control falls to 83%. Small bowel complications remain similar (despite combination with surgery) if the dose of external radiation does not exceed 4000–4500 rad/4–5 weeks. Above this dose, there is a high risk of severe complications when surgery is incorporated in treatment.

In advanced disease, there is a progressive fall in local control (61% and 51% in Stages IIb and III respectively). Increasing external radiation dose results in increasing complications. Increasing dosage above 6000 rad does not increase local control in advanced disease (Castro *et al.*, 1970) but increases the complication rate.

The incidence of para-aortic node metastases increases with stage, and failure of treatment in advanced disease is increasingly the result of distant metastases. Therefore, extending radiation to include the common iliac nodes, and even the para-aortic nodes, becomes tempting in Stages IIb and

III. However, high doses of 5000 rad or more in 5 weeks to such large volumes results in a prohibitive incidence of often fatal complications (Piver *et al.*, 1977b; El Senoussi *et al.*, 1979; Lepanto *et al.*, 1975), especially if radiation is combined with surgery. The maximum dose which can be given safely is 4500 rad at a rate of 900 rad per week (El Senoussi *et al.*, 1979).

Despite the high morbidity of para-aortic radiation, the increase in survival which can be obtained is modest and was estimated by Chism *et al.* (1975) as less than 3%. Such treatment can only be successful if para-aortic nodal metastases are small and there is a high probability of controlling the pelvic primary. However, in Stages IIb and III, local control is only 61% and 51% , respectively. Fletcher and Rutledge (1972) reported that only 25% of patients proved to have common iliac or para-aortic nodal metastases at surgery or lymphangiography were alive at 18 months. This would suggest that, at best, survival could be increased in Stages IIb or III by one-quarter of the percentage dying from extrapelvic disease (in Cardiff, 18% and 17% for Stages IIb and IIIb respectively).

Rotman *et al.* (1979) reported that extending radiation to the para-aortic nodes and delivering 4500 rad in 5 weeks did not increase survival in Stage III, and severe complications were seen in those patients also having surgery. Surprisingly, they did find that such treatment increased survival from 50% to 75% (statistically different) in Stage IIb, but this was not a randomized study. It is, on the whole, difficult to justify the morbidity of staging laparotomy, especially when combined with radiotherapy, since staging laparotomy is unlikely to contribute to increased survival in these patients and it merely increases morbidity.

Radical surgery

Radical surgery by Wertheim hysterectomy with lymphadenectomy, offers an alternative to radiotherapy in Stages I and Stage IIa. Few surgeons would contemplate dissecting tumour from the ureters or the pelvic wall in more advanced disease. Lymphadenectomy is effective for isolated nodal metastases but fails when nodes are large and multiple (Rutledge and Saski, 1979). One of the largest comparisons of surgery and radiation was reported by Masabucci *et al.* (1966) on a total of 2145 patients treated in Japan where surgery is the preferred treatment. Five-year survival was virtually identical in both stages for both treatments. Despite the selection of fitter patients for surgery, other retrospective studies have reported similar findings (Park *et al.*, 1973), including a prospective comparison (Newton, 1975) (Table 4).

Surgery offers the advantage in young women of ovarian conservation since the risk of ovarian metastases in Stage I is negligible. It is also argued that irradiation causes scarring leading to dyspareunia. However, extended hysterectomy removes 30–50% of vaginal length, which may create sexual

Table 4 Comparison of results from surgery and radiotherapy in carcinoma of the cervix. (Modified from Masabucci *et al.*, 1966)

Stage	Surgery				Radiotherapy			
	Five-year survival (No. of patients)	Morbidity			Five-year survival (no. of patients)	Morbidity		
		Urinary	Intestinal	Sexual		Urinary	Intestinal	Sexual
IB	90.5% (268/296)				88.2% (134/152)			
IIA	74.4% (198/266)	47.1%	63.9%	57.9%	68.7% (309/450)	23.5%	28.2%	37.4%

problems equal to those of radiation therapy (Rutledge and Saski, 1979). Also if lymphadenectomy reveals lymph node metastases, post-operative irradiation is usually indicated, thereby destroying ovarian function in any case. Masabucci *et al.* (1966) sent a questionnaire to 293 surgically treated and 234 irradiated patients five years after treatment and found there were more symptoms related to urinary and intestinal complications in surgical patients than in those treated with radiotherapy (see Table 4). In addition, sexual activity continued more frequently in those treated with radiation than those surgically treated and the husbands' responses were in agreement.

Combined surgery and radiotherapy

It is argued that since there is frequently histological evidence of residual tumour in the uterus and lymph nodes after radical irradiation, surgery should be combined with radiotherapy in all operable patients. Stallworthy and Wiernick (1975) reported that there was histological evidence of residual tumour in the uterus of 37% of patients six weeks after irradiation and 25% had histological evidence of nodal metastases. However, it is well known that histological evidence of tumour may persist for up to three months after radiotherapy but does not prove that the tumour is necessarily viable.

A large retrospective study with 437 patients with Stages Ib and IIa disease found that there was no difference in survival, pelvic-tumour control or complications, when surgery was combined with radiotherapy (Perez *et al.*, 1979). More recently a prospective study (Perez *et al.*, 1980) again reported no difference in survival in either stage (bulky tumours were excluded). Complications were similar in both groups, possibly because those receiving combined treatment receive only 2000 rad external pelvic radiation.

As we have seen, local control of bulky tumours (4 cm or more) is reduced in Stages Ia and IIa, and at the same time the incidence of lymph nodes and distant metastases is increased. A study of 276 patients with tumours larger than 6 cm reported that the survival rate was increased to that of non-bulky tumours when conservative hysterectomy was combined with pre-operative radium (5000 mg h) and 4000 rad in four weeks external whole-pelvis radiation (Rutledge *et al.*, 1976). However, when 5000 rad whole-pelvis radiation was used in the early part of the study, a higher incidence of fatal operative complications was seen.

Chemotherapy

In our experience, 5% of patients present with distant metastases, and 20% develop distant metastases after radical pelvic treatment. In such patients there is clearly a need for effective systemic therapy, and it would be of value to increase control in Stages IIb and III also. However, the value of current

Table 5 Results of cytotoxic chemotherapy in carcinoma of the cervix (metastatic or recurrent disease previously untreated with chemotherapy)

Drug regime		Proportion responding (complete and partial response)	Proportion with complete response	Reference
Cisplatin 50 mg/m^2 every 3 weeks		11/22 (50%)	3/22 (14%)	Thigpen *et al.*(1980)
Adriamycin 25 mg/m^2	every			
Cisplatin 50 mg/m^2	3 weeks	6/19 (32%)	2/19 (11%)	Slayton and Mladineo, (1978)

chemotherapeutic regimes remains unclear. Wasserman and Carter (1977) reviewed the response rate to single agents and reported it to be between 22 and 27% for chlorambucil, vincristine, adriamycin or mitomycin C. However, the responses were of short duration and usually in distant sites rather than in the pelvis.

Cisplatin used in doses of 50 mg/m^2 in patients with normal renal function has been suggested to give more encouraging results. Thigpen *et al.* (1980) reported three complete remissions and eight partial responses in a series of 22 patients who had received no previous chemotherapy. Combination cisplatin regimes have not been proved to yield a higher complete remission rate, and toxicity is greatly increased (Slayton and Mladineo, 1978; Lele *et al.*, 1981; Hakes *et al.*, 1981) (Table 5). At present there are insufficient data to indicate its value in terms of palliation, survival, or local control, used either alone or in combination with radiotherapy.

Hydroxyurea is the agent most studied in combination with radiotherapy. Piver *et al.* (1977a) reported significant increase in survival at two years when this agent was administered concurrently with radiotherapy in Stages IIb and IIIb.

PATIENT FACTORS AFFECTING TREATMENT CHOICE

The following factors have to be considered when selecting patients for radiotherapy or radical surgery:

Age

Patients over the age of 60 years are more likely to suffer from cardiac and respiratory disease, and present a higher operative risk. Consequently, radiotherapy is usually preferred in operable cases in this age group and the results of treatment are identical with those of surgery. Currie (1971) reported in a large series of 475 patients treated by Wertheim's hysterectomy that fit, elderly patients tolerate surgery well, but two out of seven of his post-operative deaths were from ischaemic heart disease.

In our experience, patients over 70 years who are fit enough to complete radical radiotherapy have the same likelihood of local control as do younger patients (Table 6). However, 10% were unable to complete treatment because of their frail condition, and would have been unsuitable for surgery. It appears that patients' general condition should be considered rather than age *per se*, when determining suitability for radical treatment.

Table 6 Relationship of age to local control of carcinoma of the cervix with radiotherapy

Stage	Local control four years after treatment [a]	
	70 years old or more	Less than 70 years old
Ib	6/7 (86%)	93/112 (83%)
IIa	4/6 (67%)	62/86 (76%)
IIb	5/9 (56%)	35/56 (63%)
III	17/36 (47%)	31/59 (53%)

[a] Velindre Hospital, Cardiff

Pelvic sepsis

Patients with active extrauterine pelvic sepsis tolerate radiotherapy poorly, and there is a risk of peritonitis. Such patients, if technically operable, should be treated surgically.

Previous surgery

As mentioned above, previous surgery increases the morbidity of radiotherapy. However, post-operative adhesions also make radical surgery technically difficult, and therefore this factor hardly affects selection of treatment.

Obesity

The obese patient imposes technical difficulties for the surgeon. Tissue planes are indistinct, limits of cancer are vague, and haemorrhage and trauma more likely (Rutledge and Saski, 1979). However, such patients may also develop more severe reaction to external beam treatment. This can be overcome with the use of megavoltage radiation or the use of special beam arrangements so that, on the whole, radiotherapy is to be preferred.

Hypertension and low socioeconomic state with poor nutrition have been reported to reduce survival rates in radiotherapeutically treated patients (Jenkin and Stryker 1968; Diddle *et al.*, 1956). However, such factors are likely also to reduce tolerance for radical surgery and therefore hardly affects selection of treatment.

INDIVIDUAL SELECTION OF TREATMENT

From our analysis of tumour spread, tumour biology, patient prognostic factors, and the efficacy and morbidity of treatments available, we can draw up a plan of treatment selection. In essence, this follows clinical stage, but subgroups must be stratified according to other factors.

Micro-invasive cancer

Early stromal invasion

If stromal invasion does not exceed 3 mm and there is no vascular invasion (as shown on a carefully sectioned cone biopsy), there is a minimal risk of pelvic node metastases and survival likelihood approaches 100%. Simple hysterectomy with removal of a vaginal cuff as for *in situ* cancer offers the simplest type of adequate treatment, and in this way morbidity can be kept to a minimum.

If the patient is not a good anaesthetic risk, intracavitary radiation alone is a good alternative. Hamberger *et al.* (1978) reported no local failure in a group of 41 patients treated with two 48 hour radium insertions. Serious morbidity was seen in only one patient to whom an excessive dose was delivered to the bladder base. External radiation is not necessary in view of the insignificant risk of pelvic nodal metastases, and will increase morbidity. Patients with vascular invasion or with an oat cell carcinoma should be considered as a separate group, as their risk of pelvic nodal metastases is greatly increased.

Micro-carcinoma

Simple hysterectomy is adequate to deal with the primary tumour as invasion approaches 3–5 mm. The role of lymphadenectomy is unclear. The risk of nodal metastases is 3.5% and lymphadenectomy in this good prognosis group becomes tempting, but it does not guarantee a 100% chance of cure. Lohe *et al.* (1978) found that 14 out of 26 cancer deaths among their patients and nearly 2500 cases reviewed from the literature occurred after such radical treatment.

Hamberger *et al.* (1978) reported 100% of five-year survival in patients with carcinomas 1 cm or less treated with intracavitary radiation alone. This would provide cancericidal radiation dosage only to the first line of lymph nodes, but probably only the first line of lymph nodes is at risk of involvement in the absence of vascular invasion. The good control by intracavitary radiation alone suggests that micro-carcinomas, in the absence of vascular invasion, can be effectively treated with intracavitary radiation alone, with less morbidity than would be expected from Wertheim's hysterectomy and lymphadenectomy.

Stage Ib (3 cm diameter or less)

Most patients in this category can be treated either by radical surgery or by intracavitary and external beam radiation treatment, with equal survival likelihood and similar morbidity. Patients over 60 years and obese patients are more suitable for radiotherapy.

Radiotherapy is to be preferred where possible since lymphadenectomy is unlikely to be complete in the presence of multiple pelvic node metastases. The presence of a heavy lymphocytic tumour infiltrate suggests a reduced likelihood of pelvic nodal metastases, and this is reassuring if the patient wishes to be treated surgically. Simple hysterectomy offers a means of salvage for patients who develop central local recurrence.

Stage Ib (4cm diameter or more, oat cell type or presence of vascular invasion)

More than one-third of such patients will have pelvic node metastases and therefore whole-pelvis radiotherapy is to be preferred, since lymphadenec-tomy is unlikely to be complete. There is no conclusive evidence to support the elective combination of surgery and radiotherapy for bulky tumours. Our experience shows that such tumours can frequently be controlled with radiotherapy alone, and the added morbidity of surgery is then avoided. Limiting the dose of external beam radiation to 4000 rad in 20 fractions in four weeks or the equivalent, avoids excessive morbidity if surgery proves necessary for residual tumour. Careful follow-up within the first three months after radiotherapy is necessary.

Stage IIa

In such cases, there is a greater risk of cutting through occult parametrial disease at surgery and a higher risk of pelvic nodal metastases. Therefore, radiotherapy is preferred and surgery is carried out on those with residual local disease.

Stages IIb and III

These stages offer similar problems; they are both primarily treated with radiotherapy and the main problems are poor local control and an increased incidence of extrapelvic disease. Extended radiotherapy to include para-aortic nodes has not been proved to affect survival significantly and morbidity is increased. Chemotherapy studies are needed to assess whether increased local control can be achieved when it is combined with radiotherapy and to ensure that this hoped-for advantage is not outweighed by increased morbidity.

Stage IV

Prognosis of patients with Stage IV disease is very poor indeed. In our experience, the median survival is five months. Control of symptoms with palliative radiotherapy and analgesics is the most important part of management. The use of ureterostomy in patients with bilateral obstructive uropathy appears to offer little benefit. In our experience, six patients treated in this way and subsequently followed by radiotherapy were all dead within one year.

ENDOMETRIAL CANCER

Endometrial cancer is well recognized to have a more favourable prognosis than has cervical cancer. However, an overall five-year survival of 65.4% (Kottmeier, 1979) should not invite complacency. Management, as in cervical cancer, has to be determined by the extent of tumour spread, the biology of the tumour, effectiveness of treatment, and patient fitness factors.

EXTENT OF DISEASE

Staging

Endometrial cancer invades the myometrium and may spread towards the cervix. Clinical assessment of local spread forms the basis of the FIGO staging system (Table 7). The risk of lymphatic metastases increases with stage, as in carcinoma of the cervix; however, in Stage I the incidence of nodal metastases is only 11.2%, rising to 23% in Stage II (Lewis *et al.*, 1972).

Tumour spread outside the uterus is a poor prognostic sign except where spread is confined to the ovaries. Nilson and Koller (1969) found that 19 out of 23 patients with tumour spread to the ovaries were still living at five years. Since most patients are in Stage I, pathological factors assume a greater importance in selecting treatment. The risk of spread is zero in cases with superficial invasion, rising to 36.2% in those with deep invasion (2 mm from serosa) (Lewis *et al.*, 1972).

Myometrial invasion

The depth of myometrial invasion is related to the incidence of pelvic nodal metastases. The risk appears to increase when more than one–third of the myometrium has been invaded. Pelvic lymphatic spread often means para-aortic involvement. Creasman *et al.* (1976) reported that when no myometrial invasion was present 3.6% had pelvic node metastases and 1.8% para-aortic node metastases, but with deep myometrial invasion 43% had pelvic node metastases and 21% had para-aortic node metastases. This emphasizes the limitations of pelvic treatment but, in spite of this, 36% of pelvic-node-positive patients reported by Lewis *et al.* (1972) survived five years with pelvic treatment.

BIOLOGY OF THE TUMOUR

Unlike the situation in the case of carcinoma of the cervix, tumour grade has been found to be a useful prognostic factor which is now incorporated in the FIGO system (Table 7). Poorly differentiated tumours are more likely to metastasize and have a worse prognosis (Lewis *et al.*, 1972). The risk increases from 5.5% in Stage I well differentiated tumours to 26% in the case of poorly differentiated tumours. Poorly differentiated lesions also have a high incidence of para-aortic node metastases. Creasman *et al.* (1976) found that in such patients 54% had positive pelvic nodes and as many as 46% had para-aortic node metastases. Such data suggest that pelvic treatment alone is unlikely to cure many patients with poorly differentiated lesions and most relapses will occur outside the pelvis.

The extent of myometrial invasion and tumour grade can be usefully combined to determine the risk of pelvic node metastases (Creasman *et al.*, 1976; see Figure 2), and may be useful in planning treatment. Similarly, the risk of all types of vaginal recurrence is increased with poorly differentiated tumours and increasing muscle invasion (Frick *et al.*, 1973; Ingersoll, 1971; Kagan *et al.*, 1975). Vaginal cuff recurrence probably results from transection of lymphatics containing tumour rather than from implantation at surgery (Morrow *et al.*, 1976). To date, there is no evidence that techniques aiming to reduce the risk of implantation of cells at surgery are effective in reducing vaginal recurrence rates.

Table 7 Correlation of stage of endometrial cancer and survival rate

FIGO stage	Definition (FIGO system)	Absolute five-year survival [a] (no. of patients)
I[b]	Confined to corpus	74.7% (8009)
	G1 Well differentiated	78.4% (2788)
	G2 Moderately differentiated	74.1% (1665)
	G3 Poorly differentiated	60.8% (556)
II	Spread to the cervix after arising in the corpus	55.7% (1426)
III	Spread has occurred outside the uterus	31.3% (895)
IV	Spread has extended outside the true pelvis or has obviously involved the bladder or rectum	9.2% (359)

[a] From Kottmeier (1979)
[b] Stage I is subdivided into: A—length of uterine cavity is 8 cm or less; B—length of uterine cavity is greater than 8 cm

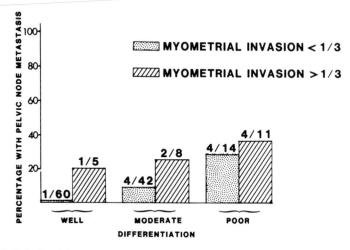

Figure 2 Relationship of pelvic node metastases to myometrial invasion and tumour grade in Stage I endometrial cancer. (Modified from Creasman *et al.*, 1976.)

EFFECTIVENESS OF TREATMENT

Treatment selection aims to decide whether surgery or radiotherapy is the better primary treatment for the individual, and whether adjuvant radiation or progestogen therapy is necessary after surgery. Treatment options available are as follows:

Surgery alone

Five-year survival of patients treated surgically is approximately 20% greater than that of patients treated with radiation alone, both in Stage I and Stage II (Kottmeier, 1979). A higher rate of intercurrent death would be expected in those selected for radiotherapy alone, because they are generally less fit and older than those selected for surgery. Nevertheless, surgery still has an advantage even when prognostically similar patients are compared.

Nilson and Koller (1969) found that in a series of 359 surgically treated patients the corrected five-year survival rate for surgery was 98% in Stage I compared with 67.5% for treatment by radiation alone. Bickenbach *et al.* (1967) found a similar advantage for surgery in 190 prognostically similar patients. It is generally agreed that surgery is to be preferred both in Stage I and Stage II as primary treatment.

The use of Wertheim hysterectomy and lymphadenectomy has not in-creased survival when compared with more conservative surgery. Jones (1975) calculated the overall survival in five reports of patients treated with radical surgery and found that the crude five-year survival rate of 77% was no greater than one would expect with less radical treatment in Stage I. In these, frequently obese patients, severe morbidity rises to between 10 and 24% with radical surgery (Schwartz and Brunschwig, 1975; Park *et al.*, 1974), and 8% will develop pulmonary emboli when treated with lymphadenectomy (Andersen and Staples, 1965). Consequently, radical surgery including lymphadenectomy has largely been abandoned.

It has been suggested that hysterectomy alone is adequate treatment in most patients with Stage I disease. Keller *et al.* (1974) found no recurrence in 63 patients with less than 50% myometrial invasion treated by this method. However, this series was relatively small and other series have revealed a small incidence of vaginal recurrence even in the presence of little or no myometrial invasion. Price *et al.* (1965) showed that, when myometrial invasion increased beyond 50%, the recurrence rate increased to 12.5% and that four out of seven Stage II cases recurred in the pelvis. There is, therefore, a place for pelvic adjuvant radiotherapy in the presence of deep myometrial invasion.

Adjuvant irradiation

Intracavitary radiation alone

The role of intracavitary radiation in preventing vaginal recurrence is well established; the incidence is reduced from the order of 10% to 2.5% (Dobbie, 1953; Gusberg *et al.*, 1960; Sala and del Regato, 1962; Wade *et al.*, 1967). Prevention is to be preferred since only one-third of patients treated for vaginal recurrence will survive five years (Reddy *et al.*, 1979; Badib *et al.*, 1969; Salazar *et al.*, 1977). Results of pre- and post-operative radium therapy are similar (Graham, 1971; Shah and Green, 1972; Monson *et al.*, 1976).

Intracavitary radiation alone is suitable for those patients with risk of vault recurrence but an insignificant risk of pelvic node metastases and for well differentiated superficial lesions. The use of pre-operative radium precludes accurate assessment of myometrial invasion, thereby limiting accurate selection of treatment on a pathological basis (Wilson *et al.*, 1980). Consequently, we prefer post-operative irradiation using a cathetron vaginal obturator (Joslin and Smith, 1971); the procedure does not need anaesthesia and can be administered as an outpatient. Corrected survival rates for those patients treated by this method treated between 1974 and 1976 is 100% and no serious morbidity was observed.

External radiation

If the tumour has penetrated more than *one* third of the myometrium, and especially if the lesion is moderately or poorly differentiated, the use of external beam therapy is logical. Joslin *et al.* (1977) reported overall five-year survival rates to be increased from 67% (280 patients) to 78% (250 patients) from the use of such treatment. However, a large controlled study involving 386 patients has not established any survival advantage for the addition of 4000 rad in 4 weeks external radiation given post-operatively (Onsrad *et al.*, 1976). Although the incidence of local recurrence in the vagina and pelvis was reduced, a greater number of patients developed distant metastases in the radiated group.

We have employed post-operative external beam radiotherapy for all patients with myometrial invasion penetrating more than one-third and for those with moderately or poorly differentiated tumours. The incidence of pelvic recurrence is low and death usually occurred from distant metastases.

Table 8 Effect of primary treatment on survival rate in endometrial cancer

Treatment	Five-year survival		
	Conservative surgery[a]	Irradiation alone[a]	Radical hysterectomy and lymphadenectomy[b]
Stage I	121/139 (87%)	90/130 (69%)	289/376 (77%)
Stage II	23/33 (70%)	15/31 (49%)	—

[a]From Bickenbach *et al.* (1967)
[b]From pooled data (Jones, 1975)

Morbidity was not greatly increased with added external radiation. Consequently, it appears that external radiation is successful in decreasing the incidence of pelvic recurrence but its effect on survival is not clear.

Adjuvant progestogen therapy

Progestogen therapy is safe and well tolerated in advanced endometrial cancer and objective response will be achieved in approximately 30% of patients (Reifenstein, 1971). It is therefore logical that its role should be explored as an adjuvant in early endometrial cancer where there is a risk of extrapelvic disease. Preliminary reports suggest that such treatment increases survival in Stage I (Bonte *et al.*, 1978), but it is not clear which prognostic groups benefit.

The high survival rates in endometrial carcinoma in the early stages mean that large numbers of patients will be needed to demonstrate statistically significant results. However, it is likely that patients with poorly differentiated tumours (responsible for most deaths) do not benefit as much as patients with well differentiated tumours. On the other hand, in patients with well differentiated superficial carcinomas it is possible that adjuvant progestogen therapy is unnecessary. Its use should be explored in pathologically more aggressive tumours where death generally results from distant metastases. This may apply especially to patients with Stage II or Stage III carcinomas.

Radiotherapy only

Radiotherapy alone is generally reserved for patients who are poor operative risks or have locally advanced disease (Stage III). Strickland (1965) reported that 31 out of 42 patients were cured with radiation alone. Nevertheless, as we have discussed, the results in large series reveal that surgery consistently produces better survival rates than does radiation alone.

External radiation combined with intracavitary treatment increases survival in those with uteri longer than 8 cm (Badib *et al.*, 1969). This is understandable since intracavitary treatment using the Machester system will provide a poor dose distribution and will not treat nodal metastases. Bonte *et al.* (1978) reported 57% survival at five years in a group of 50 patients treated with radiation alone preceded by progestogens. The results, however, are no better than those reported by Badib *et al.* (1969) from radiation alone.

Once the tumour has infiltrated the parametrium, the tumour is technically inoperable; nevertheless, approximately one-quarter of these patients can be salvaged with radical radiotherapy, treated in the same way as Stage III cancer of the cervix (Lampe, 1963; Kottmeier, 1959).

PATIENT FACTORS AFFECTING TREATMENT CHOICE

Patients with endometrial cancer are frequently obese and hypertensive and consequently poor operative risks. It is therefore tempting to refer such patients for primary radiation. However, since surgery is associated with higher survival rates, this must be the preferred treatment unless the operative risks are considered very great.

INDIVIDUAL SELECTION OF TREATMENT

Surgery is to be preferred in all patients with operable Stage I or Stage II disease. Radical radiotherapy is reserved for those who are poor operative risks or have Stage III disease. Intracavitary radiotherapy effectively reduces the risk of recurrence in those with well differentiated superficial lesions and carries minimal morbidity. There may be an advantage for the addition of external beam radiation or adjuvant progestogen therapy in these patients.

Once the tumour has invaded more than one-third of the myometrium and is less than well differentiated or Stage II, external radiation is necessary. Further investigation to establish whether progestogen therapy can reduce the incidence of distant metastases is clearly needed.

Once distant metastases have occurred, progestogen therapy offers the prospect of significant palliation for approximately one-third of the patients. At present there is no proven palliative value for non-hormonal chemotherapy in the case of endometrial cancer.

CONCLUSION

The considerable information that has been gathered on the prognostic variables and pattern of treatment failure in uterine cancer can be used to individualize treatment. Good prognosis groups can be defined which can be treated conservatively with good results and with minimum morbidity. On the other hand, poor prognosis groups can be defined where more agressive therapeutic efforts may improve results.

Endometrial cancer presents with Stage I disease in 74% of patients and over 50% are well differentiated. Overall five-year survival is consequently relatively high (65.4% of 10 720 patients) (Kottmeier, 1979). Unfortunately, only a third of patients with cervical cancer present with Stage I disease and tumours tend to be less well differentiated. Consequently, overall survival is not as good (55.7% of 21 430 patients) as in endometrial cancer.

Acknowledgements

We are indebted to Dr K.W. James and Dr Newman who kindly gave us access to clinical data on the treatment results of carcinoma of the cervix at

Velindre Hospital. We are grateful to Mrs T. Purcell for secretarial assistance.

REFERENCES

Andersen, J., and Staples, S., (1965). Survival in carcinoma of the endometrium following pelvic node dissection. *Acta Obstet. Gynecol. Scand.*, **43**, Suppl. 7, 115.

Averette, H.E., Dudan, R.C., and Ford, J.H. (1972). Exploratory celiotomy for surgical staging of cervical cancer. *Am. J. Obstet. Gynecol.*, **113**, 1090–1096.

Averette, H.E., Ford, J.H., Jr, Dudan, R., Girtanner, R.E., Hoskins, W.J., and Lutz, M.H. (1975). Staging of cervical cancer. *Clin. Obstet. Gynecol.*, **18**, 215–232.

Averette, H.E., and Jobson, V.W. (1979). The role of exploratory laparotomy in the staging and treatment of invasive cervical carcinoma. *Int. J. Radiat. Oncol., Biol. Phys.*, **5**, 2137–2138.

Averette., Nelson, J.H., Ng, A.B.P., Hoskins, J.M., Boyce, J.G., and Ford, J.H. (1976). Diagnosis and management of microinvasive (Stage Ia) carcinoma of the cervix. *Cancer*, **38**, 414–425.

Badib, A.O., Kurohara, S.S., Vongtamm, V.Y., and Webster, J.H. (1969). Evaluation of primary radiation theory in Stage I Group 2 endometrial cancer. *Radiology*, **93**, 417–421.

Barber, H.R.K., Sommers, S.C., Rotterdam, H., and Kwan, T. (1978). Vascular invasion as a prognostic factor in Stage Ib cancer of the cervix. *Obstet. Gynecol.*, **52**, 343–348.

Berry, R.J. (1980). High dose rate afterloading. In *Treatment of cancer of the uterus* (eds T.D. Bates, and R.J. Berry). Institute of Radiology. pp. 190–193.

Bickenbach, W., Lochmuller, H. Dirlich, G., Roland, G., and Thurnover, R. (1967) Factor analysis of endometrial cancer in relation to treatment. *Obstet. Gynecol.*, **29**, 632.

Black, M.M., Freeman, C., Homer, S., and Cutter, S.J. (1971). Prognostic significance of microscopic structure of gastric carcinomas and their regional nodes. *Cancer*, **27**, 703–711

Bloom, H.J., and Field J.R. (1971). Impact of tumour grade and host resistance in survival of women with breast cancer. *Cancer*, **28**, 1580–1589.

Bonte, J., de Coster, J.M., Ide, P., and Billiet, G. (1978). Hormone prophylaxis and hormone therapy in the treatment of endometrial adenocarcinoma by means of medroxy progesterone acetate. In *Endometrial cancer* (eds I.G. Brush, R.J.B. King, and R.W. Taylor). London: Balliere Tindall. Chap. 22, pp. 192–205.

Boronow, R.C. (1977). Stage I cervix cancer and pelvic node metastasis. *Am. J. Obstet. Gynecol.*, **127** (2), 135–137.

Bucksbaum, H. J. (1972). Para-aortic lymph node involvement in cervical carcinoma. *Am. J. Obstet. Gynecol.*, **113**, (7), 942–947.

Bush R.S. (1979). *Malignancies of the ovary, uterus and cervix*. London: Edward Arnold. pp. 172–173.

Castro, J.R., Philippe, I., and Fletcher, G.M. (1970). Carcinoma of the cervix treated with external irradiation alone. *Radiology*, **95**, 163–166.

Chism, S.E., Park, R.C., and Keys, H.M. (1975). Prospects of para-aortic irradiation in treatment of cancer of the cervix. *Cancer* **35**, 1505–1509.

Creasman, W.T., Boronow, R.C., Morrow, O.P., Di Saia, P.J., and Blessing, J. (1976). Adenocarcinom of the endometrium: its metastatic lymph node potential. *Gynecol. Oncol.*, **4**, 239–243.

Currie, D.W. (1971). Operative treatment of carcinoma of the cervix. *J. Obstet. Gynecol. Br. Commonw.*, **78**(5), 385–405.

Delgado, G., Chun, B., Calgar, H., and Bepko, F. (1977). Para-aortic lymphadenectomy in gynaecologic malignancies confined to the pelvis. *Obstet. Gynecol.*, **50**, 418–423.

Diddle, A.W., Doris, M., O'Connor, K.A., and Brown, B. (1956). Nutrition and irradiation of cervix cancer. *Am. J. Obstet. Gynecol.*, **71**(4), 768–775.

Dobbie, B.M. (1953). Vaginal recurrence in carcinoma of body of uterus and their prevention by radium therapy. *J. Obstet. Gynaecol. Br. Emp.*, **60**, 702–705.

El Senoussi, M.A., Fletcher, G.H., and Borlase, B.C. (1979). Correlation of radiation and surgical parameters in complications in the extended field technique for carcinoma of the cervix. *Int. J. Radiat. Oncol., Biol. Phys.*, **5**, 927–934.

Fletcher, G.H. (1973). Clinical dose response curves of human malignant epithelial tumours. *Br. J. Radiol.* **46**, I–12.

Fletcher, G.H., and Rutledge, F.W. (1972). Extended field technique in the management of cancer of the cervix. *Am. J. Roentgenol.*, **114**, 116–122.

Frick, H.C., Munnel, E.W., Benger, A.P., and Lawry, M. (1973). Carcinoma of the endometrium. *Am. J. Obstet. Gynecol.*, **115**, 663–676.

Graham, J. (1971). The value of pre-operative or post-operative treatment by radium for carcinoma of the uteric body. *Surg. Gynaecol. Obstet.*, **132**, 855·860.

Gusberg, S.B., Jones, H.C., and Tovell, H.M. (1960). Selection of treatment for corpus cancer. *Am. J. Obstet Gynecol.*, **80**, 379–480.

Hakes, T.B., Lynch, G., and Lewis, J.L. (1981). Recurrent cervix cancer treated with high dose cisplatin and bleomycin. *Proc. Am. Soc. Clin. Oncol.*, **22**, 465.

Hamberger, A.D., Fletcher, G.H., and Wharton, J.T. (1978). Results of treatment of early Stage I carcinoma of the cervix with intracavitary radium alone. *Cancer*, **41**, 980–985.

Ingersoll, F.M., (1971). Vaginal recurrence of carcinoma of the corpus. Management and prevention. *Am.J. Surg.*, **121**, 470–477.

Jenkin R.D.T., and Stryker, J.A. (1968). The influence of the blood pressure on survival in cancer of the cervix. *Br. J. Radiol.*, **41**913.

Jones. H.W. (1975). Treatment of adenocarcinoma of the endometrium. *Obstet. Gynaecol. Surg.*, **30**, (3), 147–169.

Joslin, C.A., and Smith, C.W. (1971). Post-operative radiotherapy in the management of uterine corpus carcinoma. *Clin. Radiol.*, **22**, 118–124.

Joslin, C.A., Smith, C.W., and Mallik, A. (1972). The treatment of cervix cancer using high activity sources. *Br. J. Radiol.*, **45**, 257–270.

Joslin, C.A., Vaishampayan, G.V., and Mallik, A. (1977). The treatment of early cancer of the corpus uteri. *Br. J. Radiol.*, **50**, 38–45.

Kagan, A.R., Nussbaum, H., and Ziel, H. (1975). Adenocarcinoma of the endometrium. Vaginal recurrences and mortality. *Am. J. Roentgenol.*, **123**, 567–570.

Keller, D., Kempson, R., Levine G., and McLennon, C. (1974). Management of the patient with early endometrial carcinoma. *Cancer*, **33**, 1108–1116.

Kistner, R.W., and Hertig, A.T. (1951). A correlation of histologic grade, clinical stage and radiation response in carcinoma of the cervix. *Am J. Obstet. Gynecol.*, **61**, 1293–1300.

Kottmeier, H.I. (1959). Carcinoma of the corpus uteri, diagnosis and therapy. *Am. J. Obstet. Gynecol.*, **78**, 1127–1140.

Kottmeier, H.L. (1979). *Annual report on 'Results of treatment in gynaecological cancer'*, vol. 17. Radiumhemmet, Stockholm, Sweden.

Lampe, I. (1963). Endometrial carcinoma. *Am. J. Roentgenol.*, **90**, 1011–1015.

Lele, S.B., Piver, M.S., and Barlow, J.J. (1981). Cyclophosphamide, adriamycin and cis-dichlorodiammine-platinum chemotherapy in recurrent and metastatic cervical cancer. *Proc. Am. Soc. Clin. Oncol.,* **22**, 467.

Lepanto, P., Littman, P., Mikutu, J., Davis, L., and Celebre, J. (1975). Treatment of para-aortic nodes in carcinoma of the cervix. *Cancer,* **35**, 1510–1513.

Lewis, B., Stallworthy, J.A., and Cowdell, R. (1972). Adenocarcinoma of the body of the uterus. *J. Obstet. Gynaecol. Br. Commonw.,* **77**, 343–348.

Linnell, F., and Maansson, B. (1952). Prognostic value of histologic grading of carcinoma of cervix uteri; study of 388 cases treated with radium and roentgen therapy. *Acta Radiol.,* **38**, 219–238.

Lohe, K.J., Burghanlt, E., Hillemanns, H.G., Kaufman, C., Oher, K.G., and Zander, J. (1978). Early squamous cell carcinoma of the cervix. II. Clinical results of a co-operative study in the management of 419 patients with early stromal invasion and microcarcinoma. *Gynecol. Oncol.,* **6**, 31–50.

Lukes, T.J., Butler, J.J., and Hicks, E.B. (1966). Natural history of Hodgkin's disease as related to its pathologic picture. *Cancer,* **19**, 317–344.

Masabucci, K. Tenjin, Y. Kubo, H., and Kimura, M. (1966). Five year cure rate for carcinoma of the cervix uteri. *Am. J. Obstet. Gynecol.,* **103**(4), 566–573.

Mitani, Y., Fujii, J., Michitoshi, M., Ishizu, S., and Matukado, M., (1962). Lymph node metastases of carcinoma of the uterine cervix. *Am. J. Obstet. Gynecol.,* **84** (4), 515–522.

Monson, R.R. MacMahon, B., Austin, J.H. (1976). Post-operative irradiation in carcinoma of the endometrium. *Cancer,* **31**, 630–632.

Morrow, C.P., Saia, P.J., and Townsend, D.E. (1976). The role of post-operative irradiation in the management of Stage I adenocarcinoma of the endometrium. *Am. J. Roentgenol,* **127**, 325–329.

Morton, D.G., La Gasse, L.D., Moise, J.G., Jacobs, M., and Amromin, G (1961). Pelvic lymphadenectomy following radiation in cervical cancer. *Am. J. Obstet. Gynecol.* **88**, 932–943.

Nelson, J.H., Boyce, J.M., Macaset, M., Lu, T., Bohorquez, J.F., Nicastin, A.D., and Fruchter, R. (1977). Incidence significance and follow-up of para-aortic lymph node metastases in late invasive carcinoma of the cervix. *Am. J. Obstet. Gynecol.,* **128**, (3), 336–340.

Newton, M. (1975). Radical hysterectomy or radiotherapy for Stage I cervical cancer. A prospective comparison with 5 and 10 year follow-up. *Am. J. Obstet. Gynecol.,* **123**, 535–542.

Ng, A.B.P., and Atkin, W.B. (1973). Histological cell types and DNA value in the prognosis of squamous cell cancer of the uterine cervix. *Br. J. Cancer,* **28**, 322–331.

Nilson, P.A., and Koller, O. (1969). Carcinoma of the endometrium in Ninory 1957–1960 with special reference to treatment results. *Am. J. Obstet. Gynecol.,* **105**, 1099–1109.

O'Connell, D., Howard, W., Joslin, C.A.F., Romsey, W.W., and Liversage, W.E. (1967). The treatment of uterine carcinoma using the cathetron. Part I:technique. *Br. J. Radiol.,* **40**, 882–887.

Onsrad, M., Kolstod, P., and Norman, W.T. (1976). Post-operative external pelvic irradiation in carcinoma of the corpus. Stage I: a controlled clinical trial. *Gynecol. Oncol.,* **4**, 222–231.

Park, R., Patow, W., Petty, W., and Zimmerman, E. (1974). Treatment of adenocarcinoma of the endometrium. *Gynecol. Oncol.,* **2**, 60–70.

Park, R., Patow, W., Rogers, R.E., and Zimmerman, E.A. (1973). Treatment of Stage I carcinoma of the cervix. *Obstet. Gynecol.,* **41**, 117–122.

Perez, C.A., Breaux, S., Ashim, F., Carnel, H.M., and Powers, W.E. (1979). Irradiation alone or in combination with surgery in Stage Ib and IIa carcinoma of the uterine cervix. A non-randomised comparison. *Cancer,* **43**, 1062–1072.

Perez, C.A., Comel, H.M., Kao., M.S., and Askin, F. (1980). Randomised study of pre-operative radiation and surgery or irradiation alone in the treatment of Stage Ib and IIa carcinoma of the uterine cervix. *Cancer*, **45**, 2759–2768.

Piver, M.S., and Chung, W.S. (1975). Prognostic significance of cervical lesion size and pelvic node metastases in cervical carcinoma. *Obstet. Gynecol.,* **46**, 507–510.

Piver, M.S., Barlow, J.J., Vongtuma V., and Blumenson, L. (1977a). Hydroxyurea as a radiation sensitiser in women with carcinoma of the uterine cervix. *Am. J. Obstet. Gynecol.,* **127**, 379–383.

Piver, M.S., Chung, M.S., and Barolwo, J.J. (1977b). High dose irradiation to biopsy confined aortic node metastases from carcinoma of the cervix. *Cancer*, **39**, 1243–1246.

Price, J.J., Hahn, G.A., and Rominger, C.T. (1965). Vaginal involvement in endometrial carcinoma. *Am. J. Obstet. Gynecol.,* **91**, 1060–1065.

Reagan, J.W., Hamonic, M.S., and Wertz, W.B. (1957). Analytical study of the cells in cervical squamous cell cancer. *Lab. Invest.,* **6**, 241–250.

Reagan, J.W., and Fu, Y.S. (1979). Histologic types and prognosis of cancers of the uterine cervix. *Int. J. Radiat. Oncol., Biol. Phys.,* **5**, 1015–1020.

Reddy, S., Myung-Sook Lee, and Hendrickson, F.R. (1979). Pattern of recurrences in endometrial carcinoma and their management. *Radiology*, **133**, 737–740.

Reifenstein, E.C., Jr (1971). Hydroxy progesterone cuprocite therapy in advanced endometrial cancer. *Cancer*, **27**, 485–502.

Rotman, M., Moon, S., John, M., Choi, K., and Sall, S. (1979). Extended field para-aortic radiation in cervical carcinoma: the case for prophylactic treatment. *Int. J. Radiat. Oncol., Biol. Phys.,* **5**, 2139–2141.

Rutledge, F., and Saski, J. (1979). More or less radical surgery. *Int. J. Radiat. Oncol., Biol. Phys.,* **5**, 1881–1884.

Rutledge, F.W., Wharton, J.T., and Fletcher, G.H. (1976). Clinical studies with adjunctive surgery and radiation therapy in the treatment of carcinoma of the cervix. *Cancer*, **38**, 596–602.

Sala, J.M., and del Regato, J.A. (1962). Treatment of carcinoma of the endometrium. *Radiology*, **79**, 12–17.

Salazar, O.M., Felstein, M.L., de Papp, E.W., Bonfigio, T.A., Keller, B.E., Rubin, P., and Rudolph, J.H. (1977). Endometrial carcinoma: analysis of failures with special emphasis on the use of initial pre-operative external pelvic radiation. *Int. J. Radiat. Oncol., Biol. Phys.,* **2**, 1101–1107.

Schwartz, A., and Brunschwig, A. (1957). Radical panhysterectomy and pelvic node excision for carcinoma of the corpus uteri. *Surg. Gynaecol. Obstet.,* **105**, 675–680.

Shah, C.A., and Green, T.J. (1972). Evaluation of current management of endometrial carcinoma. *Obstet. Gynaecol.,* **39**, 500–509.

Slayton, R.E., and Mladineo, J.P. (1978). Adriamycin and cis-diamminedichloroplatinum in recurrent and metastatic squamous cell carcinoma of the cervix: a pilot study. *Proc. Am. Soc. Clin. Oncol.,* **19**, 335.

Sotto, L.S.J., Graham, J.B., and Picken, J.W. (1960). Post-mortem findings in cancer of the cervix. *Am. J. Obstet. Gynecol.,* **80**, 791–796.

Stallworthy, J., and Wiernik, G. (1975). Management of cervical malignant disease—combined radiotherapy and surgery techniques. In *The cervix* (eds J.A. Jordan, and A. Singer). London: W.B. Saunders. Chap. 41.

Strickland, P. (1965). Carcinoma corpus uteri: a radical intracavitary treatment. *Br. J. Radiol.*, **16**, 112–118.

Thigpen, T., Shingleton, H., Homesley, H., Di Saia, P.J., La Gasse, L., and Blessing, J. (1980). Cisplatinum in the treatment of advanced or recurrent cervix and uterine cancer. In *Cisplatin: current studies and new developments* (eds A.W. Prestoyko, S.T. Crooke and S.K. Carter). London: Academic Press. Chap. 29, pp. 411–422.

van Nagell, J.R., Donaldson, E.S., Wood, E.G., Murayama, Y., and Utley, J. (1977). Small cell cancer of the uterine cervix. *Cancer*, **40**, 2243–2249.

van Nagell, J.R., Rayburn, W., Donaldson, E.S., Hanson, M., Gay, E.C., Yonedin, J., Marayuma, Y., and Powell, D.F. (1979). Therapeutic implications of patterns of recurrence in cancer of the uterine cervix. *Cancer*, **44**, 2354–2361.

van Nagell, J.R., Roddick, J.W., and Lowin, M. (1971). The staging of cervical cancer: inevitable discrepancies between clinical staging and pathologic findings. *Am. J. Obstet. Gynecol.*, **110**, 973–978.

Wade, M.E., Kohorn, E.I., and Morris, J.M. (1967). Adenocarcinoma of the endometrium; evaluation of pre-operative irradiation and factors influencing prognosis. *Am. J. Obstet. Gynecol.*, **99**, 869–876.

Wasserman, T.H., and Carter, S.K. (1977). The integration of chemotherapy into combined modality treatment of solid tumours. *Cancer Treat. Rev.*, **4**, 25–46.

Weiner, S., and Wizenberg, M.J. (1975). Treatment of primary adenocarcinoma of the cervix. *Cancer*, **35**, 1514–1516.

Wilson, J.F., Cox, J.D., Chahbazian, C.M., and del Regato, J.A. (1980). Time dose relationships in endometrial adenocarcinoma: importance of the interval from external pelvic irradiation to surgery. *Int. J. Radiat. Oncol., Biol. Phys.*, **6**, 597–600.

Cancer Treatment: End Point Evaluation
Edited by B.A. Stoll
© 1983 John Wiley & Sons Ltd.

Chapter

17 C.M.L. COPPIN and K.D. SWENERTON

Selective Treatment in Breast Cancer

INTRODUCTION

Breast cancer has a wide spectrum of clinical behavior. In addition to the differences between individual tumors, cellular heterogeneity probably leads to changes with time in the progeny of any one tumor, particularly under the selection pressure of systemic therapy. Currently, the different treatment options and combinations are often applied indiscriminately to each of the many variants. Such stratification of treatment as occurs tends to be based on anatomical staging of the spread of disease.

But clinical outcome depends on the result of dynamic interaction between three main components—patient, disease, and treatment. The disease itself comprises three main elements: the locoregional component, which can usually be successfully treated; the liability to develop a new primary in any remaining breast tissue; and the risk and extent of viable cancer cells disseminated beyond the range of local and regional therapeutic modalities. Although measures to control the first two of these components are clearly important, outcome is very largely determined by the systemic component of the disease (D_S). The critical underlying problem thus centers on the interaction of D_S with host and treatment (Figure 1). D_S cannot be readily eliminated in most patients, so that this interaction frequently represents a chronic process.

With time, D_S becomes more extensive and more heterogeneous, with greater risk of more virulent components arising; it also becomes less responsive to treatment because of kinetic, adaptive, and particularly mutational changes which may either pre-exist or result from treatment. Eventual-

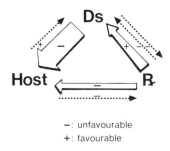

−: unfavourable
+: favourable

Figure 1 Chronic interaction of systemic component of cancer (D_S) with host and treatment. Proceeds from stage of dissemination to death or to possible cure by systemic therapy. D_S = systemic disease (extent × virulence).

ly in advanced disease, diminished host tolerance limits therapy either by general loss of functional integrity or by involvement of a therapy -limiting organ. The possibility that treatment may stimulate the disease (particularly in its occult phase) also cannot be ignored (Piro and Hellman, 1978). The diagram does not take account of supportive treatment measures, either physical or emotional.

Our basic thesis is that improved results with reduced morbidity can be obtained by taking a more selective approach using available treatment options. This requires identification of patient subsets which are defined according to the *therapeutic gain* that can be achieved from a given treatment modality. (Particularly for systemic treatment, such subsets may differ from traditional staging based solely on clinical extent). It requires the construction of specially designed controlled clinical trials which prospectively examine for factors predicting response (Carter, 1981b), and the results can then be selectively applied to individual patients.

The approach to the topic will be under the following headings:

Prognostic variables in the disease.
Predictors of response to treatment.
Selective therapy—goals and strategies.
Selective therapy in localized disease.
Selective therapy in advanced disease.

PROGNOSTIC VARIABLES IN THE DISEASE

Prognostic factors define the risk of relapse, and are essential for comparison or stratification in clinical studies (Zelen, 1975) and for assessing a patient's prognosis. They can indicate a *need* for treatment but not whether benefit is likely from treatment.

Natural history of disease

Although 90% of patients present with a cancer clinically localized to the breast and axillary lymph nodes (M_0), about 80% of the total will eventually die from the cancer (Mueller and Jeffries, 1975; Brinkley and Haybittle, 1977; Gore *et al.*, 1982), nearly all from systemic hematogenous metastases despite local control. Breast cancer is a chronic disease exhibiting a smooth mortality curve with no evidence of a discrete break-point. Although the mortality *ratio* decays exponentially, there remains a 60% excess death rate and a 20-fold increase in expected deaths from breast cancer during the 15–20 year follow-up period (Langlands *et al.*, 1979), with continuing loss at 30 years (Robbins and Berg, 1977).

The survival curve may be composed of a family of exponentials, but for simplicity one can postulate two dominant populations, one with a relative mortality of about 25% per year, and one with a mortality rate of 2.5% per year (Fox, 1979). The high-risk group has a mortality similar to untreated patients seen about a century ago, and there is some evidence that the increasing incidence of breast cancer may represent detection of more of the low-risk groups, for example by screening techniques (Fox, 1979). Survival will mainly represent the product of the risk, size, and growth rate of the systemic tumor burden, and ways of assessing these variables in the individual patient will be discussed in the subsequent sections.

Invasive ductal or lobular carcinomas begin as *in situ* lesions (Gallager, 1980). These are much more frequent than clinically appreciated (as shown in specimens from both mastectomy and autopsy), and are probably increased in proportion to the epidemiologic risk of carcinoma. The natural history of occult pre-invasive carcinomas is of major importance, as it determines the risk of second malignancy in the contralateral breast or remaining operated breast. The clinical risk is clearly far lower than the incidence of pathologically observed lesions and studies are urgently needed to identify the true risk and any measures which may modify it, including radiotherapy or hormonal manipulation.

Invasive cancers are probably initially monoclonal (Fialkow, 1976), but evolve into a range of heterogeneous clonal sublines exhibiting varying degrees of proliferative capacity, invasiveness, and response to endocrine influence, drug therapy or radiotherapy (Nowell, 1976; Parbhoo, 1981; Bruchovsky and Goldie, 1982a). After about 20 net doublings (1 mm^3 of tumor containing approximately a million cells), tumor cells may gain access to lymphatic and vascular channels as potential routes for metastases. Clinically detected lesions are usually in the 1–5 cm diameter range representing, approximately 30–37 net doublings.

The route of lymphatic metastases (as judged by distribution of involved lymph nodes) differs according to the location of the primary. For outer quadrant primaries the route is axillary alone in 74%, internal mammary alone in 5%, and both in 21%; corresponding figures for inner-central lesions are 57%, 9%, and 34% respectively (Lacour *et al.*, 1976).

After treatment of the presenting local and regional disease, there is usually a disease-free interval (DFI). Common sites of first relapse include chest wall, axillary or supraclavicular lymph nodes, and bone, or less commonly pleura, lung, liver, and brain. Relapse marks a relatively discrete point in the growth of the systemic tumor burden, although detection of metastases depends on the use and frequency of bone scan and other sensitive diagnostic procedures.

Examination of the post-relapse survival time shows it to be influenced not only by the extent of disease at relapse (reflecting the particular point in the natural history at which relapse is detected) but also by the duration of the preceeding DFI (Cutler *et al.*, 1969) and degree of differentiation of the primary (Pater *et al.*, 1981). These relationships strongly suggest that biological characteristics of the primary tumor continue to dominate subsequent events. Higher stage not only diminishes DFI but also has an independent negative effect on the post-relapse survival, suggesting a correlation of stage with tumor aggressiveness rather than with occult burden (Figure 2). This does not imply therapeutic nihilism, but stresses the importance of establishing a baseline of anticipated behavior in the individual patient.

Extent of disease

At diagnosis, clinical staging by the TNM system provides the international standard of tumor extent (Charlson and Feinstein, 1973). One of its major disadvantages is the unreliability of clinical assessment of regional lymph node involvement; there are one-third false negatives in stage N_0 and one-quarter false positives in stage N_1 (Hellman *et al.*, 1982).

Radical mastectomy provides definitive information on axillary lymph nodes, and the accuracy of information obtained by lesser procedures has been compared both pathologically and prognostically (Davies *et al.*, 1980; Rosen *et al.*, 1981). It appears that the number of positive axillary lymph nodes found by standard processing of material obtained at dissection of the lower two levels of the axilla provides sufficient prognostic accuracy (Fisher *et al.*, 1981d). In fact, the presence or absence of axillary node involvement is reliably achieved by sampling only five nodes, although more are needed for accurate placing in either the $N^{+(1-3)}$ or $N^{+(4+)}$ categories. (Pathologically negative axillary lymph nodes are here referred to as N^- and the presence and number (n) of pathologically confirmed positive axillary lymph nodes as $N^{+(n)}$.

The TNM system is also handicapped by the concept of sequential spread from breast to axilla to distant metastases (American Joint Committee for Cancer Staging, 1977) with its connotation of early or late diagnosis. The

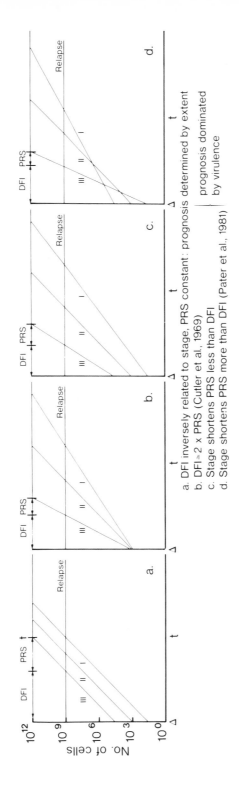

Figure 2 Possible relationships between clinical stage (I–III), occult tumor burden at diagnosis ($t = \Delta$), and doubling frequency (slope or virulence), and their effect on the disease-free interval (DFI) and post-relapse survival (PRS).

extent of disease at the time of diagnosis depends on chance discovery and on subsequent delay by patient or physician; treatment delay has been found to be associated with better, worse or no influence on prognosis (Elwood and Moorehead, 1980). The association will depend on whether a lump is regarded as malignant only if it changes in size (as in the past), or is viewed as malignant until proved otherwise. In the latter case, the extent of disease at diagnosis is likely to depend on the ratio between the rate of growth and frequency of examination.

Numerous publications have examined the relationship between extent of disease and prognosis (Rozencweig and Heuson, 1975; Henderson and Canellos, 1980). The number of positive lymph nodes is by far the strongest prognostic factor (Fisher *et al.*, 1975; Valagussa *et al.*, 1978). Although the size of primary tumor and extent of axillary involvement are positively correlated, tumor diameter is also an independent prognostic factor (Bedwani *et al.*, 1981; Fisher *et al.*, 1969; Duncan and Kerr, 1976). The level of axillary involvement is correlated with the number of lymph nodes but is not an independent factor (Smith *et al.*, 1977), while the size of axillary metastases may influence prognosis especially when the primary is less than 2 cm (Rosen *et al.*, 1981).

As with axillary node involvement, internal mammary node spread is an adverse factor principally because of correlation with distant spread (Fisher *et al.*, 1980b; Donegan, 1977). Internal mammary node involvement can largely be predicted on the basis of axillary node involvement and location of the primary (Lacour *et al.*, 1976), and internal mammary biopsy has an inconsistent yield. Lymphoscintigraphy is a promising technique which requires further evaluation before it can be incorporated into treatment decisions, and is likely to demonstrate only relatively gross disease (Ege, 1980).

In general, grouping of TNM categories has the advantage of simplifying comparisons but with some loss of resolution. The stage groupings identify lesser or greater mortality *rates* which converge beyond about 10 years to approximately 5% per year (Gore *et al.*, 1982).

Tumor biology

It is becoming clear that different breast cancers have a wide range of intrinsic behavior or aggressiveness, and that this largely determines the duration of phases in the natural history such as DFI, response duration, time to progression, and post-relapse survival. Until cure is possible in this disease, these periods of time will continue to be determined more by the disease than by treatment.

One can envisage a spectrum of tumor biology. Tumors at one end of the spectrum would be well differentiated, with a low labeling index (LI), low growth fraction, long doubling time, and possibly a lower mutation rate;

clonogenic cells might be proportionately fewer and more cohesive, accumulating a larger tumor mass before disseminating, and exhibiting relatively uniform treatment response properties. At the other end of the spectrum would be poorly differentiated tumors with a high growth fraction, high LI, short doubling time, and a tendency to progressive loss of regulatory mechanisms and consequent increased heterogeneity and risk of mutation to resistance. Metastases are likely to be selected from the most malignant end of this spectrum (Fidler and Hart, 1981) where a higher proportion of poorly cohesive clonogenic cells may metastasize when the primary is small.

Clinical observations on metastases have shown a log-normal distribution of doubling times in the range of 2–200 days (Lee, 1972). Growth rates of primary cancers have been estimated retrospectively from mammograms, and faster growing lesions were significantly more likely to metastasize (Heuser *et al.*, 1979). Some estimate of the rate of growth can be obtained from the patient's history (Charlson and Feinstein, 1974), tumor histologic grade (Boyd *et al.*, 1981b), and probably (by association) from the extent of lymph node involvement.

Urgently needed are quantitative indicators of aggressiveness which can be applied to tumor tissue at the time of diagnosis (Silvestrini *et al.*, 1981). Histologic grading of cellular or nuclear differentiation has not been sufficiently sensitive or reproducible to be helpful in the individual patient. Direct measurement of kinetic parameters has considerable appeal as a prognostic indicator (Tubiana *et al.*, 1981). Thus a high labeling index (LI) is associated with advanced stage at presentation and early relapse (Meyer and Hixon, 1979) while the mitotic index is an independent prognostic factor especially for estrogen receptor negative (ER−) tumors (Russo *et al.*, 1981).

An unexpected bonus of the ER assay was the retrospective finding of a correlation between ER positivity in the tumor with DFI and total survival, independent of TNM stage. Tumors with ER-negative cells are likely to be poorly differentiated and hyperdiploid (Olszewski *et al.*, 1981), and more likely to give rise to visceral metastases (Samaan *et al.*, 1981; Stewart *et al.*, 1981). The incidence of ER-positive tumors is greater in post-menopausal patients but appears more precisely correlated with age (Elwood and Godolphin, 1980).

There is considerable variation in the degree of prognostic influence in different series, and a better correlation may be obtained by using the absolute level of ER, not only in the positive range over 10 fmol/mg, but possibly also by stratifying the conventional negative range (Godolphin *et al.*, 1981). Using this system, ER level may have independent prognostic import at least as great as that of axillary node involvement. The obstacle is lack of international standardization of the ER assay and wide interlaboratory variation, particularly in the low range where accuracy is more likely to be critical (Cohen *et al.*, 1980).

ER is inversely related to LI, but the association is marked by a high degree of scatter (Hahnel, 1981; Bertuzzi *et al.*, 1981). ER may be merely a convenient if inaccurate kinetic marker, but the independence of ER, N^+, and LI as markers could permit more refined characterization than if they were directly linked (Silvestrini *et al.*, 1982; Hager *et al.*, 1982).

Other prognostic factors

Pathologic identification of invasion into intramammary lymphatics, blood vessels, and surrounding breast tissue identifies a relatively poor prognosis (Nealon *et al.*, 1979; Nime *et al.*, 1977; Weigand *et al.*, 1981). NSABP has identified tumor necrosis, poor tumor differentiation, primary size over 4 cm, and germinal center predominance as the best discriminants for relapse in the first five years (Fisher *et al.*, 1980c). Multicentricity carries an adverse prognosis despite mastectomy (Egan and Henson, 1982). Node-positive patients can be stratified further on the basis of clinical predictors (Kister *et al.*, 1979). In Stage III cases, short duration of symptoms and diffuse primary lesions were correlated with early appearance of distant metastases and short survival (Rubens *et al.*, 1977).

Table 1 Prognostic influence of tumor biology and extent.

(a) Estrogen receptor (Godolphin *et al.*, 1981).

ER concentration (fmol/mg cytosol protein)	≥160	10–159	2–9	≤
Three-year survival (%)	92	76	64	35
Relative risk (compared to group average)	0.38	1.14	1.71	3.10
N^- (%)	42	35	31	37

(b) Tumour and nodal extent: five-year relapse-free survival (Fisher *et al.*, 1975). Relative risk in parentheses

N/T	<2 cm	2–5 cm	>5 cm
N^-	88%(0.34)	78%(0.63)	72%(0.80)
$N^{+(1-3)}$	60%(1.14)	52%(1.37)	42%(1.66)
$N^{+(4+)}$	38%(1.77)	25%(2.14)	9%(2.60)

By stratifying into four ER ranges, an eight-fold range of risk can be identified and is independent of extent. Histologic node status in the most widely used categories defines a four-fold risk range and tumour size a two-fold range of risk.

Table 1 provides an approximation of the prognostic influence of ER level, histologic axillary node status, and tumor size. Although tumor aggressiveness may dominate natural history, curability is more likely to be related to occult systemic tumor load, a variable which cannot be quantitated at present.

PREDICTORS OF RESPONSE TO TREATMENT

The complexity of breast cancer therapy reflects the large number of available treatment options, particularly with increasing use of combined modalities. Treatment has become more selective in the sense of an improved therapeutic index (i.e. greater efficacy and less host damage), but selective treatment in different subsets of patients requires better understanding of mechanisms of action, reasons for failure, and predictors of favorable response.

Surgery

Surgery has several roles in initial management. First, it confirms the diagnosis, and this includes the use of carefully interpreted fine-needle aspirate. Secondly, it provides tumor tissue for analysis of other histopathologic features and receptor proteins (and potentially for testing in short-term culture for receptor function, LI, and chemosensitivity as dynamic predictive tests for systemic therapy). Thirdly, surgery is required to determine the presence and extent of axillary lymph node involvement, currently the most important prognostic factor. The fourth role is the removal of bulk disease to reduce the tumor burden to a size that may be more successfully dealt with by the other modalities (Surgery has the advantage that it is not liable to failure from selection of resistant cells). The fifth and traditional role of surgery is in attempting removal of microscopic spread by *en bloc* resection of normal structures including the breast, pectoral muscles, and axillary contents.

Recognition of features predicting local and distant failure after radical mastectomy resulted in clinical criteria of inoperability. Although one of the first attempts at a selective treatment approach (Haagensen, 1971), these are likely to require major revision in a combined modality setting. Radical operation is responsible for nearly all chronic post-surgical morbidity. Although providing good locoregional control, it has an unfavorable therapeutic index which is only partly mitigated by sparing of the pectoralis major or by reconstructive procedures.

Radiotherapy

Breast cancer is a moderately radiosensitive tumor, and technical advances since the introduction of supervoltage equipment now permit accurate radiation to a prescribed dose, volume, and depth. There is a direct relationship between the volume of tumor and the dose required to sterilize it (Fletcher, 1973; Hellman, 1980). Normal tissue tolerance varies with the organ and volume irradiated, but in the case of soft tissues, sterilization of minimal clinical disease is possible within moderately wide fields. Morbidity consists of erythema and minor late fibrosis. The importance of adequate dose at the primary treatment is emphasized by the difficulty of treating infield recurrence because of limited further radiation tolerance, reduced drug delivery, possible cross-resistance, and loss of ER (Janssens *et al.*, 1981).

The main role of radiotherapy has been to treat the remaining locoregional volume at risk after surgery, and appropriate selection depends on accurate prediction of the degree of risk, location of occult disease, and possibility of salvage. Irradiation is also the best form of palliation for parenchymal brain metastases and lytic lesions in weight-bearing bones. Other distant sites are usually best treated by systemic therapy.

Hormone therapy

Advances in receptor physiology have provided some insight into the mechanism of action of various additive or 'subtractive' hormonal manipulations. They all have a remarkably similar partial response rate of about 30% in advanced disease, for a median duration of about a year (Kiang, 1981), and it is believed that first-line treatments operate through ER-associated mechanisms. In pre-menopausal women, estrogen deprivation is accomplished by ovarian castration or radiation ablation, or by tamoxifen, all with low morbidity. In post-menopausal patients, tamoxifen acts as an anti-estrogen but also has a partial estrogen agonist action. It has less morbidity than diethylstilbestrol (Ingle *et al.*, 1981).

Hormonal therapy can lead to autolysis in differentiated responsive cells, but hormone-dependent stem cells are probably only suppressed. This leads to relapse on discontinuing the hormonal maneuver, or they can undergo change to an unresponsive phenotype (Bruchovsky and Goldie, 1982b). Selection of pre-existing autonomous cells is an additional reason why hormone therapy is non-curative (Sluyser, 1980), at least in advanced disease. Unlike chemotherapy, response to hormones is little affected by dose (Bruchovsky and Goldie, 1982b) or tumor burden (Coppin, 1982).

A number of clinical predictors of response to endocrine therapy have long been recognized, including long DFI, late post-menopausal status, and non-visceral disease. These have been augmented by biochemical assays of ER concentration in biopsy samples of primary or metastatic breast cancer (Byar *et al.*, 1979; Osborne and McGuire, 1981). At ER concentrations of less than about 10 fmol/mg cytosol protein, the chance of response to any hormonal manipulation is small (about 5%) and such tumors are usually referred to as ER-negative (ER−), although ER-poor would be a more accurate description. ER-rich (ER+) tumors have about a 60% response rate. There are several possible reasons for false positive or false negative results (Lippman and Thompson, 1979).

Where available, ER assay should done on all biopsied breast cancer and patients with ER− tumors should not be subjected to a probably futile hormonal trial until other modalities have failed. Assay of the primary tumor may have application to possible adjuvant therapy, and to later treatment should metastases prove inaccessible to biopsy. Future improvement in prediction of response may be obtained from the absolute ER concentration (Lippman and Allegra, 1980; Campbell *et al.*, 1981), allowance for proportion of tumor cells (Hawkins *et al.*, 1981), assay for nuclear receptor (Leake *et al.*, 1981), presence of progesterone receptor (McGuire and Horwitz, 1978), and assessment of ER function *in vivo* (Namer *et al.*, 1980) or *in vitro* (Israel and Saez, 1978). All these are likely to be positively correlated, and functional testing is probably the best if it can be done routinely.

New assay techniques may be more specific (monoclonal antibody to estrophilin; Egan and Henson, 1982) or provide insight into heterogenicity (immunofluorescence; Nenci, 1981). Immunoperoxidase ER staining has several advantages including its ability to use formalin-fixed tissue for retrospective study, and its assessment of the relative proportions of ER++ cells, ER+ cells, ER− cells, and non-malignant cells, but has not yet been correlated with hormonal responsiveness (Taylor *et al.*, 1981). Endocrine therapy selectively eliminates ER+ cells so that ER levels may fall in sequential samples (Allegra *et al.*, 1980). The predictive value of ER is claimed to decline with the number of metastatic sites (De Wys *et al.*, 1980).

A striking characteristic of hormone therapy is the ability to obtain secondary (and even subsequent) responses by further manipulations, including withdrawal of a prior inhibitory treatment. This may reflect either adaptation or selection within the ER+ cell population, an important difference with implications for combined versus sequential hormonal treatments. Sequential therapy would be less empiric if functional receptors to progestogens, androgens, corticosteroids or prolactin could be assayed at relapse, or if potentially useful hormone combinations could be predicted at presentation. Non-functional receptors might still enable targeting of compounds such as estramustine (Lippman, 1978) or ^{131}I-tamoxifen (Hellman, 1980).

Cytotoxic chemotherapy

Breast cancer is among the most chemosensitive of the common solid tumors. Many cytotoxic agents are active when used as the initial treatment for metastases, but adriamycin probably has the highest single-agent response

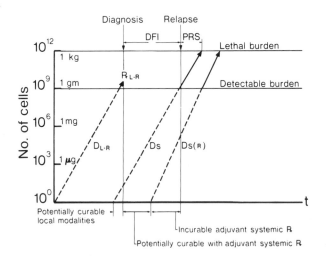

Figure 3 Potential curability according to tumour burden in hypothetical Stage II patient from inception of tumour until death. DFI = disease-free interval; PRS = post-relapse survival; D_{LR} = locoregional disease; D_S = systemic disease; $D_{S(R)}$ = systemic disease resistance to available hormono-chemotherapy (steeper slope due to continuing mutation to resistance).

rate (Hoogstraten and Fabian, 1979) and a cell-kill in combination of up to 6 logs (Blumenschein, 1979). Cytotoxic drugs have a steep dose–response relationship (Frei and Canellos, 1980), and follow first-order kinetics (fixed proportions of sensitive tumor cells are killed per treatment). Ideally, combination therapy should utilize agents which minimize cross-resistance and overlapping toxicity, and with synergistic mechanisms of action. In practice, combinations tend to be empiric and there is a need to define agents active after adriamycin response.

Agents might be brought into an alternating sequence in order to minimize the proportion of multiply-resistant cells which are the ultimate source of chemotherapy failure (Figure 3). The development of drug-resistant clonogenic cells can be minimized by using the broadest combination available at full dose, immediately on diagnosis when eradication of all systemic spread might be possible (Goldie and Coldman, 1979). Even failing cure, the early use of chemotherapy is still likely to be the most beneficial, since the resistant proportion is less, the growth fraction greater, and the host best able to tolerate maximum dose. The relative importance of dose, treatment interval, and total number of cycles to eliminate the sensitive clonogenic population is largely unknown.

No predictive factors are as yet sufficiently reliable to be of practical use in selecting optimal chemotherapy on an individual basis and only generalizations can be made. Patients are more likely to respond if tumor burden is less (Swenerton *et al.*, 1979). The likelihood and duration of complete remission is also inversely related to the bulk of metastatic tumor (Legha *et al.*, 1979). Weight loss, poor performance status, and visceral involvement are adverse factors because of their correlation with extensive disease. High drug dose and lack of prior radiotherapy are favorable factors. High tumor LI (Sulkes *et al.*, 1979) and thymidine kinase activity (Kiang *et al.*, 1982) appear to correlate better with response in visceral than in osseous disease (Fey *et al.*, 1981). On the other hand, chemotherapy may change the natural history so that at autopsy disease is more widespread and more likely to involve the CNS (Amer, 1982).

ER assay has been examined for possible chemopredictive value. Ideally, the test should be performed on a biopsy of the evaluable site immediately prior to chemotherapy and preferably at the first relapse in post-menopausal patients (chemotherapy induces hormonal changes in pre-menopausal patients). Under such circumstances, ER− tumors may have a higher response rate (Jonat and Maass, 1978; Lippman and Allegra, 1980) as noted *in vitro* (Kaufmann *et al.*, 1980), probably related to their larger growth fraction. The several contrary reports appear to be looking at ER under different circumstances.

An ER− assay is said to predict longer duration of response (Holdaway *et al.*, 1980), which is certainly at variance with the natural history. ER− tumors occasionally shift to ER+ under selection from chemotherapy (Allegra *et al.*, 1980), while ER+ tumors may remain hormone-sensitive after chemotherapy (Kiang and Kennedy, 1977).

In vitro chemosensitivity testing is becoming a realistic if difficult technique (Salmon, 1980; von Hoff *et al.*, 1981), and may be valuable in predicting macroscopic response. Its main advantage is direct observation of the clonogenic stem cell population, and its role in selective therapy will depend on the degree of biologic variation between metastases as well as its predictive reliability. For adjuvant therapy, testing of the primary tumor may not be respresentative of micrometastases (Weiss, 1980), and it may be impossible to identify small numbers of multiply-resistant cells.

Second-line chemotherapy is not usually very rewarding in advanced breast cancer, especially after a poor response to an adriamycin-containing combination. Research into this problem may spare futile and often toxic therapy trials.

Combined hormono-chemotherapy

The factors predicting frequency of response to systemic treatment are summarized in Table 2. Given the selective action of hormones on cells with functional receptors, and the greater cell-kill with cytotoxic agents in more

Table 2 Factors predicting frequency of response to systemic treatment

Prognostic factor	Cytotoxic Chemotherapy	Hormone Therapy
Disease factors		
Disease-free interval	±	+ +
Tumor grade	±	+ +
Tumor steroid receptors	±	+ +
Tumor burden	+ +	−
Site of tumor	−	−
Patient factors		
Age	−	−
Performance status	+ +	±
Treatment factors		
Dose–response	+	−
Prior response	+	+ +
Combinations better than sequential	+ +	±

rapidly dividing cells, heterogeneity suggests the use of combined therapy and this is an area of current investigation (Stoll, 1979). If hormonal and cytotoxic maneuvers lack cross-resistance and interference, the risk and number of totally resistant cells is less ($D_{S(R)}$ line in Figure 3 is shifted to the right) and even weak hormone action can markedly raise the projected cure rate (Goldie *et al.*, 1981). Predictive factors for each modality may provide some guide as to the value of combined therapy, but probably all tumors contain varying proportions of both elements.

In practice, the possible variables are too numerous to allow prediction of potential modality interactions. Different cell lines have demonstrated interference (Kiang and Kennedy, 1981) or subadditive benefit (Sluyser *et al.*, 1981). Tamoxifen induces cell cycle changes (Sutherland and Taylor, 1981) and can modify 5-fluorouracil metabolism to increase cytotoxicity (Benz and Cadman, 1981). Consequently, only clinical trials can assess the net result of concurrent versus sequential treatment in different subsets, and great interpretative care is required (Carter, 1981a). Some results will be presented in a later section.

Host factors determining prognosis

The extent to which host factors influence the natural history of breast cancer is not clear although age-related tumor properties (such as increasing ER level and decreasing LI) are presumably related to the tissue and hormonal environment in which the tumor arises. Evidence of immunologic host response (e.g. sinus histiocytosis found in reactive axillary lymphadenopathy) has not been proved to have prognostic value, despite demonstration that the regional nodes are immunologically competent (Ellis *et al.*, 1975). Lymphocyte infiltration around the tumor is associated with adverse histologic features in the tumor.

Immunodeficiency is correlated with a worse prognosis in advanced disease, but this is at least partly related to tumor burden (Hortobagyi *et al.*, 1981b), and tumor dissemination appears to be the cause rather than the result of immunosuppression (Stein *et al.*, 1976). Immunotherapy has been notable for its lack of benefit in breast cancer (Hewitt, 1980). Obesity appears to have an adverse significance (possibly due to hormonal mechanisms such as increased peripheral aromatization), but whether weight reduction has any therapeutic merit remains to be shown (Boyd *et al.*, 1981a).

The host clearly plays a major role in a different sense, namely in subjective and objective treatment tolerance. Advanced age or serious additional illness may render aggressive treatment dangerous or long-term goals not worth while (e.g. in considering adjuvant chemotherapy, life expectancy should be greater than anticipated prognosis from the cancer). The view that the elderly are more predisposed to chemotherapy toxicity appears to be largely false (Begg *et al.*, 1980) and, in general, there are no reliable predictors for subjective toxicity. Patients with a history of severe nausea of pregnancy and motion sickness may be more prone to drug-induced nausea (Swenerton, unpublished data).

The most significant host factor is compliance with treatment. When more than one treatment option is under consideration, the patient's attitude to an aggressive approach must influence the treatment decision (see Chapter 6).

SELECTIVE THERAPY—GOALS AND STRATEGIES

The very variable natural history of breast cancer raises considerable difficulties in demonstrating treatment benefit in terms of cure rate, survival gain, quality of remissions or symptomatic palliation (see opening chapters). To improve the results of treatment, early detection is critical but, unfortunately, the most malignant tumors are least likely to be recognized in a screening program. The main thrust, then, is to minimize delay between first symptom, diagnosis, and treatment, as at least a proportion of patients are at rapidly increasing risk of developing drug-resistant systemic spread (Goldie and Coldman, 1979).

Except for small tumors of low aggressiveness, it is unclear if breast cancer is curable. To demonstrate cure, patients would need to exhibit normal life expectancy and death unrelated to breast cancer or its treatment, and the cure rate would be given by the level of the plateau on the disease-specific

survival curve (see Chapter 1). An added treatment may improve the overall
cure rate by salvaging a proportion of those at risk for failure (Figure 4), a
ratio which might be described as the *proportional cure rate*. Any morbidity
affects all patients treated and can be quantitated as: risk × severity ×
duration.

In the event that cure is not possible, or at an earlier phase in a clinical
study, improved survival would be the objective. This is usually assessed by
looking for a statistically significant separation between two survival curves.
Such an approach fails to quantitate the degree of improvement and often
yields false negatives because, even in large trials, there are many subsets and
only some may achieve benefit. It is also easier to demonstrate gain in
situations where the prognosis is exceptionally poor compared to a simultaneously treated subset for whom the *proportional gain* is as great, but it may
not achieve statistical significance until a considerably longer time has
elapsed.

An approach to this problem, similar to that described above, is illustrated
in Figure 4. This can be done for different subsets, and may show equivalent
proportional gain even though the absolute improvement would be less at any
given time for a subset with a better prognosis. Because the prognosis denotes
rate of attrition, the absolute gain may be just as great, but takes longer to
achieve. The duration of study required to show clinically useful gain will

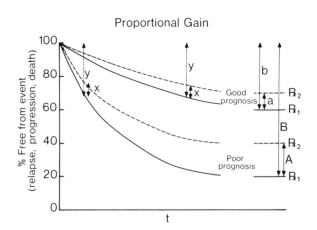

Proportional Gain

Figure 4 Proportional gain is the improvement in results generated by the application
of treatment 2 expressed in terms of the patients at risk of failure at any given time
after the comparison treatment 1. This example is drawn such that the proportional
gain is continuously 25% for both poor and good prognosis subsets for whom the
improvement in cure rate is A/B or a/b respectively. Proportional gain (x/y) may be
just as great for good prognosis as for poor prognosis patients but the same absolute
gain for the good prognosis subset takes greater time (t) to achieve.

depend on the expected course for the subset. Constant proportional gain with time suggests that survival gain may eventually translate into cure.

The majority of breast cancer patients undergo a number of therapeutic interventions between diagnosis and death; minor degrees of survival gain may be hard to demonstrate for any one component, especially as treatment sequence is rarely standardized. It is therefore often more useful to look at the interval between major events, usually expressed as median time to relapse (or time to progression). A systemic treatment would be judged by systemic (and local) events, and a local modality of treatment by local relapse or progression.

For systemic therapy of evaluable disease, objective response rates with standard criteria (Hayward *et al.*, 1977) are used for comparative purposes. Durations of response and survival reflect the behavior of unresponsive tumor cells. *Comparison of survival in responders versus non-responders is very misleading* as an index of survival gain, because response is largely determined by factors which independently influence survival, particularly tumor burden and ER status.

Non-curative treatment is often referred to as palliative, but these terms should be clearly distinguished in breast cancer where modest survival gain in advanced disease is more often the illusory goal than pure symptom relief, important though this is. Symptomatic palliation can also be prophylactic, as with post-operative irradiation or orthopedic pinning to prevent fracture. Quality of life is very hard to evaluate (see Chapter 6).

Any treatment contemplated must satisfy certain fundamental doubts:

> Treatment is unnecessary because the prognosis does not warrant it, or the situation could be salvaged at later relapse.
>
> The situation is too late for the treatment option to be beneficial.
>
> Only if greater gain is expected in relation to toxicity by use of early rather than delayed treatment is it justified to proceed.

Increasing use of combined modality treatment makes it necessary to demonstrate the effectiveness of *each* component in relation to the toxicity. The more successful the treatment, the more care is required to avoid chronic morbidity which may outlast the treatment itself. Where the gain is comparatively small, it may be difficult to distinguish whether most of it accrues to a minority group, but identification of such a subset must be the ultimate goal of selective therapy.

Adjuvant therapy commits patients to a course of treatment which is likely to be completed before there is any information as to individual outcome. This is in marked contrast to the advanced disease where response can be evaluated and treatment discontinued if ineffective, with corresponding reduction of toxicity. The main strategy in breast cancer at the present time is

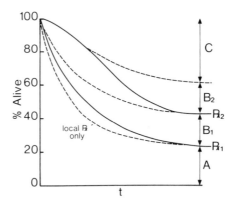

Figure 5 Adjuvant systemic therapy, major patient subsets by response: R_1 represents definitive locoregional therapy at diagnosis with optimal systemic therapy at relapse. R_2 represents optimal adjuvant systemic therapy at diagnosis with additional appropriate locoregional therapy. A = subset not requiring adjuvant therapy, systemic spread not present. B_1 = subset for which early adjuvant therapy curative. B_2 = subset for which early adjuvant therapy produces a survival gain. C = subset achieving no gain, adjuvant therapy yields no survival advantage over palliative systemic therapy.

to evaluate combination chemotherapy programs in advanced disease (for example, the use of non-cross-resistant alternating combinations) and to assess the optimal sequence of chemotherapy and hormonal therapy. Effective treatment can then be moved up into the adjuvant setting.

An assessment of the degree of gain resulting from early adjuvant therapy is presented in Figure 5. This gain accrues entirely to group B, defined retrospectively, and one cannot distinguish this for the individual patient. Factors predicting the proportional gain resulting from adjuvant treatment must be estimated from separate analysis in subsets chosen according to variables considered likely to determine response. These might include treatment delay, tolerated dose, and extent or biological properties of the original tumor.

Before discussing the management of subsets in breast cancer, it is useful to set out the overall treatment approach commonly followed. For operable cancers, two National Cancer Institute (NCI) consensus development conferences have concluded that modified radical mastectomy is appropriate standard surgery, and that this should be followed by adjuvant chemotherapy in N^+ pre-menopausal patients (Consensus Development Panel, 1979, 1980). Inoperable lesions or locoregional recurrences are usually treated with radiotherapy. Overt metastases are treated with combination chemotherapy if the tumour is ER− or if dire circumstances demand rapid response, otherwise one of a variety of hormonal manipulations is used first.

While this scheme has attractive simplicity, it is insensitive to treatment details, alternative strategies, and special situations, and in the following sections we examine current trends in *selective* treatment. In many instances, these are still in the investigational phase.

SELECTIVE THERAPY IN LOCALIZED DISEASE (LOW RISK)

Although the large majority of patients dying of breast cancer do so from systemic spread (usually with local control), a minority have disease truly curable by local measures. Increasing disease incidence but static mortality suggest that this group is enlarging and screening may be a factor in this. It is important to identify this minority to avoid overtreatment, yet to ensure local control.

This is the subset with invasive disease but in whom the risk of systemic spread is too low, or relapse too delayed, to warrant consideration of adjuvant chemotherapy. The subset comprises patients with small primary tumors, no regional spread, and low aggressiveness (as indicated by ER+ status), that is $T_{1-2}N^-M_0ER+$. Those without axillary nodes clearly require no further axillary treatment apart from adequate sampling. Controversy therefore revolves around appropriate therapy for the breast, and the simplest choice is total mastectomy, indicated at least for those tumors too large to make a lesser procedure cosmetically worthwhile (usually tumors larger than 3 cm). Whether equivalent results can be obtained with lesser surgical procedures is currently a matter of investigation.

The NSABP is comparing total mastectomy with wide excision, with or without radiotherapy in $N_0(N^+$ or $N^-)$ patients. Although wide excision alone can give good results in highly selected patients (Hermann *et al.*, 1978), at present it is reasonable to recommend that patients refusing mastectomy undergo wide excision, axillary sampling, and megavoltage radiotherapy to tissue tolerance. Radiotherapy is probably more readily standardized than limited surgery (which may range from lumpectomy, to quadrantectomy but with less satisfactory cosmetic results.) This approach yields five-year results in T_1N_0 cases which are equivalent to those of radical mastectomy (Veronesi *et al.*, 1981). Results from individual institutions are reassuring, both as regards possible long-term risks and survival (Peters, 1975; Harris *et al.*, 1981; Amalric *et al.*, 1982).

Multifocal occult *in situ* or invasive cancers are frequently found in mastectomy specimens. Pre-operative high-quality mammograms are mandatory before considering partial mastectomy (Gefter *et al.*, 1982). Multifocality itself does not necessarily require treatment as only a small proportion of these ever become invasive. A decision on prophylactic removal of breast tissue must take into account the expected lifetime risk of second malignancy on the basis of life expectancy from the first cancer, the presence of lobular carcinoma or of a family history of invasive carcinoma (e.g. in a pre-menopausal first-degree relative), and the wishes of the patient. Long-term studies will be required to assess the effect of unilateral breast radiotherapy on the incidence of second malignancy in either breast. One might predict reduced risk in the treated breast but increased risk in the contralateral breast from low-dose scatter (Boice and Monson, 1977).

It is likely that internal mammary node involvement is of similar significance to that of axillary nodes. Patients with negative nodes do not need further treatment, while positive nodes are indicators of systemic disease. The incidence of internal mammary node involvement in axillary N^- cases is low, but for inner-central lesions a parasternal radiotherapy field might reasonably be included as part of a radiotherapy program being given for other reasons.

The excellent prognosis for this overall group requires *prolonged* follow-up in randomized studies examining more conservative approaches, or additional maneuvers such as adjuvant hormonal manipulation.

SELECTIVE THERAPY IN LOCALIZED DISEASE (HIGH RISK)

This large group comprises subsets for whom the unifying feature is high risk of occult hematogenous metastases and potential benefit from adjuvant chemotherapy. This is the area where multimodality treatment interactions are most likely. Treatment selection involves consideration of several disease components, namely: the primary lesion; the remainder of the ipsilateral breast and adjacent tissues; the regional drainage to axillary and internal mammary chains; distant metastases; and management of the contralateral breast. Systemic adjuvant treatment will be discussed first because systemic treatment may also influence the need, choice, and timing of locoregional treatment.

Adjuvant hormonal therapy

Since prophylactic oophorectomy was first suggested in the 1930s, at least 17 studies of adjuvant oophorectomy or ovarian irradiation have been carried out in pre-menopausal patients without definite conclusions (Rozencweig, *et al.* 1978; Powles, 1981). Most are difficult to interpret for methodologic reasons. A recent report showed significant survival gain from oophorectomy particularly in N^+ patients, for whom crude survival was 7% better at five years and 20% better at 10 years (Bryant and Weir, 1981). Benefit was marginal for Stage I or pre-menopausal patients over the age of 50. The entry period was rather long and the randomization procedures faulty, and no information is available on the treatment at relapse.

The Toronto study of radiation ovarian ablation showed an improved DFI and a lesser improved survival (Meakin *et al.*, 1979). The addition of low-dose prednisone as a third arm in pre-menopausal patients over the age of 45 led to significant improvement in survival, and this result represents one of the few indications that combination hormonal therapy may be advantageous in breast cancer.

Only about one-third of pre-menopausal patients have ER+ tumors, and this may explain the marginal results obtained so far with ovarian ablation. There is thus a clear need for a comparison of immediate versus delayed hormonal manipulation in pre-menopausal cases stratified by ER level, and it is perhaps unfortunate that the early success of adjuvant chemotherapy may have stifled such an approach in the N^+ER+ subset. The Copenhagen study (Palshof, 1981) has demonstrated increased disease-free interval from tamoxifen in patients with ER-rich tumors, but survival data are not yet available. Tamoxifen therapy is possibly less attractive than ovarian ablation because of increase in plasma estrogens, compliance concerns, and potential for reactivation of dormant disease when the drug is discontinued.

In the post-menopausal group, tamoxifen is most often selected because of low toxicity and well documented effectiveness in advanced disease. Wallgren *et al.* (1981) have demonstrated improved three-year relapse-free survival of 80% versus 58% for controls, with greater benefit for ER+ than ER− cases. From their data it would also appear that survival is significantly improved at three years, although treatment at relapse was not described.

Adjuvant chemotherapy

Adjuvant chemotherapy is given with the aim of eradicating microscopic disease and improving the cure rate. Results of ongoing trials have been summarized (Salmon and Jones, 1981; Carter, 1980; Rozencweig *et al.*, 1978). The present generation of trials is based on three postulates—steep dose–response, first-order cell-kill kinetics, and the presence of cell sublines sensitive to different drugs. Improved results generally confirm the need to use combinations of non-cross-resistant drugs in maximum tolerated pulses. For future trial design, it is essential to examine present results for those disease or treatment factors which influence the degree of benefit so that stratification can be carried out in subsequent prospective investigations.

After a nine months course of CMFVP, 68% of $N^{+(4+)}$ women are reported to be disease-free at 12 years (Holland, 1981). The study was not randomized, but this result is remarkable in view of the expected very poor prognosis in this group. More recent studies are evaluable mainly for freedom from relapse, and in the case of the NSABP studies, the lack of accelerated relapse following completion of therapy (Fisher *et al.*, 1981c). By five years from diagnosis, prolongation of DFI has matured into overall survival gain

(Bonadonna *et al.*, 1982; Fisher *et al.*, 1980b; Senn *et al.*, 1981). Until the relapse curve flattens out, survival benefit depends to a large degree on the comparative post-relapse survival experience in the treated and control arms.

Relapse after adjuvant therapy is worth study as the patterns of drug sensitivity or sites of failure may provide insight leading to beneficial modifications. Thus, 5FU relapses can be salvaged by CMF (Chlebowski *et al.*, 1981), and early CMF relapses by adriamycin (Rossi *et al.*, 1980), but adriamycin and cyclophosphamide relapses cannot be salvaged by CMF (Wendt *et al.*, 1980), suggesting that the former combination has the broader spectrum. Late CMF relapses are still CMF-sensitive, indicating that absolute drug resistance is not the reason for failure (Rossi *et al.*, 1980). Hormone responsiveness in relapsing cases after CMF appears about the same as for previously untreated patients.

The Milan group find no significant difference in the relapse pattern after chemotherapy, with locoregional recurrence reduced in proportion, i.e. still the site of first relapse in 25% in the unirradiated N^+ group (Valagussa *et al.*, 1980). Brain metastases may become commoner (Paterson *et al.*, 1982), but would only warrant prophylactic treatment if they frequently occurred alone.

Factors modifying response

Variables related to disease, treatment, and host are being examined for their effect on the benefit from adjuvant chemotherapy (Table 3). Most results are too preliminary to provide survival data, and only randomized studies with a control arm, or a clear difference between treatment arms, can be used for comparative analysis.

The number of involved nodes has no consistent effect on gain. The weak benefit of single agents may be easier to demonstrate in $N^{+(4+)}$, but this group also gains most from multidrug combinations. Neither the Milan or the NSABP placebo-controlled studies were examined for ER status, although a retrospective immunoperoxidase assessment of stored blocks could still possibly be made. The West Midlands group showed a greater trend to improvement in ER− than in ER+ patients (Morrison *et al.*, 1981) and adjuvant chemotherapy with greater benefit for ER− cases might obliterate the expected difference in natural history (Bonadonna *et al.*, 1980; Hilf *et al.*, 1980). Studies demonstrating greater benefit for pre-menopausal ER+ patients may be indicative of the hormonal effects of chemotherapy (Stephens *et al.*, 1982), but ER− cases can clearly benefit too (Knight *et al.*, 1981).

There is some support for the use of drug combinations. The potential for cardiotoxicity with adriamycin requires the demonstration of superior results before its inclusion in adjuvant regimens; preliminary results indicate that adriamycin-based combinations reduce the early relapse rate (Misset *et al.*,

Table 3 Adjuvant chemotherapy: factors known or suspected to improve response

Factors	Example reference
1 *Disease*	
(a) Fewer +ve nodes (CMF)	Bonadonna *et al*. (1982)
(b) More +ve nodes (thiotepa)	Fisher *et al*. (1975)
(cyclophosphamide)	Nissen-Meyer *et al*. (1982)
(c) ER− (controversial: see text)	
2 *Treatment*	
(a) Cytotoxic	
(i) More drugs (esp. $N^{+(10+)}$,	
post-menopausal)	
CMFVP[a] > CMF	Tormey *et al*. (1981b)
CMF > melphalan	Howat *et al*. (1981)
PMF = PF > melphalan	Fisher *et al*. (1981b)
(ii) Adriamycin: AVCF > CMF	Misset *et al*. (1982)
(iii) Less delay: cyclophosphamide	Nissen-Meyer *et al*. (1982)
(FAC — no effect: see text)	Buzdar *et al*. (1981b)
(b) Delayed radiotherapy ($N^{+(1-3)}$)	Allen *et al*. (1981)
(immediate radiotherapy adverse)	Cooper *et al*. (1981)
(c) Surgery	
(unknown: increases labelling	
index in mice)	
3 *Host*	
(a) Dose	Bonadonna and Valagussa
	(1981)
(b) Premenopausal status	Fisher *et al*. (1981b)
	Bonadonna *et al*. (1982)

[a] Prednisone may permit higher chemotherapy dosage in addition to adrenal suppression (Rose and Davis, 1980)

1982). In view of the relationship between dose and number of agents, an alternating strategy might be better (Goldie *et al*., 1982).

Delays of only a few weeks in initiating chemotherapy may abolish benefit, at least with peri-operative single-agent cyclophosphamide (Nissen-Meyer *et al*., 1982), perhaps reflecting rapid mutation to resistance, or possibly a transient rise in growth fraction after removal of the primary as noted in mouse metastases (Gunduz *et al*., 1979). (Comparison of immediately pre-operative with immediately post-operative chemotherapy might distinguish these possibilities.) Radiotherapy prior to chemotherapy may produce deleterious effect by delay and by leading to reduction of the first, apparently critical, drug doses (Cooper *et al*., 1981). For example, the use of delayed dose escalation with CMF appears to yield inferior results compared to other studies (Hubay *et al*., 1981), although one report (Buzdar *et al*., 1981b) suggests that slight delays are less critical in combination programs which may diminish the chance of resistance developing ($D_{S(R)}$ in Figure 3 displaced to the right).

The optimal duration of therapy is unknown, but in view of the comparatively small difference in results between the best peri-operative treatment and prolonged combination therapy, and the importance of early dosage, it may be preferable to use short, more intensive treatment (Henderson *et al.*, 1982; Jungi *et al.*, 1981; Tancini *et al.*, 1982). The most important host factor is dose tolerance, usually determined by marrow reserve. The Milan group found a steep dose–benefit correlation retrospectively; only a small proportion received full dose, mainly because of a 50% dose reduction for a leukocyte count less than 4000/mm^3. In view of the lethality of the disease and the short duration of leukopenia, treatment could be intensified without undue risk. Erratic gut absorption suggests that oral medications are best avoided, unless automatic and rapid dose escalation is employed (Carpenter *et al.*, 1981).

These observations raise the question of what to do in the presence of neutropenia at the usual three-week treatment interval. The first option is to extend the interval. The next is to look at the granulocyte count between cycles which may suggest reasonable safety in pressing the higher dose. Another is the use of agents such as prednisone. Failing these, it is very questionable whether 50% doses should continue to be administered or written into protocols. In addition, it would not be surprising if near-maximal benefit could be obtained from as few as four full-dose cycles. Adjuvant radiotherapy should be delayed to avoid any possibility of dose reduction.

Host effects of adjuvant chemotherapy

Acute and chronic toxicity may differ for the various agents commonly employed. The most prominent immediate manifestations of toxicity are usually nausea, vomiting, and alopecia (Glass *et al.*, 1981). They tend to be less with chlorambucil, melphalan, methotrexate or 5FU, and greater with cyclophosphamide and adriamycin. It is acute hematologic toxicity which exerts a dose-limiting effect.

Neutropenia is rarely sufficiently severe or prolonged to result in septic complications, but some patients show cumulative loss of regenerative capacity, and chronic mild neutropenia may continue for at least two years beyond the end of treatment (Goodyear *et al.*, 1981). These effects are more prominent with melphalan and chlorambucil, both of which can permanently reduce the stem cell population. This not only limits the intensity and duration of useful treatment, but also reduces the capacity for retreatment in the event of relapse. A more worrying aspect is the experimental observation of chronically increased stem cell cycling which may be related to the marked incidence of leukemia with low-dose melphalan administration in mice (Hellman, 1980). Long-term monitoring for second malignancies is essential, especially leukemia and second primary breast cancers.

Combination chemotherapy undoubtedly has a detrimental influence on quality of life during treatment (Palmer *et al.*, 1980; McArdle *et al.*, 1979). Anxiety, depression, and sexual difficulties are common (Maguire *et al.*, 1980), and emotional stress may be generated by the patient's desire to discontinue therapy against pressures to continue. Duration of treatment is probably a greater cause of distress that is its intensity (Jungi *et al.*, 1981).

Chemotherapy frequently induces primary ovarian failure. The incidence of amenorrhoea is related to age over 40, and to the intensity of the treatment. However, this is unlikely to be the major mechanism of action of chemotherapy in pre-menopausal patients as adjuvant oophorectomy alone has little effect on prognosis, and outcome in the NSABP studies was better in the younger patients who experienced less frequent ovarian suppression (Fisher *et al.*, 1979). The marked effects of dose and delay on outcome are also more characteristic of a direct effect by chemotherapy, and the so far unconfirmed advantage to ER− patients would also support this. In addition, post-menopausal patients show gain at equivalent dose levels (Bonadonna and Valagussa, 1981). The likelihood is that late pre-menopausal patients with ER+ tumors derive significant benefit from both modes of action.

Combined adjuvant hormono-chemotherapy

The addition of tamoxifen to melphalan and 5FU (PFT vs. PF) prolongs DFI in post-menopausal patients approximately in proportion to the ER level (Fisher *et al.*, 1981a), but is statistically significant only for $N^{+(4+)}$ cases. However, the proportional gain over placebo (Figure 4) in the DFI at two years was 22% for PF and 70% for PFT (Fisher *et al.*, 1980b, 1981a), compared to about 50% proportional gain for tamoxifen alone (Wallgren *et al.*, 1981). Determined in this manner, the gain was virtually identical for $N^{+(1-3)}$ compared to $N^{+(4+)}$ cases. This suggests the possibility of an additive effect on DFI, but clearly these results are very preliminary. The study of Hubay *et al.* (1981) is difficult to interpret because of the doubtful efficacy of the chemotherapy control arm, but the addition of tamoxifen did prolong the DFI.

In pre-menopausal patients, there is a slightly adverse effect from the addition of tamoxifen to melphalan and 5FU (Fisher *et al.*, 1981a). The incidence of ER+ cases would be highest in the late pre-menopausal group, those most likely to be experiencing cytotoxic ovarian suppression. Tamoxifen might be unable to add benefit for these, or alternatively, the modalities may be competing.

Locoregional management

Control of the primary tumor and regional nodes is necessary for good-quality survival and emphasis is on how to reduce morbidity (both functional and cosmetic) without loss of therapeutic effectiveness. There is a trend to modification of the Halsted radical mastectomy by sparing the pectoralis major (Vana *et al.*, 1981) and a randomized comparison of results supports this for Stages I and II (Turner *et al.*, 1981). The addition of post-operative radiotherapy can reduce the incidence of local and regional recurrences (Rozencweig *et al.*, 1978) but in view of the useful salvage rate from delayed radiotherapy, its morbidity must be carefully considered. Adjuvant axillary and supraclavicular radiotherapy would seem clearly indicated for cases with clinically involved nodes, but low dosage to unremoved involved nodes gives poor control and a higher mortality rate (Atkins *et al.*, 1972).

About one-third of N_0 patients are N^+, yet only 11% relapse in the axilla in the first five years after simple mastectomy alone (Fisher *et al.*, 1980a), with the possibility of salvage by node dissection and radiotherapy. This relapse frequency might be further reduced by clearance of the lower and middle axilla, and by adjuvant chemotherapy. Therefore the role of post-operative radiotherapy as a routine requires re-evaluation, and, it is clear that radiotherapy should be delayed if chemotherapy is also to be given.

While treatment of the axillary contents has not been very rewarding, there is somewhat more encouragement for treatment of the internal mammary chain. Either surgical (Lacour *et al.*, 1976) or radiotherapeutic treatment (Host and Brennhovd, 1977) of these nodes appears to confer benefit specifically in the high-risk group (that is, patients with inner and central primary lesions and positive axillary nodes). However, it is disturbing to note that the NSABP results of total mastectomy and apparently adequate post-operative radiotherapy are showing an adverse trend in exactly this subset compared to those treated by radical mastectomy in which the internal mammary nodes are untreated (Fisher *et al.*, 1981e). Fletcher and Montague (1978) have emphasized the importance of an *accurate* technique particularly for the internal mammary chain, but the NSABP group were unable to associate the location of recurrence with technical errors (Fisher *et al.*, 1980a).

SELECTIVE THERAPY IN ADVANCED DISEASE

Advanced disease includes metastatic or inoperable disease at the time of diagnosis, or disease recurring sometime after the completion of primary treatment. Such patients have a disease burden of the order of 10^9–10^{10} systemic tumor cells, a number beyond our ability to eradicate with currently available treatment. However, long-term survival may be observed in a small proportion of cases (Abramowitz, 1982).

Patient assessment

A prerequisite to selecting treatment is to evaluate the urgency of the clinical situation—the sites of disease involvement, the rate of disease progression, and the general health of the patient. Disease in a functionally critical site is the first priority in any plan of therapy. An estimate of the disease aggressiveness can be made from the temporal pattern of symptoms, the rapidity of growth of measured lesions, the DFI and the ER status. Patients with a DFI of more than two years who bear ER+ tumors have a more indolent course to their disease.

Other medical problems, either tumor-related (Davis and Tormey, 1981) or not tumor-related must also be taken into consideration. It is important to measure parameters of disease extent, and it may be useful to leave a local marker lesion undisturbed to facilitate monitoring. Non-specific indicators of tumor activity such as carcinoembryonic antigen (CEA) may sometimes help to assess response to systemic therapy, achievement of maximal remission, or early relapse.

Hormone therapy

Emerging data suggest that the traditional hormonal treatment sequence is changing (Hayward, 1980) and that the very similar response rates and durations obtained with most therapies favours the use of the least toxic, tamoxifen, as first line therapy. Sequential hormone therapy can be used as long as objective responses are obtained although there is a tendency to diminishing response rate and duration. In pre-menopausal patients, tamoxifen can predict oophorectomy response (Pritchard *et al.*, 1980). Medical adrenalectomy with aminoglutethimide would be used as second line therapy in preference to ablative surgery, because of its low and reversible morbidity (Santen *et al.*, 1981).

Chemotherapy

In general, combination chemotherapy results in a more rapid onset of response, higher response rates, more complete responses, and a longer time to treatment failure compared to sequential single-agent therapy (Canellos *et al.*, 1976; Smalley *et al.*, 1976; Carmo-Pereira *et al.*, 1980). However, combination chemotherapy of advanced breast cancer remains palliative and overall improvement in long-term survival is unproven (Chlebowski *et al.*, 1979). Adriamycin-based combinations provide higher response rates and improved survival than do the others (Bull *et al.*, 1978) and a reduction in the number of patients who progress primarily (Smalley, 1981). CMF therapy could be used as a first alternative for those in whom adriamycin is contra-indicated. Sequential single-agent treatment could be reserved for those unable to tolerate combination regimens.

The optimal duration of chemotherapy in the advanced disease is unknown. The usual practice is to continue cyclic therapy until relapse but it may be that, in patients with incurable disease, equivalent benefit could be achieved with short-duration induction treatment, and the overall morbidity greatly decreased by shortening the treatment period. Post-induction maintenance chemotherapy regimens appear to have only limited value (Tormey *et al.*, 1981a; Hortobagyi *et al.*, 1981a).

Hormono-chemotherapy

The question of relative efficacy of combined or sequential hormonochemotherapy is largely unresolved. For example, Stoll (1981) suggests hormone therapy be administered prior to chemotherapy, but Brunner and Cavalli (1981) caution that primary hormone therapy may impede the efficacy of chemotherapy by diminishing proliferative activity. Available clinical data indicate that combination hormono-chemotherapy may be superior to cytotoxic therapy alone (Lloyd *et al.*, 1979; Ahmann *et al.*, 1981; Engelsman, 1981) but these studies were not stratified according to ER status.

Comparisons of hormone therapy with early or delayed additional chemotherapy demonstrate improved response rate, response duration, and survival time for early combined treatment (Ahmann *et al.*, 1977; Priestman *et al.*, 1978; Falkson *et al.*, 1979). Once again, patients were not stratified according to ER level. However, the greatest benefit accrues to young women with rapidly progressive visceral (and presumably ER-poor) disease. This benefit may be secondary not to combined modality effects but to a decreased rate of primary progression and increased time to progression afforded by the chemotherapy element. No benefit is derived by adding CMF chemotherapy in tamoxifen repsonders (Glick *et al.*, 1980).

It is important to emphasize that delay is likely to compromise the efficacy of chemotherapy (Ahmann *et al.*, 1977) but less likely to compromise hormone responsiveness. This would suggest that chemotherapy be given initially, for a predetermined, but as yet undefined, time. Cytotoxic agents could be continued in the subset demonstrating chemotherapy response and tolerable toxicity while hormone therapy could then be added in the ER+ subset. In this manner, the more toxic treatment component would only be continued if benefit were being achieved. At relapse, if the tumour remained ER+, secondary hormonal therapy could be instituted.

Special situations

Patients who achieve remissions with combination chemotherapy relapse most often at the site of initial metastatic involvement and also in the central nervous system (Legha *et al.*, 1979). Data are available to suggest that consolidative therapy with radiation and/or surgery to overt sites of metastases can prolong the duration of response (Nervi *et al.*, 1979; Buzdar *et al.*, 1982). Since nearly all patients with locally advanced inoperable tumors have occult systemic disease of considerable extent, those with ER+ tumors might be managed initially with tamoxifen followed by consolidating small field radiotherapy and surgery (Bedwinek *et al.*, 1982). Patients with inflammatory carcinoma (most of whom will be ER−) have a desperate prognosis (Bozzetti *et al.*, 1981) but survival might be marginally improved with initial combination chemotherapy (Buzdar *et al.*, 1981a) and radiotherapy (Rubens *et al.*, 1980).

Patients with locoregional recurrence which can be eradicated occasionally do not develop overt systemic spread (Chu *et al.*, 1976; Donegan, 1979). Since a further proportion will have minimal systemic spread, it suggests the possibility of improved survival from combination chemotherapy, hormone therapy and standard local measures (Nervi *et al.*, 1979).

CONCLUSION

The large majority of patients developing breast cancer will die of their disease because of spread beyond the local site, and are thus candidates for surgery in one form or another, prophylactic or palliative radiotherapy, hormonal manipulation, and chemotherapy. Selective treatment is therefore not so much a problem of selecting modalities, as one of timing, sequencing, and extent. Because of the disseminated and heterogeneous nature of the disease, simultaneous use of modalities carries the greatest potential for benefit, but also the greatest possibility of damage because of interference, synergistic morbidity, or difficulty in identifying an inactive or harmful component.

An attempt to illustrate selective management is presented in Figure 6, whose approach should be compared with that of standard therapy (Consensus Development Panel, 1979, 1980). After diagnosis, clinical assessment of locoregional extent guides the process of systemic screening and surgical planning. The tumor is excised if practicable, with removal of the breast if lesser surgery is not feasible. (The value of the resected tumor for laboratory evaluation of biological properties will be vitiated by pre-operative use of other modalities). An axillary sampling procedure is done simultaneously. Inoperable disease is managed with systemic therapy according to ER status.

A decision on adjuvant chemotherapy should be made in the immediate post-operative phase, and the N⁻ER+ subset without adverse pathologic features can be excluded on the basis of low risk. (No other subset can yet be excluded on the basis of insufficient gain, as optimal therapy with available agents has not yet been defined.) All tumors are likely to contain a mix of ER− and ER+ stem cells and ER− cells are presumed to be killed only by

A CONSECUTIVE APPROACH

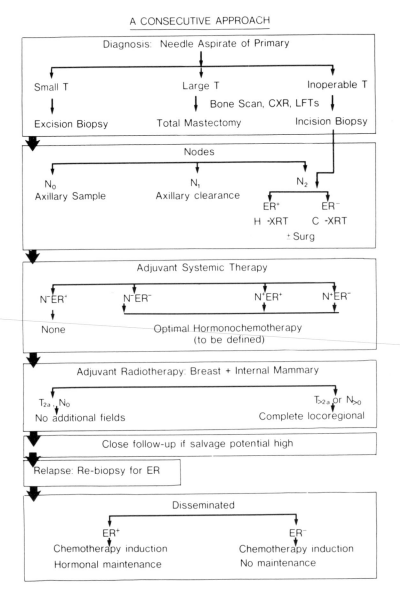

Figure 6 Current clinical investigation is leading toward a series of selection steps such as these. A consecutive approach identifies the least investigation and treatment resulting in the most potential individual gain by separate consideration of the primary, regional, and systemic components of breast cancer. T = primary tumor; CXR = chest x-ray; LFTs = liver function tests; $N_{0,1,2}$ = clinical axillary node status; $N^{-,+}$ = pathological axillary node status, either negative or positive; H = hormone therapy; C = chemotherapy; XRT = radiotherapy; $ER^{-,+}$ = estrogen receptor level, either poor or rich.

intensive broad-spectrum chemotherapy. The best way of eliminating (as opposed to suppressing) ER+ stem cells is unknown and requires elucidation in advanced disease trials. The use of hormonal priming before chemotherapy has potential but may have disadvantages. Recent results suggest that adjuvant hormonal therapy should consist of ovarian ablation with low dosage prednisone for pre-menopausal patients, and tamoxifen for post-menopausal cases.

Adjuvant chemotherapy should be used with minimum delay, with maximum dosage in the first as well as in subsequent cycles. Most regimens still tend to err on the 'safe' side, which may be a fatal mistake. Urgently requiring confirmation is the suspicion that a 50% dose reduction (and perhaps lesser reductions also) results in loss of most cytotoxic benefit.

After completion of primary therapy, close follow-up is still essential in patients who had not been given adjuvant chemotherapy or radiotherapy, as localized recurrence could still be salvaged in this group. Relapses after adjuvant therapy of any type should be carefully assessed for DFI and location, and also for ER and chemosensitivity changes (clinical or *in vitro*).

In disseminated disease, the role of chemotherapy and hormone interaction requires further investigation. Chemotherapy may best be used first, even in ER+ cases, while the hormone-insensitive component is smallest, and then hormone therapy may be added in ER+ chemotherapy responders and continued as maintenance. Chemotherapy could be continued if primarily effective and tolerated, although the useful duration of chemotherapy in advanced disease may be much shorter than the clinical time to response and stabilization. This approach should be tested against the traditional hormone-to-chemotherapy sequence, both for benefit and overall morbidity.

With chemotherapy, our main responsibility is to identify non-responders. In advanced disease this goal is relatively easy but often badly done, as careful and repeated observation of response parameters must be actively pursued. In the case of adjuvant therapy, groups of patients who do not benefit can only be detected by comparative analysis.

Acknowledgements

We greatly appreciate the support and thoughtful suggestions of the members of the Breast Tumour Group and Department of Advanced Therapeutics of the Cancer Control Agency of British Columbia. Our special gratitude is due to Mrs Joan McGee for her invaluable help and patience in preparing this manuscript.

REFERENCES

Abramowitz, J.W. (1982). Long term complete remissions from chemotherapy and hormonal therapy in breast cancer patients (Abstract). *Proc. Am. Soc. Clin. Oncol.*, 76 (C294).

Ahmann, D.L., O'Connell, M.J., Hahn, R.G., Bisel, H.F., Lee, R.A., and Edmonson, J.H. (1977). An evaluation of early or delayed adjuvant chemotherapy in premenopausal patients with advanced breast cancer undergoing oophorectomy. *New Engl. J. Med.,* **297**, 356.

Ahmann, F.R., Jones, S.E., Moon, T.E., Davis, S.L., and Salmon, S.E. (1981). Improved survival of patients with advanced breast cancer treated with adriamycin–cyclophosphamide plus tamoxifen (TAC) (Abstract). *Am. Assoc. Clin. Res.,* **22**, 148 (586).

Allegra, J.C., Barlock, A., Huff, K.K., and Lippman, M.E. (1980). Changes in multiple or sequential estrogen receptor determinations in breast cancer. *Cancer,* **45**, 792.

Allen, H., Brooks, R., Jones, S.E., Chase, E., Heusinkveld, R.S., Giordano, G.F., Ketchel, S.J., Jackson, R.A., Davis, S., Moon, T.E., and Salmon, S.E. (1981). Adjuvant treatment for Stage II (node positive) breast cancer with adriamycin–cyclophosphamide (AC) ± radiotherapy (XRT). In *Adjuvant therapy of cancer,* vol. 3. (eds S.E. Salmon and S.E. Jones). London: Grune and Stratton. p. 453.

Amalric, R., Santamaria, F., Robert, F., Seigle, J., Altschuler C., Kurtz, J.M., Spitalier, J.M., Brandone, H., Ayme, Y., Pollet, J.F., Burmeister, R., and Abed, R. (1982). Radiation therapy with or without primary limited surgery for operable breast cancer: a 20-year experience at the Marseilles Cancer Institute. *Cancer,* **49**, 30.

Amer, M.H. (1982). Chemotherapy and pattern of metastases in breast cancer patients. *J. Surg. Oncol.,* **19**, 101.

American Joint Committee for Cancer Staging (1977). Philosophy of classifications and staging by the TNM system. *Manual for staging of cancer.* p. 1.

Atkins, Sir H., Hayward, J.L., Klugman, D.J., and Wayte, A.B. (1972). Treatment of early breast cancer: a report after ten years of a clinical trial. *Br. Med. J.,* **2**, 423.

Bedwani, R., Vana, J., Rosner, D., Schmitz, R.L., and Murphy, G.P. (1981). Management and survival of female patients with 'minimal' breast cancer: as observed in the long-term and short-term surveys of the American College of Surgeons. *Cancer,* **47**, 2769.

Bedwinek, J., Rao, D.V., Perez, C., Lee, J., and Fineberg, B. (1982). Stage III and localized Stage IV breast cancer: irradiation alone vs. irradiation plus surgery. *Int. J. Radiat. Oncol.,* **8**, 31.

Begg, C.B., Cohen, J.L., and Ellerton, J. (1980). Are the elderly predisposed to toxicity from cancer chemotherapy? *Cancer Clin. Trials,* **3**, 369.

Benz, C., and Cadman, E. (1981). Modulation of 5-fluorouracil metabolism and toxicity via estrogen receptor *Proc. Cancer Res. Treat.,* **1**, 61.

Bertuzzi, A., Daidone, M.G., Di Fronzo, G., and Silvestrini, R. (1981). Relationship among estrogen receptors, proliferative activity and menopausal status in breast cancer. *Breast Cancer Res. Treat.,* **1**, 253.

Blumenschein, G.R. (1979). Tumor burden killed by adriamycin-combination therapy in metastatic breast cancer. *Adjuvant Ther.,* **11**, 71.

Boice, J.D., Jr., and Monson, R.R. (1977). Breast cancer in women after repeated fluoroscopic examinations of the chest *J. Nat. Cancer Inst.,* **59**, 823.

Bonadonna, G., and Valagussa, P. (1981). Dose–response effect of adjuvant chemotherapy in breast cancer. *New Engl. J. Med.,* **304**, 10.

Bonadonna, G., Valagussa, P., Rossi, A., Tancini, G., Brambilla, Marchini, S., and Veronesi, U. (1982). Multimodal therapy with CMF in resectable breast cancer with positive axillary nodes: the Milan Institute experience. *Recent Results Cancer Res.,* **80**, 149.

Bonadonna, G., Valagussa, P., Tancini, G., and Di Fronzo, G. (1980). Estrogen-receptor status and response to chemotherapy in early and advanced breast cancer. *Cancer Chemother. Pharmacol.*, **4**, 37.

Boyd, N.F., Campbell, J.E., Germanson, T., Thomson, D.B., Sutherland, D.J., and Meakin, J.W. (1981a) Body weight and prognosis in breast cancer. *J. Nat. Cancer Inst.*, **67**, 785.

Boyd, N.F., Meakin, J.W., Hayward, J.L., and Brown, T.C. (1981b). Clinical estimation of the growth rate of breast cancer. *Cancer*, **48**, 1037.

Bozzetti, F., Saccozzi, R., De Lena, M., and Salvadori, B. (1981). Inflammatory cancer of the breast: analysis of 114 cases. *J. Surg. Oncol.*, **18**, 355.

Brinkley, D., and Haybittle, J.L. (1977). The curability of breast cancer. *World J. Surg.*, **1**, 287.

Bruchovsky, N., and Goldie, J.H. (eds) (1982a). *Durg and Hormone resistance in neoplasia*. Boca Raton: CRC Press. (in press).

Bruchovsky, N., and Goldie, J.H. (1982b). Basis for the use of drug and hormone combinations in the treatment of endocrine related cancer. In *Drug and hormone resistance in neoplasia* (eds N. Bruchovsky, and J.H. Goldie. Boca Raton. CRC Press. Chapter 14. (in press).

Brunner, K.W., and Cavalli, F. (1981). Combination endocrine/cytotoxic therapy in breast cancer. In *Hormonal management of endocrine-related cancer* (ed B.A. Stoll). London: Lloyd-Luke (Medical Books). p. 220.

Bryant, A.J.S., and Weir, J.A. (eds) (1981). Prophylactic oophorectomy in operable instances of carcinoma of the breast. *Surg., Gynaecol. Obstet.*, **153**, 660.

Bull, J., Tormey, D.C., Li, S.-H., Carbone, P.P., Falkson, G., Blom, J., Perlin, E and Simon, R. (1978). A randomized comparative trial of adriamycin versus methotrexate in combination drug therapy. *Cancer*, **41**, 1649.

Buzdar, A., Blumenschein, G., Montague, E., Powell, K., Hortobagyi, G., and Yap. H. (1982). Regional consolidative therapy following systemic chemotherapy in metastatic breast cancer. *Proc. Am. Soc. Clin. Oncol.*, **1**, 74.

Buzdar, A.U., Montague, E.D., Barker, J.L., Hortobagyi, G.N., and Blumenschein, G.R. (1981a). Management of inflammatory carcinoma of the breast with combined modality approach—an update. *Cancer*, **47**, 2537.

Buzdar, A., Smith, T., and Blumenschein, G. (1981b). Effect of timing of initiation of adjuvant chemotherapy on disease-free interval in operable breast cancer (Abstract). *Breast Cancer Res. Treat.*, **1**, 16.

Byar, D.P., Sears, M.E., and McGuire, W.L. (1979). Relationship between estrogen receptor values and clinical data in predicting the response to endocrine therapy for patients with advanced breast cancer. *Eur. J. Cancer*, **15**, 299.

Campbell, F.C., Blamey, R.W., Elston, C.W., Morris, A.H., Nicholson, R.I., Griffiths, K., and Haybittle, J.L. (1981). Quantitative oestradiol receptor values in primary breast cancer and response of metastases to endocrine therapy. *Lancet* **ii**, 1317.

Canellos, G.P., Pocock, S.J., Taylor, S.G., Sears, M.E., Klaasen, D.J., and Band, P.R. (1976). Combination chemotherapy for metastatic breast carcinoma: prospective comparison of multiple drug therapy with L-phenylalanine mustard. *Cancer*, **38**, 1882.

Carmo-Pereira, J., Costa, F.O., and Henriques, E. (1980). Single-drug vs. combination cytotoxic chemotherapy in advanced breast cancer: a randomized study. *Eur. J. Cancer Res.*, **16**, 1621.

Carpenter, J.T., Maddox, W.A., Laws, H.L., Wirtschafter, D.D., and Soong, S.J. (1981). The importance of leukopenia in breast cancer adjuvant therapy with melphalan (MPL) (Abstract). *Proc. Am. Soc. Clin. Oncol.*, **22** (C-434).

Carter, S.K. (1980). Surgery plus adjuvant chemotherapy—a review of therapeutic implications. 1. Breast cancer. *Cancer Chemother. Pharmacol.*, **4**, 147.

Carter, S.K. (1981a). The interpretation of trials: combined hormonal therapy and chemotherapy in disseminated breast cancer. *Breast Cancer Res. Treat.* **1**, 43.

Carter, S.K. (1981b). Predictors of response and their clinical evaluation. *Cancer Chemother. Pharmacol.*, **7**, 1.

Charlson, M.E., and Feinstein, A.R. (1973). An analytic critique of existing systems of staging for breast cancer. *Surgery*, **73**, 579.

Charlson, M.E., and Feinstein, A.R. (1974). The auxometric dimension: a new method for using rate of growth in prognostic staging of breast cancer. *J. Am. Med. Assoc.*, **228**, 180.

Chlebowski, R.T., Irwin, L.E., Pugh, R.P., Sadoff, L., Hestorff, R., Wiener, J.M., and Bateman, J.R. (1979). Survival of patients with metastatic breast cancer treated with either combination or sequential chemotherapy. *Cancer Res.*, **39**, 4503.

Chlebowski, R.T., Weiner, J.M., Luce, J., Hestorff, R., Lang, J.E., Reynolds, R., Godfrey, T., Ryden, V.M., and Bateman, J.R. (1981). Significance of relapse after adjuvant treatment with combination chemotherapy or 5-fluorouracil alone in high-risk breast cancer. *Cancer Res.*, **41**, 4399.

Chu, F.C.H., Lin, F-J., Kim, J.H., Huh, S.H., and Garmatic, C.J. (1976). Locally recurrent carcinoma of the breast: results of radiation therapy. *Cancer*, **37**, 2677.

Cohen, J.L., Gelman, R., and Raam, S. (1980). A blinded study of inter- and intra-laboratory variations in the performance of estrogen receptor (ER) (Abstract) assay. *Proc. Am. Soc. Clin. Oncol.*, **21** (C-29).

Consensus Development Panel (1979). Treatment of primary breast cancer: management of local disease. *New Engl. J. Med.*, **301,** 340.

Consensus Development Panel (1980). *Adjuvant chemotherapy of breast cancer.* Amsterdam: Excerpta Medica. p. 1.

Cooper, M.R., Rhyne, A.L., Muss, H.B., Ferree, C., Richards, F.II., White, D.R., Stuart, J.J., Jackson, D.V., Howard, V., Shore, A., and Spurr, C.L. (1981). A randomized comparative trial of chemotherapy and irradiation therapy for Stage II breast cancer. *Cancer*, **47**, 2833.

Coppin, C.M.L. (1982). The treatment of advanced prostatic cancer with drugs and hormones. In *Drug and hormone resistance in neoplasia* (eds N. Bruchovsky, and J.H. Goldie). Boca Raton: CRC Press. Chap. 11. (in press).

Cutler, S.J., Asire, A.J., and Taylor, S.G. (1969). Classification of patients with disseminated cancer of the breast. *Cancer*, **24**, 861.

Davies, G.C., Millis, R.R., and Hayward, J.D. (1980). Assessment of axillary lymph node status. *Ann. Surg.*, **192**, 148.

Davis, T.E., and Tormey, D.C. (1981). Special problems in the management of advanced breast cancer. In *Breast cancer* (eds B. Hoogstraten, and R.W. McDivitt). Boca Raton: CRC Press. p.245.

De Wys, W.D., Allegra, J.C., Simon, R., and Lippman, M.E. (1980). A proposed model for the prediction of response to endocrine therapy in breast cancer from the estrogen receptor status of one site and the number of metastatic sites. *Cancer Res.*, **40**, 2423.

Donegan, W.L. (1977). The influence of untreated internal mammary metastases upon the course of mammary cancer. *Cancer*, **39**, 533.

Donegan, W.L. (1979). Local and regional recurrence. In *Cancer of the breast*, 2nd edn (eds W.L. Donegan and J.S. Spratt, Jr). London: W.B. Saunders.

Duncan, W., and Kerr, G.R. (1976). The curability of breast cancer. *Br. Med. J.*, **2**, 781.

Egan, M.L., and Henson, D.E. (1982). Monoclonal antibodies and breast cancer. *J. Natl Cancer Inst.*, **68**, 338.

Ege, G.N. (1980). Radiocolloid lymphoscintigraphy in neoplastic disease. *Cancer Res.*, **40**, 3065.

Ellis, R.J., Wernick, G., Zabriskie, J.B., and Goldman, L.I. (1975). Immunologic competence of regional lymph nodes in patients with breast cancer. *Cancer*, **35**, 655.

Elwood, J.M., and Godolphin, W. (1980). Oestrogen receptors in breast tumours: associations with age, menopausal status and epidemiological and clinical features in 735 patients. *Br. J. Cancer*, **42**, 635.

Elwood, J.M., and Moorehead, W.P. (1980). Delay in diagnosis and long-term survival in breast cancer. *Br. Med. J.*, **280**, 1291.

Engelsman, E. (1981). The status of EORTC trials of combined Nolvadex and chemotherapy. *Rev. Endocrine-Related Cancer*, Suppl. 8, 45.

Falkson, G., Falkson, H.C., Glidewell, O., Weinberg, V., Leone, L., and Holland, J.F. (1979). Improved remission rates and remission duration in young women with metastatic breast cancer following combined oophorectomy and chemotherapy: a study by cancer and leukemia group B. *Cancer*, **43**, 2215.

Fey, M.F., Brunner, K.W., and Sonntag, R.W. (1981). Prognostic factors in metastatic breast cancer. *Cancer Clin. Trials*, **4**, 237.

Fialkow, P.I. (1976). Clonal origin of human tumours. *Biochim. Biophys. Acta*, **458**, 283.

Fidler, I.J., and Hart, I.R. (1981). The origin of metastatic heterogeneity in tumours. *Eur. J. Cancer*, **17**, 487.

Fisher, B., Montague, E., Redmond, C., Deutsch, M., Brown, G.R., Zauber, A., Hanson, W.F., Wong, A., and Other NSABP Investigators (1980a). Findings from NSABP protocol no. B-04—Comparison of radical mastectomy with alternative treatments for primary breast cancer. I. Radiation compliance and its relation to treatment outcome. *Cancer*, **46**, 1.

Fisher, B., Redmond, C., Fisher, E.R., and Participating NSABP Investigators (1980b). The contribution of recent NSABP clinical trials of primary breast cancer therapy to an understanding of tumor biology—an overview of findings. *Cancer*, **46**, 1009.

Fisher, B., Redmond, C., Brown, A., and Participating NSABP Investigators (1981a). Treatment of primary breast cancer with chemotherapy and tamoxifen. *New Engl. J. Med.* **305**, 1.

Fisher, B., Redmond, C., Wolmark, N., and Participating NSABP Investigators (1981b). Breast cancer studies of the NSABP: an editorialized overview. In *Adjuvant therapy of cancer*, vol.3 (eds S.E. Salmon, and S.E. Jones. London: Grune and Stratton. p.359.

Fisher, B., Redmond, C., Wolmark, N., and Wieand, H.S. (1981c). Disease-free survival at intervals during and following completion of adjuvant chemotherapy: the NSABP experience from three breast cancer protocols. *Cancer*, **48**, 1273.

Fisher, B., Sherman, B., Rockette, H., Redmond, C., Margolese, R., and Fisher, E.R. (1979). L-Phenylalanine mustard (L-PAM) in the management of premenopausal patients with primary breast cancer. Lack of assocation of disease-free survival with depression of ovarian function. *Cancer*, **44**, 847.

Fisher, B., Slack, N.H., Bross, I.D., and Cooperating Investigators (1969). Cancer of the breast: size of neoplasm and prognosis. *Cancer*, **24**, 1071.

Fisher, B., Slack, N., Katrych, D., and Wolmark, N. (1975). Ten year follow-up results of patients with carcinoma of the breast in a cooperative clinical trial evaluating surgical adjuvant chemotherapy. *Surg., Gynaecol. Obstet.*, **140**, 528.

Fisher, B., Wolmark, N., Bauer, M., Redmond, C., and Gebhardt, M. (1981d). The accuracy of clinical nodal staging and of limited axillary dissection as a determinant of histologic nodal status in carcinoma of the breast. *Surg., Gynaecol. Obstet.*, **152**, 765.

Fisher, B., Wolmark, N., Redmond, C., Deutsch, M., Fisher, E.R., and Participating NSABP Investigators (1981e). Findings from NSABP protocol no. B-04: Comparison of radical mastectomy with alternative treatments. II. The clinical and biologic significance of medial-central breast cancers. *Cancer*, **48**, 1863.

Fisher, E.R., Redmond, C., and Fisher, B. (1980c). Pathologic findings from the National Surgical Adjuvant Breast Project (protocol no.4). VI. Discriminants for five-year treatment failure. *Cancer*, **46**, 908.

Fletcher, G.H. (1973). Clinical dose–response curves of human malignant epithelial tumours. *Br. J. Radiol.*, **46**, 1.

Fletcher, G., and Montague, E.D. (1978). Does adequate irradiation of the internal mammary chain and supraclavicular nodes improve survival rates? *Int. J. Radiat. Oncol.*, **4**, 481.

Fox, M.S. (1979). On the diagnosis and treatment of breast cancer. *J. Am. Med. Assoc.*, **241**, 489.

Frei, III, E., and Canellos, G.P. (1980). Dose: a critical factor in cancer chemotherapy. *Am. J. Med.*, **69**, 585.

Gallager, H.S. (1980). The developmental pathology of breast cancer. *Cancer*, **46**, 905.

Gefter, W.B., Friedman, A.K., and Goodman, R.L. (1982). The role of mammography in evaluating patients with early carcinoma of the breast for tylectomy and radiation therapy. *Radiology*, **142**, 77.

Glass, A., Wieand, H.S., Fisher, B., Redmond, C., Lerner, H., Wolter, J., Shibata, H., Plotkin, D., Foster, R., Margolese, R., Wolmark, N., and Other NSABP Investigators (1981). Acute toxicity during adjuvant chemotherapy for breast cancer: the National Surgical Adjuvant Breast and Bowel Project (NSABP) experience from 1717 patients receiving single and multiple agents. *Cancer Treat. Rep.*, **65**, 363.

Glick, J.H., Creech, R.H., Torri, S., Holroyde, C., Brodovsky, H., Catalano, R.B., and Varano, M. (1980) Tamoxifen plus sequential CMF: Chemotherapy versus tamoxifen alone in postmenopausal patients with advanced breast cancer: a randomized trial. *Cancer*, **45**, 735.

Godolphin, W., Elwood, J.M., and Spinelli, J.J. (1981). Estrogen receptor quantitation and staging as complementary prognostic indicators in breast cancer: a study of 583 patients. *Int. J. Cancer*, **28**, 677.

Goldie, J.H., Bruchovsky, N., Coldman, A.J., and Gudauskas, G.A. (1981). Steroid receptors in adjuvant hormonal therapy for breast cancer. *Can. J. Surg.*, **24**, 290.

Goldie, J.H., and Coldman, A.J. (1979). A mathematic model for relating the drug sensitivity of tumors to their spontaneous mutation rate. *Cancer Treat. Rep.*, **63**, 1727.

Goldie, J.H., Coldman, A.J., and Gudauskas, G.A. (1982). Rationale for the use of alternating non-cross-resistant chemotherapy. *Cancer Treat. Rep.*, **66**, 439.

Goodyear, M.D.E., Mackay, I.R., and Russell, I.S. (1981). Delayed recovery of peripheral blood cell numbers after adjuvant cytotoxic chemotherapy for Stage II breat cancer. *Cancer Chemother. Pharmacol.*, **7**, 37.

Gore, S., Langlands, A., Pocock, S., and Kerr, G. (1982). Natural history of breast cancer. *Recent Results Cancer Res.*, **80**, 134.

Gunduz, N., Fisher, B., and Saffer, E.A. (1979). Effect of surgical removal on the growth and kinetics of residual tumor. *Cancer Res.*, **39**, 3861.

Haagensen, C.D. (1971). *Diseases of the breast* London: W.B. Saunders.

Hager, J.C., Furmanski, P., Heppner, G.H., Roi, L., Brennan, M.J., Rich, M.A., and the Breast Cancer Prognostic Study Associates (1982). Correlation between elevated preoperative CEA levels and early recurrence in breast cancer patients (Abstract). *Proc. Am. Assoc. Clin. Res.,* (566).

Hahnel, R. (1981). Oestrogen receptor status, breast cancer growth and prognosis. *Rev. Endocrine-Related Cancer,* **8**, 5.

Harris, J.R., Levene, M.B., and Hellman, S. (1981). Radiation therapy as primary treatment for early carcinoma of the breast. In *Breast cancer* (eds B. Hoogstraten, and R.W. McDivitt). Boca Raton: CRC Press p.185.

Hawkins, R.A., Black, R., Steele, R.J.C., Dixon, J.M.J., and Forrest, A.P.M. (1981). Oestrogen receptor concentration in primary breast cancer and axillary node metastases. *Breast Cancer Res. Treat.,* **1**, 245.

Hayward, J.L. (1980). The changing role of endocrine therapy in the management of advanced breast cancer. In *Breast cancer: experimental and clinical aspects* (eds H.T. Mouridsen, and T. Palshof). Oxford: Pergamon Press. p.81.

Hayward, J.L. Rubens, R.D., Carbone, P.P., Heuson, J.C., Kumaoka, S., and Segaloff, A. (1977). Assessment of response to therapy in advanced breast cancer. A project of the programme on clinical oncology of the International Union Against Cancer, Geneva, Switzerland. *Br. J. Cancer,* **35**, 292.

Hellman, S. (1980). Improving the therapeutic index in breast cancer treatment: The Richard and Hinda Rosenthal Foundation Award Lecture. *Cancer Res.,* **40**, 4335.

Hellman, S., Harris, J.R., Canellos, G.P., and Fisher, B. (1982). Cancer of the breast. In *Cancer: principles and practice of oncology* (eds V.T. De Vita, Jr, S. Hellman, and S.A. Rosenberg). Toronto: J.B. Lippincott. p. 914.

Henderson, I.C., and Canellos, G.P. (1980). Cancer of the breast. The past decade. *New Engl. J. Med.,* **302**, 17, 78.

Henderson, I.C., Gelman, R., Parker, L.M., Skarin, A.T., Mayer, R.J., Garnick, M.B., Canellos, G.P., and Frei, E., III, (1982). 15 vs. 30 weeks of adjuvant chemotherapy for breast cancer patients with a high risk of recurrence: a randomized trial (Abstract). *Proc. Am. Soc. Clin. Oncol.,* (C-290).

Hermann, R.E., Esselstyn, C.B., Jr, and Crile, G., Jr (1978). Conservative surgical treatment of potentially curable breast cancer. In *The breast* (eds H.S. Gallager, H.P. Leis, R.K. Snyderman, and J.A. Urban). Saint Louis: C.V. Mosby. p. 219.

Heuser, L., Spratt, J.S., and Polk, H.C., Jr, (1979). Growth rates of primary breast cancers. *Cancer,* **43**, 1888.

Hewitt, H.B. (1980). Immunotherapy of Cancer: an underview. *Mod. Med. Can.,* **35**, 1352.

Hilf, R., Feldstein, M.L., Savlov, E.D., Gibson, S.L., and Seneca, B. (1980). The lack of relationship between estrogen receptor status and response to chemotherapy. *Cancer,* **46**, 2797.

Holdaway, I.M., Mountjoy, K.G., Harvey, V.J., Allen, E.P., and Stephens, E.J. (1980). Clinical applications of receptor measurements in breast cancer. *Br. J. Cancer,* **41**, 136.

Holland, J.F. (1981). Adjuvant chemotherapy for breast cancer. *Surg. Clin. N. Am.,* **61**, 1361.

Hoogstraten, B., and Fabian, C. (1979). A reappraisal of single drugs in advanced breast cancer. *Cancer Clin. Trials,* **2**, 101.

Hortobagyi, G.N., Blumenschein, G.R., Buzdar, A.U., Yap, H.Y., Schell, F.C., Barnes, B.C., and Burges, M.A. (1981a). Combination chemoimmunotherapy with FAC–BCG for metastatic breast cancer: the impact of CMF maintenance chemotherapy. *J. Surg. Oncol.,* **18**, 163.

Hortobagyi, G.N., Smith, T.L., Swenerton, K.D., Legha, S.S., Buzdar, A.U., Blumenschein, G.R., Gutterman, J.U., and Hersh, E.M. (1981b). A prognostic value of prechemotherapy skin tests in patients with metastatic breast carcinoma. *Cancer*, **47**, 1369.

Host, H., and Brennhovd, I.O. (1977). The effect of post-operative radiotherapy in breast cance.r *Int. J. Radiat. Oncol.*, **2**, 1061.

Howat, J.M.T., Hughes, R., Durning, P., George, W.D., Sellwood, R.A., Bush, H., Phadke, K., Grafton, C., and Crowther, D. (1981). A controlled clinical trial of adjuvant chemotherapy in operable cancer of the breast. In *Adjuvant therapy of cancer*, vol. 3 (eds S.E. Salmon, and S.E. Jones). London: Grune and Stratton. p. 371.

Hubay, C.A., Pearson, O.H., Marshall, J.S., Stellato, T.A., Rhodes, R.S., DeBanne, S.M., Rosenblatt, J., Mansour, E.G., Hermann, R.E., Jones, J.C., Flynn, W.J., Eckert, C., McGuire, W.L., and 27 Participating Investigators (1981). Adjuvant therapy of Stage II breast cancer: 48 month follow-up of a prospective randomized clinical trial. *Breast Cancer Res. Treat.*, **1**, 77.

Ingle, J.N., Ahmann, D.L., Green, S.J., Edmonson, J.H., Bisel, H.F., Kvols, L.K., Nichols, W.C., Creagan, E.T., Hahn, R.G., Rubin, J., and Frytak, S. (1981). Randomized clinical trial of diethylstilbestrol versus tamoxifen in postmenopausal women with advanced breast cancer. *New Engl. J. Med.*, **304**, 16.

Israel, N., and Saez, S. (1978). Relation between steroid receptor content and the response to hormone addition in isolated human breast cancer cells in short-term culture. *Cancer Res.*, **38**, 4314.

Janssens, J.P., Teuwen, D., Bonte, J., Drochmans, A., Goddeeris, P., Lauwerijns, J.M., and De Loecker, W. (1981). Effect of radiotherapy on steroid receptors in breast cancer. *Lancet*, **ii**, 1108.

Jonat, W., and Maass, H. (1978). Some comments on the necessity of receptor determination in human breast cancer. *Cancer Res.*, **38**, 4305.

Jungi, W.F., Alberto, P., Brunner, K.W., Cavalli, F., Barrelet, L., and Senn, H. (1981). Short- or long-term adjuvant chemotherapy for breast cancer. In *Adjuvant therapy of cancer*, vol. 3 (eds S.E. Salmon, and S.E. Jones). Grune and Stratton. p. 395.

Kaufmann, M., Klinga, K., Runnebaum, B., and Kubli, F. (1980). *In vitro* adriamycin sensitivity test and hormonal receptors in primary breast cancer. *Eur. J. Cancer*, **16**, 1609.

Kiang, D.T. (1981). Breast cancer: methods and results of endocrine therapy. In *Hormonal management of endocrine-related cancer*. (ed. B.A. Stoll). Lloyd-Luke (Medical Books). London: p. 64.

Kiang, D.T., and Kennedy, B.J. (1977). Factors affecting estrogen receptors in breast cancer. *Cancer*, **40**, 1571.

Kiang, D.T., and Kennedy, B.J. (1981). Chemoendocrine therapy in advanced breast cancer. *Breast Cancer Res. Treat.*, **1**, 105.

Kiang, D.T., Zhang, H-J., and Kennedy, B.J. (1982). Use of thymidine kinase activity in predicting chemotherapy response of breast cancer (Abstract). *Proc. Am. Soc. Clin. Oncol.*, (C-341).

Kister, S., Aroesty, J., Rogers, W., Huber, C., Willis, K., Morrison, P., Shangold, G., and Lincoln, T. (1979). An analysis of predictor variables for adjuvant treatment of breast cancer. *Cancer Chemother. Pharmacol.*, **2**, 147.

Knight, W.A., III, Clark, G.M., Osborne, C.K., and McGuire, W.L. (1981). Intensive chemotherapy for estrogen receptor negative, Stage II breast cancer. In

Adjuvant therapy of cancer, vol.3 (eds S.E. Salmon and S.E. Jones). London: Grune and Stratton. p. 321.

Lacour, J., Bucalossi, P., Cacers, E., Jacobelli, G., Koszarowski, T., Le, M., Rumeau-Rouquette, C., and Veronesi, U. (1976). Radical mastectomy versus radical mastectomy plus internal mammary dissection: five year results of an international cooperative study. *Cancer,* **37**, 206.

Langlands, A.O., Pocock, S.J., Kerr, G.R., and Gore, S.M. (1979). Long-term survival of patients with breast cancer: a study of the curability of the disease. *Br. Med. J.,* **2**, 1247.

Leake, R.E., Laing, L., Calman, K.C., MacBeth, F.R., Crawford, D., and Smith, D.C. (1981). Oestrogen-receptor status and endocrine therapy of breast cancer: response rates and status stability. *Br. J. Cancer,* **43**, 59.

Lee, Y.-T.N. (1972). The lognormal distribution of growth rates of soft tissue metastases of breast cancer. *J. Surg. Oncol.,* **18**, 81.

Legha, S.S., Buzdar, A.U., Smith, T.L., Hortobagyi, G.N., Swenerton, K.D., Blumenschein, G.R., Gehan, E.A., Bodey, G.P., and Freireich, E.J. (1979). Complete remissions in metastatic breast cancer treated with combination drug therapy. *Ann. Intern. Med.,* **91**, 847.

Lippman, M. (1978). Summary of additional presentations from the workshop on the use of steroids as carriers of cytotoxic agents in breast cancer. *Cancer Treat. Rep.,* **62**, 1259.

Lippman, M., and Allegra, J.C. (1980). Quantitative estrogen receptor analyses: the response to endocrine and cytotoxic chemotherapy in human breast cancer and the disease-free interval. *Cancer,* **46**, 2829.

Lippman, M.E., and Thompson, E.B. (1979). Pitfalls in the interpretation of steroid receptor assays in clinical medicine. In *Steroid receptors and the management of cancer,* vol. 1 (eds E.B. Thompson, and M.E. Lippman. Boca Raton: CRC Press. p.235.

Lloyd, R.E., Jones, S.E., and Salmon, S.E. (1979). Comparative trial of low-dose adriamycin plus cyclophosphamide with or without additive hormonal therapy in advanced breast cancer. *Cancer,* **43**, 60.

McArdle, C.S., Cooper, A.F., Morran, C., Russell, A.R., and Smith, D.C. (1979). The emotional and social implications of adjuvant chemotherapy in breast cancer. In *Adjuvant therapy of cancer,* vol. 2 (eds S.E. Jones and S.E. Salmon). London: Grune and Stratton. p. 319.

McGuire, W.L., and Horwitz, K.G. (1978). Progesterone receptors in breast cancer. In *Hormones, receptors, and breast cancer* (ed W.L. McGuire) New York: Raven Press. p.43.

Maguire, G.P., Tait, A., Brooke, M., Thomas, C., Howat, J.M.T., and Sellwood, R.A. (1980). Psychiatric morbidity and physical toxicity associated with adjuvant chemotherapy after mastectomy. *Br. Med. J.,* **281**, 1179.

Meakin, J.W., Allt, W.E.C., Beale, F.A., Brown, T.C., Bush, R.S., Clark, R.M., Fitzpatrick, P.J., Hawkins, N.V., Jenkin, R.D.T., Pringle, J.F., Reid, J.G., Rider, W.D., Hayward, J.L., and Bulbrook, R.D. (1979). Ovarian irradiation and prednisone therapy following surgery and radiotherapy for carcinoma of the breast. *Can. Med. Assoc. J.,* **120**, 1221.

Meyer, J.S., and Hixon, B. (1979). Advanced stage and early relapse of breast carcinomas associated with high thymidine labelling indices. *Cancer Res.,* **39**, 4042.

Misset, J.L., Delgado, M., Plagne, R., Belpomme, D., Guerrin, J., Fumoleau, P.,

Metz, R., and Mathe, G. (1982). Three year results of a randomized trial comparing CMF to adriamycin, vincristine, cyclophosphamide, and 5-fluorouracil (AVCF) as adjuvant therapy for operated N+ breast cancer. A 'Group Inter-France' trial (Abstract). *Proc. Am. Soc. Clin. Oncol.,* (C-325).

Morrison, J.M., Howell, A., Grieve, R.J., Monypenny, I.J., Minawa, A., and Waterhouse, J.A. (1981). The West Midlands Oncology Association trials of adjuvant chemotherapy for operable breast cancer. In *Adjuvant therapy of cancer,* vol.3 (eds S.E. Salmon, and S.E. Jones). London: Grune and Stratton. p. 403.

Mueller, C.B., and Jeffries, W. (1975). Cancer of the breast: its outcome as measured by the rate of dying and causes of death. *Ann. Surg.,* **182**, 334.

Namer, M., Lalanne, C., and Baulieu, E.-E. (1980). Increase of progesterone receptor by tamoxifen as a hormonal challenge test in breast cancer. *Cancer Res.,* **40**, 1750.

Nealon, T.F., Jr, Nkongho, A., Grossi, C., and Gillooley, J. (1979). Pathologic identification of poor prognosis stage I ($T_1N_0M_0$) cancer of the breast. *Ann. Surg.,* **190**, 129.

Nenci, I. (1981). Estrogen receptor cytochemistry in human breast cancer: status and prospects. *Cancer,* **48**, 2674.

Nervi, C., Arcangeli, G., Concolino, F., and Cortese, M. (1979). Improved survival with combined modality treatment for stage IV breast cancer. *Int. J. Radiat. Oncol., Biol. Phys.,* **5**, 1317.

Nime, F.A., Rosen, P.P., Thaler, H.T., Ashikari, R., and Urban, J.A. (1977). Prognostic significance of tumor emboli in intramammary lymphatics in patients with mammary carcinoma. *Am. J. Surg. Pathol.,* **1**, 25.

Nissen-Meyer, R., Kjellgren, K., and Mansson, B. (1982). Adjuvant chemotherapy in breast cancer. *Recent Results Cancer Res.,* **80**, 142.

Nowell, P.C. (1976). The clonal evolution of tumor cell populations: acquired genetic lability permits stepwise selection of variant sublines and underlies tumor progression. *Science,* **194**, 23.

Olszewski, W., Darzynkiewicz, Z., Rosen, P.P., Schwartz, M.K., and Melamed, M.R. (1981). Flow cytometry of breast carcinoma: 1. Relation of DNA ploidy level to histology and estrogen receptor. *Cancer,* **48**, 980.

Osborne, C.K., and McGuire, W.L. (1981). The use of steroid hormone receptors in the management of patients with breast cancer. In *Breast cancer* (eds B. Hoogstraten, and R.W. McDivitt). Boca Raton: CRC Press. p. 155.

Palmer, B.V., Walsh, G.A., McKinna, J.A., and Greening, W.P. (1980). Adjuvant chemotherapy for breast cancer: side effects and quality of life. *Br. Med. J.,* **281**, 1594.

Parbhoo, S. (1981). Morphological and biological heterogeneity in breast cancer. *Rev. Endocrine-Related Cancer,* **8**, 23.

Palshof, T. (1981). Adjuvant endocrine therapy in the management of primary breast cancer. *Rev. Endocrine-Related Cancer,* Suppl. 7, 65.

Pater, J.L., Mores, D., and Loeb, M. (1981). Survival after recurrence of breast cancer. *Can. Med. Assoc. J.,* **124**, 1591.

Paterson, A.H.G., Agarwal, M., Lees, A., Hanson, J., and Szafran, O. (1982). Brain metastases in breast cancer patients receiving adjuvant chemotherapy. *Cancer,* **49**, 651.

Peters, M.V. (1975). Cutting the 'gordian knot' in early breast cancer. *Ann. R. Coll. Physicians Surgeons Can.,* **8**, 186.

Piro, A.J., and Hellman, S. (1978). Effect of primary treatment modality on the metastatic pattern of mammary carcinoma. *Cancer Treat. Rep.*, **62**, 1275.

Powles, T. (1981). Adjuvant endocrine therapy. In *Adjuvant therapy of cancer*, vol.3 (eds S.E. Salmon and S.E. Jones). London: Grune and Stratton. p. 305.

Pritchard, K.I., Thomson, D.B., Myers, R.E., Sutherland, D.J.A., Mobbs, B.C., and Meakin, J.W. (1980). Tamoxifen therapy in premenopausal patients with metastatic breast cancer. *Cancer Treat. Rep.*, **64**, 787.

Priestman, T., Baum, M., Jones, V., and Forbes, J. (1978). Treatment and survival in advanced breast cancer. *Br. Med. J.*, **2**, 1673.

Robbins, G.F., and Berg, J. (1977). Curability of patients with invasive breast carcinoma based on a 30–year study. *World J. Surg.*, **1**, 284.

Rose, D.P., and Davis, T.E. (1980). Effects of adjuvant chemohormonal therapy on the ovarian and adrenal function of breast cancer patients. *Cancer Res.*, **40**, 4043.

Rosen, P.P., Saigo, P.E., Braun, D.W., Weathers, E., Fracchia, A.A., and Kinne, D.W. (1981). Axillary micro- and macrometastases in breast cancer: prognostic significance of tumor size. *Ann. Surg.*, **194**, 585.

Rossi, A., Tancini, G., Marchini, S., and Bonadonna, G. (1980). Response to secondary treatment after surgical adjuvant CMF for breast cancer (Abstract). *Proc. Am. Assoc. Clin. Res.*, **21**, (760).

Rozencweig, M., and Heuson, J.-C. (1975). Breast cancer: prognostic factors and clinical evaluation. In *Cancer therapy: prognostic factors and criteria of response* (ed M.J. Staquet). New York: Raven Press. p.139.

Rozencweig, M., Heuson, J.S., von Hoff, D.D., Mattheiem, W.H., Davis, H.L., and Muggia, F.M. (1978). Breast cancer. In *Randomized trials in cancer: a critical review by sites* (ed M.J. Staquet) New York: Raven Press. p. 231.

Rubens, R.D., Armitage, P., Winter, P.J., Tong, D., and Hayward J.L. (1977). Prognosis in inoperable stage III carcinoma of the breast. *Eur. J. Cancer*, **13**, 805.

Rubens, R.D., Sexton, S., Tong, D., Winter, P.J., Knight, R.K., and Hayward, J.L. (1980). Combined chemotherapy and radiotherapy for locally advanced breast cancer. *Eur. J. Cancer*, **16**, 351.

Russo, J., Fine, G., Husain, M., Krickstein, H., Robbins, T., Rosenberg, B., Brooks, S., Ownby, H., Roi, L., Miller, J., Furmanski, P., Brennan, M.J., and Rich, M.A. (1981). Tumour grade, lymph node status and estrogen receptor as predictors of early recurrence of human breast cancers (Abstract). *Proc. Am. Assoc. Clin. Res.*, **22**, (577).

Salmon, S.E. (1980). Consideration of tumor stem cells in adjuvant therapy. *Rev. Endocrine-Related Cancer*, Suppl. 4, 1.

Salmon, S.E., and Jones, S.E. (eds) (1981). *Adjuvant therapy of Cancer*, vol. 3. London: Grune and Stratton. pp. 305–492.

Samaan, N.A., Buzdar, A.U., Aldinger, K.A., Schultz, P.N., Yang, K.-P., Romsdahl, M.M., and Martin, R. (1981). Estrogen receptor: a prognostic factor in breast cancer. *Cancer*, **47**, 554.

Santen, R.J., Worgul, T.J., Samojlik, E., *et al.* (1981). A randomised trial comparing surgical adrenalectomy with aminoglutethimide plus hydrocortisone in women with advanced breast cancer. *New Engl. J. Med.*, **305**, 545.

Senn, H., Jungi, W.F., and Amgwerd, R. (1981). Chemo(immuno)therapy with LMF+BCG in node-negative and node-positive breast cancer. In *Adjuvant therapy of cancer*, vol. 3 (eds S.E. Salmon and S.E. Jones). London: Grune and Stratton. p. 385.

Silvestrini, R., Daidone, M.G., and Bertuzzi, A. (1982). Prognostic importance of proliferative activity alone or in combination with estrogen receptors in node-negative breast cancers (Abstract). *Proc. Am. Soc. Clin. Oncol.,* **1**, (C-322).

Silvestrini, R., Daidone, M.G., and Gentili, C. (1981). Biologic characteristics of breast cancer and their clinical relevance. In *Commentaries on research in breast disease,* Vol. 2 (eds R. D. Bulbrook, and D.J. Taylor). New York: Alan R. Liss. p. 1.

Sluyser, M. (1980). The emergence of hormone-independent cells in hormone-dependent breast cancer. In *Cell biology of breast cancer* (eds C. McGrath, M.J. Brennan and M.A. Rich). London: Academic Press. p. 173.

Sluyser, M., De Goeij, C.C.J., and Evers, S.G. (1981). Combined endocrine therapy and chemotherapy of mouse mammary tumours. *Euro. J. Cancer,* **17**, 155.

Smalley, R.V. (1981). The management of disseminated breast cancer. In *Principles of cancer treatment* (eds S.K. Carter, E. Glatstein and R.B. Livingston). London: McGraw-Hill. p. 327.

Smalley, R.V., Murphy, S., Huguley, C.M., Jr, and Bartolucci, A.A. (1976). Combination versus sequential five-drug chemotherapy in metastatic carcinoma of the breast. *Cancer Res.,* **36**, 3911.

Smith, J.A., III, Gamez-Araujo, J.J., Gallager, H.S., White, E.C., and McBride, C.M. (1977). Carcinoma of the breast: analysis of total lymph node involvement versus level of metastasis. *Cancer,* **39**, 527.

Stein, J.A., Adler, A., Efraim, S.B., and Maor, M. (1976). Immunocompetence, immunosuppression, and human breast cancer. 1. An analysis of their relationship by known parameters of cell-mediated immunity in well-defined clinical stages of disease. *Cancer,* **38**, 1171.

Stephens, R.B., Abeloff, M.D., Mellits, E.D., and Baker, R.R. (1982). The role of estrogen receptor status in predicting the response of carcinoma of the breast to adjuvant chemotherapy. *Surg., Gynecol. Obstet.,* **154**, 200.

Stewart, J.F., King, R.J.B., Sexton, S.A., Millis, R.R., Rubens, R.D., and Hayward, J.L. (1981). Oestrogen receptors, sites of metastatic disease and survival in recurrent breast cancer. *Eur. J. Cancer,* **17**, 449.

Stoll, B.A. (1979). Prospects for combined endocrine–cytotoxic treatment in breast cancer. *Rev. Endocrine-Related Cancer,* February, 29.

Stoll, B.A. (1981). Breast cancer: rationale for endocrine therapy. In *Hormonal management of endocrine related cancer* (ed B.A. Stoll). London: Lloyd-Luke Medical. p. 77.

Sulkes, A., Livingston, R.B., and Murphy, W.K. (1979). Tritiated thymidine labeling index and response in human breast cancer. *J. Natl. Cancer Inst.,* **62**, 513.

Sutherland, R.L., and Taylor, D.W. (1981). Effect of tamoxifen on the cell cycle kinetics of cultured human mammary carcinoma cells. *Rev. Endocrine-Related Cancer,* Suppl. 8, 17.

Swenerton, K.D., Legha, S.S., Smith, T., Hortobagyi, G.N., Gehan, E.A., Yap, H.-Y., Gutterman, J.U., and Blumenschein, G.R. (1979). Prognostic factors in metastatic breast cancer treated with combination chemotherapy. *Cancer Res.,* **39**, 1552.

Tancini, G., Bonadonna, G., Marchini, S., Bajetta, E., Valagussa, P., and Veronesi, U. (1982). Adjuvant CMF in breast cancer: comparative 5-year results of 12 vs. 6 cycles (Abstract). *Proc. Am. Soc. Clin. Oncol.,* **1**, (C-333).

Taylor, C.R., Cooper, C.L., Kurman, R. J., Goebelsmann, U., and Markland, F.S. (1981). Detection of estrogen receptor in breast and endometrial carcinoma by the immunoperoxidase technique. *Cancer,* **47**, 2634.

Tormey, D.C., Holland, J.F., Weinberg, V., Weiss, R., Falkson, G., Glidewell, O., Leone, L., and Perloff, M. (1981a) 5-Drug vs. 3-drug ± MER postoperative chemotherapy for mammary carcinoma. In *Adjuvant therapy of cancer*, vol.3 (eds S.E. Salmon and S.E. Jones). London: Grune and Stratton. p. 377.

Tormey, D.C., Kline, J., Davis, T.E., Love, R.R., and Carbone, P.P. (1981b). Short term intensive chemohormonotherapy in metastatic breast carcinoma (Abstract). *Proc. Am. Assoc. Clin. Oncol., 22*, (C-440).

Tubiana, M., Pejovic, M.J., Renaud, A., Contesso, G., Chavaudra, N., Gioanni, J., and Malaise, E.P. (1981). Kinetic parameters and the course of the disease in breast cancer. *Cancer, 47*, 937.

Turner, L., Swindell, R., Bell, W.G.T., Hartley, R.C., Tasker, J.H., Wilson, W.W., Alderson, M.R., and Leck, I.M. (1981). Radical versus modified radical mastectomy for breast cancer. *Ann. R. Coll. Surgeons Engl., 63*, 239.

Valagussa, P., Bonadonna, G., and Veronesi, U. (1978). Patterns of relapse and survival following radical mastectomy: analysis of 716 consecutive patients. *Cancer, 41*, 1170.

Valagussa, P., Tess, J.D.T., Rossi, A., Tancini, G., and Bonadonna, G. (1980). Has adjuvant CMF altered the patterns of first recurrence in operable breast cancer with N+? (Abstract). *Proc. Am. Soc. Clin. Oncol., 22*, (C-375).

Vana, J., Bedwani, R., Mettlin, C., and Murphy, G.P. (1981). Trends in diagnosis and management of breast cancer in the U.S.: from the surveys of the American College of Surgeons. *Cancer, 48*, 1043.

Veronesi, U., Saccozzi, R., Del Vecchio, M., Banfi, A., Clemente, C., De Lena, M., Gallus, G., Greco, M., Luini, A., Marubini, E., Muscolino, G., Rilke, F., Salvadori, B., Zecchini, A., and Zucali, R. (1981). Comparing radical mastectomy with quandrantectomy, axillary dissection, and radiotherapy in patients with small cancers of the breast. *New Engl. J. Med., 305*, 6.

von Hoff, D.D., Sandbach, J., Osborne, C.K., Metelmann, C., Clark, G.M., O'Brien, M., and the South Central Texas Human Tumour Cloning Group (1981). Potential and problems with growth of breast cancer in a human tumor cloning system. *Breast Cancer Res. Treat., 1*, 141.

Wallgren, A., Baral, E., Glas, U., Kaigas, M., Karnstrom, L., Nordenskjold, B., Theve, N.-O., Wilking, N., and Silfversward, C. (1981). Adjuvant breast cancer treatment with tamoxifen and combination chemotherapy in postmenopausal women. In *Adjuvant therapy of cancer,* vol.3 (eds S.E. Salmon and S.E. Jones). London: Grune and Stratton. p. 345.

Weigand, R.A., Russo, J., Zuzga, L., Isenberg, W.M., Horowitz, S.B., Furmanski, P., Rich, M.A., and the Breast Cancer Prognostic Study Associates (1981). Blood vessel invasion in primary breast carcinomas as an indicator of early recurrence (Abstract). *Proc. Am. Assoc. Clin. Res., 22*, (590).

Weiss, L. (1980). Cancer cells in primary tumours and their metastases. In *Cell biology of breast cancer* (eds C. McGrath, M.J. Brennan and M.A. Rich). London: Academic Press. p.189.

Wendt, A.G., Jones, S.E., and Salmon, S.E. (1980). Salvage treatment of patients relapsing after breast cancer adjuvant chemotherapy. *Cancer Treat. Rep., 64*, 269.

Zelen, M. (1975). Importance of prognostic factors in planning therapeutic trials. In *Cancer therapy: prognostic factors and criteria of response* (ed M.J. Staquet). New York: Raven Press. p.1.

Cancer Treatment: End Point Evaluation
Edited by B.A. Stoll
© 1983 John Wiley & Sons Ltd.

Chapter

18 CAROL S. PORTLOCK

Selective Treatment in Lymphoma

The management of patients with non-Hodgkin's lymphoma is rapidly evolving. There are few standard approaches and many treatments remain investigational and controversial. Nonetheless, it is important to develop strategies for selecting the optimal therapeutic regimen for the patient and for evaluating the relative benefits of those treatments available. Histopathology and staging are the major factors which have been evaluated for their prognostic significance, but other factors also distinguish 'good-risk' from 'poor-risk' patients.

HISTOPATHOLOGY

Prior to any consideration of treatment one must have available adequate pathologic material and excellent histopathologic interpretation. The largest body of clinical information is based on the Rappaport classification (see Table 1) (Rappaport *et al.* 1956). This classification identifies both architectural and cytological characteristics of the malignant lymph node

Table 1 The Rappaport histopathologic classification.

Cytology	Architecture[a]	
	Nodular	Diffuse
Lymphocytic, well differentiated	NLWD	DLWD
Lymphocytic, poorly differentiated	NLPD	DLPD
Mixed lymphocytic and histiocytic	NML	DML
Histiocytic	NHL	DHL

[a] For abbreviations see text

431

which have prognostic significance. A nodular pattern is associated with a more favorable prognosis than a diffuse architecture; and a lymphocytic cytology is more favorable than a histiocytic cytology, while a mixed lymphocytic–histiocytic cytology is intermediate.

Using the Rappaport classifiction, Jones *et al.* (1973a) identified four histopathologic subtypes which appeared to have a favorable prognosis in spite of advanced disease at presentation—well differentiated lymphocytic lymphomas of the nodular (NLWD) or diffuse (DLWD) type, nodular poorly differentiated lymphocytic lymphoma (NLPD), and nodular mixed lymphocytic–histiocytic lymphoma (NML)—and four with unfavorable prognoses often in spite of localized disease—histiocytic lymphomas of the nodular (NHL) or diffuse (DHL) type, diffuse poorly differentiated lymphocytic lymphoma (DLPD), and diffuse mixed lymphocytic histiocytic lymphoma (DML). The median survival time for the favorable histologies was approximately eight years as compared to less than 18 months for the unfavorable subtypes.

In spite of its clinical utility, the Rappaport classification has been criticized on several grounds. First, it requires expert pathologic interpretation and sometimes is difficult to reproduce. Secondly, it simply describes the morphologic and cytologic appearance of the involved lymph node and does not consider the functional or immunologic origins and characteristics of the malignant cells. Thirdly, some of the terminology is incorrect when applied to the malignant cell population. Jaffe *et al.* (1977) and other workers have clearly demonstrated that the malignant lymphocytes of nodular lymphoma are derived from follicular B lymphocytes and that many of the 'histiocytic' lymphomas are, in fact, wholly of lymphocytic origin. Moreover, the mixed lymphocytic–'histiocytic' cytology of Rappaport represents an admixture of small and large malignant lymphocytes, and the 'poorly differentiated' lymphocyte is derived instead from a transformed cell.

Unlike the Rappaport classification, the classification proposed by Lukes and Collins (1974) attempts to account for the immunologic origin of the malignant cell population. It relies upon morphologic identification of malignant B and T cell neoplasms relating morphologic characteristics to alterations in lymphocyte transformation. Approximately 10 subtypes of non-Hodgkin's lymphomas are defined using this classification. Almost 70% are composed of B cell diseases, while 30% are of null cell, T cell or rarely histocytic origin. Unfortunately, there is much less clinical experience with the Lukes–Collins classification than with that of Rappaport. Nevertheless, there are several important prognostic features of both classifications which have been identified and these will be discussed later.

Although the prognosis for many patients with non-Hodgkin's lymphomas has improved dramatically since the clinicopathologic correlations made by Jones *et al.* in 1973, the 'favorable' and 'unfavorable' groupings remain valid.

Recently a large multi-institutional study has reproduced the Rappaport, Lukes–Collins, and other classifications and has defined three prognostic groups. Based on these data, a compromise classification has been recommended by an expert international panel of pathologists, subdividing the non-Hodgkin's lymphomas into three major pathologic groups: low-grade, intermediate-grade, and high-grade lymphomas. The low-grade lymphomas are those previously termed favorable by Jones *et al.*, and the intermediate- and high-grade lymphomas are those previously termed unfavorable. For the purposes of discussing treatment strategies, however, the Rappaport classification remains the most useful, and the two prognostic subgroups identified by Jones *et al.* are more appropriately termed 'indolent' and 'aggressive'.

Using the Rappaport classification, approximately half of the lymphomas have a nodular architecture and half a diffuse one. The most common histologic subtypes are NLPD and DHL, each representing 30% of cases. Another 30% are either NML or DLPD and the remaining 10% are NHL, DLWD or DML. NLWD is a rare histologic subtype and some pathologists question its existence. Patients with non-Hodgkin's lymphomas have a median age of 50–60 years in most series. The indolent histologies are rarely diagnosed during the first two decades of life, whereas diffuse lymphomas are the rule among pediatric patients. The sex distribution is equal in the indolent histologies while there is a slight male preponderance in the aggressive subtypes.

STAGING

The Ann Arbor staging system (Carbone *et al.*, 1971) developed for use in Hodgkin's disease has been adapted to the non-Hodgkin's lymphomas. Although it is clinically useful, it does have several shortcomings when applied to the non-Hodgkin's lymphomas. First, with localized presentations, site and bulk of disease are not considered. Secondly, extranodal presentations are grouped together in Stage IV and, as discussed later, the sites and extent of extranodal involvement may have prognostic importance. Thirdly, the influence of systemic symptoms on prognosis is much less evident in the non-Hodgkin's lymphomas than in Hodgkin's disease. In spite of its limitations, however, thorough staging is a necessity in patient evaluation and management.

Non-invasive staging usually includes the following: a complete history and physical examination, complete blood count and platelet count, Coombs' test if anemic, serum protein electrophoresis, liver function tests with alkaline phosphatase, renal function studies, and radiologic examinations of the chest and abdomen. The chest x-ray yields positive information in only 15–20% of patients and is most often abnormal in those with aggressive histologies. Full lung tomography aids in delineating previously identified abnormalities but is not of additional value if the chest x-ray is normal. An intravenous pyelogram may reveal asymptomatic ureteral deviation or obstruction but it does not adequately evaluate the presence of retroperitoneal adenopathy. On the other hand, the bipedal lymphogram accurately identifies iliac and para-aortic adenopathy and may be followed serially to evaluate disease activity and response to treatment.

Mesenteric adenopathy is not identified by lymphography. This is of particular importance in patients with indolent lymphomas, where almost 50% with normal lymphograms will be found to have mesenteric disease if subjected to laparotomy (Goffinet *et al.*, 1977). Mesenteric involvement occurs in less than 10% of patients with aggressive histologies and a normal lymphogram. Ultrasonography and computerized tomography can be of value in identifying abdominal lymph node masses not opacified by lymphography. However, these methods rely upon abnormalities of lymph node size and are not necessarily diagnostic. Other studies such as bone survey, bone scan, liver–spleen scan, gastrointestinal series, and ^{67}Ga scan provide little additional information unless there is prior suspicion of pathology in that organ.

The clinical stage is determined by these non-invasive procedures. Approximately 50–75% of patients with indolent histologies will have clinical Stage III disease, less than 10% will be Stage I or IV, and the remainder will be Stage II. For those with aggressive histologies, approximately 15% will be clinical Stage I, 30% Stage II, 30% Stage III, and 20% Stage IV. Although clinical staging provides useful information about disease extent, it is not adequate for thorough patient evaluation, nor does it allow for a meaningful comparison of treatment results.

Following complete pathologic staging, fewer than 5% of patients are found to have a lesser extent of disease than that determined by clinical staging. On the other hand, more than 50% of those with indolent histologies and 25% with aggressive subtypes are found to have more advanced disease following pathologic staging. Most of these changes are from clinical Stage III to pathologic Stage IV disease, usually on the basis of a positive bone marrow examination. The incidence of bone marrow involvement varies according to histology, with positive biopsies obtained in more than 50% of those with indolent histologies and in less than 30% with aggressive subtypes.

Other invasive procedures such as percutaneous liver biopsy, peritoneoscopy and staging laparotomy are of limited value (Chabner *et al.*, 1976). In those patients with a normal lymphogram and negative bone marrow examination, hepatic involvement is demonstrated in less than 5%. Likewise, in this setting, less than 10% of patients with aggressive histologies will be found to have mesenteric and/or splenic disease if taken to laparotomy. By contrast, almost 50% of those with indolent lymphomas and a normal lymphogram and bone marrow will be found to have mesenteric and/or splenic disease at laparotomy (Goffinet *et al.*, 1977). Nonetheless, staging laparotomy is rarely indicated and its use depends upon the plan and effectiveness of treatment.

CONSIDERATIONS IN THE CHOICE OF TREATMENT

The non-Hodgkin's lymphomas are highly treatable malignancies with a myriad of available therapies. Choosing among them requires consideration of such factors as histology, disease extent, thoroughness of initial staging, and the goals and effectiveness of treatment. Potential therapeutic options are outlined in Tables 2 and 3.

Table 2 Treatment approaches in the indolent non-Hodgkin's lymphomas.

Stages I and II	Regional field irradiation
	Total lymphoid irradiation
	Radiation therapy/chemotherapy
Stage III	Total lymphoid irradiation
	Radiation therapy/chemotherapy
Stages II and IV	Single alkylating agent chemotherapy
	Combination chemotherapy
	Whole-body irradiation
	Chemotherapy/radiation therapy
	Deferred initial therapy
	Local field irradiation

Table 3 Treatment approaches in the aggressive non-Hodgkin's lymphomas.

Stages I and II	Regional irradiation
	Total lymphoid irradiation
	Radiation therapy/chemotherapy
	Combination chemotherapy
Stages III and IV	Combination chemotherapy
	Chemotherapy/radiation therapy

In order to judge the relative value of the therapies listed, one must consider the following:

(1) Complete response (CR) rate. In order to be meaningful, the CR rate must be pathologically (pCR), not clinically, defined. This requires that the patient's pathologic stage be determined prior to therapy and

again upon its conclusion. If 'systematic restaging' is not performed then undetected occult disease may persist when treatment is discontinued prematurely. As one might expect, this is a common cause of treatment failure.

(2) The time required to achieve CR. If a prompt response to treatment is necessary, then regimens such as single alkylating agent therapy which require many months to achieve CR are inappropriate.

(3) Duration of complete remission. The disease-free interval is calculated from the date of the pathologically documented complete response (pCR) or the conclusion of all therapy to the date of relapse. Another interval which is often used is 'progression-free' survival, calculated from the initiation of all treatment to relapse. If the latter interval is used, the remission duration may appear much longer than it actually is since some treatment programs require a year or more to complete.

'Cure' is often defined as a disease-free interval exceeding two years. This appears to be relatively valid for patients with aggressive histologies where most relapses occur within the first two years following treatment. However, for those with indolent lymphomas, relapse may occur as late as 5, 10 or more years after therapy. Consequently, the demonstration of cure in the indolent lymphomas requires a much longer period of observation than most studies provide.

(4) Survival. Actuarial survival is calculated from the date of first treatment to death. End-results in the indolent lymphomas require more than 10 years of observation, and few studies have such data available.

(5) Acute toxicities. If treatment approaches appear comparable in terms of the above parameters, then morbidities of therapy may become decisive. Included among the many host toxicities are intensity and duration of treatment, cost, and psychological impact.

(6) Chronic and/or delayed toxicities. Such toxicities as myelosuppression may be apparent at the conclusion of therapy and persist as a chronic problem. Other effects may be delayed by several years, such as the development of second malignancies or aseptic necrosis of the femoral head. Most current treatments do not have adequate follow-up to assess the relative risk of such complications.

(7) Ability to salvage patients at relapse. If a therapeutic regimen does not result in cure, then it becomes important to assess the ability to deliver second-line treatment. For example, initial therapies which result in chronic myelosuppression might limit subsequent salvage attempts. These considertions are particularly relevant to patients with indolent lymphomas where the initial disease-free interval may be short but survival long, even in the presence of active disease. Under these circumstances, effective second-line palliative therapy is of great importance.

Even though the above parameters are of primary importance in the evaluation of therapeutic regimens, it is necessary to recognize that, in addition, a multitude of prognostic factors may influence treatment results. (Some of these factors will be discussed in detail later.) Therefore, when comparing data, the possible heterogeneity of the treated groups must be taken into consideration.

TREATMENT CONSIDERATIONS: Stages I and II

Because of the diversity of the non-Hodgkin's lymphomas and their varied presentations and prognoses, treatment approaches may differ stage for stage according to histology. For Stage I or II disease, radiation therapy is usually employed. However, there are few data available to answer the questions of necessary radiation dose and field size for curative intent. Utilizing 4000 rad or more in patients with clinical Stage I and II, Fuks and Kaplan (1973) reported excellent local disease control in patients with nodular lymphoma. On the other hand, local recurrences were documented in approximately 15–30% of the fields at risk when this same dose was applied to patients with diffuse lymphomas. Also, in both groups, relapse was often seen in unirradiated lymph nodes and extranodal sites even when good local control was achieved.

Jones *et al.* (1973b) subsequently reported a retrospective series of clinically staged patients who received at least 3000–4000 rad to the involved regions. The median disease-free survival was five years for clinical Stage I NLPD and NML and 3.5 years for clinical Stage II. Patients with DHL had a median disease-free survival of only two years with clinical Stage I and six months with clinical Stage II disease. For NLPD and NML it appeared that extended field or total lymphoid irradiation improved disease-free survival as compared to involved field treatment, whereas for DHL the more extended fields conferred no additional benefit. Nonetheless, in a prospectively randomized trial comparing involved field to total lymphoid irradiation in patients with pathological Stage I and II indolent lymphomas, no significant differences were noted in treatment results (Rosenberg, 1982). Actuarial freedom from progression and survival were both greater than 75% at 10 years among the 20 patients studied.

A similar prospective trial has not been performed in patients with aggressive histologies. Retrospective studies have usually lumped Stages I and II DHL together and most patients have been clinically staged. However, Sweet and Golomb (1980) have recently reported their experience in 28 pathologically staged (PS) patients who received 4000 rad regional or total irradiation. Only one of 14 patients with PS I or I_E (extranodal) disease has relapsed with a median relapse-free survival and actuarial survival of 53+ months. For the 14 patients with PS II or II_E disease, on the other hand, the median relapse-free survival was only 14 months and median survival 18 months. The difference between the outcomes of PS I and II patients was highly significant. The authors concluded that PS I disease is curable in most cases with radiation alone, whereas that is not the case with PS II or II$_E$. They suggested that combined modality or chemotherapy alone might be more effective.

Data to support the use of the latter approaches are scanty but very encouraging. Miller and Jones (1979) have reported their experience with combination chemotherapy in 23 patients with localized aggressive lymphomas. Fifteen received chemotherapy alone and eight combined chemotherapy and radiation. All achieved complete remission and there was only one relapse with a median follow-up of 27+ months. Others (Cabanillas *et al.*, 1980) have recently confirmed these excellent results using combination chemotherapy alone in patients with Stage I and II aggressive lymphomas. Combined chemotherapy and irradiation regimens have usually employed chemotherapy following radiation therapy and the results of such trials are less impressive. Whether 'adjuvant' irradiation delivered concurrently or following chemotherapy can improve the results of chemotherapy alone awaits prospective study.

Since localized indolent lymphomas are rare and the results of radiation therapy so good, little is known about the efficacy of chemotherapy or combined modality therapy in this setting. Monfardini *et al.*, (1980) have recently reported the results of a prospectively randomized trial comparing regional irradiation (11 patients) to radiation followed by combination chemotherapy (15 patients). At five years, relapse-free survival was 55% for RT and 63% for RT + CT ($p = 0.60$), and survival was 62% and 93% respectively ($p = 0.10$).

TREATMENT RECOMMENDATIONS: Stages I and II

Although conclusions must be drawn from small numbers and relatively short follow-up, it appears that regional irradiation alone is the treatment of choice for patients with PS I and II indolent lymphomas. The results of such treatment (>75% progression-free at 10 years) suggest that these patients may have the potential for cure, although a pattern of late relapse is characteristic of these histologies. Without pathologic staging (which may require staging laparotomy), those who are clinical Stage I or II have a high likelihood of undetected subdiaphragmatic disease involving mesenteric lymph nodes and/or spleen. Under these circumstances, regional irradiation may have only palliative intent since subdiaphragmatic disease will remain untreated. However, there are no data to suggest that any modality, including total lymphoid irradiation, has curative potential for those patients with Stage III indolent lymphomas. Consequently, more extended-field approaches are probably not justified in clinical Stage I and II patients and may not provide superior palliative benefit as compared to regional irradiation alone.

Treatment recommendations for localized aggressive lymphomas are more difficult to specify because the very favorable experience reported with combination chemotherapy remains preliminary. For patients with pathologic Stage I, particularly supradiaphragmatic presentations, radiation therapy alone appears to be the treatment of choice. In addition, it is probably unnecessary to deliver more extended-field treatment than regional irradiation. The results of such therapy (>90% disease-free at 4+ years) suggest that these patients have a high likelihood of cure, particularly since most relapses occur during the first one to two years after treatment. Extranodal Stage I (I_E) presentations have an equally good prognosis. However, it is especially important in these cases to rule out other extranodal or lymph node disease that would change both stage and therapy. Since the results of radiation alone are so good in patients with Stage I disease, there is no place for combination chemotherapy. 'Poor-risk' patients with Stage I aggressive lymphomas should be managed like those with Stage II disease. (A discussion of prognostic factors and the definition of 'poor risk' will be presented later).

Although the reports of combination chemotherapy in Stage II patients are preliminary, results are so superior (>90% disease-free at 36+ months) to those reported for radiation alone (25–50% disease-free at 60 months) that chemotherapy must be considered the treatment of choice. In addition, it appears that the efficacy of combination chemotherapy relies upon its prompt use as initial therapy rather than as an adjuvant following irradiation. Moreover, the role of radiation therapy as an adjuvant to chemotherapy or in a combined modality regimen is yet to be defined.

TREATMENT CONSIDERATIONS: INDOLENT HISTOLOGIES, Stages III and IV

Unlike Hodgkin's disease, there is little experience with radiation therapy alone for Stage III non-Hodgkin's lymphomas. Instead, most studies have lumped patients with Stage III and IV disease together, treated them similarly, and analyzed the data as a single group. Glatstein *et al.* (1976) have reported their experience with total lymphoid irradiation (>3500 rad) in patients with Stage III lymphomas. At five years the relapse-free survival was 43% for patients with nodular lymphoma and 28% for those with diffuse histologies; at 10 years, 33% of patients with nodular disease remained relapse-free. Actuarial survival at five years was 75% for the nodular lymphomas and 39% for the diffuse. The majority of relapses in both groups occurred in lymph nodes; and those with nodular lymphoma relapsed primarily in unirradiated nodal sites. The authors suggested that better end-results might be obtained by including Waldeyer's ring as well as the epitrochlear and mesenteric regions in the usual total lymphoid portals. This approach has yet to be tested prospectively.

Chemotherapy is of major importance in the treatment of patients with Stage III and IV lymphomas, since many drugs are highly effective as single agents and as part of combination chemotherapy regimens. In a retrospective study of single-agent chemotherapy, Jones *et al.* (1973a) reported that both a nodular architecture and a lymphocytic cytology were associated with a significantly greater response rate and survival as compared to the diffuse or histiocytic lymphomas. The clinical complete response rate was 48% in patients with NLPD and only 5% for those with DHL. Likewise, actuarial median survival was greater for patients with NLPD (60+ months) as compared to those with DHL (7.5 months). Response and survival results for patients with the other histologic subtypes were distributed between these two extremes. Since their report, other groups have observed similar response and survival correlations utilizing combination chemotherapy. Schein *et al.* (1974) treated 80 patients with cyclophosphamide, vincristine, prednisone (CVP), nitrogen mustard, vincristine, procarbazine, prednisone (MOPP) or cyclophosphamide, vincristine, procarbazine, prednisone (C-MOPP) and documented significantly more pCRs in those with nodular lymphomas (NLPD 60%, NML 71%) as compared to those with diffuse histologies (DLWD 50%, DLPD 22%, DML none, DHL 35%). Median survival also demonstrated the influence of histologic subtype (NLPD 40+ months, DHL 6 months).

Although chemotherapy is pivotal to the management of patients with Stage III and IV disease, there are fundamental differences in the approach to patients with indolent lymphomas and those with aggressive histologies. For patients with indolent disease, it has not yet been established that combination chemotherapy is superior to single alkylating agent therapy. Approximately 40–80% of patients can achieve pathologically documented complete remissions employing either regimen. The Stanford group (Hoppe *et al.*, 1981) has prospectively compared daily single alkylating agent vs CVP vs CVP–total lymphoid irradiation–CVP in 63 patients with Stage IV disease; and in a second trial, daily single alkylating agent vs CVP vs whole-body irradiation in 51 patients with Stage III and IV disease. In both three-armed studies, pCR rates (65% vs 83% vs 70%; and 64% vs 81% vs 71%), median relapse-free survivals (36 vs 36 vs 48 months; and 36 vs 36 vs 12 months), and actuarial survivals (>65% at 6 years; and >80% at 4 years) were not significantly different. In both trials, the time required to achieve complete remission was longest for daily single alkylating agent therapy (12–24 months). Acute toxicities were least for patients who received single alkylating agent or whole-body irradiation, and greatest for those who received CVP or combined CVP plus total lymphoid irradiation. Chronic hematologic depression was observed in some of those who received combined modality therapy or whole-body irradiation. Two other prospective trials have compared single alkylating agent therapy to CVP, and neither has shown a significant benefit for the drug combination (Kennedy *et al.*, 1978; Lister *et al.*, 1978).

Drug combinations other than CVP have been studied without prospective comparison to single alkylating agent therapy. Most have revealed similar results to those described above for CVP. One exception has been the experience at the National Cancer Institute using MOPP or C-MOPP in patients with NML. Rather than a pattern of continuous late relapse, Anderson *et al.*, (1977) have reported that 79% were disease-free at 90+ months. However, with longer follow-up, late relapses have been observed and the median remission duration has now been reached at six years (Longo *et al.*, 1981). Even though the appearance of late relapses suggests the inability to cure such patients, the median remission duration remains significantly longer than that observed with CVP or single alkylating agent therapy. However, in a recent prospective comparison of C-MOPP to cyclophosphamide, prednisone (CP) and BCNU, cyclophosphamide, vincristine, prednisone (BCVP) in patients with NML, no significant differences were noted (Glick *et al.*, 1981). For 18 patients treated with C-MOPP, the pCR rate was 61%, the median disease-free interval 16.5 months, and median survival 41 months.

Since none of the above therapies for indolent lymphoma appear to offer the potential for cure, many have asked whether it is necessary to initiate treatment at all. It is characteristic for these diseases to present as asymptomatic lymphadenopathy which may wax and wane without treatment. In fact, in spite of Stage III or IV extent, the majority of patients have no threatening disease at diagnosis, and thus no specific need for the initiation of palliative therapy. In a retrospective series reported by Portlock and Rosenberg (1979), 44 such patients were closely followed without initiation of treatment until it was required. The median treatment-free interval was 31 months for all patients, and significant differences according to histologic subtype were noted. The median time to initiation of palliative therapy was nine months for patients with NML as compared to 32 months for NLPD and 8+ years for DLWD. On the other hand, actuarial survival did not differ significantly according to histology, with a median survival of 10 years for all patients.

The potential benefits of deferring initial therapy in patients with indolent lymphomas who are asymptomatic and clinically well include some of the following:

(1) The patient may experience a prolonged treatment-free period.
(2) The patient will not be exposed to agents which might later produce tumour cell resistance.

(3) The patient may experience spontaneous disease regression (Kriko-rian *et al.*, 1980). The frequency of spontaneous regression is not known. Of the 44 patients reported by Portlock and Rosenberg, seven developed spontaneous regressions: three were clinically complete (21+ to 60+ months' duration) and four were partial (6 to 34 months' duration).

(4) Palliative therapy can be appropriately chosen at the time disease progression occurs.

(5) The indolent lymphomas may evolve to a more aggressive histologic subtype which has curative potential.

Histologic evolution has been documented both at relapse (Cullen *et al.*, 1979; Jones *et al.*, 1979a) and at autopsy (Rappaport *et al.*, 1956; Risdall *et al.*, 1979). There is loss of the nodular architecture and the appearance of increasing numbers of large cells. At relapse, such evolution connotes a poor response to salvage chemotherapy and a shortened survival. Whether histologic transformation occurs in untreated patients and whether the resultant aggressive histologies are curable with combination chemotherapy is not known.

The potential hazards of withholding initial treatment include:

(1) The patient must have close follow-up so that the disease can be monitored.

(2) The patient must be able to accept the uncertainty of remaining untreated.

(3) The disease may progress in threatening sites, even with close follow-up.

(4) The results of treatment may be compromised by disease progression during the observation period.

(5) The lymphoma may evolve to an aggressive histology which responds poorly to treatment.

In spite of these potential disadvantages, deferring initial treatment still appears to be a reasonable option in the management of patients with advanced indolent lymphomas. Certainly the survival results of the selected patients reported by Portlock and Rosenberg are comparable to any systemic therapy tested to date.

Factors which should be considered in choosing a deferred treatment approach include the following:

(1) Histopathology. An aggressive histologic subtype precludes deferral of therapy. Patients with NLPD and DLWD may remain treatment-free for three or more years whereas the majority of patients with NML will require therapy during the first year of observation.

(2) Stage. Treatment deferral is appropriate only for those with Stage III or IV disease.

(3) Sites of disease. Lymphadenopathy may be locally bulky or in a threatening site (such as retroperitoneal adenopathy causing ureteral obstruction).

(4) Pace of disease. Rapid progression may indicate histologic evolution. Treatment deferral would be inappropriate.

(5) Systemic symptoms. Symptoms are correlated with advanced disease and usually require systemic palliation.

(6) Age. Should the young patient have treatment deferred?

(7) General medical condition.

(8) Morbidities of therapy.

(9) Psychological make-up. Is the patient reliable? Can the patient tolerate the anxiety of a no-treatment approach?

(10) Anticipated benefits of treatment. Initiating palliative therapy in the asymptomatic patient with NLPD or DLWD probably accomplishes little. On the other hand, for patients with NML deferral of treatment offers few a long treatment-free period, whereas C-MOPP may produce a prolonged and unmaintained complete remission.

TREATMENT CONSIDERATIONS: AGGRESSIVE HISTOLOGIES, Stages III and IV

Unlike the disappointing experience in the indolent lymphomas, combination chemotherpy has been dramatically successful in the treatment of aggressive histologies. Rather than a complete response rate of 5% as seen with single-agent treatment of DHL, many groups have reported complete response rates of more than 40% with combination chemotherapy. Moreover, in contrast to the rapidly progressive and invariably fatal course of DHL when treated with single agents, prolonged disease-free survival and probable cure is the rule among complete responders treated with combination chemotherapy. In addition, rather than the characteristic pattern of continuous late relapse from complete remission observed in the indolent lymphomas, relapse following pathologically documented complete response is uncommon in DHL and usually occurs within the first two years after discontinuing treatment.

In addition to survival, the relative efficacy of treatment regimens for DHL must consider both complete response rate and remission duration. If patients with DHL are pathologically restaged at the conclusion of all treatment, as many as 25% with clinical complete remissions will be found to have residual microscopic disease. Consequently if treatment is discontinued prematurely, such clinical complete responders with occult disease will later relapse; and few, if any, will be salvaged. Several drug programs appear to be comparable in terms of pCR rate, remission duration and survival, including MOPP, C-MOPP, bleomycin, adriamycin, cyclophosphamide, vincristine, prednisone (BACOP) (Fisher *et al.*, 1977), cyclophosphamide, adriamycin, vincristine, prednisone (CHOP) (Jones *et al.*, 1979b), and cyclophosphamide, vincristine, methotrexate with leucovorin rescue, cytarabine (COMLA) (Sweet *et al.*, 1980). The pCR rate for Stage III disese is approximately 60–80% whereas that for Stage IV is less than 25%. Combined chemotherapy/irradiation approaches, debulking surgery, and maintenance chemotherapy have not been shown significantly to improve the results of chemotherapy alone. In most series where patients are pathologically restaged, few complete responders relapse after discontinuation of all therapy. Therefore, the pathologic CR rate closely reflects the rate of cure.

Lymphomatous meningitis has become a more frequently recognized site of relapse in clinical complete responders with DHL. This complication has been reported in as many as 30% of relapsing patients and is correlated with the presence of bone marrow involvement (Bunn, 1976). Regimens that contain drugs which penetrate the blood–brain barrier, such as methotrexate, appear to show a decreased incidence of meningeal lymphoma. However, it is not known whether central nervous system prophylaxis is warranted in DHL.

All of the most commonly used regimens for advanced DHL have acceptable toxicity. The most important parameter in choosing among them is that the physician be familiar with its use and capable of delivering intensive chemotherapy. Since a partial remission confers no survival benefit, palliation is not a realistic goal. All patients must be treated with the intent to cure.

The chemotherapy experience with other aggressive histologies is limited. In most series, NHL is lumped together with DHL and not analyzed separately, whereas DML is not even reported. A retrospective study by Osborne *et al.* (1980) reported that the results of chemotherapy in advanced NHL appeared comparable to those for DHL (seven of 11 patients achieved pCR and long-term disease-free survival following combination chemotherapy). On the other hand, DML appears to respond poorly to chemotherapy and few patients achieve long-term complete remission. In most reports DLPD is comprised of several diseases (diffuse lymphocytic lymphoma of intermediate differentiation (DLID), lymphoblastic lymphoma, and DLPD), making the analysis of treatment results meaningless. Complete response rates of 22–80% have been reported and some patients appear to have prolonged remissions. Lymphoblastic lymphoma is a distinct clinicopathologic entity characterized by a male predominance, mediastinal mass, and a predilection for bone marrow and meningeal involvement either at presentation or relapse. Patients with this disease should receive intensive chemotherapy and central nervous system prophylaxis, even if they present with what appears to be localized lymphoma. With such treatment, prolonged complete remissions appear to be possible (Weinstein *et al.*, 1979).

TREATMENT RECOMMENDATIONS: Stages III and IV

The principles of management for patients with advanced non-Hodgkin's lymphomas are similar, regardless of histology. First, a realistic goal of treatment must be defined: is it cure, prolonged disease-free survival or palliation? If prolonged disease-free survival or cure is the goal of therapy, then it is important to identify the extent of disease with thorough pretreatment staging. Chemotherapy must be delivered intensively and consistently, closely monitoring disease parameters. Once a clinical complete remission is achieved (requiring at least six months of treatment), then all staging studies which were positive at the initiation of therapy should be repeated. Chemotherapy must not be discontinued prematurely prior to a pathologically documented complete response. For patients with indolent histologies, a pCR may require 6–18 months of chemotherapy; for those with aggressive histologies, 6–9 months. Following the documentation of pCR, an additional 2–4 courses of chemotherapy are usually administered to patients with indolent histologies, whereas all drugs are discontinued for those with aggressive lymphomas. Maintenance chemotherapy offers no additional benefit.

When the goal of management is palliation, one must ask if the patient requires any therapy at all. It is unrealistic and potentially hazardous to defer the treatment of patients with aggressive histologies. Prompt and intensive chemotherapy is indicated for all patients. On the other hand, patients with indolent histologies may be closely followed without initiation of therapy if their disease is clinically asymptomatic and not threatening. The selection of palliative treatment depends upon the sites of disease and their rate of progression. For patients with indolent lymphomas, this may require local irradiation with or without chemotherapy, chemotherapy alone, or whole-body irradiation. For those with aggressive histologies, this invariably requires combination chemotherapy with or without local irradiation to bulky sites. Whenever systemic treatment is delivered, the intent should be to achieve pCR and then to discontinue therapy as outlined above. Unnecessary continuous treatment should be avoided if possible so that chronic myelosup-pression and other host toxicities can be minimized.

PROGNOSTIC FACTORS

The treatment recommendations discussed above are derived from relatively homogeneous and favorable groups of patients. In addition to histopathology and stage, a host of other factors have been evaluated for their prognostic significance in the non-Hodgkin's lymphomas. They are best utilized in identifying patients as either 'good risk' or 'poor risk' when selecting therapy and determining possible therapeutic outcome. In general, a more intensive treatment approach is indicated for patients who are considered 'poor risk'.

(1) Age. Age greater than 50–65 years has been reported to influence prognosis adversely for patients with indolent histologies (Qazi *et al*, 1976; Rudders *et al.*, 1979). No effect has been noted for patients with aggressive disease (Fisher *et al.*, 1977).

(2) Sex. No effect (Rudders *et al.*, 1979; Fisher *et al.*, 1977).

(3) Constitutional symptoms. Systemic symptoms adversely influence prognosis for patients with indolent histologies but not for those with aggressive disease (Rudders *et al.*, 1979; Fisher *et al.*, 1977).

(4) Prior irradiation. There appears to be no influence of prior irradiation on the prognosis of patients with indolent histologies (Rudders *et al.*, 1979), whereas it is an adverse prognostic factor for those with aggressive lymphomas (Fisher *et al.*, 1977).

(5) Prior chemotherapy. For all histologies, prior chemotherapy predicts a poorer treatment outcome.

(6) Extranodal sites. For patients with indolent lymphomas, involvement of extranodal sites other than bone marrow or liver has been associated with a poor prognosis (Bagley *et al.*, 1972). On the other hand, patients with DHL involving skin have a complete response rate comparable to those with Stage III disease (60–80%), whereas those with gastrointestinal tract or bone marrow disease respond poorly if at all (Fisher *et al.*, 1977).

(7) Tumor bulk. This parameter has not been evaluated in indolent histologies. Tumors with aggressive histologies larger than 10 cm are reported to respond poorly to chemotherapy or combined modality programs (Fisher *et al.*, 1977).

(8) Nodular tumor architecture. Conflicting data are available on the clinical significance of lymphomas which have varying degrees of tumor nodularity. Three studies (Butler *et al.*, 1975; Patchefsky *et al.*, 1974; Colbey *et al.*, 1980) have concluded that the greater the nodular component, the better the prognosis; and three studies (Rudders *et al.*, 1979; Cox *et al.*, 1974; Warnke *et al.*, 1977) have shown no significant influence on prognosis as long as the lymphoma has a nodular architecture.

(9) Tumor cell morphology. Histologic subclassification of DHL has been reported to identify prognostic groups with favorable and unfavorable responses to chemotherapy (Strauchen *et al.*, 1978).

(10) Mitotic rate. In lymphocytic lymphoma, more than 30 mitoses per 20 high-power fields has been associated with a poorer survival (Evans *et al.*, 1978).

(11) Surface immunoglobulins. The absence of surface immunoglobulin in a morphologically identified B cell lymphoma is reported to connote an unfavorable prognosis (Bloomfield *et al.*, 1979). Among patients with small cleaved follicular center cell lymphomas (SCFCC), those

with IgD/C_3^1 positive tumors appear to have a more favorable prognosis (median survival of 58 months) as compared to those with IgD/C_3^1 negative tumors (median survival 30 months) (Rudders *et al.*, 1981). (12) Response to treatment. In all histologies, complete responders have significantly longer survival than partial and non-responders (Anderson *et al.*, 1977).

CONCLUSION

The selection of therapy for patients with non-Hodgkin's lymphomas is dependent upon a multifactorial approach. On the one hand there are aggressive histologies which require prompt and intensive treatment with the possibility of cure; and on the other there are indolent histologies which may require no specific therapy at diagnosis and whose treatment offers no potential for cure. The challenge for the clinician is to evaluate carefully all parameters and to develop a plan of management that determines when, and if, treatment is necessary and then maximizes the effectiveness of therapy when it is indicated.

Acknowledgements

Supported by grant CA 08341–16 from the National Institutes of Health.

REFERENCES

Anderson, T., Bender, R.A., Fisher, R.I., *et al.* (1977). Combination chemotherapy in non-Hodgkin's lymphoma: results of long-term follow-up. *Cancer Treat. Rep.*, **61**, 1057–1066.

Bagley, C.M., Jr, DeVita, V.T., Jr, Berard, C.W., *et al.* (1972). Advanced lymphosarcoma—intensive cyclical combination chemotherapy with cyclophosphamide, vincristine, and prednisone. *Ann. Intern. Med.*, **76**, 227–234.

Bloomfield, C.D., Gajl-Peczalska, K.J., Frizzera, G., *et al.* (1979). Clinical utility of lymphocyte surface markers combined with the Lukes–Collins histologic classification in adult lymphoma. *New Engl. J. Med.*, **301**, 512–518.

Bunn, P.A., Jr, Schein, P.S., Banks, P.M., and DeVita, V.T., Jr (1976). Central nervous system complications in patients with diffuse histiocytic and undifferentiated lymphoma: leukemia revisited. *Blood*, **47**, 3–10.

Butler, J.J., Stryker, J.A., and Shullenberger, C.C. (1975). A clinicopathological study of stages I and II non-Hodgkin's lymphomata using the Lukes–Collins classification. *Br. J. Cancer*, **31**, 208–216.

Cabanillas, F., Bodey, G.P., and Freireich, E.J. (1980). Management with chemotherapy only of stage I and II malignant lymphoma of aggressive histologic types. *Cancer*, **46**, 2356–2359.

Carbone, P.P., Kaplan, H.S., Musshoff, K., Smithers, D.W., and Tubiana, M. (1971). Report of the committee on Hodgkin's disease staging classification. *Cancer Res.*, **31**, 1860–1861.

Chabner, B.A., Johnson, R.E., Young, R.C., *et al.* (1976). Sequential nonsurgical and surgical staging of non-Hodgkin's lymphomas. *Ann. Intern. Med.,* **85,** 149–154.

Colbey, T.V., Hoppe, R.T., and Burke, J.S. (1980). Nodular lymphoma: clinicopathologic correlations of parafollicular small lymphocytes and degree of nodularity. *Cancer,* **45,** 2364–2367.

Cox, J.D., Koehl, R.H., Turner, W.M., *et al.* (1974). Malignant lymphoid tumors of lymph nodes in the adult. *Arch. Pathol. Lab. Med.,* **97,** 22–28.

Cullen, M.H., Lister, T.A., Brearley, R.L., *et al.* (1979). Histological transformation of non-Hodgkin's lymphoma. A prospective study. *Cancer,* **44,** 645–651.

Evans, H.L., Butler, J.J., and Youness, E.L. (1978). Malignant lymphoma, small lymphocytic type: a clinicopathologic study of 84 cases with suggested criteria for intermediate lymphocytic lymphoma. *Cancer,* **41,** 1440–1455.

Fisher, R.I., DeVita, V.T., Johnson, B.L., *et al.* (1977). Prognostic factors for advanced diffuse lymphoma following treatment with combination chemotherapy. *Am. J. Med.,* **63,** 177–182.

Fuks, Z., and Kaplan, H.S. (1973). Recurrence rates following radiation therapy of nodular and diffuse malignant lymphomas. *Radiology,* **108,** 675–684.

Glatstein, E., Fuks, Z., Goffinet, D.R., *et al.* (1976). Non-Hodgkin's lymphomas of stage III extent: is total lymphoid irradiation appropriate treatment? *Cancer,* **37,** 2806–2812.

Glick, J.H., Barnes, J.M., Ezdinli, E.Z., Berard, C.W., Orlow, E.L., and Bennet, J.M. (1981). Nodular mixed lymphoma: results of a randomized trial failing to confirm prolonged disease-free survival with COPP chemotherapy. *Blood,* (in press).

Goffinet, D.R., Warnke, R., Dunnick, N.R., *et al.* (1977). Clinical and surgical (laparotomy) evaluation of patients with non-Hodgkin's lymphomas. *Cancer Treat. Rep.,* **61,** 981–992.

Hoppe, R.T., Kushlan, P., Kaplan, H.S., Rosenberg, S.A., and Brown, B.W. (1981). The treatment of advanced stage favorable histology non-Hodgkin's lymphoma: a preliminary report of a randomized trial comparing single agent chemotherapy, combination chemotherapy, and whole body irradiation. *Blood,* **58,** 592–598.

Jaffe, E.S., Braylan, R.C., and Nanba, K., *et al.* (1977). Functional markers: a new perspective on malignant lymphomas. *Cancer Treat. Rep.,* **61,** 953–962.

Jones, R., Young, R.C., Berard, C.W., *et al.* (1979a). Histologic progression in non-Hodgkin's lymphoma (NHL). Implications for survival and clinical trials (Abstract). *Proc. Am. Soc. Clin. Oncol.,* **20,** 353.

Jones, S.E., Fuks, Z., Bull, M., *et al.* (1973a). Non-Hodgkin's lymphomas: IV. Clinicopathologic correlation in 405 cases. *Cancer,* **31,** 806–823.

Jones, S.E., Fuks, Z., Kaplan, H.S., *et al.* (1973b). Non-Hodgkin's lymphomas: V. Results of radiotherapy. *Cancer,* **32,** 682–691.

Jones, S.E., Grozea, P.N., Metz, E.N., *et al.* (1979b). Superiority of adriamycin-containing combination chemotherapy in the treatment of diffuse lymphoma: a Southwest Oncology Group study. *Cancer,* **43,** 417–425.

Kennedy, B.J., Bloomfield, C.D., Kiang, D.T., *et al.* (1978). Combination versus successive single agent chemotherapy in lymphocytic lymphoma. *Cancer,* **41,** 23–28.

Krikorian, J.G., Portlock, C.S., Cooney, D.P., and Rosenberg, S.A. (1980). Spontaneous regression of non-Hodgkin's lymphoma. A report of nine cases. *Cancer,* **46,** 2093–2099.

Lister, T.A., Cullen, M.H., Beard, M.E.J., *et al.* (1978). Comparison of combined and single-agent chemotherapy in non-Hodgkin's lymphoma of favourable histological type. *Br. Med. J.,* **1**, 533–537.

Longo, D., Hubbard, S., Wesley, M., Jaffe, E., Chabner, B., DeVita, V., and Young, R. (1981). Prolonged initial remission in patients with nodular mixed lymphoma (NML) (Abstract). *Proc. Am. Soc. Clin. Oncol.,* **22**, 521.

Lukes, R.J., and Collins, R.D. (1974). Immunologic characterization of human malignant lymphomas. *Cancer,* **34**, 1488–1503.

Miller, T.P., and Jones, S.E. (1979). Chemotherapy or chemotherapy with adjuvant radiotherapy for localized diffuse lymphoma. In *Adjuvant therapy of cancer, vol.2* (eds S.E. Jones, and S.E. Salmon). New York: Grune and Stratton. pp. 155–162.

Monfardini, S., Banfi, A., Bonadonna, G., Rilke, F., Milani, F., Valagussa, P., and Lattuada, A. (1980). Improved five year survival after combined radiotherapy–chemotherapy for stage I–II non-Hodgkin's lymphoma. *Int. J. Radiat. Oncol., Biol. Phys.,* **6**, 125–134.

Osborne, C.K., Norton, L., Young, R.C., Garvin, A.J., Simon, R.M., Berard, C.W., Hubbard, S., and DeVita, V.T., Jr (1980). Nodular histiocytic lymphoma: an aggressive nodular lymphoma with potential for prolonged disease-free survival. *Blood,* **56**, 98–103.

Patchefsky, A.S., Brodovsky, H.S., Menduke, H., *et al.* (1974). Non-Hodgkin's lymphomas: a clinicopathologic study of 293 cases. *Cancer,* **34**, 1173–1186.

Portlock, C.S., and Rosenberg, S.A. (1979). No initial therapy for stage III and IV non-Hodgkin's lymphomas of favorable histologic types. *Ann. Intern. Med.,* **90**, 10–13.

Qazi, R., Aisenberg, A.C., and Long, J.C. (1976). The natural history of nodular lymphoma. *Cancer,* **37**, 1923–1927.

Rappaport, H., Winter, W.J., and Hicks, E.B. (1956). Follicular lymphoma—a re-evaluation of its position in the scheme of malignant lymphoma, based on a survey of 253 cases. *Cancer,* **9**, 792–821.

Risdall, R., Hoppe, R.T., and Warnke, R. (1979). Non-Hodgkin's lymphoma. A study of the evolution of the disease based upon 92 autopsied cases. *Cancer,* **44**, 529–542.

Rosenberg, S. A. (1982). Is intensive treatment of favorable non-Hodgkin's lymphoma necessary? In *Controversies in oncology* (ed P.H. Wiernik). New York: John Wiley & Sons. pp.45–60.

Rudders, R.A., Ahl, T.A., Jr. DeLellis, R.A., Begg, C.B., *et al.* (1981). Surface marker identification of a subset of small cleaved follicular center cell lymphomas (SCFCC) with a highly favorable prognosis (Abstract) *Proc. Am. Soc. Clin. Oncol.,* **22**, 516.

Rudders, R.A., Kaddis, M., DeLellis, R.A., *et al.* (1979). Nodular non-Hodgkin's lymphoma (NHL): factors influencing prognosis and indications for aggressive treatment. *Cancer,* **43**, 1643–1651.

Schein, P.S., Chabner, B.A., Canellos, G.P., Young, R.C., Berard, C., and DeVita, V.T., Jr (1974). Potential for prolonged disease-free survival following combination chemotherapy of non-Hodgkin's lymphoma. *Blood,* **43**, 181–189.

Strauchen, J.A., Young, R.C., DeVita, V.T., Jr, Anderson, T., Fantone, J.C., and Berard, C.W. (1978). Clinical relevance of the histopathological subclassification of diffuse 'histiocytic' lymphoma. *New Engl. J. Med.,* **229**, 1382–1387.

Sweet, D.L., and Golomb, H.M. (1980). The treatment of histiocytic lymphoma. *Semin. Oncol.* **7** (3), 210–217.

Sweet, D.L., Golomb, H.M., Ultmann, J.E., Miller, J.B., Stein, R.S., Lester, E.P., Mintz, U., Bitran, J.D., Streuli, R.A., Daly, K., and Roth, N.O. (1980).

Cyclophosphamide, vincristine, methotrexate with leucovorin rescue, and cytarabine (COMLA) combination sequential chemotherapy for advanced diffuse histiocytic lymphoma. *Ann. Intern. Med.,* **92,** 785–790.

Warnke, R.A., Kim, H., Fuks, Z., *et al.* (1977). The coexistence of nodular and diffuse patterns in nodular non-Hodgkin's lymphomas: significance and clinicopathologic correlation. *Cancer,* **40,** 1229–1233.

Weinstein, H.J., Vance, Z.B., Jaffe, N., Buell, D., Cassady, J.R., and Nathan, D.G. (1979). Improved prognosis for patients with mediastinal lymphoblastic lymphoma. *Blood,* **53,** 687–694.

Cancer Treatment: End Point Evaluation
Edited by B.A. Stoll
© 1983 John Wiley & Sons Ltd.

Chapter

19 G.R. GILES and D.R. DONALDSON

Selective Treatment in Gastric Carcinoma

Gastric cancer has recently shown a decrease in mortality rate in the United Kingdom, in common with the pattern in the USA. The incidence of gastric cancer is markedly higher in other parts of the world, notably Japan, Iceland, Finland, and some areas of South America, and it is suggested that there are two different types of gastric carcinoma, possibly with a different aetiology. The diffuse, undifferentiated type has a somewhat higher frequency and is more common in females and younger patients. The intestinal type (well differentiated) seems to be more common in the high-risk areas around the world and in older patients, and may be an end-stage of early gastric cancer.

FACTORS AFFECTING PROGNOSIS

The prognosis of gastric cancer depends primarily upon its resectability rate, and this depends on the degree of local invasion and the development of metastasis. In the 1950s, Brookes *et al.* (1965) found that 63.5% of patients with gastric cancer underwent exploration, but in the more recent report of Lundh *et al.* (1974), 91% of patients were thought worthy of laparotomy. Yet the resection rate during that interval has increased only marginally, from 42.5% to 50%, and the number of patients undergoing radical resection with curative intent has increased from only 26.5% to 28%. There must be unknown pathological and clinical features which are important in prognosis because of the wide variability in survival rates reported around the world—overall five-year survival rates range from 1.4 to 27.7%.

Gastric cancer is relatively rare below the age of 30 years and increases in incidence up to the sixth decade. Survival rates are unaffected by age, given that a curative resection has been carried out, but the length of symptoms prior to the procedure does influence the survival time. Patients with symptoms for more than six months have a *better* prognosis (45–50%) than those in whom the symptoms have existed for less than six months (30–35%) (Thomas, 1973).

Survival and also resectability rates of the tumour relate particularly to the site of the primary tumour. The resectability rate of patients with antropyloric cancers is relatively high and this is reflected in the overall prognosis. With carcinomas of the body, cardia or fundus, only 10–12% of patients survive to five years, compared with 45–50% for carcinomas of the antrum and body.

This difference also reflects the size of the tumour at the time of primary diagnosis and treatment, and it can be shown that, as the size of the primary tumour increases, survival rates decrease from over 50% for tumours of less than 3 cm, to 17% when the tumour is greater than 9 cm in diameter. Carcinomas of the cardia and fundus are notorious for not producing symptoms until a large size is reached, unless a chance diagnosis is made. The size of the primary tumour can be related to the presence of lymph node involvement.

Carcinomas of the stomach are classified into three types—the intestinal type, diffuse type, and mixed type as described by Lauren (1965). There is a slight bias in favour of the intestinal type in terms of survival, though this rarely achieves statistical significance in a European study. Lymph node involvement and serosal invasion appear more frequent with the diffuse type of carcinoma than with the intestinal type. When these factors are taken into account, it becomes evident that the major factor affecting prognosis is the degree of infiltration of the gastric wall and its subsequent lymph node involvement.

The lymph node status of the tumour specimen reflects the prognosis, with an overall five-year cure rate of approximately 55% for those with negative lymph nodes, compared with 15–20% for those patients with positive nodes. Survival rates decrease as the number of involved nodes increases, and especially when nodes distant to the primary tumour, or situated around the common hepatic artery or aorta, are involved (Table 1). These factors are important when consideration is given (*vide infra*) to the type of surgery to be performed.

No one factor acts independently, and the final prognosis can be measured by a multifactorial analysis of these pathological factors. Nazakato *et al.* (1979) were able to give an individual prognosis on the basis of nine pathological criteria. The seemingly paradoxical fact that patients with a long history of symptoms have a better prognosis than those with a short history may have a pathological basis and may represent the period of symptomatology from an early gastric cancer before it becomes invasive.

It is clear that the best information concerning prognosis comes from

Table 1 Sites of lymph node involvement in gastric carcinoma

	Sites of nodes		
	N_1 lymph nodes	N_2 lymph nodes	N_3 lymph nodes
Carcinoma of antropyloric region	Lesser curvature Greater curvature Suprapyloric region Infrapyloric region	Left gastric artery Common hepatic artery Coeliac axis Right paraoesophageal	Splenic hilus Splenic artery Root of mesentery Hepatoduodenal ligament Left paraoesophageal
Carcinoma of body	Lesser curvature Greater curvature Suprapyloric region Infrapyloric region Right paraoesophageal	Left paraoesophageal Left gastric artery Common hepatic artery Coeliac axis Splenic hilus Splenic artery	Posterior surface of pancreas Root of mesentery Hepatoduodenal ligament
Carcinoma of cardia and fundus	Right and left paraoesophageal Lesser curvature Greater curvature	Left gastric artery Common hepatic artery Coeliac axis Splenic hilus Suprapyloric region Infrapyloric region	Hepatoduodenal ligament Posterior surface of pancreas Root of mesentery Intrathoracic, paraoesophageal and diaphragmatic nodes
Whole stomach (linitis plastica)	Lesser curvature Greater curvature Right and left para-oesophageal Infrapyloric region	Left gastric artery Coeliac axis Splenic artery Splenic hilus	Root of mesentery Hepatoduodenal ligament

careful weighing of such factors as tumour size and site, and the results of careful pathological examination including histology. However, since many patients do not benefit from laparotomy or resection and have an extremely short post-operative survival time, there is need for prognostic assessment pre-operatively.

There is growing evidence that some tumour markers may provide such prognostic information. Although pre-operative raised carcinoembryonic antigen (CEA) levels have been judged to carry a poor prognosis in colonic cancer, only a weak association has been found between survival with gastric cancer and CEA level (Freeman et al., 1979). Analysis of acute phase reactant proteins may prove more useful. In an analysis of 104 patients with gastric cancer, Rashid et al. (1982) found that the median survival of patients having raised CEA and antichymotrypsin levels was only five weeks compared with 64 weeks for a group of patients in whom both proteins were normal. The patients with a raised level of only one of the protein markers had a median survival of 15 weeks.

If this type of testing becomes more widely available, and if the prognosis can be assessed by the use of markers, then those patients not requiring palliative surgery for relief of symptoms might be spared a laparotomy. In many cases this merely confirms the inoperable nature of the primary tumour, and confirmation of the diagnosis and extent could be achieved by gastroscopy and laparoscopy.

CHOICE OF TREATMENT FOR EARLY GASTRIC CANCER

Early gastric cancer (EGC) is defined as a carcinoma confined to the gastric mucosa or submucosa, regardless of the presence of metastatic involvement of lymph glands. If we assume that by detecting and treating early gastric cancer we will prevent it becoming invasive, then ultimately the mortality from gastric cancer must fall. Such an effect will take several decades to be effective. In Japan many centres report that 30% of diagnosed gastric cancers are of the non-invasive type, but this is the result of massive investment in gastric screening of asymptomatic patients. In the UK and Europe, we should set our sights more modestly and attempt to increase the rate of diagnosis of EGC from 1% to 10%.

In the treatment of EGC it must be recognized that the condition is one of true malignancy but with limited depth of infiltration. It cannot be considered a precancerous state or an extremely low-grade malignancy. This is shown by the fact that lymph node metastases are found in 3–4% of mucosal cancers and in more than 20% of patients where the infiltration has reached the submucosa but not the muscle. Furthermore, there have been several reports of both local and distant recurrence after surgery for EGC.

How much of the stomach needs be removed? The main debate concerns the need for total gastrectomy, which provides the most complete lymph node dissection particularly from the region of the tail of pancreas and splenic hilum. It also removes the whole gastric mucosa and cannot be followed by a recurrence in the gastric stump—a complication which is reported in the long term in 4–5% of patients (Domellof and Janugar, 1977). However, a total gastrectomy is not indicated where the EGC has been accurately located in the prepyloric region alone, or in a gastric polyp with early malignancy. Nor can it be justified in patients in a poor nutritional state or in the aged patient. In these circumstances, a partial gastrectomy, local excision or endoscopic polypectomy may be appropriate.

For the younger patient, a radical subtotal gastrectomy (R_2) or total gastrectomy (R_3) has been shown to have an acceptably low hospital mortality rate (4–5%) in experienced centres. The radical nature of the procedure is justified on the basis that, in terms of cancer cure, it achieves a high success rate in general. It should also be noted that the presence of lymph node metastases does not necessarily affect the prognosis in the same manner as with invasive gastric cancer, and some series have 100% five-year survival despite lymph node involvement. It is interesting that the overall five-year survival results of EGC in European series do not seem as good as those from Japanese centres (65% compared with 90%).

CHOICE OF TREATMENT OF INVASIVE GASTRIC CANCER

Radical surgical treatment

Radical ('curative') surgical treatment gives the best chance of survival for patients with invasive gastric cancer. A subtotal gastrectomy has been the standard procedure for advanced gastric carcinoma, with appropriate dissection of surrounding tissues. The approach is most suited to carcinomas arising in the gastric antrum (40–50%), and requires that at least 6 cm clearance of macroscopically normal stomach is achieved proximal to the lesion. It is also necessary to remove the first 3 cm of duodenum beyond the pylorus.

For carcinomas in the body of the stomach, it is unlikely that the resection margins will be clear of tumour unless a total gastrectomy is carried out, although for lesions in the upper third of the stomach the position is less clear. Current practice is to perform a total gastrectomy with some form of oesophagojejunal anastomosis for all carcinomas of the cardia, fundus or body where such a procedure seems feasible.

The question arises whether a total gastrectomy can be justified in terms of operative mortality and subsequent survival. The early attempts at this procedure, beginning in the 1940s and extending into the next decade, reported an operative mortality varying from 12.8% to 33% (Lewin, 1960; Rush *et al.*, 1960; Bittner *et al.*, 1978). This compares with an operative mortality of about 5% for subtotal gastrectomy.

In Marshall's review of nearly 250 total gastrectomies performed at the Lahey Clinic (Marshall, 1957), he came to the conclusion that, whilst the operative mortality was steadily decreasing, total gastrectomy could not be justified unless the long-term survival also showed the same type of improvement. As only 14.1% of patients lived for five years, there was no convincing evidence that total gastrectomy should be the routine operation for gastric cancer. Similarly, Rush *et al.* (1960), analysing the experience at Johns Hopkins Hospital in Baltimore, found a five-year survival after total gastrectomy of only 9%, whereas after subtotal gastrectomy it was 25%.

Nevertheless, the more recent results of Japanese surgical centres (Kajitani and Takagi, 1979) do suggest that total gastrectomy can be performed with a low operative mortality and with apparent improvement in survival. The resurgence of interest in total gastrectomy results from the observation that the involvement of lymph nodes with gastric cancer need not necessarily be an overriding prognostic factor, provided that the tumour is not widely invading the serosal surface of the stomach. The radical operation allows a careful dissection of lymph node groups and has led to the categorization of gastrectomies into R_1, R_2 or R_3 resections:

> R_1 resections are limited and remove only perigastric lymph nodes.
>
> R_2 resections remove the primary tumour and perigastric lymph nodes directly draining the tumour together with intermediate groups of nodes around the coeliac axis and splenic artery.
>
> R_3 gastrectomy requires removal of nodes from around the aorta and hepatic artery, and may also involve contiguous excision of the distal pancreas and spleen (in the majority) and, in some patients, the excision of involved colon or liver lobe.

The initial reports were not encouraging, for the operative mortality was high, and in the final analysis (Gilbertson, 1969) of 1983 patients operated on in Minnesota, this radical approach did not effectively extend the five- or 10-year survival rate. However, Kajitani and Takagi (1979) also reported on 2533 apparently curative gastrectomies in which the standard procedure was a R_2 gastrectomy. The overall five-year survival for this group was 55%. Frozen section on the N_2 nodes was carried out at the time of surgery and, if positive, an R_3 procedure was undertaken removing the nodes around the hepatic artery and para-aortic regions, and in the case of an antral cancer, at the splenic hilum. The five-year survival for an R_3 resection was 22% with a 5% operative mortality. Though there were survivors of extensive procedures involving contiguous pancreatic, colonic and liver resections, survival was significantly extended only if the R_3 nodes proved to be negative.

More recent reports from Japan give a detailed analysis of the lymph node involvement for the various subgroups and sites of primary tumour (Jinnai, 1978; Kodama *et al.*, 1981). However, if these recent results are compared with historical controls undergoing more limited surgery, the conclusions are not completely satisfactory. An overall improvement in five-year survival for patients with serosal involvement from 18% with simple resection to 45% with extended lymph node dissection is reported. In those patients with lymph node involvement, five-year survival increases from 18% to 39% for simple and extended resection respectively. This may be due, in part, to a very low current operative mortality of 1.7% and to a more careful clinical and pathological staging of the resected specimens.

Role of adjuvant chemotherapy

Although surgery alone is a satisfactory treatment for early gastric cancer, the results obtained by surgical resection of invasive gastric cancers are clearly less satisfactory, with 50% (or less) five-year survival following surgery of curative intent. Additional treatment is required if these survival statistics are to be improved.

Adjuvant chemotherapy for gastric cancer has been attempted for well over two decades. Early studies involved the use of thiotepa as an adjuvant to surgical resection of gastric cancer (Dixon *et al.*, 1971) and a further study was reported by the Veterans' Association Cooperative Surgical Adjuvant Group (1965) also using thiotepa. There appeared to be no improvement in overall survival by the use of this agent, and in some groups, particularly those in whom a splenectomy had been carried out, the survival rates were distinctly reduced.

However, the use of single cytotoxic agents has been reported in some studies to be effective in prolonging survival, particularly those reported from Japan by Imanaga and Nakazato (1977) and Nakajima *et al.* (1978), in both instances using mitomycin C. Nakajima's study of 207 patients treated with mitomycin C plus surgery compared with 230 patients undergoing surgery alone is noteworthy. Overall, there were no significant differences in survival rate at five and 10 years when comparing patients treated with or without chemotherapy. However, significant improvement in survival rate was observed after mitomycin C in patients with both serosal involvement and lymph node involvement, while there were no advantages from the use of mitomycin C for patients without metastatic disease in the nodes or with superficial cancers. Nevertheless, the overall death rate due to cancer was 37.7% in the treated group and 46.6% in the control group at five years, and 42% and 51.1% at 10 years.

The use of 5-fluorouracil as an adjuvant cytotoxic agent was reported by Franz and Cruz (1977) who studied 156 patients with gastric cancer. They observed a feature common to many adjuvant studies, in that there was early improvement in survival which did not persist for five years. Thus at one year, 46.7% were alive after surgery alone as compared with 73.9% after surgery plus chemotherapy, and at two years the comparative figures were 40% and 47%. By three years the difference had narrowed and there was no difference found at four and five years respectively. Although Kovach *et al.* (1974) had reported that BCNU plus 5-FU was an effective combination for advanced gastric cancer, Lawton *et al.* (1981), using an identical combination of drugs for patients after incomplete resection of gastric cancer, found no improvement in survival.

With the experience gained from the treatment of disseminated gastric cancer, attention has turned to the use of the FAM regimen in adjuvant trials and we await the outcome of the trials. It is disappointing that the British Stomach Cancer Group trial using 5-FU and mitomycin, has not yet shown evidence of improved survival, though the final analysis awaits publication.

Role of adjuvant radiotherapy

There appear to be three possible approaches. First, the stomach and surrounding tissues can be irradiated pre-operatively as suggested by Hoshi (1968), who gave doses of 2000 rad without apparently affecting the incidence of intra-operative bleeding and post-operative complications. The resected specimens showed evidence of a favourable connective tissue reaction, especially at the serosal surface, but the incidence of lymph node metastases was not apparently reduced.

Secondly, radiotherapy may be administered at operation. Abe *et al.* (1975) used doses of 2000–3500 rad as a single treatment. Two of seven patients who had undergone surgery survived five years, which would seem encouraging but not conclusive evidence of an adjuvant effect. The technical difficulties of delivering treatment make it unlikely to have a widespread use in clinical practice.

Thirdly, as over half the patients with recurrent cancer have a recurrence locally in the field of surgery, the logical use of radiotherapy is as a post-operative treatment to the gastric bed. There is evidence too that the radiosensitivity of gastric cancer can be enhanced by combination with chemotherapy. An EORTC trial of radiotherapy combined with short- or long-term 5-FU administration is reported by Goffin and Machin (1979) and suggests that radiotherapy with long-term chemotherapy was perhaps slightly superior; however, the study does not include a surgery-alone group.

The report of Cohen *et al.* (1981) also suggests that long-term chemotherapy (18 months) gives equivalent results to the combination of radiotherapy (3000 rad) plus chemotherapy, where there was an actuarial five-year survival rate of 57% after curative surgery. However, patients receiving combination therapy were significantly younger than those patients receiving chemotherapy alone and it was found that patients under the age of 50 years survive significantly longer, irrespective of the type of treatment.

CHOICE OF TREATMENT FOR ADVANCED GASTRIC CANCER

Palliative surgical treatment

Many advanced cancers are ulcerated and obstructing and, even though the cancer may be disseminated, gastric resection may offer relief of symptoms. Unfortunately, many advanced tumours require a total or proximal gastrectomy for removal of the primary tumour and this cannot be justified because of the very high operative mortality and morbidity. A subtotal gastrectomy can be justified in the presence of metastases but not if it requires extensive *en bloc* resection of adherent structures, e.g. colon, pancreas, liver. Distal obstruction can also be relieved by a gastroenterostomy but stenosing neoplasms at the cardia pose more of a problem. A Mousseau–Barbin or Celestin tube can be placed operatively or an Alkinson tube positioned endoscopically after dilatation of the lesion, but palliation is not completely achieved.

Role of radiotherapy for locally advanced cancer

Early reports from the Mayo Clinic (Moertel *et al.*, 1969) showed that the use of radiation doses of 3500–4000 rad in the case of locally advanced tumours did not significantly extend survival beyond a median of five months, which is similar to that of untreated controls. It was also reported subsequently by the same group (Moertel *et al.*, 1979) that no patient survived beyond 15 months. It has been argued that the radiation doses used in these early studies were too low, and 4500–6000 rad would be required to sterilize the field (Wieland and Hymmen, 1970). However, exposures of this magnitude would lead to severe side-effects on the irradiated non-resected stomach and on the surrounding structures, particularly kidneys, pancreas, and spinal cord.

Fast-neutron therapy has been reported as showing excellent regression of tumour in 39 patients (Catterall *et al.*, 1975), and in 10 patients out of 14 who came ultimately to necropsy there was no macroscopic evidence of tumour, though it persisted histologically. Pain, dysphagia, vomiting, and bleeding were reported to be relieved and side-effects were apparently few. This type of radiation therapy is available only on a limited scale and requires further evaluation. It is unlikely to be helpful in patients with extensive disease outside the radiation fields. However, it was suggested that some inoperable tumours were converted to a more favourable state enabling subsequent resection of the primary tumour.

Chemotherapy for locally advanced or disseminated cancer

5-Fluorouracil has been extensively investigated as a single agent, and objective response rates of between 5 and 20% have been recorded for advanced gastric cancer. There have been some studies suggesting that the use of Ftorafur at doses of 800 to 1200 mg daily can achieve response rates of 24.7% (Furue *et al.*, 1975).

The second most commonly used drug in advanced gastric cancer has been mitomycin C. Various doses have been tried, varying between 4 and 10 mg/m^2 every two to three weeks. The dose-limiting factor of this drug is cumulative haematological and renal cytotoxicity, and, in particular, a very low platelet count is common. Objective response rates have been reported to be just over 20%. The initial work for this investigation has been carried out within Japanese centres.

The nitrosourea group of drugs has been extensively investigated and overall has yielded the relatively low response rate of approximately 10%. Of the three most commonly available drugs, BCNU seems to have been the most effective. More recently, adriamycin has been recognized to have distinct clinical activity against advanced gastric cancer and the response rate overall from a number of collected series is of the order of 15%.

The two-drug combinations that have been thoroughly tested use 5-fluorouracil in combination with either mitomycin C, BCNU or adriamycin. The reported objective response rates have varied between 15 and 30%. A similar range of responses has been obtained with three-drug combinations which have utilized mitomycin C plus 5-fluorouracil and another drug such as adriamycin, prednisone, chromamycin or cytosine arabinoside. It is the combination of 5-fluorouracil, adriamycin and mitomycin C (FAM) which is currently thought to be the most efficacious in the management of advanced gastric cancer (Table 2).

Table 2 The FAM regimen of cytotoxic chemotherapy

5-Fluorouracil	500 mg/m^2 on days 1,8,21, and 28
Adriamycin	30 mg/m^2 on days 1, and 21
Mitomycin C	10 mg/m^2 on day 1

It has to be recognized that evidence of an objective response does not necessarily predict prolonged survival. In patients with untreated advanced gastric cancer, the average survival is 3 to 3.5 months and the average survival of patients treatment with mitomycin C alone is almost identical. In those patients who had an objective response, however, the median survival time has been extended to five months while that of non-responders was only 2.4 months. Similarly the median survival rate of responders to the FAM regimen may be 7–8 months and that of non-responders only 3–4 months.

In an analysis by Moertel *et al.* (1979), the range of survival for some 517 patients entered into four different randomized trials (organized by the Gastrointestinal Tumour Study Group and the Eastern Co-operative Group) ranged from only 16 up to 36 weeks. Long-term survival is very unusual and, while it is important that the clinical investigation groups continue their vital work, the general surgeon and physician may reflect on the report of Saito and Yokoyama (1975) who collected reports on 4020 patients with advanced gastric cancer treated by chemotherapy and found that the median survival time of responders from the commencement of treatment was 108 days (median), and that of non-responders was 48 days. Only 31 (0.8%) survived two years.

Combined radiotherapy and chemotherapy for locally advanced cancer

In the initial report of Moertel *et al.* (1969), half of the patients were randomly selected to receive 5-FU in addition to radiotherapy and these patients had a median survival of 14 months compared with 6 months for those patients receiving radiation alone. It is interesting that three of the 25 patients in the combined therapy group survived five years.

A more recent study has compared a group of patients treated with methyl-CCNU and 5-FU, with patients receiving 5000 rad given in two courses of 2500 rad over three weeks and separated by a two-week rest interval. In addition, 5-FU (500 mg/m^2) was given on the first three days of each course of radiation treatment. After the courses of radiation were completed, the patients were placed on the same chemotherapy regimen as in the alternative arm.

At first sight it appears that the patients in the combined modality group were at a disadvantage, for the median survival of the chemotherapy group was 70 weeks compared with 35 weeks in the combined modality group (Schein and Novak, 1980). It is interesting, however, that there appeared to be a plateau of 20% survival at 2–4 years in the combined modality group, whereas the patients in the chemotherapy group continued to die in this period.

Whilst these are modest effects, it does suggest that the combination of radiotherapy and chemotherapy does have a prolonged biological effect on the tumour. If the early deaths from toxicity with this combined treatment could be countered by nutritional and haematological support, and if the side-effect of upper abdominal irradiation could be contained, then there might be a role for this treatment, particularly if it allowed a safe resection of the primary tumour subsequently. For it remains a fact that surgical resection of the primary tumour, even if incomplete, continues to improve survival statistics. Furthermore, when the development of new chemotherapy regimens for disseminated gastric cancer begin to show increased evidence of objective responses, then the combination of chemotherapy, radiotherapy, and surgical excision may ultimately prove to be the optimal method of management for locally advanced gastric cancer.

REFERENCES

Abe, M., Takahashi, M., Yabumoto, E., Onoyama, Y, Torizuko, K., Tobe, T., and Mori, K. (1975). Techniques, indication and results of intraoperative radiotherapy of advanced cancers. *Radiology*, **116**, 693–702.

Bittner, R., Beger, H.G., Krass, E., and Gogler, H. (1978). Magencarzinochirugie auch bei über 70 jahrigen? *Arch. Chir.,* **344**, 293–307.

Brookes, V.S., Waterhouse, J.A., and Dowell, D.J. (1965). Carcinoma of the stomach: a 10 year survey of results and of factors affecting prognosis. *Br. Med. J.,* **1**, 1577–1580.

Catterall, M., Kingsley, D., Lawrence, G., Grainger, J., and Spencer, J. (1975). The effects of fast neutrons on inoperable carcinoma of the stomach. *Gut,* **16**, 150–156.

Cohen, Y., Zidan, J., and Robinson, E. (1981). Adjuvant therapy of stomach cancer: a non-randomised study. In *Diagnosis and treatment of upper gastrointestinal tumors* (eds M. Friedman, M. Ogawa and D. Kisner). Amsterdam, Oxford, Princeton: Excerpta Medica. pp. 274–285.

Dixon, W.J., Longmire, W.P., and Holden, W.D. (1971). Use of triethylthophosphoramide as an adjuvant to the surgical resection of gastric and colorectal carcinoma. *Am. J. Surg.,* **173**, 26–34.

Domellof, L., and Janugar, K.-G. (1977). The risk of gastric carcinoma after partial gastrectomy. *Am. J. Surg.,* **134**, 581–584.

Franz, J.L., and Cruz, A.B. (1977). The treatment of gastric carcinoma with combined resection and chemotherapy. *J. Surg. Oncol.,* **9**, 131–137.

Freeman, J.G., Latner, A.L., Turner, G.A., and Venables, C.W. (1979). CEA in gastric cancer. *Lancet,* **i**, 210–212.

Furue, H., Nakao, I., Kanko, T., Yokoyama, T., and Furukawa, K. (1975). Chemotherapy of gastric cancer. *Cancer Chemother.,* **2**, 351–356.

Gilbertson, V.A. (1969). Results of treatment of stomach cancer. *Cancer,* **23**, 1305–1308.

Goffin, J.C., and Machin, D. (1979). Treatment of patients with gastric cancer by surgery, radiotherapy and chemotherapy: preliminary results of an EORTC randomised study. In *Recent results in cancer research* (eds G. Bonnadonna, G. Mathe, and S.E. Salmon). Berlin, Heidelberg, New York: Springer-Verlag. pp. 208–211.

Hoshi, H. (1968). Histologic study on the effect of preoperative irradiation of gastric cancer. *Tohoku, J. Exp. Med.,* **96**, 293–311.

Imanaga, H., and Nazakato, H. (1977). Results in surgery for gastric cancer and the effect of adjuvant mitomycin C on cancer recurrence. *World. J. Surg.,* **1**, 213–218.

Jinnai, D. (1978) Evaluation of extended radical operation for gastric cancer with regard to lymph node metastasis and follow-up results. *Gann. Monogr.* **3**, 225–294.

Kajitani, T., and Takagi, K. (1979). Cancer of the stomach at Cancer Institute Hospital. *(Gann. Monogr) Cancer Res.,* **22**, 77–94.

Kodama, Y., Sugimach, K., Soejima, K., Matsusaka, T., and Inokudhi, K. (1981). Evaluation of extensive lymph node dissection for carcinoma of the stomach. *World J. Surg.,* **5**, 241–248.

Kovach, J.S., Moertel, C.J., and Schutt, A.J. (1974). A controlled study of combined 1,3-Bis, (2-Chloroethyl)-1-Nitrosoaurea and 5-Fluorouracil therapy for advanced gastric and pancreatic cancer. *Cancer,* **33**, 563–575.

Lauren, P. (1965). The two histological main types of gastric carcinoma. Diffuse and so-called intestinal type carcinoma. An attempt at a histoclinical classification. *Acta. Pathol. Microbiol. Scand.,* **64**, 31–37.

Lawton, J.O., Giles, G.R., Hall, R., Bird, G.G., and Matheson, T. (1981). Chemotherapy following palliative resection of gastric cancer. *Br. J. Surg.,* **68**, 397–399.

Lewin, E. (1960). Gastric cancer. *Acta Chir. Scand.,* Suppl. 2, 62.

Lundh, G., Burn, J.I., Kolig, G., Richard, C.A., Thomson, J.W.W., van Elk, P.J., and Oszacki, J. (1974). A cooperative International study of gastric cancer. *Ann. Roy. Coll. Surg. Engl.*, **54**, 219–228.

Marshall, S.F. (1957). Total versus radical partial resection for cancer of the stomach. *Surg. Gynecol. Obstet.*, **104**, 497–489.

Moertel, C.G., Childs, D.S., Reitemeier, R.J., Colby, M.Y., and Holbrook, M.A. (1969). Combined 5-fluorouracil and supervoltage radiation therapy of locally unresectable gastrointestinal cancer. *Lancet*, **ii**, 865–867.

Moertel, C.G., O'Connell, M.J., and Lavin, P.T. (1979). Chemotherapy of gastric carcinoma. *Proc. Am. Soc. Clin. Oncol.* 288.

Nakajima, T., Fukami, A., Ohashi, I., and Kajitani, T. (1978). Long-term follow-up study of gastric cancer patients treated with surgery and adjuvant chemotherapy with mitomycin C. *Int. J. Clin. Pharmacol.*, **16**, 209–217.

Nakazato, H., Kato, K., Goto, M., and Matsubara, Y. (1979). A statistical trial on evaluation for the prognosis of gastric cancer. In *Gastric cancer* (eds Ch. Herfarth, and P. Schlag). Berlin, Heidelberg, New York: Springer-Verlag. pp. 187–203.

Rashid, S.A., O'Quigley, J., Axon, A.T.R., and Cooper, E.H. (1982). Plasma protein profiles and prognosis in gastric cancer. *Br. J. Cancer*, **45**, 390–394.

Rush, B.F., Brown, M.W. and Ravitch, M.M. (1960). Total gastrectomy: an evaluation of its use in the treatment of gastric cancer. *Cancer*, **13**, 645–648.

Saito, T., and Yokoyama, M. (1975). Evaluation of chemotherapy from a viewpoint of survival of patients with gastric cancer. *Cancer Chemother.*, **2**, 25–32.

Schein, P.S., and Novak, J. (1980). Combined modality therapy versus chemotherapy alone for locally unresectable gastric cancer. *Proc. Am. Soc. Clin. Oncol.*, **21**, 419.

Thomas, E. (1973). Current thought on factors that influence prognosis of gastric cancer. *Med. J. Aust.*, **2**, 821–825.

Veterans' Association Cooperative Surgical Adjuvant Study Group (1965). Use of thiotepa as an adjuvant to the surgical management of carcinoma of the stomach. *Cancer*, **18**, 291–298.

Wieland, C., and Hymmen, U. (1970). Megavolttherapie maligner Neoplasien des Magens. *Strahlentherapie*, **140**, 20–26.

Cancer Treatment: End Point Evaluation
Edited by B.A. Stoll
© 1983 John Wiley & Sons Ltd.

Chapter

20 G. R. GILES and S. H. LEVESON

Selective Treatment in Colorectal Carcinoma

Of this group of tumours, about 40% are situated in the rectum and the remainder are distributed throughout the colon, particularly the sigmoid region, followed by right colon, left colon, transverse colon, and flexures. The incidence of carcinoma of the colon and rectum in relation to the sexes is approximately equal but the death rate from colonic carcinoma is significantly higher in females (11:7) whereas the death rate from carcinoma of the rectum is slightly higher in the male population (6:5).

Approximately 50% of patients are over the age of 60 at the time of diagnosis of colorectal cancer, although carcinoma of the rectum appears at an earlier age in women than men. However, colorectal carcinomas are not infrequently found in patients under the age of 20 years.

FACTORS AFFECTING THE PROGNOSIS

Age plays an important role in survival rates. Very elderly patients have a somewhat lower survival rate at five years, not only because of recurrent disease but also because of a lower resectability rate and a higher peri-operative mortality. Nevertheless, Jensen *et al.* (1970) point out that, in patients surviving a radical operation for carcinoma of the colon, the survival rates over the age of 70 are only slightly inferior to those for patients under the age of 70 years.

It is interesting that a history of symptoms for six months or more is a *favourable* prognostic sign in terms of length of survival (Slaney, 1971). Although the age, general physical status, and the existence of concurrent disease are of major importance in determining the ultimate prognosis of patients with colorectal cancer, the most important factors relate to the pathological nature of the growth.

Size

While small sessile tumours give rise to metastases more quickly than polypoidal growths, the size of the tumour base affects the prognosis. Whittaker and Goligher (1976) found that rectal growths which occupied three-quarters or more of the circumference of the bowel had a significantly worse prognosis than those occupying one-half or less. Similarly, patients with obstructing tumours of the colorectum had a five-year survival rate approximately one-half of that of patients with non-obstructing tumours (Copelands, *et al.* 1968; Minister, 1964).

Site

Carcinomas of the right colon may reach a large size before producing sufficient symptoms to bring them to clinical notice, yet the survival rates after curative excision are better than those for carcinomas of the left colon and transverse colon where obstruction occurs more commonly. Carcinomas arising in the rectosigmoid and rectum have the worst overall prognosis, and the survival rate decreases as the level of the lower edge of the tumour approaches the anal margin.

Local invasion

There is an inverse relationship between the extent of local invasion by colorectal cancers and the five-year survival rate, with a marked decrease in survival following penetration of the muscularis propria. Where it is possible to quantify the degree of spread through the muscularis propria, slight spread is associated with 65% five-year survival rate, moderate spread with 45%, and extensive spread with only 25% survival. Nodal metastases are only infrequently found unless the carcinoma has spread by continuity into the pericolic fat, but thereafter lymph node metastases occur in a progressive manner from pericolic nodes (C_1) to nodes abutting the main mesenteric vessels (C_2). Once these nodes are involved, the overall survival rate falls to about 30%.

Grade of malignancy

Histological grading of colorectal cancer reveals that 20% of all tumours are low-grade, 60% are average, and 20% are high-grade. Furthermore, it is possible to relate the grade of malignancy to the extent of direct venous and lymphatic spread and to the levels of circulating carcinoembryonic antigen (CEA). It is also possible to relate the histological grading to the five-year survival rate. Low-grade tumours show about 80%, average-grade 60%, and high-grade tumours 25% five-year survival rates.

However, the high-grade category has various subtypes within it: anaplastic tumours, poorly differentiated tumours, undifferentiated tumours with a limited tendency to tubule formation, and signet ring cell carcinomas. While purely anaplastic tumours have almost no five-year survivors, those retaining a degree of tubule formation may be associated with survival rates up to 30% (Morson, 1965).

The use to which such pathological data can be put is twofold. First, it may identify a group of patients with a marked tendency towards local recurrence. Bad prognostic features would be extensive spread through the muscularis propria and a high-grade malignancy. Where possible, therefore, anastomoses should not be made through the area of excision, and this may mean either abdominoperineal excision of the rectum or Hartmann's procedure rather than an anterior resection. Such patients may also be more appropriately treated by local radiotherapy either prior to or in the post-operative period (*vide infra*). Secondly, the pathological data identify a group of patients who are at high risk of metastatic spread, and these may therefore be candidates for adjuvant therapy in the form of chemotherapy.

PREMALIGNANT LESIONS

Certain disorders predispose to the development of invasive cancer, and increasing recognition of this fact has arisen because of wider application of colonoscopy and mucosal biopsy. Thus, it may be possible to predict in an individual the development of colorectal cancer or diagnose it at an earlier pathological stage.

Ulcerative colitis

There is a seven-fold increased risk of colonic cancer in patients with colitis, while in those patients with extensive colitis, the risk is 30 times that in the control population. The risk of carcinoma is in the range of 1 in 80 to 1 in 100 per patient year (Lennard-Jones *et al.*, 1977). There is also a relationship between pre-cancer of the rectal and colonic epithelium and the subsequent development of cancer. The high-risk group of patients with ulcerative colitis are those having a history greater than 10 years and those in whom the inflammation involves most or all of the colon.

Some surgeons advocate prophylactic colectomy in all patients that meet these criteria—either a full proctocolectomy or a colectomy with ileorectal anastomosis, but since not all patients develop colonic cancer, this policy has considerable disadvantages. The question arises, therefore, whether there are any means of identifying those patients likely to develop carcinoma. While the report of Morson and Pang (1967) suggested that the development of colonic cancer could be expected if a rectal biopsy showed epithelial dysplasia, it soon became apparent that pre-cancerous changes in the colonic mucosa quite commonly spared the rectum entirely, even in the presence of developed cancers at a more proximal level.

With the development of long fibreoptic colonoscopes, it is possible to examine the colon more completely and to biopsy multiple sites. A carcinoma is usually visible macroscopically as a polyp, as a very low elevated lesion, or as an ulcer. Similarly, dysplasia can be seen either colonoscopically or on x-ray as a slightly elevated lesion. Studies of excised specimens and colonoscopic biopsies have shown that approximately one-third of patients with pre-cancer or severe epithelial dysplasia in the proximal colon had normal rectal biopsies, but about 30% of patients with epithelial dysplasia of the rectal mucosa undergoing colectomy already had cancer and some of these had already metastasized.

It must be concluded that suspicious areas of colitic colon should be biopsied, and if dysplasia is present the colon should be removed, as carcinoma is commonly present at the base of dysplastic mucosa. Although colonoscopic screening has not yet proved to be an accurate security measure for patients in high-risk groups, it is suggested that patients with quiescent colitis should be followed every two years by full colonoscopic examination and biopsy. Survival rates after surgical treatment for carcinoma complicating colitis are similar to those of colorectal cancer without colitis. The question is still open as to whether the patient with mild or moderate dysplasia should have a colectomy.

Familial polyposis

The symptoms from multiple polyps within the colon of these families normally arise about puberty, and carcinoma of the colon arising from the polyps appears to be diagnosed most frequently about 15 years after the start of symptoms, when the patients are in early adult life. Since the average age of death of patients with familial polyposis is of the order of 40 years, it is clear that it represents a considerable risk to the individual patient. Cases are on record in which the malignant transformation took place before the age of 20 years and it seems appropriate that these patients should undergo some form of colectomy about the age of 15 years.

In most instances, this will take the form of a total colectomy with preservation of the rectum. Thereafter careful sigmoidoscopic examination and fulguration of the remaining rectal polyps should be performed. Having diagnosed such a case, it is important to investigate the family further and to counsel the affected members concerning the future generations. It is unlikely that individuals of the family who have not developed polyps by the age of 14 will have inherited polyposis.

CANCER IN INDIVIDUAL COLONIC POLYPS

The increasing use of flexible endoscopes has allowed the widespread removal of polyps from the colon without recourse to open colotomy. The advantage to the patient is considerable, particularly as 30% of these patients develop a second polyp within five years (Henry *et al.*, 1975). However, a problem is that 5–20% of polyps are found to contain invasive cancer or carcinoma *in situ*. The potential for malignant transformation can be predicted and is related to:

(1) the size of the polyp—less than 1 cm, 1.3% 1–2 cm, 9.5%; greater than 2 cm, 46.0%
(2) the histological features—tubular (adenomatous), 4.8%; tubulovillous, 22.5%; villous, 40.7%
(3) the degree of cellular dysplasia—mild, 5.7%; moderate, 18.0%; severe, 34.5%.

What is the management when a polyp has been removed and is found to contain invasive cancer? Invasion is defined as penetration of tumour cells through the basement membrane and into the lamina propria (Okike *et al.*, 1977). It is known that lymphatic vessels are not present superficial to the lamina propria (Fenoglio *et al.*, 1973). It is generally agreed that intramucosal cancer or carcinoma *in situ* does not metastasize and that provided local treatment is complete, no further resection is needed. However, when histological examination shows carcinoma at the cut edge of the polyp, it is considered that more extensive colectomy is necessary. This situation arises more commonly when the polyp is found to be sessile.

The main area of controversy is in the management of adenomas containing early invasive cancer but with an apparent free margin of clearance. It was suggested by Shatney *et al* (1974) on the basis of 59 cases that polypectomy is sufficient, provided that the cancer is limited to the head of the adenoma, does not invade the pedicle, is not highly undifferentiated, and shows no evidence of lymphatic invasion within the polyp. However, Wolff and Shinya (1975) found that, of 11 of 33 patients who underwent colonic resection after removal of a polyp with invasive cancer, three had local residual disease though none had lymphatic metastases. A similar study of nine patients by Contsoftides *et al.* (1978) revealed local residual disease in four patients and one had lymph node metastases.

Finally, Colacchio *et al.* (1981) studied 24 patients undergoing colonic resection for polyps with invasive cancer; no local residual disease was found but six patients had lymph node metastases. They did not find the criteria outlined by Shatney *et al.* (1974) to be useful in defining those patients who might be managed conservatively. Nevertheless, it would seem that the dangers of poorly differentiated cancers, lymphatic invasion, sessile tumours or the occurrence of the cancer in close proximity to the line of resection are real, and that residual cancer may be removed in these high-risk patients by colonic resection.

THE SCOPE OF SURGERY FOR CARCINOMA OF THE COLORECTUM

Colonic cancer

It is generally recognized that a primary colonic cancer should be excised where possible, irrespective of the presence of distant metastases, since palliation is best achieved by these means. Circumstances exist where even palliative excision may not be possible and this could result from gross fixity to surrounding vital structures due to malignant infiltration. Since a proportion of patients will have inflammatory adhesions to surrounding viscera, trial dissection is required to confirm inoperability.

The extent of resection required for carcinomas of the colon is determined by the concept that it is necessary to remove the surrounding lymph nodes which run alongside the colic vessels supplying that particular segment of colon. In order to remove these lymph glands, the colonic vessels are normally transected near their origin from the mesenteric artery. Thus by devitalizing the colon, it becomes necessary to perform the anastomosis at a level where the viability is not compromised.

Rectal cancer

Two modalities of treatment offer hope of cure at this site: surgery and radiotherapy; and the choice depends on anatomical factors as well as on the pathological nature of the tumour itself. As far as surgery is concerned, two choices are possible: one involves the use of abdominoperineal excision of the rectum and anal canal while sphincter-saving resections are based on the concept that the lymphatic spread of rectal cancer is mainly in an upward direction, and that spread through the anal canal to the inguinal nodes is relatively rare.

The selection of the individual type of treatment for a rectal cancer is dependent largely on the position of the growth within the rectum. It is now recognized that, providing that the excision can be carried out at a level approximately 3 cm below the primary growth without stretching the rectum, then adequate lines of clearance are obtained. Thus, carcinomas lying in the lower rectum 3–7 cm from the anal verge require an abdominoperineal excision of the rectum. Carcinomas of the upper rectum, 11–15 cm, may be treated by anterior resection. Carcinomas of the middle rectum, 7–11 cm, may under certain circumstances be treated by rectal excision with sphincter preservation.

Consideration must also be given to the pathological nature of the lesion. With malignant change within a segment of a large villous papilloma, it may be possible to accept a lesser margin of clearance. Conversely, carcinomas in which the biopsy has shown a highly anaplastic tumour are probably best treated by abdominoperineal excision of the rectum since they prove to be highly invasive. Attempts to anastomose the colon and lower rectum within the pelvis are likely to be followed by recurrent tumour growing directly into the lumen producing further symptoms.

FACTORS INVOLVED IN THE MANAGEMENT OF SMALL CANCERS OF THE RECTUM

Small tumours are commonly found in the very elderly and relatively unfit patient and may occasionally occur in patients who refuse rectal excision. What then are the alternative types of treatment? Small tumours which are lightly fixed to the rectal wall may be excised locally, and may be reached through the anus or by the trans-sphincteric approach described by Mason (1972). The tumour requires to be excised with a margin of healthy tissue, and, provided that no more than one-half of the circumference is involved, it is generally possible to effect a closure without significant stenosis. Should the operative specimen later show spread outside the bowel wall, consideration is given to rectal excision.

An alternative approach is described by Papillon (1973) using endocavitary radiation. This technique is applied by the introduction of a probe into the rectum which is able to deliver a high dose of radiation (2000 rad/min) and is applied sequentially to different parts of the surface of the tumour. The patient receives between three and five treatments over four to six weeks on an outpatient basis, and it is calculated that each small tumour will receive between 9000 and 15000 rad.

It seems applicable only to very carefully selected tumours which must be completely accessible in all parts, and in the lower 10–12 cm of rectum. The size of the growth must be relatively small and ideally the tumour will have a sessile morphology rather than being of an infiltrating type. Papillon has reported that of 103 patients treated by local endocavitary irradiation 70% were alive at five years and free from disease. This suggests that this type of growth, being a small, well-differentiated, exophytic carcinoma, is unlikely to be associated with widespread lymphatic metastases, and clearly in the elderly unfit patient, this treatment may be the method of choice.

An alternative approach is that of electrocoagulation, a technique originally introduced by Strauss *et al.* (1935) and reinvestigated by Madden and
Kandalaft (1971) and Crile and Turnbull (1972). The entire surface of the
tumour is diathermied and then scraped off to expose the underlying and
untreated parts of the tumour. Several sessions over intervals of two to three
weeks are necessary in order to achieve a satisfactory local control. The
technique is occasionally complicated by the development of haemorrhage,
and rarely by a perforation into the peritoneal cavity. Survival rates of 50% or
more are possible for patients with invasive cancer as opposed to pedunculated neoplasms and since many patients are poor-risk, this technique clearly
has advantages.

SURVIVAL AFTER SURGERY

The overall survival from carcinoma of the colorectum is appallingly low, and
Slaney (1971) found that approximately 20% of patients survived five years.
These statistics obviously include a proportion of patients who present late in
the course of disease or with widespread metastatic disease at the time of their
primary treatment.

The failure rates after curative treatment for carcinoma of the right colon,
transverse colon, left colon, and rectosigmoid neoplasms are 25.5, 12.5, 15,
and 45% respectively. It is possible to relate the incidence of failure closely to
the clinical and pathological staging of the neoplasm at the time of excision.
Using the modification by Astler Coller of Dukes' classification, the failure
rate for mucosal cancer (Stage A) is 12%, for penetration into the muscle wall
but not through the muscle wall (B_1) is 12%, for spread to the pericolic nodes
is 33%, spread through the muscle wall into the pericolic fat (B_2) is 37%, and
spread to the more proximal nodes and to residual nodes (C_2, C_3) is 59%.

It is thus interesting that local spread (B_2 lesions) is a more serious
consequence than spread to the immediate pericolic lymph nodes. This
discriminatory power of the pathological staging applies to both right and left
sides of the colon, yet carcinoma of the rectosigmoid apparently confined to
the mucosa and submucosa (Dukes' A) has a significantly worse prognosis
than elsewhere in the colon.

ADJUVANT TREATMENT OF COLORECTAL CANCER

Since disease-free survival following apparently curative resection of colorectal cancer is poor, it warrants an investigation of alternative or additional
forms of treatment, particularly where there is evidence of breakthrough of
the cancer through the bowel wall and evidence of spread to regional lymph
nodes (B and C cases). Adjuvant therapy is in the process of being evaluated
and it must be said immediately that there are no firm indications for the

application of additional therapy on an individual patient basis. Nevertheless, patients with significant lymph node involvement identify themselves as a subset of patients who do require effective additional treatment in order to improve their chance of survival.

Adjuvant studies take many years to unfold and the results currently available are drawn from studies that were initiated a decade ago. They largely involve the use of a single cytotoxic agent, namely thiotepa or 5-fluorouracil. These agents have been given a variety of dose schedules and for a variable period of time (Rousselot *et al.*, 1972; Higgins *et al.*, 1975).

Most reports suggest that adjuvant cytotoxic therapy may achieve a modest gain in survival for patients undergoing curative resection where the tumour has penetrated the bowel wall and where lymph nodes have been shown to be positive. This applies more particularly to rectal cancer rather than to cancer elsewhere in the colon. The improved results have often not appeared until the third, fourth or fifth year post-operatively. It would also seem that this modest gain in survival (approximately 10% overall) has not been bought at the expense of excess morbidity or toxicity from the cytotoxic agent. Where the agents have been started in the peri-operative period, there does not seem to have been any increased frequency of post-operative complications or mortality. It is however interesting that in one series at least, patients made leukopaenic from the cytotoxic therapy did rather better than those who maintained a normal blood count, though as yet this study has not shown that these patients have done better in terms of long-term survival (Grage, 1979).

In the case of radiotherapy, there is no controlled study in which neo-plasms, arising at sites other than the rectosigmoid, have been evaluated in a randomized fashion. The studies have various dosage schedules, so that trials are not comparable from one institution to another, but it does seem that the use of pre-operative radiotherapy in doses which range from 2500 to 4000 rad improves the five-year survival modestly (10%) and, in particular, reduces the incidence of local recurrence in rectal cancer. This improvement seems confined to male patients and to those in whom the cancer is in the mid or lower rectum. This may be related to the use of a perineal portal of radiation. There does not seem to be any advantage to patients with cancers lying in the upper rectum who are treated by anterior resection or sigmoid colectomy. Apart from these points, the only other patients likely to benefit from the use of pre-operative radiotherapy are those who appear to have a fixed cancer and who are ultimately to go on and have surgical excision. This subset of paitents has been identified by the MRC as worthy of study in their second radiotherapy trial.

Many patients undergoing an attempt at curative resection do in fact have occult hepatic metastases at the time of operation (Finlay *et al.*, 1982) and they may represent up to 30% of the total. Suspecting this, Taylor *et al.* (1977) have used the portal vein as a means of perfusing the liver with

5-fluorouracil in the peri-operative period, giving 1 g intraportally for seven days. There was no increase in post-operative infection rate nor in the length of hospital stay in the 154 patients treated in the randomized study. During a two-year median follow-up period, 23 patients died in the control group, five with multiple liver metastases and eight with generalized and liver metastases. In the perfusion group, one patient had liver metastases alone, one liver metastases and local recurrence while four others had local recurrence only. It will be interesting to see whether or not the use of this treatment in patients with liver metastases detected only by CT scanning will prove to be effective.

RADICAL SURGERY FOR THE TREATMENT OF LOCALLY ADVANCED COLORECTAL CANCER

Many of the patients who ultimately die of colorectal cancer die from uncontrolled localized pelvic disease which may lead to bowel obstruction, bleeding, renal failure, and sepsis. A small percentage have no evidence of liver metastasis or systemic involvement, and this group could theoretically benefit from extensive surgery to prevent or correct these complications. Total pelvic exenteration performed in selected patients has been proved to have both palliative and curative potential (Ledesma *et al.*, 1981). Removal of involved adjacent organs such as the vagina, uterus, bladder or prostate has been proved effective in controlling local disease and improving symptoms.

Recently the 20-year experience was published by the Roswell Park Group. The patient group comprised 17 Dukes' stage B and 8 Dukes' stage C patients. Patients with overt dissemination were not submitted to exenterative procedures. The overall post-operative mortality rate in the series was 10% and morbidity was described as minimal. The Dukes' classification correlated well with the survival rate. Of the 17 patients with stage B disease, eight were alive at five years and nine patients died, of whom two were cancer-free at the time of death. Only two of eight patients with stage C disease were alive with no detectable tumour at five years.

From this study, it would appear that by careful selection, locally advanced sigmoid cancers which are invading the bladder, uterus, ovaries or vagina can be excised with some hope of long-term control. It has to be recognized that the relatively excellent results come from a highly specialized institution where this type of surgery can be performed with a low morbidity.

SECOND-LOOK SURGERY

The concept of 'second-look' surgery in colorectal cancer has been stimulated by the work of Wangensteen and his group (1951). The intention was to re-explore patients who had had a supposedly curative resection, but in whom metastases were present in the resected lymph nodes, i.e. Dukes' C tumours.

The second-look procedure was carried out approximately six months after the initial operation, whilst patients were still asymptomatic and had no clinical or radiological evidence of recurrent disease. At the second operation, the entire operative field was inspected and any residual cancer removed, if possible. Further laparotomies were carried out at intervals of six months to a year in patients in whom residual cancer was removed, and these procedures were repeated until no residual cancer was evident or until inoperable progression of disease had occurred. The results of this series are largely anectodal but it did demonstrate that some patients could safely undergo reoperation for excision of residual cancer, and some patients could be classified as long-term survivors.

Based on these findings, Griffen *et al.* (1964) reported on 98 patients with colon cancer who were submitted to second-look surgery. Of the total, 62 were found to be negative at second operation and 41 of these remained alive and well, 25 surviving for more than five years. The remaining 36 patients were positive at reoperation, but, as a result of repeated surgery, all were alive and well at the last second-look. The series included also 44 patients with carcinoma of the rectum, of whom 24 had a negative second-look. In this negative group there was one operative death, seven deaths from recurrent disease, and nine deaths which were unrelated to cancer. In the 20 patients with a positive second-look operation, there were two operative deaths, 16 recurrent cases, and two patients were finally converted to a negative status.

Questions which arise from these reports are: Is it a justifiable use of surgical time? Does it alter the natural history of the recurrent disease? None of these trials have been mounted in a randomized prospective fashion and it is difficult to evaluate their worth in answering these questions. No one can doubt the logic of performing second-look surgery on cancer patients who have become symptomatic. Studies have been published (Ellis, 1974) which show that completely benign conditions can mimic recurrences: stricture of colonic anastomoses, adhesions, sterile abscesses, and internal hernias are all prone to occur in these patients post-operatively, and can occur at some considerable time from the initial operation. If the detection of recurrent cancer can be accomplished before it has progressed too far (e.g. by the use of markers), then a selected group of patients may benefit from second-look surgery.

CARCINOEMBRYONIC ANTIGEN (CEA) IN THE MANAGEMENT OF COLORECTAL CANCER

CEA levels are elevated in 60–65% of all cases of colorectal cancer (NIH Consensus Statement, 1981). Elevations in CEA tend to be indicators of more advanced disease and are associated with a group of patients who have a poor prognosis. The levels of circulating CEA depend on several factors which include tumour mass, stage, degree of differentiation, site, dissemination, and the functional status of the liver:

Tumour stage

Levels are elevated in 80% of patients with hepatic metastases, but only in 20% of patients with Dukes' stage A tumours.

Tumour site

The highest serum levels are produced by left-sided colonic tumours, whilst levels are on average lower in right-sided and rectal carcinomata.

Specificity

CEA may be found in increased concentration in the serum of patients with cancer of non-colorectal origin, especially in gastric and breast cancer. Elevated levels may also be present in a number of non-malignant conditions. CEA is mainly cleared by the liver, and hence patients with some degree of hepatic functional impairment such as cirrhosis, obstructive jaundice, liver abscess, and pancreatitis may all have elevated levels. Abnormally high levels may be associated with smoking as well as with inflammatory bowel disease.

Plasma CEA levels may be an indicator of the adequacy of excision in colorectal cancer and patients who maintain elevated serum levels post-operatively are more likely to have residual malignant disease. However, a single post-operative normal result does not exclude the presence of residual tumour and, if CEA is to be used to monitor tumour recurrence, serial assays are required (Sugarbaker *et al.*, 1976b).

CEA in the detection of recurrent cancer

The role of CEA in the detection of early recurrent cancer has been studied in great detail. Sorokin *et al.* (1974) prospectively studied 102 patients who had undergone potentially curative resections for colorectal cancer. Eighteen patients showed CEA elevations greater than 2.5 ng/ml and six of these showed a progressive rise and subsequently developed recurrent cancer. Similar studies have been reported by Holyoke *et al.* (1976), Mach *et al.* (1974), and Mackay *et al.* (1974). In all these series, the CEA elevations preceded clinical recurrence by between two and 18 months. Sugarbaker *et al.* (1976b) stress that a careful symptom review is also necessary, since some cases of recurrent cancer did not produce any elevations in plasma CEA.

From these series it would seem that, in order to provide significant information, the serum CEA must be elevated pre-operatively and must either remain elevated or rise after an initial fall. In such patients, the assay may find a place in defining an 'at risk' group who could benefit from some form of adjuvant treatment, but there are still major drawbacks. Between 20 and 30% of patients with known recurrences do not show any CEA elevation (Sugarbaker *et al.*, 1976a) while other patients, apparently disease-free, show transient rises in their serum CEA levels (Rittgers *et al.*, 1978).

The relation between CEA level and time, site, and extent of recurrence has been evaluated in 358 patients with colorectal cancer (Wanebo *et al.*, 1978b). Recurrence rates were higher in patients with Dukes' B and C lesions who had pre-operative CEA levels higher than 5 ng, and there appeared to be a linear inverse correlation between pre-operative levels and estimated mean time to recurrence in patients with Dukes' B and C lesions. These ranged from 30 months for a level of 2 ng/ml to 9.8 months for a level of 70 ng/ml. In patients with Dukes' C lesion the median time to recurrence was 13 months if pre-operative levels were higher than 5 ng/ml, and 28 months if they were lower. Pre-operative CEA levels in patients with resectable Dukes' B and C cancers provide additional criteria for allocating these patients to groups at high or low risk to recurrence.

CEA and second-look surgery

If CEA elevations may antedate clinical recurrence in a proportion of patients, the next question is whether the resectability rate and survival times could be influenced by the performance of laparotomy based on CEA elevation. Martin *et al.*, (1977) have performed second-look surgery on 32 patients based primarily on the presence of rising serial CEA measurements. They found resectable localized disease in 13 (41%) of patients, one of whom survived five years following the second operation. Recurrence was not clinically apparent pre-operatively in any of the patients submitted to second-look surgery. In this group, three patients (9%) underwent negative laparotomy on the basis of their elevated CEA levels. The report on this trial concluded that, having excluded benign causes for elevation of CEA, re-exploration was indicated if two consecutive CEA levels were elevated significantly above the post-operative baseline value.

Staab *et al.* (1978) have combined computerized serial CEA measurement and clinical diagnostic methods to select 30 patients for second-look surgery. They attempted to distinguish between localized and diffuse recurrences based on the rate of rise of plasma CEA levels. A slowly rising CEA level could usually be correlated with a local recurrence, whereas a rapidly rising CEA could generally be correlated with distant metastases, predominantly in the liver. The results of these studies would suggest, therefore, that second-look surgery should be initiated on the basis of rising CEA levels. Steele *et al.*

(1980) have recommended that chemotherapy without second-look surgery would be beneficial in patients with a CEA rise of greater than 2.1 ng/ml in 30 days.

The question still remains whether second-look surgery based on CEA change will increase resectability and, more especially, increase survival. In a recently published study (Attiyeh and Stearns, 1981), patients underwent second-look procedures in the presence of rising CEA levels. Liver metastasis was evident in 18 patients, seven of whom underwent resection. Local abdominal disease was present in 15 patients, of whom nine underwent 'curative' resection. Although the resectability rates of those patients with lower CEA levels was higher than in the group with higher levels, only 19% of patients who underwent 'second-look' procedures were disease-free with a median follow-up of 15 months. There was a significantly increased survival in those patients who had their second resection for 'cure'. It would appear therefore that monitoring levels may provide an indication of early 'curable' recurrence, but whether second-look surgery will make any impact on survival when based on CEA elevation alone is still in doubt.

CEA and chemotherapy

Lawton *et al.* (1980) have investigated plasma CEA levels and their relationship to disease progression. Forty-three patients were studied, who were known to have residual disease after resection of the primary colonic tumour. Serial CEA estimations tended to correlate with disease progression and also tended to correlate with chemotherapy-induced regression and indeed with increased survival. This group have suggested that CEA may find clinical application in the monitoring of responses to chemotherapy.

A much larger series has been published by Shani *et al.* (1978) who have assessed serial CEA measurement in following the clinical course of patients with metastatic colorectal cancer receiving chemotherapy. In a study of 263 patients, there appeared to be a general relationship between plasma CEA and clinical tumour measurements, though there were discordant correlations in a significant number of patients. Changes in CEA did not correlate with survival although there was a general correlation with disease progression. This latter correlation was roughly comparable to that of serum alkaline phosphatase in evaluating the recurrence and progression of liver metastases. In general, therefore, in monitoring chemotherapeutic responses, the currently used plasma CEA assay probably does not contribute significantly to the information which may be obtained by clinical and biochemical examination.

CEA and radiotherapy

The possible value of monitoring radiation therapy, has been studied by Sugarbaker *et al.* (1976a). CEA assays were performed in 16 patients receiving pre-operative radiation therapy for primary rectal cancer or recurrent colorectal cancer. Radiation therapy of localized colorectal cancer reliably reduced previously elevated circulating titres. Significant decreases of elevated CEA titres with accumulating doses of radiation indicated that the bulk of the CEA-producing tumour was within the radiation treatment portal. Radiation therapy failed to lower the CEA values when there was disseminated disease. A rebound in CEA levels strongly suggested that the initial fall of CEA did not presage long term control.

SELECTIVE TREATMENT FOR ADVANCED COLORECTAL CANCER

It may be debatable whether any treatment is justifiable when colorectal cancer has recurred locally or spread to distant sites. It is our contention that some patients with localized disease may benefit from further aggressive surgery and a small number of patients with disseminated disease may benefit from chemotherapy.

Selective treatment of hepatic metastases

It is unfortunately not uncommon for overt hepatic metastases to be detected at the time of operation for a primary colorectal neoplasm. In almost all cases it is still advisable to remove the primary lesion for palliative purposes and many patients will continue to live for two years, and a small number for four or five years, in relative comfort. Massive involvement of the liver (estimated to be greater than 60%) is usually associated with survival of only a few weeks and it may therefore be more appropriate in this situation to leave the primary growth.

However, some metastases are apparently localized to one part of the liver, or seem to be solitary. Brunschwig (1961) reported on some 14 patients undergoing either right or left hepatic lobectomy for liver deposits due to cancer of the colorectum. The longest period of survival was only 27 months. However, if the deposits are genuinely limited, then a limited wedge excision or segmental resection is much more successful.

In a report from Wilson and Adson (1976) on some 60 patients treated at the Mayo Clinic, 40 patients were found to have solitary metastases and 20 to have multiple deposits. In 39 of these patients the metastases were removed by wedge excision, in 10 patients segmental resection was necessary, and in 11 a full standard hepatic lobectomy was carried out. Analysis of pathological data revealed that 80% of the primary tumours were recorded as well differentiated but over 50% had lymph node metastases. No patient with multiple metastases survived five years, but 15 of the 36 patients with single metastasis and followed for five years or more were alive, and eight were alive without recurrence 10 years or more after operation. Wanebo *et al.* (1978a) have also described a 28% five-year survival rate in some 27 patients with colorectal cancer treated by resection of the bowel and removal of the liver metastasis by local excision in 13, wedge resection in 10 and hepatic lobectomy in four.

Provided that the tumour is pathologically relatively non-aggressive and is clearly localized to the bowel and its immediate lymph nodes, then a direct surgical attack on the liver metastases from colorectal cancer seems to be a worthwhile procedure. With the current availability of CT scanning, it should prove possible to detect those patients who already have non-palpable metastases in the liver, and should define accurately the patients who might benefit from this procedure. It is clear that the best results are obtained where the simplest form of liver resection proves possible.

Selective chemotherapy for disseminated and locally recurrent colorectal cancer

The interest in chemotherapy for colorectal cancer defies justification in terms of results so far. Clinical trials first defined the activity of a single drug, and then that of a combination of active drugs in an attempt to improve clinical efficacy. That some of the drugs were not used optimally in the early trials was illustrated by Ansfield *et al.* (1977) who reported that the objective efficacy of 5-FU could be doubled by appropriate administration of the drug.

There is some evidence that the site of metastatic deposits may affect response. For example, it has been reported that the response rate of lung metastases from colorectal cancer to fluorinated pyrimidines was only 6% compared with a rate of 24% for liver metastases and 32% for unspecified intra-abdominal masses. Cutaneous and subcutaneous nodules are also relatively resistant. In addition, patients with a massive tumour load or a decreased performance status are less likely to respond than patients with smaller tumour masses.

Provided that the patient is symptomatic but not confined to bed, a course of chemotherapy can be justified and the response assessed at 4–6 weeks. This objective assessment has its importance in deciding whether further treatment can be justified. The duration of the response is usually short, as is also the median survival, but a more prolonged survival is occasionally possible. For example, 60% of patients with metastatic colorectal cancer who had an objective response to 5-FU survived one year compared with 20% of those who did not respond (Moertel, 1968). At the present time, patients with evidence of progression after one or two courses are probably better served by symptomatic treatment than by ringing the changes in chemotherapy schedules.

CONCLUSION

The selection of treatment for gastrointestinal cancer in an individual patient usually takes place at the time of primary treatment. Surgery remains the most appropriate treatment at this time, but the decision to operate and the extent of the surgical procedure depend upon the pathological extent of the primary cancer and the presence and site of metastatic deposits.

The overall results of treatment for gastrointestinal cancer are exceedingly poor, mostly because of the advanced nature of many neoplasms at the time of diagnosis. Though schemes for earlier diagnosis are of great interest, it may be equally appropriate to channel research efforts into those individuals most at risk and into preventive measures.

Selection of patients for adjuvant treatment (chemotherapy or radiotherapy) is based upon the premise that, as a group, most patients do poorly with surgical treatment alone. There are, as yet, no discriminatory factors which will detect those patients who will benefit from adjuvant treatment of any form. However the signs are there; useful gains in survival are attainable for groups of patients with colorectal cancer given chemotherapy, and other groups of patients with rectal cancer given radiotherapy.

REFERENCES

Ansfield, F.J., Klotz, J., Nealon, T., Raminez, G., Minton, J., Hill, G., Wilson, W., Davis, H., Jr, and Cornell, G. (1977) A phase II study comparing the clinial utility of four regimens of 5-fluorouracil—a preliminary report. *Cancer*, **39**, 34–40.

Attiyeh, F.F., and Stearns, M.W. (1981). Second-look laparotomy based on CEA elevations in colorectal cancer. *Cancer*, **47**, 2199–2125.

Brunschwig, A. (1961). Radical surgical management of cancer of the colon spread to tissues and organs beyond the colon. *Dis. Colon Rectum*, **4**, 83–89.

Colacchio, T.A., Forde, K.A., and Scantlebury, V.P. (1981). Endoscopic polypectomy: inadequate treatment for invasive colorectal carcinoma. *Ann. Surg.*, **194**, 704–707.

Contsoftides, T., Sivak, M.V., and Benjamin, S.P. (1978). Colonoscopy and the management of polyps containing invasive carcinoma. *Ann. Surg.*, **188**, 638–641.

Copelands, E.M., Miller, L.D., and Jones R.S. (1968). Prognostic factors in carcinoma of the colon and rectum. *Am. J. Surg.*, **116**, 875–879.

Crile, G., Jr, and Turnbull, R.B., Jr (1972). The role of electrocoagulation in the treatment of carcinoma of rectum. *Surg., Gynecol. Obstet.*, **135**, 391–396.

Ellis, H. (1974). 'Second-look' surgery for suspected recurrences in cancer of the large bowel. *Cancer Treat. Rev.*, **1**, 205–220.

Fenoglio, C.M., Kaye, G.I., and Lane, N. (1973). Distribution of human colonic lymphatics in normal, hyperplastic and adenomatous tissue. Its relationship to metastasis from small carcinomas in pedunculated polyps. *Gastroenterology*, **64**, 51–66.

Finlay, I.G., Meek, D.R., Gray, H.W., Duncan, J.G., and McCardle, C.S. (1982). Incidence and detection of occult hepatic metastases in colorectal carcinoma. *Br. Med. J.*, **284**, 803–806.

Grage, T.B. (1979). Adjuvant chemotherapy for large bowel cancer. An optimistic appraisal. *Minnesota Med.*, **62**, 511–513.

Griffen, W.O., Gilbertson, V.A., and Wangensteen, O.H. (1964). 'Second-look' surger. *Natl Cancer Inst. Monogr.*, no.24.

Henry, L.G., Condon, R.E., and Schulte, W.J. (1975). Risk of recurrence of colon polyps. *Ann. Surg.*, **182**, 511–514.

Higgins, G.A., Humphrey, E., Juter, G.L., Leveen, H.H., McGaughan, J., and Keehn, R.J. (1975). Adjuvant chemotherapy in the surgical treatment of large bowel cancer. *Cancer*, **38**, 1461–1467.

Holyoke, E.D., Reynoso, G., and Chu, M. (1976). Carcinoembryonic antigen in patients with carcinoma of the digestive trace. In *Embryonic and fetal antigens in cancer*, vol.2 (eds Anderson, Coggin, Cole, and Holleman). AEC Report CONF-720208. Springfield, VA: Dept of Commerce. pp. 215–219.

Jensen, H.E., Nielsen, J., and Balsley, I. (1970). Carcinoma of the colon in old age. *Ann. Surg.*, **171**, 107–111.

Lawton, J.O., Giles, G.R., and Cooper, E.H. (1980). Evaluation of CEA in patients with known residual disease after resection of colonic carcinoma. *J. R. Soc. Med.*, **73**, 23–28.

Ledesma, E.J., Bruno, S., and Mittelman, A. (1981). Total pelvic exenteration in colorectal disease. *Ann. Surg.*, **194**, (6), 701–703.

Lennard-Jones, J.E., Morson, B.C., and Ritchie, J.K. (1977). *Gastroenterology*, **73**, 1280–1289.

Mach, J.P., Jaeger, P.M., Betholet, M.M., Ruegsegger, C.A., Loosli, R.M., and Pettarel, J. (1974). Detection of recurrence of large bowel carcinoma by radioimmunoassay of circulating CEA. *Lancet*, **ii**, 535–540.

Mackay, A.M., Patel, S., Canter, S., Stevens, U., Laurence, D.J.R., Cooper, E.H., and Neville, A.M. (1974). Role of serial plasma CEA assays in detection of recurrent and metastatic colorectal carcinoma. *Br. Med. J.*, **1**, 383–385.

Madden, J.R., and Kandalaft, S. (1971). Electrocoagulation in the treatment of cancer of rectum: a continuing study. *Ann. Surg.*, **174**, 530–565.

Martin, E.W., James, K.J., Hurtubise, P.E., Catalano, P., and Minton, J.P. (1977). The use of CEA as an indicator for gastrointestinal tumor recurrence and second-look procedures. *Cancer*, **39**, 440–446.

Mason, A.Y. (1972). Transsphincteric exposure of the rectum. *Ann. R. Coll. Surgeons Engl.*, **51**, 320–327.

Minister, J.J. (1964). Comparison of obstructing and non-obstructing carcinoma of the colon. *Cancer*, **17**, 242–248.

Moertel, C.G., and Reitemeier, R.J. (1969). Advanced gastrointestinal cancer. *Clinical Management and Chemotherapy*. New York: Harper and Row.

Morson, B.C. (1965). Notes on the pathology of carcinoma of the large intestine. *Natl Cancer Inst. Monogr.*, no.25.

Morson, B.C., and Pang, L.S.C. (1967). Rectal biopsy as an aid to cancer control in ulcerative colitis. *Gut*, **8**, 423–434.

NIH Consensus Statement (1981). *Br. Med. J.*, **242**, 373–374.

Okike, N., Weiland, L.H., and Anderson, M.J. (1977). Stromal invasion of cancer in pedunculated adematous colorectal polyps; significiance for surgical management. *Arch. Surg.*, **122**, 527–530.

Papillon, J. (1973). Endocavitary irradiation of early rectal cancer for cure: a series of 123 cases. *Proc. R. Soc. Med.*, **66**, 1179–1181.

Rittgers, R.A., Steele, G., Zamcheck, N., Loewenstein, M.S., Sugarbaker, P.H., Mayer, R.J., Lokich, J.J., Maltz, J., and Wilson, R.E. (1978). Transient carcinoembryonic antigen (CEA) elevations following resection of colorectal cancer: a limitation in the use of CEA levels as an indicator for second look surgery. *J. Natl Cancer Inst.,* **61**, 315–318.

Rousselot, L.M., Cole, D.R., Grossi, C.E., Conte, A.J., Gonzalez, E.M., and Pasternack, B.S. (1972). Adjuvant chemotherapy with 5-fluorouracil in surgery for colorectal cancer. *Dis. Colon Rectum,* **15**, 169–174.

Shani, A., O'Connell, M.J., and Moertel, C.G. (1978). Serial plasma carcinoembryonic antigen measurements in the management of metastatic colorectal cancer. *Ann. Intern. Med.,* (1974). **88**, 627–630.

Shatney, C.H., Lober, P.H., and Gilbertsen, W.A. (1974). The treatment of pedunculated adenomatous polyps with focal cancer. *Surg., Gynecol. Obstet.,* **139**, 845–850.

Slaney, G. (1971). Results of treatment of carcinoma of the colon and rectum. In *Modern trends in surgery,* vol.3 (ed W.I. Irvine). London: Butterworths. p. 197.

Sorokin, J.J., Sugarbaker, P.H., Zamcheck, N., Pisik, M., Kuplink, H.Z., and Moore, F.D. (1974). Serial CEA assays: use in detection of recurrence following resection of colon cancer. *J. Am. Med. Assoc.,* **228**, 49–53.

Staab, H.J., Auderer, F.A., Stumpf, E., and Fischer, R. (1978). Slope analysis of post-operative CEA time course and its possible application as an aid in diagnosis of disease in gastrointestinal cancer. *Am. J. Surg.,* **136**, 322–327.

Steele, G., Zamcheck, N., Wilson, R.E., Mayer, R., Lokich, J., Ran, P., and Maltz, J. (1980). Results of CEA-initiated 'second look' surgery for recurrent colorectal cancer. *Am. J. Surg.,* **139**, 544–548.

Strauss, A.A., Strauss, S.F., Crawford, R.A., and Strauss, H.A. (1935). Surgical diathermy of carcinoma of the rectum: its clinical end results. *J. Am. Med. Assoc.,* **104**, 1480–1486.

Sugarbaker, P.H., Bloomer, W.D., Corbett, E.D., and Chaffey, J.T. (1976a). Carcinoembryonic antigen monitoring of radiation therapy for colorectal cancer. *Am. J. Roentgenol.,* **127**, 641–644.

Sugarbaker, P.H., Zamcheck, N., and Moore, F.D. (1976b). Assessment of serial carcinomembryonic antigen CEA assays in postoperative detection of recurrent colorectal carcinoma. *Cancer,* **38**, 2310–2315.

Taylor, I., Brooman, P., and Rowling, J.T. (1977). Adjuvant liver perfusion in colorectal cancer: initial results of a clinical trial. *Br. Med. J.,* **2**, 1320–1322.

Wanebo, H.J., Rao, B., Pinsky, C.M., Hoffmann, R.G., Stearns, M., Schwartz, M.K., and Oettgen, H.F. (1978a). Preoperative carcinoembryonic antigen as a prognostic indicator in colorectal cancer. *New Engl. J. Med.,* **299**, 448–451.

Wanebo, H.J., Stearns, M., and Schwartz, M.K. (1978b). The use of CEA as an indicator of early recurrence as a guide to a selected second-look procedure in patients with colorectal cancer. *Ann. Surg.,* **188**, 481–492.

Wangensteen, O.H., Lewis, F.J., and Tongen, L.A. (1951). The 'second-look' in cancer surgery. *Lancet,* **ii**, 303–305.

Whittaker, M., and Goligher, J.C. (1976). The prognosis after surgical treatment for carcinoma of the rectum. *Br. J. Surg.,* **63**, 384–388.

Wilson, S.M. and Adson, M.A. (1976). Surgical treatment of hepatic metastases from colorectal causes. *Arch. Surg.,* **111**, 329–334.

Wolff, W.I., and Shinya, H. (1975). Definitive treatment of malignant polyps of the colon. *Ann. Surg.,* **182**, 516–524.804

Chapter

21 DAVID F. PAULSON

Selective Treatment in Prostatic Cancer

INTRODUCTION

When comparing different treatment regimens for carcinoma of the prostate, it is essential that the disease in the patients in the treatment groups should be not only of comparable anatomic extent but also of similar biologic characteristics. The following discussion on the selection of treatment for the individual patient will be under the headings of;

Treatment selection based on disease extent.
End-points for evaluating treatment of local and regional disease.
Prognostic variables influencing the course of disseminated disease.
Criteria of response in disseminated disease.

TREATMENT SELECTION BASED ON DISEASE EXTENT

Staging of prostatic adenocarcinoma in the patient has two major purposes; first to determine the anatomic extent of the disease so that treatment can be selected for the individual and, secondly, so that patient groups being compared should have a similar disease status. This section will examine our methods of assessing the extent of the disease, beginning with distant sites of metastasis and then progressively focusing onto the primary site. Initially, therefore, we will look at distant parenchymal and bone metastases, then at disease in the regional nodes, and finally at the extent of the local disease.

Distant metastases

Prostatic adenocarcinoma classically produces osteoblastic lesions in bone which are readily identified in routine radiographs. However, as demonstrated by the Uro-Oncology Research Group (Paulson and Uro-Oncology Research Group, 1979), detection of bone metastases in prostatic cancer is markedly improved by radioisotopic bone scanning. In this study, 356 patients found to be free of bone metastasis on the basis of radiographs were assigned to a preliminary staging process (Table 1). Subsequently they were submitted to radioisotopic bone scanning with 99-technetium medronate and it was reported that 20% of patients regarded as free of bone metastasis in radiographs showed evidence of such metastasis in the isotopic bone scan (Table 2). As would be expected, the discovery of metastasis by the skeletal scan was increased with greater local spread.

Elevated serum acid phosphatase levels in the presence of normal bone radiographs were a pointer to isotope scan-positive disease. Of the patients with biopsy-proven cancer, negative radiographs but elevated levels of serum acid phosphatase (Stage IVa), 35% showed bone involvement in the isotope scan. Only long-term follow-up will determine how many of the patients with elevated serum acid phosphatase levels but *negative* scans had occult bone metastases, but preliminary observations already indicate more metastases developing in this group than in those with normal acid phosphatase levels.

The use of routine skeletal radiographic survey is unnecessary in the clinical evaluation of patients with prostatic adenocarcinoma. Only 4% of patients have metastases in bone sites not encompassed by either the plain film of the abdomen and pelvis, or by a routine chest radiograph. The clinician is justified in proceeding directly to isotopic bone scanning when patients fail to

Table 1 Preliminary stage classification in prostatic cancer

Stage	AJC classification	Local lesion	Prostatic acid phosphatase	Bone metastases by x-ray
IA	$T_0N_xM_0$	Not palpable, focal	Not elevated	No
Ib	$T_0N_xM_0$	Not palpable, diffuse	Not elevated	No
II	$T_{1-2}N_xM_0$	Confined to prostate	Not elevated	No
III	$T_3N_xM_0$	Local extension	Not elevated	No
IVa	$T_{any}N_xM_0$	Any	Elevated	No
IVb	$T_{any}N_{1-4}M_0$ [a]	Any	Any	No
IVc	$T_{any}N_{any}M_1$	Any	Any	Yes

[a] IVb patients could not be assigned a stage classification until after node dissection as this category was reserved for patients with lymph node extension.

Table 2 Positive isotopic bone scan in relation to the preliminary staging

Preliminary stage	No. of patients	Bone scan	
		Positive	Negative
Ia	31	3 (10%)	28 (90%)
Ib	51	4 (10%)	47 (92%)
II	101	20 (20%)	81 (80%)
III	79	19 (24%)	60 (75%)
IVa	94	33 (35%)	61 (65%)
IVc	69	65 (94%)	4 (6%)

show metastases in these routine screening films, because approximately 20% of these patients will show bone involvement in the isotopic scan (Kane and Paulson 1977; Paulson and Uro-Oncology Research Group, 1979).

Lymph node metastases

The identification of lymph node metastases in prostatic carcinoma depends on pedal lymphangiogram and staging pelvic lymphadenectomy. (Ardinno and Glucksman, 1962; Whitmore *et al.*, 1974; McCullough *et al.*, 1974; McLaughlin *et al.*, 1976; Wilson *et al.*, 1977, Freiha and Salzman, 1977; Paulson and Uro-Oncology Research Group, 1979). Lymphatic spread of prostatic carcinoma occurs primarily through the vessels which leave the posterior aspect of the prostate with subsequent extension to the hypogastric (primary), obturator (secondary), external iliac (tertiary), and presacral (quaternary) lymphatics (Smith, 1966; Flocks *et al.*, 1975; Golimbu *et al.*, 1979). The nodes readily opacified by pedal lymphangiogram are those of the tertiary areas of prostatic drainage, the external iliac, common iliac, and peri-aortic lymphatics, and this explains the relatively low false positive rates observed when the lymphangiograms are subsequently confirmed by pelvic lymphadenectomy (Castellino *et al.*, 1973; Cerny *et al.*, 1975; Ray *et al.*, 1976; Freiha *et al.*, 1979). The relatively high incidence of false negative lymphangiograms results mainly from the difficulty in visualizing nodes of the hypogastric and obturator lymphatics (those lymphatics usually involved in early disease extension) by pedal lymphangiography.

Recognizing this problem, surgeons have resorted to staging pelvic lymphadenectomy to establish the presence or absence of positive pelvic disease. (Ardinno and Glucksman, 1962; Whitmore *et al.*, 1974; McCullough *et al.*, 1974; McLaughlin *et al.*, 1976; Wilson *et al.*, 1977, Freiha and Salzman, 1977; Paulson and Uro-Oncology Research Group, 1979). The limits of the dissection vary, some authors advocating dissection even to the bifurcation of

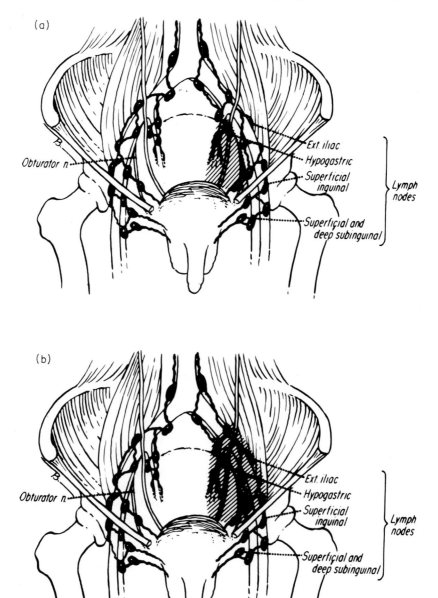

Figure 1 (a) Area of nodal drainage removed by limited lymphadenectomy as advocated by Paulson and Uro-Oncology Research Group (1979). (b) Area of nodal drainage removed by more extensive lymphadenectomy as advocated by Wilson *et al.* (1977)

Table 3 Lymph node metastasis shown by lymphangiography in relation to preliminary staging

Preliminary stage	No. of patients	Lymph nodes	
		Positive	Negative
Paulson and Uro-Oncology Research Group (1979)			
Ia	3	0 (0 %)	3 (100%)
Ib	29	8 (28%)	21(72%)
II	52	16 (30%)	36 (70%)
III	26	10 (39%)	16 (61%)
IVa	19	11 (58%)	8 (42%)
Wilson *et al.* (1977)			
A–1	27	1(4 %)	26(96%)
A–2	24	6 (25%)	18 (75%)
B–1	62	10 (16%)	52 (84%)
B–2	55	14 (25%)	41 (75%)
C	32	19 (59%)	13 (41%)

aorta, but accumulated data indicate that extending the area of dissection does not significantly improve the identification of patients with nodal disease. The data published by the Uro-Oncology Research Group accurately reflect the incidence of positive nodes in patients subjected to limited pelvic lymphadenectomy (Figure 1 and Table 3). The more extensive node dissection (Wilson *et al.*, 1977) does not increase the incidence of positive nodes found in relation to clinical stage, but may be associated with the development of troublesome leg and genital edema in those who subsequently received full pelvic external beam radiotherapy. (Barzell *et al.*, 1977; Bagshaw, 1978; Carlton, 1978; Pistenma *et al.*, 1979; Whitmore *et al.*, 1979).

Presacral node dissection as advocated by Golimbu *et al.* (1979) also adds little to the identification of metastatic disease. Only two out of 30 patients with prostatic adenocarcinoma who were subjected to an extensive pelvic lymphadenectomy (which included both presacral and presciatic nodes) showed presacral or presciatic nodal metastases when there was not also involvement of the external iliac, obturator, or external iliac nodes.

There also seems little justification to dissect the peri-aortic nodes to detect nodal spread when the pelvic lymph nodes are negative. The Uro-Oncology Research Group study demonstrated that the paralumbar (peri-aortic) nodal groups were involved in 12 of 54 (22%) patients when the external and internal iliac nodes were positive, but of 54 patients with negative pelvic lymph nodes, none had positive peri-aortic nodes. This substantiates the previous report of Spellman *et al.* (1977) that peri-aortic nodal metastases occur only when the pelvic nodes are involved.

We have mentioned above some attempts made to identify the presence of pelvic lymph node extension without resorting to pelvic lymphadenectomy. Pedal lymphangiography is associated with false positive and false negative rates which preclude its use as an accurate guide. Elevation of the serum acid phosphatase level in patients with a negative isotopic bone scan is associated with an increased likelihood of finding positive pelvic lymph nodes at lymphadenectomy but is not sufficiently reliable to exclude the need for node dissection in this subpopulation (Table 4).

Table 4 Relationship of raised level of serum acid phosphatase to node extension

Acid Phosphatase	Bone scan	Node biopsy	
		Positive	Negative
Uro-Oncology	Research Group (unpublished)		
Normal	Negative	32 (25%)	95 (75%)
Elevated	Negative	27 (64%)	15 (36%)
Freiha *et al.* (1979)			
Normal	Negative	7 (25%)	21 (75%)
Elevated	Negative	29 (54%)	25 (46%)

Gleason's histopathology 'sum' on the primary prostatic tumor may permit the clinician to predict the presence or absence of positive pelvic lymph nodes in a significant number of patients. Gleason *et al.* (1974) documented a system of histopathologic grading based upon the glandular pattern of the tumor growth at low magnification (40–100×). The Uro-Oncology Research Group classified all primary prostatic biopsies in this way, and in 110 cases the five growth patterns were recognized and numbered in order of increasing histologic malignancy. The predominant and secondary patterns of growth were identified and their numerical sums were combined to provide a final overall grade of between 2 and 10 (Table 5).

Those patients who had a low Gleason sum of 2–5 had a 14% probability of pelvic lymph node disease while those with a sum of 9 or 10 had a 100% probability of having positive nodes. The presence of a normal or an elevated acid phosphatase level in the serum did not enhance discrimination. Twelve patients did not have a Gleason sum assigned due to insufficient tissue, and the incidence of positive nodes in this group was 33%. In a second study comprising 144 patients (Kramer *et al.*, 1980), 93% who had a Gleason sum of 8, 9 or 10 demonstrated regional nodal metastases (Table 6) and no patient with a Gleason sum of 2, 3 or 4 had nodal metastases. As might be anticipated, the incidence of positive nodes in those patients with intermediate Gleason sums of 5, 6 or 7 increased progressively (Table 7).

Table 5 Relationship of Gleason sum to node biopsy in prostatic cancer Uro-Oncology Research Group, in press)

Gleason sum	Node biopsy Positive	Node biopsy Negative	No. of patients
2–5	13.9%	86.1%	36
6	32.4%	67.6%	34
7	49.9%	50.1%	21
8	75.0%	25.0%	12
9–10	100.0%	0%	7
No diagnosis	33.3%	66.7%	12

$\chi^2 = 28.2$
$p = 0.0005$

Table 6 Gleason sum as a predictor of nodal metastatic disease in prostatic cancer (Kramer *et al.*, 1980)

Pelvic lymphadenectomy	No. of patients	Gleason sum (2,3,4)	(5,6,7)	(8,9,10)
Positive	53	0/31 (0%)	26/84 (31%)	27/29 (93%)
Negative	91	31/31 (100%)	58/84 (69%)	2/29 (7%)

Table 7 Relationship of Gleason sum to surgical stage of disease (Kramer *et al.*, 1980)

Surgical stage	No. of patients	2	3	4	5	6	7	8	9	10
A–1	5	1	4							
A–2	22		1	6	8	6	1			
B	67	2	5	22	19	17	2			
C	37	1	1	3	10	4	15	3		
D	97				2	13	30	28	22	2

These data would indicate that the histologic grading of prostatic carcinoma using the Gleason classification system predicts the presence or absence of node disease with an accuracy that approaches that of pelvic lymphangiography. It provides an alternative method for selecting a patient's treatment without resorting to pelvic lymphangiography.

Accurate staging of the extent of disease involves definition of the anatomic structures involved by the malignancy. Given the accuracy of the staging procedures which are available today, the classic staging of prostatic cancer based on the definition of extent of disease by the letters A, B, C or D should be replaced by the TNM system which accurately reflects (1) the size and local extent of the local lesion, (2) the presence or absence and number of regional and distant lymph nodes, and (3) the presence or absence of metastatic disease involving distant parenchymal or bone structures. This then provides a rational method for treatment selection based on disease extent.

END-POINTS FOR EVALUATING TREATMENT OF LOCAL AND REGIONAL DISEASE

The following report is of a study of (a) the relative impact of radical prostatectomy or external beam radiotherapy in the control of prostatic adenocarcinoma confined to the prostate gland and (b) the relative value of external beam radiation therapy versus delayed endocrine therapy in patients with node-positive prostatic adenocarcinoma but no identified bone metastases. The study not only establishes the importance of defining the extent of the disease but also identifies criteria other than survival time for identifying the impact of treatment. In the study all patients presenting with newly diagnosed, previously untreated, biopsy proven, prostatic adenocarcinoma were staged by rectal examination, by colorometric serum prostatic acid phosphatase, by radioisotopic bone scanning, and by pelvic lymphadenectomy.

Patients with disease confined within the anatomic boundaries of the prostate by rectal examination (clinical stage A_2 or clinical stage B $(T_1-_2N_0M_0)$) who had no elevation of serum prostatic acid phosphatase (King–Armstrong units), no detectable metastatic disease involving the skeleton, and no lymph node extention were randomly assigned to either radical prostatectomy or megavoltage radiation therapy (Paulson *et al.*, 1982a). Patients with only an isolated focus of adenocarcinoma in the prostate were excluded from this trial as were patients with clinical stage C disease that extended beyond the anatomic confines of the prostate itself.

Patients staged as above but identified as having adenocarcinoma in the pelvic nodes in addition, were randomly assigned to either delayed endocrine therapy (bilateral orchiectomy, diethylstilbestrol 3 mg daily, or both) or extended field megavoltage irradiation (Paulson *et al.*, 1982b). Elevation of the serum acid phosphatase level did not exclude patients from trial. Patients assigned to delayed endocrine therapy received no treatment until symptomatic evidence of disease progression was noted, and the mere presence of spread did not qualify for such treatment. Patients assigned to extended field radiation therapy were treated as in the above trial with the exception that the peri-aortic lymph nodes to the level of the L–1 vertebra were included. Serum biochemical profiles with acid phosphatase determination, Karnofsky performance rating, and physical examination were obtained at each follow-up, with chest x-rays and isotopic bone scans at six-month intervals.

The impact of treatment was assessed using first evidence of treatment failure as the end-point. In the group assigned to either radical prostatectomy or radiation therapy, treatment failure was identified as acid phosphatase elevation evident on two consecutive follow-ups, or by the appearance of bone or distant parenchymal metastases with or without concomitant acid phosphatase elevation. Although many of the patients receiving radiation underwent serial transrectal needle biopsy, the histopathological identification of cancer in the prostate after radiation did not signify treatment failure for the purpose of assessing treatment efficacy.

In the group assigned to external beam radiation therapy with extended fields versus delayed endocrine therapy, first evidence of treatment failure was again the end-point of the study, but progressive elevation of acid phosphatase alone in a patient who entered with elevated acid phosphatase levels did not constitute failure. In both groups, curves representing non-perimetric estimates of survival and time to first evidence of treatment failure were generated using the Kaplan and Meier (1958) method. Censored values representing patients without evidence of treatment failure at the time of last follow-up are noted by several vertical tricks in Figure 2. The treatment

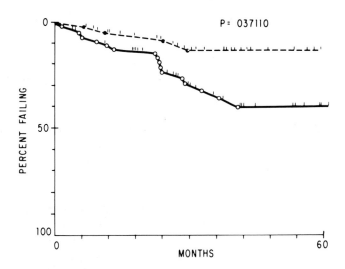

Figure 2 Time to failure for patients receiving radical surgery (broken line) versus patients receiving regional radiation therapy (solid line). Vertical ticks represent patients without evidence of treatment failure at time of last follow-up. The closed and open circles represent patients who demonstrated treatment failure.

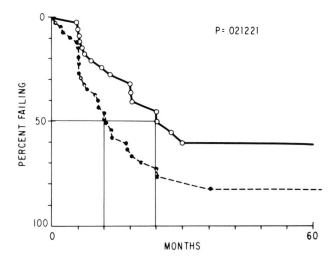

Figure 3 Time to failure for patients receiving endocrine therapy (broken line) versus patients receiving extended field radiation therapy (solid line).

efficacy between subgroups was tested for difference by the Cox–Mantel test (Cox, 1972).

Fifty-six patients received regional radiation and 41 received radical surgery. An analysis of time-to-failure curves in these two treatment groups (Figure 2) suggested that radical surgery possessed a distinct advantage over radiation therapy, significant at the 0.037 level. Thirty-six patients received delayed endocrine therapy and 41 received extended field irradiation therapy. When the two populations were analyzed for first evidence of disease spread (Figure 3), the median time to failure for patients receiving extended field radiation therapy was 23.9 months compared to only 12.2 months for patients assigned to delayed endocrine therapy ($p=0.02$).

These two randomized trials clearly indicate the necessity for accurate anatomic staging of the disease in patients entered into therapeutic trials. The poor control rates previously attributed to both regional radiation and surgery may very well be due to the failure of previous single-modality studies to define the extent of disease accurately (Vickery and Kerr, 1963; Walsh, 1980; Perez *et al.*, 1980). It is possible that malignant disease confined to a single organ site can be controlled effectively, and the inability to show this conclusively in earlier studies may be due to lack of accuracy in defining the extent of the disease before treatment was assigned.

Radioisotopic bone scan and pelvic lymphadenectomy will demonstrate metastatic disease in over 40% of patients with Stage A_2 or B cancer who show no elevation in the serum acid phosphatase level and no radiographic evidence of bone metastases (Paulson and Uro-Oncology Research Group, 1979). Studies of treatment efficacy in these stages which do not apply these staging maneuvers prior to treatment are adversely biasing their analyses. Errors which could be introduced by using a treatment designed for a single organ site when the disease has already spread to regional nodes are shown in the second of the above studies (Paulson *et al.*, 1982b). The presence of nodal metastases enhances the risk for a patient under treatment, irrespective of the nature of the treatment.

Another trial involved 44 patients with regional node metastases and negative isotopic bone scans and positive pelvic nodes who were assigned to treatment with either radical prostatectomy, external beam radiation therapy (5000 rad) to the full pelvis and peri-aortic lymph nodes with a 2000 rad boost to the prostate, or to delayed endocrine therapy (Kramer *et al.*, 1981). The time to first evidence of treatment failure was similar for all groups (Figure 4). An eight-months difference in the time to failure (statistically not significant) could be identified in patients having only one positive lymph node as compared with those having more than one positive lymph node (Figure 5).

The majority of patients with positive nodes fail their applied treatment in less than two years. The use of time to first evidence of treatment failure as the end-point for evaluation of treatment efficacy in prostatic carcinoma therefore seems reasonable when the patient population is aged and liable to die from intercurrent, non-malignant disease. It is reasonable also in a disease which survival may be affected by subsequent treatment using endocrine therapy, radiation or chemotherapy. It is obvious that the use of a second treatment distorts assessment of survival following the initial treatment.

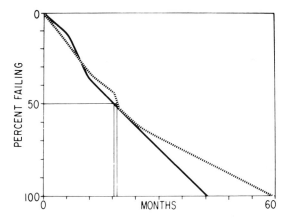

Figure 4 Time to failure for patients receiving radical surgery (solid line) versus patients receiving either delayed endocrine therapy or extended field radiation therapy (broken line).

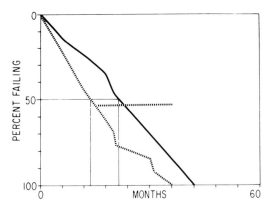

Figure 5 Time to failure for patients with one positive node (solid line) or more than one positive node (broken line). See text for details of trial.

PROGNOSTIC VARIABLES INFLUENCING THE COURSE OF DISSEMINATED DISEASE

Individual patients with disseminated prostatic carcinoma of apparently identical histologic type and similar stage may demonstrate different survival times and patterns of disease. These differences are due to host factors or to the biologic characteristics of the individual tumor in each patient. Identification of those factors which influence survival is important in the comparison of treatment modalities, and it is necessary to identify the major prognostic variables in order to stratify patients for randomized clinical trials.

A study was undertaken to define the responsiveness of patients with endocrine-unresponsive metastatic carcinoma of the prostate to a multi-agent chemotherapy program (Berry *et al.*, 1979; Paulson *et al.*, 1979). The historical, physical, and biochemical variables which were associated with good or poor prognosis in patients receiving this treatment served to identify specific stratification indices. Eighty-eight patients with endocrine-unresponsive Stage IV disseminated prostatic carcinoma were treated by combination cytotoxic chemotherapy including melphalan, methotrexate, 5-fluorouracil, vincristine, and prednisone.

All patients were followed through the entire course of their illness and were continued on therapy until the occurrence of disease progression, drug intolerance, toxicity or death. Progression was identified as increase in bone pain, progressive weight loss, or an increase in measurements of tumor masses. Secondary therapy utilized intravenous estrogen, diethylstilbestrol phosphate or single-agent chemotherapy in a few patients.

The variables assayed and their prognostic impact on the disease course are identified in Table 8. No difference in survival could be found between the 64

Table 8 Prognostic impact of host/tumor variables in prostatic cancer (Berry *et al.*, (1979)

Variable	Group A (number)		Median survival (weeks)	Group B (number)		Median survival (weeks)	p value
Race	White	(64)	39.2	Black	(22)	44.2	0.789
Age	>65	(43)	28.8	<65	(45)	57.0	0.014
Prior radiation	No	(39)	39.0	Yes	(49)	39.6	0.653
Sites of metastases	Bone + other organ	(22)	28.9	Bone only	(63)	45.6	0.012
Malignant pleural effusion	Yes	(9)	24.5	No	(79)	41.9	0.041
Liver scan	Abnormal	(13)	27.0	Normal	(75)	40.3	0.058
LDH	>200 U	(53)	29.1	≤200 U	(35)	62.7	0.003
SGOT	> 50 U	(21)	27.2	≤ 50 U	(67)	48.5	0.006
Alkaline phosphatase	>110 U	(71)	35.4	≤110 U	(17)	75.9	0.013
Acid phosphatase	>5 U	(32)	26.5	≤ 5 U	(56)	51.7	0.010

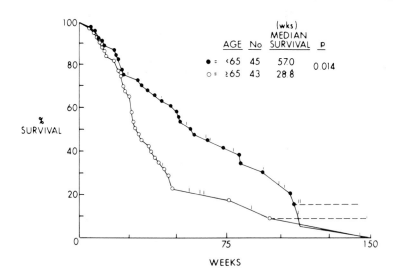

Figure 6 Effect of stratification by age on survival in trial of combination therapy in
disseminated disease.

white and the 22 black patients. Patients older than 65 years of age had a
significantly shorter survival than those aged 65 or younger (Figure 6). The
duration of the disease prior to chemotherapy was not associated with any
statistically significant difference in survival, although patients with a duration of disease or less than one year tended to have a longer survival after
chemotherapy. There was no difference in survival for patients with or
without prior radiation. Dose modification and the toxicity of the chemotherapy program was identical in both groups. There was no statistically significant difference between the survival of patients having had orchiectomy and
those not having had prior orchiectomy.

All patients had widely disseminated disease. Eighty-five of the 88 patients
had bone metastases (84 with positive scan, 72 with positive x-rays, and only
one with positive x-rays and a negative scan). Twenty-two of these 85 patients
had metastases in soft tissues (lung, liver, and/or lymph nodes) in addition to
bone metastases. The patients who had soft tissue metastases as well as bone
metastases had a decreased survival compared with patients who had only
bone metastases (Figure 7).

Hemoglobin less than 10 mg% was associated with a shortened survival
time. Abnormality of serum LDH or SGOT levels was significantly associated
with a shortened survival. If both LDH and SGOT levels were abnormal, the
association was even greater ($p=0.002$), although the median survival was
about the same as if either alone was abnormal (27.2 weeks). Any initial

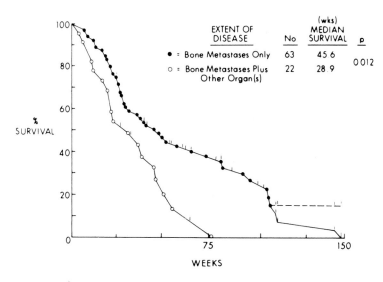

Figure 7 Effect of stratification by anatomic distribution of disease on survival in trial of combination chemotherapy in disseminated disease.

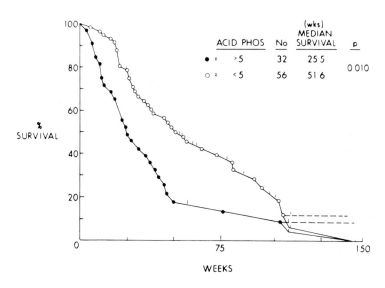

Figure 8 Effect of stratification by acid phosphatase level in trial of combination chemotherapy in disseminated disease.

elevation of serum alkaline phosphatase level was associated with a decreased survival. Sixty-eight of 88 patients had an elevated acid phosphatase level as performed by the colorometric assay, but only when the acid phosphatase was initially greater than twice normal (0.5 units) could a significantly shorter survival be identified (Figure 8).

This study indicates that there are prognostic factors other than therapy which influence the course of patients with endocrine-unresponsive metastatic prostatic carcinoma. When future randomized clinical trials are designed, these prognostic factors should be used either to stratify patients for treatment groups or to determine that a single treatment group is not heavily weighted with patients who have adverse prognostic factors.

CRITERIA OF RESPONSE IN DISSEMINATED DISEASE

Metastatic prostatic adenocarcinoma presents a problem in the evaluation of treatment response as few patients have measurable soft tissue disease, and those patients who do have soft tissue disease appear to be atypical because they seem to have a worse prognosis than do most patients with only bone metastases. It may be useful to examine an alternative approach to the evaluation of therapy in metastatic prostatic adenocarcinoma on the basis of arbitrary criteria of response.

For example, 67 of the 85 patients in the multi-agent chemotherapy program outlined above had elevated levels of acid phosphatase prior to

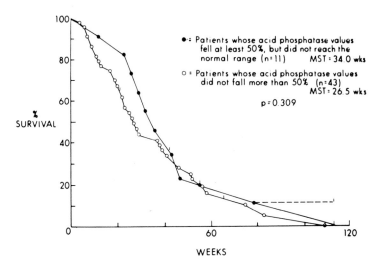

Figure 9 Survival if no normalization of acid phosphatase level in trial of combination chemotherapy in disseminated disease.

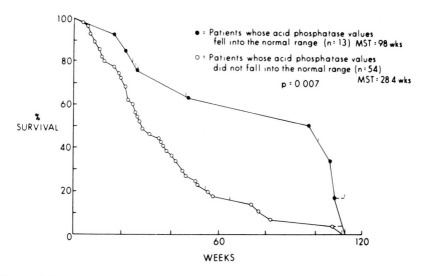

Figure 10 Survival if normalization of acid phosphatase level in trial of combination chemotherapy in disseminated disease.

therapy, and a comparison was made between the duration of survival in those patients whose acid phosphatase level fell more than 50% (but not to normal) and in those whose level did not fall by 50%. Eleven patients had values which fell more than 50% but not to normal, and their median survival time (MST) was 34.0 weeks as compared to the MST of 26.5 weeks for those whose values did not fall by 50% (p=0.309) (Figure 9). However, the 13 patients with elevated levels of acid phosphatase which fell to normal showed a median survival time of 98.0 weeks as compared to an MST of 28.4 weeks for all of the other patients with elevated values which had not fallen to normal (p=0.007) (Figure 10). Prolonged survival was thus noted only in that group of patients whose elevated acid phosphatase levels fell to normal.

Seventy patients had elevated levels of serum alkaline phosphatase before treatment. Twelve patients whose alkaline phosphatase levels fell by more than 50% but not to normal had an MST of 32.0 weeks as compared to an MST of 25.1 weeks for those whose values did not fall by 50% ($p = 0.44$) (Figure 11). The MST for the 12 patients whose elevated values fell to normal was 75.1 weeks; it was 27.7 weeks for all patients with initially elevated enzyme levels that did not return to normal ($p = 0.012$) (Figure 12). It would appear that a fall in an elevated alkaline phosphatase level was associated with prolonged survival only if the enzyme levels returned to normal. However, prolonged survival could not be correlated with return to normal of elevated levels of CEA or of LDH.

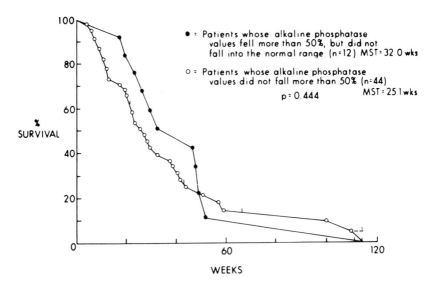

Figure 11 Survival if no normalization of alkaline phosphatase level in trial of combination chemotherapy in disseminated disease.

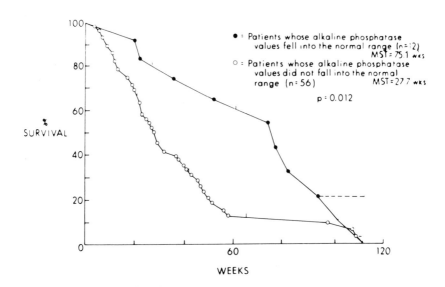

Figure 12 Survival if normalization of alkaline phosphatase level in trial of combination chemotherapy in disseminated disease.

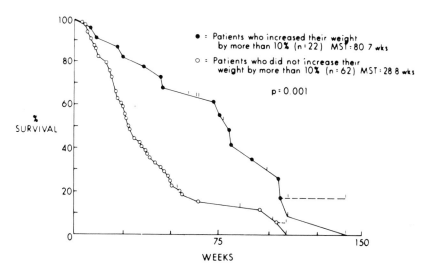

Figure 13 Survival if weight gain of 10% in trial of combination chemotherapy in disseminated disease.

Twenty-two patients increased their weight by 10% or more over their on-study weight. Edema was eliminated as a cause of increased weight. These 22 patients had a MST of 79.9 weeks as compared to a MST of 30.1 weeks for patients who did not increase their weight by more than 10% ($p = 0.001$) (Figure 13). One patient who did not receive prednisone because of a peptic ulcer nevertheless increased his weight by 10%.

Of the patients under study, 25 had soft tissue disease, either pulmonary, liver, or lymph node metastases, and seven of these had physically measurable tumor nodules. Three of these seven showed a greater than 50% reduction in measurable tumor mass and this was associated with a return to normal of raised alkaline or acid phosphatase levels, and a greater than 10% weight gain. The four without tumor shrinkage demonstrated no reduction in alkaline or acid phosphatase levels or weight gain. Decrease in bone pain by either one or two pain levels was not associated with prolongation of survival. Improvement in the performance status by at least one level was not associated with prolongation of survival.

CONCLUSION

The data would indicate that biochemical and physiologic indicators of response to chemotherapy do exist and that these can be correlated with prolongation of survival and a reduction in the size of soft tissue lesions. The identification of objective indicators of response to treatment eliminates the need to use subjective response criteria in prostatic cancer. In conclusion, the studies described above confirm the necessity for accurate evaluation of the anatomic extent of disease and for identification of specific risk factors which can distort analysis of the treatment response.

Acknowledgements

Supported in part by funds provided by the CURED Committee, the MacHarg Endowment, the Sunderlin Endowment, the Medical Research Service of the Veterans Administration Hospital, and NIH Grant No. CA14236.

REFERENCES

Ardinno, L.J. and Glucksman, M.A. (1962). Lymph node metastases in early carcinoma of the prostate. *J. Urol.*, **88**, 91.

Bagshaw, M.A. (1978). Radiation therapy for cancer of the prostate. In *Genitourinary cancer* (eds D.G. Skinner, and J.B. deKernion). Philadelphia: W.B. Saunders. p. 360.

Barzell, W., Bean, M.A., Hilaria, B.S., and Whitmore, W.F., Jr (1977). Prostatic adenocarcinoma: relationship of grade and local extent to the pattern of metastases. *J. Urol.*, **118**, 278.

Berry, W.R., Laszlo, J., Cox, E., Walker, A., and Paulson, D.F. (1979). Prognostic factors in metastatic and hormonally unresponsive carcinoma of the prostate. *Cancer*, **44** (2), 763–775.

Carlton, C.E., Jr (1978). Radioactive isotope implantation for cancer of the prostate. In *Genitourinary cancer* (eds D.G. Skinner, and J.B. deKernion). Philadelphia: W.B. Saunders. p. 385.

Castellino, R.A., Ray, G., Blank, N., Govan, D., and Bagshaw, M. (1973). Lymphangiography in prostatic carcinoma: preliminary observation *J. Am. Med. Assoc.*, **223**, 877.

Cerny, J.C., Farah, R., Rian, R., and Weckstein, M.L. (1975). An evaluation of lymphangiography in staging carcinoma of the prostate. *J. Urol.*, **113**, 367.

Cox, D.R. (1972). Regression models and life tables. *J.R. Stat. Soc.*, **34**, 187–202.

Flocks, R.H., Culp, D., and Porto, R. (1975). Lymphatic spread from prostatic cancer. *J. Urol.*, **81**, 194.

Freiha, F.S., Pistenma, D.A., and Bagshaw, M.A. (1979). Pelvic lymphadenectomy for staging prostatic carcinoma: is it always necessary? *J. Urol.*, **122**, 176.

Freiha, F.S., and Salzman, J. (1977). Surgical staging of prostatic cancer: transperitoneal versus extraperitoneal lymphadenectomy. *J. Urol.*, **118**, 616.

Gleason, D.F., Mellinger, G.T., and the Veterans Administration Cooperative Urological Research Group (1974). Prediction of prognosis for prostatic adenocarcinoma by combined histological grading and clinical staging. *J. Urol.*, **111**, 58.

Golimbu, M., Morales, P., Al-Askari, S., and Brown, J. (1979). Extended pelvic lymphadenectomy for prostatic cancer. *J. Urol.*, **121**, 617.

Kane, R.D., and Paulson, D.F. (1977). Radioisotopic bone scanning characteristics of metastatic skeletal deposits of prostatic adenocarcinoma. *J. Urol.*, **117**, 618.

Kaplan, E.L., and Meier, P. (1958). Non-parametric estimation from incomplete observations. *J. Am. Stat. Assoc.*, **53**, 457–480.

Kramer, S.A., Cline W.A., Jr, Farnham, R., Carson, C.C., Cox, E.B., Hinshaw, W., Glenn, J.F., and Paulson, D.F., (1981). Prognosis of patients with stage D prostatic adenocarcinoma. *Urology*, **125**, 817–820.

Kramer, S.A., Spahr, J., Brendler, C.B., Glenn, J.F., and Paulson, D.F. (1980). Experience with Gleason histopathologic grading in prostatic cancer. *J. Urol.*, **124**, 223.

McCullough, D.L., Prout, G.R., Jr, and Daly, J.J. (1974). Carcinoma of the prostate and lymphatic metastases. *J. Urol.*, **111**, 65.

McLaughlin, A.P., Saltzstein, S.L., McCullough, D.L., and Gittes, R.F. (1976). Prostatic carcinoma: incidence and location of unsuspected lymphatic metastases. *J. Urol.*, **115**, 89.

Paulson, D.F., Berry, W.R., Cox, E.B., Walker, A., and Laszlo, J. (1979). Treatment of metastatic endocrine-unresponsive carcinoma of the prostate gland with multiagent chemotherapy: indicators of response to therapy. *J. Natl Cancer Inst.*, **63**, 615.

Paulson, D.F., Cline, W.A. Jr, Hinshaw, W., and Uro-Oncology Research Group (1982b). Extended field radiation therapy versus delayed hormonal therapy in node positive prostatic adenocarcinoma. *J. Urol.* (submitted for publication).

Paulson, D.F., Lin, G.H., Hinshaw, W., and Uro-Oncology Research Group (1982a). Radical surgery versus radiotherapy for stage A_2 and stage B $(T_{1-2}N_0M_0)$ adenocarcinoma of the prostate. *J. Urol.* (submitted for publication).

Paulson, D.F., and Uro-Oncology Research Group (1979). The impact of current staging procedures in assessing disease extent of prostatic adenocarcinoma. *J. Urol.*, **121**, 300.

Perez, C.A., Walz, B.J., Zivnuska, F.R., Pilepich, M., Prasad, K., and Bauer, W. (1980). Irradiation of carcinoma of the prostate localized to the pelvis: analysis of tumor response and prognosis. *Int. J. Radiat. Oncol., Biol. Phys.*, **6**, 555–563.

Pistenma, D.A., Bagshaw, M.A., and Freiha, F.S. (1979). Extended field radiation therapy for prostatic adenocarcinoma: status report of a limited prospective trial. In *Cancer of the genitourinary tract* (eds T.R. Johnson and E. Samuels). New York: Raven Press. p. 229.

Ray, G.R., Pistenma, D.A., Castellino, R.A., Kempson, R.L., Meares, E., and Bagshaw, M.A. (1976). Operative staging of apparently localized adenocarcinoma of the prostate: results in fifty unselected patients. I. Experimental design and preliminary results. *Cancer*, **38**, 73.

Smith, M.J.V. (1966). The lymphatics of the prostate. *Invest. Urol.*, **3**, 439.

Spellman, M.L., Costellino, R.A., Ray, G.R., Pistenma, D.A., and Bagshaw, M.A. (1977). An evaluation of lymphangiography in localized carcinoma of the prostate. *Radiology*, **125**, 737.

Vickery, A.L., Jr, and Kerr, W.S., Jr (1963). Carcinoma of the prostate treated by radical prostatectomy. A clinicopathological survey of 187 cases followed for 5 years and 148 cases followed for 10 years. *Cancer*, **16**, 1598–1608.

Walsh, P.C. (1980). Radical prostatectomy for the treatment of localized prostatic carcinoma. *Urol. Clin. N. Am.*, **7**, (3), 273.

Whitmore, W.F., Batata, M., and Hilaris, B. (1979). Prostatic irradiation: Iodine 125 implantation. In *Cancer of the genitourinary tract* (eds T.R. Johnson and E. Samuels). New York: Raven Press. p. 195.

Whitmore, W.F., Jr, Hilaris, B., Grabstald, H., and Batata, M. (1974). Implantation of ^{125}I in prostatic cancer. *Surg. Clin. N. Am.*, **54**, 887.

Wilson, C.S., Dahl, D.S. and Middleton, R.G. (1977). Pelvic lymphadenectomy for the staging of apparently localized prostatic cancer. *J. Urol.*, **117**, 197.

Index